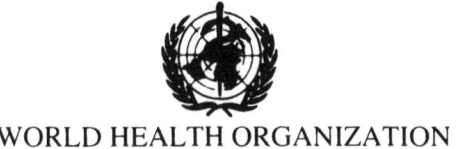

WORLD HEALTH ORGANIZATION

INTERNATIONAL AGENCY FOR RESEARCH ON CANCER

IARC MONOGRAPHS
ON THE
EVALUATION OF CARCINOGENIC
RISKS TO HUMANS

*Human Immunodeficiency Viruses and
Human T-Cell Lymphotropic Viruses*

VOLUME 67

This publication represents the views and expert opinions
of an IARC Working Group on the
Evaluation of Carcinogenic Risks to Humans,
which met in Lyon,

11–18 June 1996

1996

IARC MONOGRAPHS

In 1969, the International Agency for Research on Cancer (IARC) initiated a programme on the evaluation of the carcinogenic risk of chemicals to humans involving the production of critically evaluated monographs on individual chemicals. The programme was subsequently expanded to include evaluations of carcinogenic risks associated with exposures to complex mixtures, life-style factors and biological agents, as well as those in specific occupations.

The objective of the programme is to elaborate and publish in the form of monographs critical reviews of data on carcinogenicity for agents to which humans are known to be exposed and on specific exposure situations; to evaluate these data in terms of human risk with the help of international working groups of experts in chemical carcinogenesis and related fields; and to indicate where additional research efforts are needed.

This project is supported by PHS Grant No. 5-UO1 CA33193-15 awarded by the United States National Cancer Institute, Department of Health and Human Services. Additional support has been provided since 1986 by the European Commission.

©International Agency for Research on Cancer, 1996

IARC Library Cataloguing in Publication Data

Human immunodeficiency viruses and human T-cell lymphotropic viruses /
  IARC Working Group on the Evaluation of
  Carcinogenic Risks to Humans (1996 : Lyon,
  France).

  (IARC monographs on the evaluation of carcinogenic
  risks to humans ; 67)

  1. Acquired Immunodeficiency Syndrome – congresses 2. Oncogenic Viruses – congresses 3. T-Lymphocytes – congresses I. IARC Working Group on the Evaluation of Carcinogenic Risks to Humans II. Series

  ISBN 978-9-2832126-76   (NLM Classification: W 1)
  ISSN 0250-9555

Publications of the World Health Organization enjoy copyright protection in accordance with the provisions of Protocol 2 of the Universal Copyright Convention.

All rights reserved. Application for rights of reproduction or translation, in part or in toto, should be made to the International Agency for Research on Cancer.

Distributed by IARC*Press* (Fax: +33 04 72 73 83 02; E-mail: press@iarc.fr)
and by the World Health Organization Distribution and Sales,
CH-1211 Geneva 27 (Fax: +41 22 791 4857)

PRINTED IN THE UNITED KINGDOM

CONTENTS

NOTE TO THE READER 1

LIST OF PARTICIPANTS 3

PREAMBLE
    Background 7
    Objective and Scope 7
    Selection of Topics for Monographs 8
    Data for Monographs 9
    The Working Group 9
    Working Procedures 9
    Exposure Data 10
    Studies of Cancer in Humans 12
    Studies of Cancer in Experimental Animals 15
    Other Data Relevant to an Evaluation of Carcinogenicity and Its Mechanisms ...18
    Summary of Data Reported 19
    Evaluation 21
    References 25

THE MONOGRAPHS

Human immunodeficiency viruses 31
    1. Exposure data 31
        1.1 Structure, taxonomy and biology 31
            1.1.1 Structure 31
            1.1.2 Taxonomy 32
            1.1.3 Phylogeny 33
                (a) Phylogenetic relationship of HIV-1 and HIV-2 to other
                     retroviruses 33
                (b) Relationship of HIV-1 and HIV-2 isolates to one another 36
                     (i) Genotypes 36
                     (ii) Antigenic diversity 37
            1.1.4 Host range 37
            1.1.5 Cell tropism 37
            1.1.6 Target tissues 38
                (a) Lymphoid tissue 38
                (b) Central nervous system 38
                (c) Gastrointestinal tract 38

1.1.7 The HIV-1 and HIV-2 genome and gene products 38
    (i)   Structural proteins (Gag, Pol, Env) 39
    (ii)   Regulatory proteins (Tat, Rev) 39
    (iii) Accessory proteins (Nef, Vif, Vpr, Vpu) 40
1.1.8 Replication 41
1.2 Methods of detection 41
  1.2.1 Antibody tests 41
    (a) ELISA 42
    (b) Western blot analysis 43
    (c) Indeterminate HIV antibody results 43
    (d) Undetectable HIV antibody 43
    (e) Diagnosis of HIV infection in infants 43
    (f) Detection of antibodies in saliva 44
  1.2.2 Direct detection of HIV 44
    (a) Viral culture 44
    (b) p24 Antigen 44
    (c) Detection of viral genomes 45
    (d) HIV quantification 45
1.3 Epidemiology of HIV infection 46
  1.3.1 HIV transmission 46
    (a) Sexual contact 46
    (b) Blood contact 47
    (c) Mother-to-child transmission 48
    (d) Other modes of transmission 48
  1.3.2 Geographical distribution 48
    (a) Global estimates and projections 49
    (b) United States and Canada 51
    (c) Caribbean 51
    (d) Latin America 52
    (e) Sub-Saharan Africa 52
    (f) Europe 52
    (g) Asia 52
    (h) Oceania 54
    (i) Middle East 54
1.4 Clinical description of non-neoplastic disorders 54
  1.4.1 Seroconversion syndrome 54
  1.4.2 Immunological decline 55
  1.4.3 Non-AIDS-defining manifestations of HIV infection 57
    (a) Classification of HIV disease 57
    (b) Non-AIDS illness 58
    (c) Time to AIDS 59
  1.4.4 AIDS manifestations 59
  1.4.5 Long-term non-progressors 60
  1.4.6 Human immunodeficiency virus type 2 (HIV-2) 61

CONTENTS

- 1.5 Control and prevention 61
  - 1.5.1 Behavioural prevention 61
  - 1.5.2 Screening 62
  - 1.5.3 Treatment 63
  - 1.5.4 Prospects for vaccines 64
  - 1.5.5 Other approaches 64
- 2. Studies of cancer in humans 64
  - 2.1 Kaposi's sarcoma 65
    - 2.1.1 Pathology and clinical disease 65
      - (a) Clinical disease in HIV-seronegative individuals 65
      - (b) Clinical disease in HIV-seropositive individuals 65
    - 2.1.2 Descriptive epidemiology of Kaposi's sarcoma 66
      - (a) Demographic variations: age and sex 66
      - (b) Geographical variations 66
      - (c) Temporal changes 68
    - 2.1.3 Descriptive epidemiological studies 68
      - (a) Studies in men in relation to marital status 68
      - (b) Linkage studies between AIDS and cancer registries 70
    - 2.1.4 Analytical studies 70
      - (a) Cohort studies 70
      - (b) Case–control studies 71
      - (c) Analytical studies of the relationship between degree of immunosuppression and Kaposi's sarcoma among HIV infected persons 71
    - 2.1.5 Factors influencing the occurrence of Kaposi's sarcoma in HIV infected persons 72
      - (a) Behavioural cofactors 72
        - (i) Descriptive studies 72
        - (ii) Analytical studies 78
      - (b) Infectious cofactors 79
        - (i) Human herpesvirus 8 79
        - (ii) Cytomegalovirus 85
        - (iii) Other infectious agents 86
      - (c) Genetic susceptibility 86
      - (d) Miscellaneous factors 87
    - 2.1.6 Human immunodeficiency virus type 2 88
  - 2.2 Non-Hodgkin's lymphoma 88
    - 2.2.1 Description of the clinical disease and pathology 88
      - (a) Classification of AIDS-related lymphomas 89
        - (i) Systemic non-Hodgkin's lymphomas 89
        - (ii) Body cavity-based lymphoma 90
        - (iii) Primary lymphoma of the brain 90
        - (iv) Multicentric Castleman's disease 91
      - (b) Phenotypic and genotypic features 91

2.2.2 Descriptive epidemiology of non-Hodgkin's lymphoma 91
(a) Cancer registry data 92
(b) Cohort data 93
2.2.3 Role of immunosuppression 94
2.2.4 Co-factors 95
(a) Demographic 95
(b) Geographic 95
(c) Behavioural 95
(d) Infections 99
(i) Epstein–Barr virus 99
(ii) HHV-8 102
(iii) HHV-6 102
(e) Zidovudine and other therapy 103
2.2.5 HIV-2 and non-Hodgkin's lymphoma 103
2.3 Cervical, anal and other cancers 103
2.3.1 Cervical intraepithelial neoplasia and invasive cancer 104
(a) Precancerous lesions 104
(i) Association with HIV 104
(ii) Association with HIV and HPV 108
(iii) HIV, HPV and $CD4^+$ T-cell counts 109
(iv) Progression of disease and treatment of CIN lesions 111
(b) Invasive cervical cancer 111
(i) Case series 111
(ii) Prognosis 112
(iii) Descriptive epidemiology 112
(iv) Case–control studies 113
2.3.2 Anorectal intraepithelial neoplasia and invasive cancer 114
(a) Precancerous lesions 114
(i) Association with HIV 114
(ii) Association with HIV and HPV 114
(iii) HIV, HPV and $CD4^+$ T-cell count 117
(iv) Progression of disease 119
(b) Invasive anal cancer 120
(i) Case reports and series 120
(ii) Prognosis 120
(iii) Descriptive epidemiology 120
2.3.3 Hodgkin's disease 121
(a) Distribution of histological types 122
(i) Hodgkin's disease in HIV-uninfected persons 122
(ii) Hodgkin's disease in HIV-infected persons 122
(iii) Prognosis 124
(b) Descriptive epidemiology 124
(c) Cohort studies 125
(d) Cofactors 126

	2.3.4	Testicular cancer	126
		(a) Case reports and series	126
		(b) Descriptive and cohort studies	127
	2.3.5	Non-melanoma cancers of the skin	128
		(a) Case reports and series	128
		(b) Descriptive and cohort studies	128
	2.3.6	Conjunctival tumours	129
		(a) Case reports	129
		(b) Descriptive study	130
		(c) Case–control studies	130
	2.3.7	Leiomyosarcoma	130
		(a) Case reports and series	130
		(b) Descriptive studies	131
		(c) Cofactors	131
	2.3.8	Other cancers	131

3. Studies of cancer in animals 133
   3.1 HIV-1 and HIV-2 133
   3.2 Lymphomas in non-human primates 134
       3.2.1 Occurrence of lymphomas in nonhuman primates infected with simian immunodeficiency virus 134
       3.2.2 Pathological and molecular features of lymphoma 135
       3.2.3 Other neoplastic conditions 135
       3.2.4 Cofactors in SIV oncogenesis 135
   3.3 Feline immunodeficiency virus infection in cats 136
       3.3.1 Occurrence of lymphosarcomas in FIV infection 137
       3.3.2 Pathological and molecular features of lymphosarcoma ...138
4. Other data relevant to an evaluation of carcinogenesis and its mechanisms 138
   4.1 Immunity and cancer 138
       4.1.1 Types of cancer seen in non-HIV-associated human immunodeficiency 139
       4.1.2 Time of onset of cancers in non-HIV-associated immunodeficiency 146
       4.1.3 Similarities and differences between AIDS and transplantation-associated tumours 148
             (a) In immunity 148
             (b) In cancer types 149
             (c) In onset 149
       4.1.4 Occurrence of other viruses in malignancies associated with non-HIV immunosuppression 150
       4.1.5 Mechanisms by which immune dysfunction may contribute to the genesis of cancer 150
             (a) Activation of oncogenic viruses with immunosuppression ...150
             (b) Stimulation and hyperreactivity of remaining cells in immunosuppressed persons 150

4.2 Kaposi's sarcomas 151
    4.2.1 Cell biology of Kaposi's sarcoma lesions 151
        (a) Origins of Kaposi's sarcoma spindle cells 151
        (b) Vascular lesions induced by Kaposi's sarcoma cell cultures
            in nude mice 152
        (c) Growth factors involved in the proliferation of spindle cells .. 153
            (i) Fibroblast growth factors 153
            (ii) Platelet-derived growth factor 154
        (d) Clonality of Kaposi's sarcoma and chromosomal
            abnormalities 154
    4.2.2 The role of HIV-1 Tat in the development of Kaposi's sarcoma
          lesions 154
    4.2.3 An infectious agent as a cause of Kaposi's sarcoma 156
    4.2.4 The role of human herpesvirus 8 157
        (a) Genomic organization and relationship to other primate
            herpesviruses 157
        (b) In-vivo tropism and association with Kaposi's sarcoma 157
4.3 Non-Hodgkin's lymphomas and other lymphoproliferative disorders 158
    4.3.1 Pathological models of lymphomagenesis 158
        (a) HIV infection of lymphoid tissues and polyclonal B-cell
            hyperplasia 160
            (i) Pathological changes in HIV-infected lymphoid
                follicles 161
            (ii) Destruction of follicular centres and B-cell
                hyperplasia 161
            (iii) Chronic antigen stimulation 162
            (iv) Presence of HIV in tumour cells 162
        (b) Oligoclonal B-cell proliferation 162
            (i) Immunosuppression 163
            (ii) Cytokines 163
        (c) Genetic abnormalities 165
            (i) c-myc 165
            (ii) BCL-6 166
            (iii) ras 166
            (iv) p53 166
            (v) 6q Deletions 168
            (vi) Chromosome 1q abnormalities 168
    4.3.2 Lymphotropic viruses 168
        (a) EBV 168
        (b) HHV-6 172
        (c) HHV-8 173
    4.3.3 Conclusion 173
4.4 Cofactors in anal and cervical carcinomas and other cancers 174

            4.4.1 The role of HPV in the molecular pathogenesis of anogenital
                   cancers in immunocompetent patients 175
                   (a) Status and level of HPV DNA in the natural history of
                        infection 175
                   (b) Expression of HPV proteins in the natural history of
                        infection 175
                   (c) Molecular mechanisms of transforming activity of HPV 176
                        (i)   Intrinsic properties of high-risk HPV E6 and E7 176
                        (ii) Regulation of E6 and E7 expression 176
            4.4.2 Interactions between HIV and HPV 177
                   (a) Effects of HIV-related immunosuppression on HPV
                        replication and HPV-associated anogenital lesions 178
                   (b) HIV Tat stimulation of cytokines and their role in genital
                        lesions 178
                   (c) Possible effect of HIV-1 Tat on HPV E6/E7 expression 178
5. Summary of data reported and evaluation 179
    5.1 Exposure data 179
    5.2 Human carcinogenicity data 180
    5.3 Animal carcinogenicity data 181
    5.4 Other relevant data and mechanistic considerations on HIV-1-associated
         neoplasms 182
    5.5 Evaluation 183
6. References 183

Human T-cell lymphotropic viruses 261
1. Exposure data 261
    1.1 Structure, taxonomy and biology 261
         1.1.1 Structure 261
         1.1.2 Taxonomy and phylogeny 261
         1.1.3 Host range 263
         1.1.4 Related non-human primate viruses 264
         1.1.5 Target tissue (*in vitro* and *in vivo*) 266
         1.1.6 Genomic structure and properties of gene products 266
         1.1.7 Other genes encoded by the open reading frames I, II and III
                in the HTLV-I pX region 267
    1.2 Methods of detection 268
         1.2.1 Serological detection of specific antibodies 268
         1.2.2 Detection and characterization of viral nucleic acids 269
         1.2.3 Isolation of HTLV-I and HTLV-II 270
         1.2.4 Sero-indeterminate HTLV-I western blots 270
         1.2.5 Seronegative HTLV-I-infected individuals 271
    1.3 Epidemiology of HTLV infection 271
         1.3.1 HTLV-I transmission 271
                (a) Mother-to-child transmission 271

            (b)   Sexual transmission 272
            (c)   Transmission by blood 273
      1.3.2 Animal models of HTLV-I transmission 274
      1.3.3 Geographical distribution of HTLV-I 274
      1.3.4 HTLV-I prevalence and demographic features of HTLV-I
            infection 277
      1.3.5 Epidemiology of tropical spastic paraparesis/HTLV-I-associated
            myelopathy 277
      1.3.6 Natural history of HTLV-I primary infection 279
      1.3.7 Molecular epidemiology of HTLV-I 279
      1.3.8 HTLV-II epidemiology 280
   1.4 Clinical description of non-neoplastic disorders 280
      1.4.1 HTLV-I infection 280
            (a)   Tropical spastic paraparesis/HTLV-I associated
                  myelopathy 280
            (b)   Uveitis 282
            (c)   Other inflammatory diseases 283
                  (i)   Infective dermatitis 283
                  (ii)   Polymyositis 283
                  (iii) Alveolitis 284
                  (iv)   Arthritis (HTLV-I-associated arthropathy) 284
                  (v)   Thyroiditis 285
                  (vi)   Sjögren's syndrome 285
            (d)   Immune suppression 285
      1.4.2 HTLV-II infection 285
      1.4.3 HTLV/HIV co-infection 286
   1.5 Control and prevention 286
2. Studies of cancer in humans 287
   2.1 T-cell malignancies 287
      2.1.1 HTLV-I infection and adult T-cell leukaemia/lymphoma 287
            (a)   Clinical description 287
                  (i)   Distribution by subtype 287
                  (ii)   Laboratory findings 289
                  (iii) Histological characteristics 290
                  (iv)   Genetic studies 291
                  (v)   Prognosis 292
                  (vi)   Prevention of ATLL 292
            (b)   Epidemiology 292
                  (i)   Geographical distribution 293
                  (ii)   Age- and sex-distribution of ATLL 294
                  (iii) Cohort studies 297
                  (iv)   Case–control studies on co-factors 297
      2.1.2 HTLV-I infection and cutaneous T-cell lymphomas 300
      2.1.3 HTLV-II infection 301

		2.2	Other malignancies	302
		2.2.1	HTLV-I	302
			(a) Case reports and case series	302
			(b) Cohort studies	303
			(c) Case–control studies	303
		2.2.2	HTLV-II	306
3.	Studies of cancer in animals			306
	3.1	HTLV-I in animal models		306
		3.1.1	Non-human primates	306
		3.1.2	Other models	308
	3.2	STLV-I in non-human primates		308
		3.2.1	STLV-I-associated lymphomas	308
		3.2.2	Pathological and molecular aspects	310
	3.3	Bovine leukaemia virus in sheep and cattle		311
		3.3.1	Disorders induced by BLV	313
			(a) Cattle	314
			(b) Sheep	314
		3.3.2	Pathological and molecular aspects	314
			(a) Cattle	314
			(b) Sheep	315
			(c) Mechanistic studies	316
		3.3.3	Vaccination trials	316
4.	Other data relevant to an evaluation of carcinogenesis and its mechanisms			316
	4.1	General observations on retroviral oncogenesis		316
	4.2	Host factors		317
		4.2.1	The role of the HLA system in HTLV-I infection	317
		4.2.2	Immune surveillance and escape	318
			(a) Antibodies	318
			(b) T-cells	318
		4.2.3	Host genetic factors required during the transition to ATLL	318
	4.3	Viral factors		320
		4.3.1	Proviral load and clonal integration of HTLV-I infection	320
		4.3.2	The role of Tax in cellular transformation/immortalization	321
			(a) Transforming/immortalizing properties of HTLV-I Tax *in vitro*	321
			(i) Immortalizing effects on T-cells *in vitro*	321
			(ii) Transforming effect of Tax on fibroblasts cultures *in vitro*	321
			(b) Tumorigenic properties of *tax* in transgenic mice	321
		4.3.3	Pathways of Tax-mediated transactivation of cellular genes	324
		4.3.4	Differences between HTLV-I-transformed T-cells and ATLL cells	327
		4.3.5	The role of other viral and host cell proteins in lymphocyte stimulation and leukaemogenesis	328

        4.3.6 Differences between HTLV-I and HTLV-II 330
5. Summary of data reported and evaluation 330
    5.1 Exposure data 330
    5.2 Human carcinogenicity data 331
    5.3 Animal carcinogenicity data 332
    5.4 Molecular mechanisms of leukaemogenesis 332
    5.5 Evaluation 333
6. References 334

ABBREVIATIONS 391

SUPPLEMENTARY CORRIGENDA TO VOLUMES 1–66 395

CUMULATIVE INDEX TO THE *MONOGRAPHS* SERIES 397

NOTE TO THE READER

The term 'carcinogenic risk' in the *IARC Monographs* series is taken to mean the probability that exposure to an agent will lead to cancer in humans.

Inclusion of an agent in the *Monographs* does not imply that it is a carcinogen, only that the published data have been examined. Equally, the fact that an agent has not yet been evaluated in a monograph does not mean that it is not carcinogenic.

The evaluations of carcinogenic risk are made by international working groups of independent scientists and are qualitative in nature. No recommendation is given for regulation or legislation.

Anyone who is aware of published data that may alter the evaluation of the carcinogenic risk of an agent to humans is encouraged to make this information available to the Unit of Carcinogen Identification and Evaluation, International Agency for Research on Cancer, 150 cours Albert Thomas, 69372 Lyon Cedex 08, France, in order that the agent may be considered for re-evaluation by a future Working Group.

Although every effort is made to prepare the monographs as accurately as possible, mistakes may occur. Readers are requested to communicate any errors to the Unit of Carcinogen Identification and Evaluation, so that corrections can be reported in future volumes.

IARC WORKING GROUP ON THE EVALUATION OF CARCINOGENIC RISKS TO HUMANS: HUMAN IMMUNODEFICIENCY VIRUSES AND HUMAN T-CELL LYMPHOTROPIC VIRUSES

Lyon, 11–18 June 1996

LIST OF PARTICIPANTS

Members[1]

C. Bangham, Department of Immunology, St Mary's Hospital Medical School, Praed Street, London W2 1NY, United Kingdom

P. Biberfeld, Immunopathology Laboratory, Karolinska Institute, 171 76 Stockholm, Sweden

R.J. Biggar, Viral Epidemiology Branch, National Cancer Institute, EPN/434, 6130 Executive Boulevard, Rockville, MD 20852, USA (*Co-Chairman*)

F.M. Buonaguro, Division of Viral Oncology, Istituto Nazionale per lo Studio e la Cura dei Tumori, Fondazione G. Pascale, via Mariano Semmola, 80131 Naples, Italy

A. Burny, Faculty of Agronomic Sciences, UER Biologie moléculaire et Physiologie animale, avenue Maréchal Juin, 13, Bâtiment 92, 5030 Gembloux, Belgium

J.J. Callanan, Department of Agriculture and Food, Regional Veterinary Laboratory, Model Farm Road, Cork 4, Ireland

A. Carbone, Division of Anatomy Pathology, Aviano Cancer Centre, via Pedemontana Occidentale 12, 33081 Aviano PN, Italy

S. Franceschi, Epidemiology Unit, Aviano Cancer Centre, Via Pedemontana Occidentale 12, 33081 Aviano PN, Italy

G. Franchini, Laboratory of Tumor Cell Biology, National Cancer Institute, Building 37, Room 6A01, Bethesda, MD 20892-4255, USA

A. Gessain, Unité d'Epidémiologie des Virus Oncogènes, Institut Pasteur, 28 rue du Dr Roux, 75724 Paris Cédex 15, France

---

[1] Unable to attend: V. Beral, Cancer Epidemiology Unit, Imperial Cancer Research Fund, University of Oxford, Gibson Building, The Radcliffe Infirmary, Oxford OX2 6HE, United Kingdom; E. Katongole-Mbidde, Uganda Cancer Institute, PO Box 3935, Kampala, Uganda

S.D. Holmberg, Division of HIV/AIDS, Centers for Disease Control and Prevention, 1600 Clifton Road NE, Mailstop E-45, Atlanta, GA 30333, USA

G.B. Hubbard, Southwest Foundation for Biomedical Research, Department of Laboratory Animal Medicine, PO Box 760549, San Antonio, TX 78245-0549, USA

J. Kaldor, National Centre in HIV Epidemiology and Clinical Research, St. Vincent's Hospital Medical Centre, 2nd Floor, 376 Victoria Street, Darlinghurst, Sydney NSW 2010, Australia

F.-J. Kaup, German Primate Centre, Kellnerweg 4, 37077 Göttingen, Germany

E. Matutes, Academic Department of Haematology and Cytogenetics, Royal Marsden Hospital, Fulham Road, London SW3 6JJ, United Kingdom

M.O. McClure, Department of Genito-Urinary Medicine and Communicable Diseases, St Mary's Hospital Medical School, Praed Street, London W2 1NY, United Kingdom

M. Melbye, Danish Epidemiology Science Centre, State Serum Institute, 5 Artillerivej, 2300 Copenhagen S, Denmark

N. Mueller, Department of Epidemiology, Harvard School of Public Health, 677 Huntington Avenue, Boston, MA 02115, USA

R. Newton, Cancer Epidemiology Unit, Imperial Cancer Research Fund, University of Oxford, Gibson Building, The Radcliffe Infirmary, Oxford OX2 6HE, United Kingdom

C.S. Rabkin, Viral Epidemiology Branch, National Cancer Institute, 6130 Executive Boulevard, EPN/434, Rockville, MD 20852, USA

T.F. Schulz, Department of Medical Microbiology and Genito-Urinary Medicine, Division of Genito-Urinary Medicine, Royal Liverpool University Hospital, Prescot Street, Liverpool L7 8XP, United Kingdom

F. Sitas, National Cancer Registry, South African Institute for Medical Research, PO Box 1038, Johannesburg 2000, South Africa

K. Tajima, Division of Epidemiology, Aichi Cancer Center Research Institute, 1-1 Kanokoden, Chikusa-ku, Nagoya 464, Japan

G. Taylor, Department of Communicable Diseases, Winston Churchill Wing, St. Mary's Hospital Medical School, Praed Street, London W2 1NY, United Kingdom

R.A. Weiss, Chester Beatty Laboratories, Institute of Cancer Research, Fulham Road, London SW3 6JB, United Kingdom (*Co-Chairman*)

Secretariat

P. Boffetta, Unit of Environmental Cancer Epidemiology
J. Cheney (*Editor*)
E. Lynge, Danish Cancer Society, Strandboulevarden 49, Copenhagen, Denmark
D. McGregor, Unit of Carcinogen Identification and Evaluation
A. Meneghel, Unit of Carcinogen Identification and Evaluation
D. Mietton, Unit of Carcinogen Identification and Evaluation
H. Nakazawa, Unit of Multistage Carcinogenesis
C. Partensky, Unit of Carcinogen Identification and Evaluation (*Technical Editor*)

PARTICIPANTS

I. Rajower, Programme of Epidemiology for Cancer Prevention
J. Rice, Unit of Carcinogen Identification and Evaluation
S. Ruiz, Unit of Carcinogen Identification and Evaluation
J. Wilbourn, Unit of Carcinogen Identification and Evaluation (*Responsible Officer*)
J. Ziegler, International Agency for Research on Cancer

Secretarial assistance

M. Lézère
J. Mitchell
S. Reynaud

IARC MONOGRAPHS PROGRAMME ON THE EVALUATION OF CARCINOGENIC RISKS TO HUMANS[1]

PREAMBLE

1. BACKGROUND

In 1969, the International Agency for Research on Cancer (IARC) initiated a programme to evaluate the carcinogenic risk of chemicals to humans and to produce monographs on individual chemicals. The *Monographs* programme has since been expanded to include consideration of exposures to complex mixtures of chemicals (which occur, for example, in some occupations and as a result of human habits) and of exposures to other agents, such as radiation and viruses. With Supplement 6 (IARC, 1987a), the title of the series was modified from *IARC Monographs on the Evaluation of the Carcinogenic Risk of Chemicals to Humans* to *IARC Monographs on the Evaluation of Carcinogenic Risks to Humans*, in order to reflect the widened scope of the programme.

The criteria established in 1971 to evaluate carcinogenic risk to humans were adopted by the working groups whose deliberations resulted in the first 16 volumes of the *IARC Monographs series*. Those criteria were subsequently updated by further ad-hoc working groups (IARC, 1977, 1978, 1979, 1982, 1983, 1987b, 1988, 1991a; Vainio *et al.*, 1992).

2. OBJECTIVE AND SCOPE

The objective of the programme is to prepare, with the help of international working groups of experts, and to publish in the form of monographs, critical reviews and evaluations of evidence on the carcinogenicity of a wide range of human exposures. The *Monographs* may also indicate where additional research efforts are needed.

The *Monographs* represent the first step in carcinogenic risk assessment, which involves examination of all relevant information in order to assess the strength of the available evidence that certain exposures could alter the incidence of cancer in humans. The second step is quantitative risk estimation. Detailed, quantitative evaluations of epidemiological data may be made in the *Monographs*, but without extrapolation beyond

---

[1] This project is supported by PHS Grant No. 5-UO1 CA33193-15 awarded by the United States National Cancer Institute, Department of Health and Human Services. Since 1986, the programme has also been supported by the European Commission.

the range of the data available. Quantitative extrapolation from experimental data to the human situation is not undertaken.

The term 'carcinogen' is used in these monographs to denote an exposure that is capable of increasing the incidence of malignant neoplasms; the induction of benign neoplasms may in some circumstances (see p. 17) contribute to the judgement that the exposure is carcinogenic. The terms 'neoplasm' and 'tumour' are used interchangeably.

Some epidemiological and experimental studies indicate that different agents may act at different stages in the carcinogenic process, and several different mechanisms may be involved. The aim of the *Monographs* has been, from their inception, to evaluate evidence of carcinogenicity at any stage in the carcinogenesis process, independently of the underlying mechanisms. Information on mechanisms may, however, be used in making the overall evaluation (IARC, 1991a; Vainio *et al.*, 1992; see also pp. 23–25).

The *Monographs* may assist national and international authorities in making risk assessments and in formulating decisions concerning any necessary preventive measures. The evaluations of IARC working groups are scientific, qualitative judgements about the evidence for or against carcinogenicity provided by the available data. These evaluations represent only one part of the body of information on which regulatory measures may be based. Other components of regulatory decisions may vary from one situation to another and from country to country, responding to different socioeconomic and national priorities. **Therefore, no recommendation is given with regard to regulation or legislation, which are the responsibility of individual governments and/or other international organizations.**

The *IARC Monographs* are recognized as an authoritative source of information on the carcinogenicity of a wide range of human exposures. A survey of users in 1988 indicated that the *Monographs* are consulted by various agencies in 57 countries. About 4000 copies of each volume are printed, for distribution to governments, regulatory bodies and interested scientists. The Monographs are also available from the International Agency for Research on Cancer in Lyon and via the Distribution and Sales Service of the World Health Organization.

3. SELECTION OF TOPICS FOR MONOGRAPHS

Topics are selected on the basis of two main criteria: (a) there is evidence of human exposure, and (b) there is some evidence or suspicion of carcinogenicity. The term 'agent' is used to include individual chemical compounds, groups of related chemical compounds, physical agents (such as radiation) and biological factors (such as viruses). Exposures to mixtures of agents may occur in occupational exposures and as a result of personal and cultural habits (like smoking and dietary practices). Chemical analogues and compounds with biological or physical characteristics similar to those of suspected carcinogens may also be considered, even in the absence of data on a possible carcinogenic effect in humans or experimental animals.

The scientific literature is surveyed for published data relevant to an assessment of carcinogenicity. The IARC information bulletins on agents being tested for carcinogenicity (IARC, 1973–1996) and directories of on-going research in cancer epidemiology (IARC, 1976–1994) often indicate exposures that may be scheduled for future meetings. Ad-hoc working groups convened by IARC in 1984, 1989, 1991 and 1993 gave recommendations as to which agents should be evaluated in the IARC Monographs series (IARC, 1984, 1989, 1991b, 1993).

As significant new data on subjects on which monographs have already been prepared become available, re-evaluations are made at subsequent meetings, and revised monographs are published.

4. DATA FOR MONOGRAPHS

The *Monographs* do not necessarily cite all the literature concerning the subject of an evaluation. Only those data considered by the Working Group to be relevant to making the evaluation are included.

With regard to biological and epidemiological data, only reports that have been published or accepted for publication in the openly available scientific literature are reviewed by the working groups. In certain instances, government agency reports that have undergone peer review and are widely available are considered. Exceptions may be made on an ad-hoc basis to include unpublished reports that are in their final form and publicly available, if their inclusion is considered pertinent to making a final evaluation (see pp. 23–25). In the sections on chemical and physical properties, on analysis, on production and use and on occurrence, unpublished sources of information may be used.

5. THE WORKING GROUP

Reviews and evaluations are formulated by a working group of experts. The tasks of the group are: (i) to ascertain that all appropriate data have been collected; (ii) to select the data relevant for the evaluation on the basis of scientific merit; (iii) to prepare accurate summaries of the data to enable the reader to follow the reasoning of the Working Group; (iv) to evaluate the results of epidemiological and experimental studies on cancer; (v) to evaluate data relevant to the understanding of mechanism of action; and (vi) to make an overall evaluation of the carcinogenicity of the exposure to humans.

Working Group participants who contributed to the considerations and evaluations within a particular volume are listed, with their addresses, at the beginning of each publication. Each participant who is a member of a working group serves as an individual scientist and not as a representative of any organization, government or industry. In addition, nominees of national and international agencies and industrial associations may be invited as observers.

6. WORKING PROCEDURES

Approximately one year in advance of a meeting of a working group, the topics of the monographs are announced and participants are selected by IARC staff in consultation with other experts. Subsequently, relevant biological and epidemiological data are collected by IARC from recognized sources of information on carcinogenesis, including data storage and retrieval systems such as MEDLINE and TOXLINE, and EMIC and ETIC for data on genetic and related effects and reproductive and developmental effects, respectively.

For chemicals and some complex mixtures, the major collection of data and the preparation of first drafts of the sections on chemical and physical properties, on analysis, on production and use and on occurrence are carried out under a separate contract funded by the United States National Cancer Institute. Representatives from industrial associations may assist in the preparation of sections on production and use. Information on production and trade is obtained from governmental and trade publications and, in some cases, by direct contact with industries. Separate production data on some agents may not be available because their publication could disclose confidential information. Information on uses may be obtained from published sources but is often complemented by direct contact with manufacturers. Efforts are made to supplement this information with data from other national and international sources.

Six months before the meeting, the material obtained is sent to meeting participants, or is used by IARC staff, to prepare sections for the first drafts of monographs. The first drafts are compiled by IARC staff and sent, before the meeting, to all participants of the Working Group for review.

The Working Group meets in Lyon for seven to eight days to discuss and finalize the texts of the monographs and to formulate the evaluations. After the meeting, the master copy of each monograph is verified by consulting the original literature, edited and prepared for publication. The aim is to publish monographs within six months of the Working Group meeting.

The available studies are summarized by the Working Group, with particular regard to the qualitative aspects discussed below. In general, numerical findings are indicated as they appear in the original report; units are converted when necessary for easier comparison. The Working Group may conduct additional analyses of the published data and use them in their assessment of the evidence; the results of such supplementary analyses are given in square brackets. When an important aspect of a study, directly impinging on its interpretation, should be brought to the attention of the reader, a comment is given in square brackets.

7. EXPOSURE DATA

Sections that indicate the extent of past and present human exposure, the sources of exposure, the people most likely to be exposed and the factors that contribute to the exposure are included at the beginning of each monograph.

Most monographs on individual chemicals, groups of chemicals or complex mixtures include sections on chemical and physical data, on analysis, on production and use and on occurrence. In monographs on, for example, physical agents, occupational exposures and cultural habits, other sections may be included, such as: historical perspectives, description of an industry or habit, chemistry of the complex mixture or taxonomy.

Monographs on biological agents have sections on structure and biology, methods of detection, epidemiology of infection and clinical disease other than cancer.

For chemical exposures, the Chemical Abstracts Services Registry Number, the latest Chemical Abstracts Primary Name and the IUPAC Systematic Name are recorded; other synonyms are given, but the list is not necessarily comprehensive. For biological agents, taxonomy and structure are described, and the degree of variability is given, when applicable.

Information on chemical and physical properties and, in particular, data relevant to identification, occurrence and biological activity are included. For biological agents, mode of replication, life cycle, target cells, persistence and latency and host response are given. A description of technical products of chemicals includes trades names, relevant specifications and available information on composition and impurities. Some of the trade names given may be those of mixtures in which the agent being evaluated is only one of the ingredients.

The purpose of the section on analysis or detection is to give the reader an overview of current methods, with emphasis on those widely used for regulatory purposes. Methods for monitoring human exposure are also given, when available. No critical evaluation or recommendation of any of the methods is meant or implied. The IARC publishes a series of volumes, *Environmental Carcinogens: Methods of Analysis and Exposure Measurement* (IARC, 1978–93), that describe validated methods for analysing a wide variety of chemicals and mixtures. For biological agents, methods of detection and exposure assessment are described, including their sensitivity, specificity and reproducibility.

The dates of first synthesis and of first commercial production of a chemical or mixture are provided; for agents which do not occur naturally, this information may allow a reasonable estimate to be made of the date before which no human exposure to the agent could have occurred. The dates of first reported occurrence of an exposure are also provided. In addition, methods of synthesis used in past and present commercial production and different methods of production which may give rise to different impurities are described.

Data on production, international trade and uses are obtained for representative regions, which usually include Europe, Japan and the United States of America. It should not, however, be inferred that those areas or nations are necessarily the sole or major sources or users of the agent. Some identified uses may not be current or major applications, and the coverage is not necessarily comprehensive. In the case of drugs, mention of their therapeutic uses does not necessarily represent current practice nor does it imply judgement as to their therapeutic efficacy.

Information on the occurrence of an agent or mixture in the environment is obtained from data derived from the monitoring and surveillance of levels in occupational environments, air, water, soil, foods and animal and human tissues. When available, data on the generation, persistence and bioaccumulation of the agent are also included. In the case of mixtures, industries, occupations or processes, information is given about all agents present. For processes, industries and occupations, a historical description is also given, noting variations in chemical composition, physical properties and levels of occupational exposure with time and place. For biological agents, the epidemiology of infection is described.

Statements concerning regulations and guidelines (e.g., pesticide registrations, maximal levels permitted in foods, occupational exposure limits) are included for some countries as indications of potential exposures, but they may not reflect the most recent situation, since such limits are continuously reviewed and modified. The absence of information on regulatory status for a country should not be taken to imply that that country does not have regulations with regard to the exposure. For biological agents, legislation and control, including vaccines and therapy, are described.

8. STUDIES OF CANCER IN HUMANS

(a) Types of studies considered

Three types of epidemiological studies of cancer contribute to the assessment of carcinogenicity in humans — cohort studies, case–control studies and correlation (or ecological) studies. Rarely, results from randomized trials may be available. Case series and case reports of cancer in humans may also be reviewed.

Cohort and case–control studies relate individual exposures under study to the occurrence of cancer in individuals and provide an estimate of relative risk (ratio of incidence or mortality in those exposed to incidence or mortality in those not exposed) as the main measure of association.

In correlation studies, the units of investigation are usually whole populations (e.g., in particular geographical areas or at particular times), and cancer frequency is related to a summary measure of the exposure of the population to the agent, mixture or exposure circumstance under study. Because individual exposure is not documented, however, a causal relationship is less easy to infer from correlation studies than from cohort and case–control studies. Case reports generally arise from a suspicion, based on clinical experience, that the concurrence of two events — that is, a particular exposure and occurrence of a cancer — has happened rather more frequently than would be expected by chance. Case reports usually lack complete ascertainment of cases in any population, definition or enumeration of the population at risk and estimation of the expected number of cases in the absence of exposure. The uncertainties surrounding interpretation of case reports and correlation studies make them inadequate, except in rare instances, to form the sole basis for inferring a causal relationship. When taken together with case–control and cohort studies, however, relevant case reports or correlation studies may add materially to the judgement that a causal relationship is present.

Epidemiological studies of benign neoplasms, presumed preneoplastic lesions and other end-points thought to be relevant to cancer are also reviewed by working groups. They may, in some instances, strengthen inferences drawn from studies of cancer itself.

(b) Quality of studies considered

The Monographs are not intended to summarize all published studies. Those that are judged to be inadequate or irrelevant to the evaluation are generally omitted. They may be mentioned briefly, particularly when the information is considered to be a useful supplement to that in other reports or when they provide the only data available. Their inclusion does not imply acceptance of the adequacy of the study design or of the analysis and interpretation of the results, and limitations are clearly outlined in square brackets at the end of the study description.

It is necessary to take into account the possible roles of bias, confounding and chance in the interpretation of epidemiological studies. By 'bias' is meant the operation of factors in study design or execution that lead erroneously to a stronger or weaker association than in fact exists between disease and an agent, mixture or exposure circumstance. By 'confounding' is meant a situation in which the relationship with disease is made to appear stronger or weaker than it truly is as a result of an association between the apparent causal factor and another factor that is associated with either an increase or decrease in the incidence of the disease. In evaluating the extent to which these factors have been minimized in an individual study, working groups consider a number of aspects of design and analysis as described in the report of the study. Most of these considerations apply equally to case–control, cohort and correlation studies. Lack of clarity of any of these aspects in the reporting of a study can decrease its credibility and the weight given to it in the final evaluation of the exposure.

Firstly, the study population, disease (or diseases) and exposure should have been well defined by the authors. Cases of disease in the study population should have been identified in a way that was independent of the exposure of interest, and exposure should have been assessed in a way that was not related to disease status.

Secondly, the authors should have taken account in the study design and analysis of other variables that can influence the risk of disease and may have been related to the exposure of interest. Potential confounding by such variables should have been dealt with either in the design of the study, such as by matching, or in the analysis, by statistical adjustment. In cohort studies, comparisons with local rates of disease may be more appropriate than those with national rates. Internal comparisons of disease frequency among individuals at different levels of exposure should also have been made in the study.

Thirdly, the authors should have reported the basic data on which the conclusions are founded, even if sophisticated statistical analyses were employed. At the very least, they should have given the numbers of exposed and unexposed cases and controls in a case–control study and the numbers of cases observed and expected in a cohort study. Further tabulations by time since exposure began and other temporal factors are also important. In a cohort study, data on all cancer sites and all causes of death should have been given, to reveal the possibility of reporting bias. In a case–control study, the effects of investigated factors other than the exposure of interest should have been reported.

Finally, the statistical methods used to obtain estimates of relative risk, absolute rates of cancer, confidence intervals and significance tests, and to adjust for confounding should have been clearly stated by the authors. The methods used should preferably have been the generally accepted techniques that have been refined since the mid-1970s. These methods have been reviewed for case–control studies (Breslow & Day, 1980) and for cohort studies (Breslow & Day, 1987).

(c) *Inferences about mechanism of action*

Detailed analyses of both relative and absolute risks in relation to temporal variables, such as age at first exposure, time since first exposure, duration of exposure, cumulative exposure and time since exposure ceased, are reviewed and summarized when available. The analysis of temporal relationships can be useful in formulating models of carcinogenesis. In particular, such analyses may suggest whether a carcinogen acts early or late in the process of carcinogenesis, although at best they allow only indirect inferences about the mechanism of action. Special attention is given to measurements of biological markers of carcinogen exposure or action, such as DNA or protein adducts, as well as markers of early steps in the carcinogenic process, such as proto-oncogene mutation, when these are incorporated into epidemiological studies focused on cancer incidence or mortality. Such measurements may allow inferences to be made about putative mechanisms of action (IARC, 1991a; Vainio et al., 1992).

(d) *Criteria for causality*

After the quality of individual epidemiological studies of cancer has been summarized and assessed, a judgement is made concerning the strength of evidence that the agent, mixture or exposure circumstance in question is carcinogenic for humans. In making its judgement, the Working Group considers several criteria for causality. A strong association (a large relative risk) is more likely to indicate causality than a weak association, although it is recognized that relative risks of small magnitude do not imply lack of causality and may be important if the disease is common. Associations that are replicated in several studies of the same design or using different epidemiological approaches or under different circumstances of exposure are more likely to represent a causal relationship than isolated observations from single studies. If there are inconsistent results among investigations, possible reasons are sought (such as differences in amount of exposure), and results of studies judged to be of high quality are given more weight than those of studies judged to be methodologically less sound. When suspicion of carcinogenicity arises largely from a single study, these data are not combined with those from later studies in any subsequent reassessment of the strength of the evidence.

If the risk of the disease in question increases with the amount of exposure, this is considered to be a strong indication of causality, although absence of a graded response is not necessarily evidence against a causal relationship. Demonstration of a decline in risk after cessation of or reduction in exposure in individuals or in whole populations also supports a causal interpretation of the findings.

Although a carcinogen may act upon more than one target, the specificity of an association (an increased occurrence of cancer at one anatomical site or of one morphological type) adds plausibility to a causal relationship, particularly when excess cancer occurrence is limited to one morphological type within the same organ.

Although rarely available, results from randomized trials showing different rates among exposed and unexposed individuals provide particularly strong evidence for causality.

When several epidemiological studies show little or no indication of an association between an exposure and cancer, the judgement may be made that, in the aggregate, they show evidence of lack of carcinogenicity. Such a judgement requires first of all that the studies giving rise to it meet, to a sufficient degree, the standards of design and analysis described above. Specifically, the possibility that bias, confounding or misclassification of exposure or outcome could explain the observed results should be considered and excluded with reasonable certainty. In addition, all studies that are judged to be methodologically sound should be consistent with a relative risk of unity for any observed level of exposure and, when considered together, should provide a pooled estimate of relative risk which is at or near unity and has a narrow confidence interval, due to sufficient population size. Moreover, no individual study nor the pooled results of all the studies should show any consistent tendency for relative risk of cancer to increase with increasing level of exposure. It is important to note that evidence of lack of carcinogenicity obtained in this way from several epidemiological studies can apply only to the type(s) of cancer studied and to dose levels and intervals between first exposure and observation of disease that are the same as or less than those observed in all the studies. Experience with human cancer indicates that, in some cases, the period from first exposure to the development of clinical cancer is seldom less than 20 years; latent periods substantially shorter than 30 years cannot provide evidence for lack of carcinogenicity.

9. STUDIES OF CANCER IN EXPERIMENTAL ANIMALS

All known human carcinogens that have been studied adequately in experimental animals have produced positive results in one or more animal species (Wilbourn *et al.*, 1986; Tomatis *et al.*, 1989). For several agents (aflatoxins, 4-aminobiphenyl, azathioprine, betel quid with tobacco, BCME and CMME (technical grade), chlorambucil, chlornaphazine, ciclosporin, coal-tar pitches, coal-tars, combined oral contraceptives, cyclophosphamide, diethylstilboestrol, melphalan, 8-methoxypsoralen plus UVA, mustard gas, myleran, 2-naphthylamine, nonsteroidal oestrogens, oestrogen replacement therapy/steroidal oestrogens, solar radiation, thiotepa and vinyl chloride), carcinogenicity in experimental animals was established or highly suspected before epidemiological studies confirmed the carcinogenicity in humans (Vainio *et al.*, 1995). Although this association cannot establish that all agents and mixtures that cause cancer in experimental animals also cause cancer in humans, nevertheless, **in the absence of adequate data on humans, it is biologically plausible and prudent to regard agents and mixtures for which there is sufficient evidence (see p. 22) of carcinogenicity in experimental animals as if they presented a carcinogenic risk to humans**. The possibility that a given agent may cause cancer through a species-specific mechanism which does not operate in humans (see p. 25) should also be taken into consideration.

The nature and extent of impurities or contaminants present in the chemical or mixture being evaluated are given when available. Animal strain, sex, numbers per group, age at start of treatment and survival are reported.

Other types of studies summarized include: experiments in which the agent or mixture was administered in conjunction with known carcinogens or factors that modify carcinogenic effects; studies in which the end-point was not cancer but a defined precancerous lesion; and experiments on the carcinogenicity of known metabolites and derivatives.

For experimental studies of mixtures, consideration is given to the possibility of changes in the physicochemical properties of the test substance during collection, storage, extraction, concentration and delivery. Chemical and toxicological interactions of the components of mixtures may result in nonlinear dose–response relationships.

An assessment is made as to the relevance to human exposure of samples tested in experimental animals, which may involve consideration of: (i) physical and chemical characteristics, (ii) constituent substances that indicate the presence of a class of substances, (iii) the results of tests for genetic and related effects, including genetic activity profiles, DNA adduct profiles, proto-oncogene mutation and expression and suppressor gene inactivation. The relevance of results obtained, for example, with animal viruses analogous to the virus being evaluated in the monograph must also be considered. They may provide biological and mechanistic information relevant to the understanding of the process of carcinogenesis in humans and may strengthen the plausibility of a conclusion that the biological agent under evaluation is carcinogenic in humans.

(a) Qualitative aspects

An assessment of carcinogenicity involves several considerations of qualitative importance, including (i) the experimental conditions under which the test was performed, including route and schedule of exposure, species, strain, sex, age, duration of follow-up; (ii) the consistency of the results, for example, across species and target organ(s); (iii) the spectrum of neoplastic response, from preneoplastic lesions and benign tumours to malignant neoplasms; and (iv) the possible role of modifying factors.

As mentioned earlier (p. 9), the *Monographs* are not intended to summarize all published studies. Those studies in experimental animals that are inadequate (e.g., too short a duration, too few animals, poor survival; see below) or are judged irrelevant to the evaluation are generally omitted. Guidelines for conducting adequate long-term carcinogenicity experiments have been outlined (e.g., Montesano *et al.*, 1986).

Considerations of importance to the Working Group in the interpretation and evaluation of a particular study include: (i) how clearly the agent was defined and, in the case of mixtures, how adequately the sample characterization was reported; (ii) whether the dose was adequately monitored, particularly in inhalation experiments; (iii) whether the doses and duration of treatment were appropriate and whether the survival of treated animals was similar to that of controls; (iv) whether there were adequate numbers of animals per group; (v) whether animals of both sexes were used; (vi) whether animals were allocated randomly to groups; (vii) whether the duration of observation was adequate; and (viii) whether the data were adequately reported. If available, recent data on the incidence of specific tumours in historical controls, as well as in concurrent controls, should be taken into account in the evaluation of tumour response.

When benign tumours occur together with and originate from the same cell type in an organ or tissue as malignant tumours in a particular study and appear to represent a stage in the progression to malignancy, it may be valid to combine them in assessing tumour incidence (Huff *et al.*, 1989). The occurrence of lesions presumed to be preneoplastic may in certain instances aid in assessing the biological plausibility of any neoplastic response observed. If an agent or mixture induces only benign neoplasms that appear to be end-points that do not readily undergo transition to malignancy, it should nevertheless be suspected of being a carcinogen and requires further investigation.

(*b*) *Quantitative aspects*

The probability that tumours will occur may depend on the species, sex, strain and age of the animal, the dose of the carcinogen and the route and length of exposure. Evidence of an increased incidence of neoplasms with increased level of exposure strengthens the inference of a causal association between the exposure and the development of neoplasms.

The form of the dose–response relationship can vary widely, depending on the particular agent under study and the target organ. Both DNA damage and increased cell division are important aspects of carcinogenesis, and cell proliferation is a strong determinant of dose–response relationships for some carcinogens (Cohen & Ellwein, 1990). Since many chemicals require metabolic activation before being converted into their reactive intermediates, both metabolic and pharmacokinetic aspects are important in determining the dose–response pattern. Saturation of steps such as absorption, activation, inactivation and elimination may produce nonlinearity in the dose–response relationship, as could saturation of processes such as DNA repair (Hoel *et al.*, 1983; Gart *et al.*, 1986).

(*c*) *Statistical analysis of long-term experiments in animals*

Factors considered by the Working Group include the adequacy of the information given for each treatment group: (i) the number of animals studied and the number examined histologically, (ii) the number of animals with a given tumour type and (iii) length of survival. The statistical methods used should be clearly stated and should be the generally accepted techniques refined for this purpose (Peto *et al.*, 1980; Gart *et al.*, 1986). When there is no difference in survival between control and treatment groups, the Working Group usually compares the proportions of animals developing each tumour type in each of the groups. Otherwise, consideration is given as to whether or not appropriate adjustments have been made for differences in survival. These adjustments can include: comparisons of the proportions of tumour-bearing animals among the effective number of animals (alive at the time the first tumour is discovered), in the case where most differences in survival occur before tumours appear; life-table methods, when tumours are visible or when they may be considered 'fatal' because mortality rapidly follows tumour development; and the Mantel-Haenszel test or logistic regression, when occult tumours do not affect the animals' risk of dying but are 'incidental' findings at autopsy.

In practice, classifying tumours as fatal or incidental may be difficult. Several survival-adjusted methods have been developed that do not require this distinction (Gart *et al.*, 1986), although they have not been fully evaluated.

10. OTHER DATA RELEVANT TO AN EVALUATION OF CARCINOGENICITY AND ITS MECHANISMS

In coming to an overall evaluation of carcinogenicity in humans (see pp. 23–25), the Working Group also considers related data. The nature of the information selected for the summary depends on the agent being considered.

For chemicals and complex mixtures of chemicals such as those in some occupational situations and involving cultural habits (e.g., tobacco smoking), the other data considered to be relevant are divided into those on absorption, distribution, metabolism and excretion; toxic effects; reproductive and developmental effects; and genetic and related effects.

Concise information is given on absorption, distribution (including placental transfer) and excretion in both humans and experimental animals. Kinetic factors that may affect the dose–response relationship, such as saturation of uptake, protein binding, metabolic activation, detoxification and DNA repair processes, are mentioned. Studies that indicate the metabolic fate of the agent in humans and in experimental animals are summarized briefly, and comparisons of data from humans and animals are made when possible. Comparative information on the relationship between exposure and the dose that reaches the target site may be of particular importance for extrapolation between species. Data are given on acute and chronic toxic effects (other than cancer), such as organ toxicity, increased cell proliferation, immunotoxicity and endocrine effects. The presence and toxicological significance of cellular receptors is described. Effects on reproduction, teratogenicity, fetotoxicity and embryotoxicity are also summarized briefly.

Tests of genetic and related effects are described in view of the relevance of gene mutation and chromosomal damage to carcinogenesis (Vainio *et al.*, 1992). The adequacy of the reporting of sample characterization is considered and, where necessary, commented upon; with regard to complex mixtures, such comments are similar to those described for animal carcinogenicity tests on p. 16. The available data are interpreted critically by phylogenetic group according to the end-points detected, which may include DNA damage, gene mutation, sister chromatid exchange, micronucleus formation, chromosomal aberrations, aneuploidy and cell transformation. The concentrations employed are given, and mention is made of whether use of an exogenous metabolic system *in vitro* affected the test result. These data are given as listings of test systems, data and references; bar graphs (activity profiles) and corresponding summary tables with detailed information on the preparation of the profiles (Waters *et al.*, 1987) are given in appendices.

Positive results in tests using prokaryotes, lower eukaryotes, plants, insects and cultured mammalian cells suggest that genetic and related effects could occur in mammals. Results from such tests may also give information about the types of genetic effect produced and about the involvement of metabolic activation. Some end-points described are clearly genetic in nature (e.g., gene mutations and chromosomal aberrations), while others are to a greater or lesser degree associated with genetic effects (e.g., unscheduled DNA synthesis). In-vitro tests for tumour-promoting activity and for cell transformation may be sensitive to changes that are not necessarily the result of genetic alterations but that may have specific relevance to the process of carcinogenesis. A critical appraisal of these tests has been published (Montesano et al., 1986).

Genetic or other activity manifest in experimental mammals and humans is regarded as being of greater relevance than that in other organisms. The demonstration that an agent or mixture can induce gene and chromosomal mutations in whole mammals indicates that it may have carcinogenic activity, although this activity may not be detectably expressed in any or all species. Relative potency in tests for mutagenicity and related effects is not a reliable indicator of carcinogenic potency. Negative results in tests for mutagenicity in selected tissues from animals treated *in vivo* provide less weight, partly because they do not exclude the possibility of an effect in tissues other than those examined. Moreover, negative results in short-term tests with genetic end-points cannot be considered to provide evidence to rule out carcinogenicity of agents or mixtures that act through other mechanisms (e.g., receptor-mediated effects, cellular toxicity with regenerative proliferation, peroxisome proliferation) (Vainio et al., 1992). Factors that may lead to misleading results in short-term tests have been discussed in detail elsewhere (Montesano et al., 1986).

When available, data relevant to mechanisms of carcinogenesis that do not involve structural changes at the level of the gene are also described.

The adequacy of epidemiological studies of reproductive outcome and genetic and related effects in humans is evaluated by the same criteria as are applied to epidemiological studies of cancer.

Structure–activity relationships that may be relevant to an evaluation of the carcinogenicity of an agent are also described.

For biological agents — viruses, bacteria and parasites — other data relevant to carcino-genicity include descriptions of the pathology of infection, molecular biology (integration and expression of viruses, and any genetic alterations seen in human tumours) and other observations, which might include cellular and tissue responses to infection, immune response and the presence of tumour markers.

11. SUMMARY OF DATA REPORTED

In this section, the relevant epidemiological and experimental data are summarized. Only reports, other than in abstract form, that meet the criteria outlined on p. 9 are considered for evaluating carcinogenicity. Inadequate studies are generally not summarized: such studies are usually identified by a square-bracketed comment in the preceding text.

(a) Exposure

Human exposure to chemicals and complex mixtures is summarized on the basis of elements such as production, use, occurrence in the environment and determinations in human tissues and body fluids. Quantitative data are given when available. Exposure to biological agents is described in terms of transmission, and prevalence of infection.

(b) Carcinogenicity in humans

Results of epidemiological studies that are considered to be pertinent to an assessment of human carcinogenicity are summarized. When relevant, case reports and correlation studies are also summarized.

(c) Carcinogenicity in experimental animals

Data relevant to an evaluation of carcinogenicity in animals are summarized. For each animal species and route of administration, it is stated whether an increased incidence of neoplasms or preneoplastic lesions was observed, and the tumour sites are indicated. If the agent or mixture produced tumours after prenatal exposure or in single-dose experiments, this is also indicated. Negative findings are also summarized. Dose–response and other quantitative data may be given when available.

(d) Other data relevant to an evaluation of carcinogenicity and its mechanisms

Data on biological effects in humans that are of particular relevance are summarized. These may include toxicological, kinetic and metabolic considerations and evidence of DNA binding, persistence of DNA lesions or genetic damage in exposed humans. Toxicological information, such as that on cytotoxicity and regeneration, receptor binding and hormonal and immunological effects, and data on kinetics and metabolism in experimental animals are given when considered relevant to the possible mechanism of the carcinogenic action of the agent. The results of tests for genetic and related effects are summarized for whole mammals, cultured mammalian cells and nonmammalian systems.

When available, comparisons of such data for humans and for animals, and particularly animals that have developed cancer, are described.

Structure–activity relationships are mentioned when relevant.

For the agent, mixture or exposure circumstance being evaluated, the available data on end-points or other phenomena relevant to mechanisms of carcinogenesis from studies in humans, experimental animals and tissue and cell test systems are summarized within one or more of the following descriptive dimensions:

(i) Evidence of genotoxicity (structural changes at the level of the gene): for example, structure–activity considerations, adduct formation, mutagenicity (effect on specific genes), chromosomal mutation/aneuploidy

(ii) Evidence of effects on the expression of relevant genes (functional changes at the intracellular level): for example, alterations to the structure or quantity of the product of a proto-oncogene or tumour-suppressor gene, alterations to metabolic activation/-inactivation/DNA repair

(iii) Evidence of relevant effects on cell behaviour (morphological or behavioural changes at the cellular or tissue level): for example, induction of mitogenesis, compensatory cell proliferation, preneoplasia and hyperplasia, survival of premalignant or malignant cells (immortalization, immunosuppression), effects on metastatic potential

(iv) Evidence from dose and time relationships of carcinogenic effects and interactions between agents: for example, early/late stage, as inferred from epidemiological studies; initiation/promotion/progression/malignant conversion, as defined in animal carcinogenicity experiments; toxicokinetics

These dimensions are not mutually exclusive, and an agent may fall within more than one of them. Thus, for example, the action of an agent on the expression of relevant genes could be summarized under both the first and second dimensions, even if it were known with reasonable certainty that those effects resulted from genotoxicity.

12. EVALUATION

Evaluations of the strength of the evidence for carcinogenicity arising from human and experimental animal data are made, using standard terms.

It is recognized that the criteria for these evaluations, described below, cannot encompass all of the factors that may be relevant to an evaluation of carcinogenicity. In considering all of the relevant scientific data, the Working Group may assign the agent, mixture or exposure circumstance to a higher or lower category than a strict interpretation of these criteria would indicate.

(a) Degrees of evidence for carcinogenicity in humans and in experimental animals and supporting evidence

These categories refer only to the strength of the evidence that an exposure is carcinogenic and not to the extent of its carcinogenic activity (potency) nor to the mechanisms involved. A classification may change as new information becomes available.

An evaluation of degree of evidence, whether for a single agent or a mixture, is limited to the materials tested, as defined physically, chemically or biologically. When the agents evaluated are considered by the Working Group to be sufficiently closely related, they may be grouped together for the purpose of a single evaluation of degree of evidence.

(i) Carcinogenicity in humans

The applicability of an evaluation of the carcinogenicity of a mixture, process, occupation or industry on the basis of evidence from epidemiological studies depends on the variability over time and place of the mixtures, processes, occupations and industries. The Working Group seeks to identify the specific exposure, process or activity which is considered most likely to be responsible for any excess risk. The evaluation is focused as narrowly as the available data on exposure and other aspects permit.

The evidence relevant to carcinogenicity from studies in humans is classified into one of the following categories:

Sufficient evidence of carcinogenicity: The Working Group considers that a causal relationship has been established between exposure to the agent, mixture or exposure circumstance and human cancer. That is, a positive relationship has been observed between the exposure and cancer in studies in which chance, bias and confounding could be ruled out with reasonable confidence.

Limited evidence of carcinogenicity: A positive association has been observed between exposure to the agent, mixture or exposure circumstance and cancer for which a causal interpretation is considered by the Working Group to be credible, but chance, bias or confounding could not be ruled out with reasonable confidence.

Inadequate evidence of carcinogenicity: The available studies are of insufficient quality, consistency or statistical power to permit a conclusion regarding the presence or absence of a causal association, or no data on cancer in humans are available.

Evidence suggesting lack of carcinogenicity: There are several adequate studies covering the full range of levels of exposure that human beings are known to encounter, which are mutually consistent in not showing a positive association between exposure to the agent, mixture or exposure circumstance and any studied cancer at any observed level of exposure. A conclusion of 'evidence suggesting lack of carcinogenicity' is inevitably limited to the cancer sites, conditions and levels of exposure and length of observation covered by the available studies. In addition, the possibility of a very small risk at the levels of exposure studied can never be excluded.

In some instances, the above categories may be used to classify the degree of evidence related to carcinogenicity in specific organs or tissues.

(ii) *Carcinogenicity in experimental animals*

The evidence relevant to carcinogenicity in experimental animals is classified into one of the following categories:

Sufficient evidence of carcinogenicity: The Working Group considers that a causal relationship has been established between the agent or mixture and an increased incidence of malignant neoplasms or of an appropriate combination of benign and malignant neoplasms in (a) two or more species of animals or (b) in two or more independent studies in one species carried out at different times or in different laboratories or under different protocols.

Exceptionally, a single study in one species might be considered to provide sufficient evidence of carcinogenicity when malignant neoplasms occur to an unusual degree with regard to incidence, site, type of tumour or age at onset.

Limited evidence of carcinogenicity: The data suggest a carcinogenic effect but are limited for making a definitive evaluation because, e.g., (a) the evidence of carcinogenicity is restricted to a single experiment; or (b) there are unresolved questions regarding the adequacy of the design, conduct or interpretation of the study; or (c) the agent or mixture increases the incidence only of benign neoplasms or lesions of uncertain neoplastic potential, or of certain neoplasms which may occur spontaneously in high incidences in certain strains.

Inadequate evidence of carcinogenicity: The studies cannot be interpreted as showing either the presence or absence of a carcinogenic effect because of major qualitative or quantitative limitations, or no data on cancer in experimental animals are available.

Evidence suggesting lack of carcinogenicity: Adequate studies involving at least two species are available which show that, within the limits of the tests used, the agent or mixture is not carcinogenic. A conclusion of evidence suggesting lack of carcinogenicity is inevitably limited to the species, tumour sites and levels of exposure studied.

(b) *Other data relevant to the evaluation of carcinogenicity and its mechanisms*

Other evidence judged to be relevant to an evaluation of carcinogenicity and of sufficient importance to affect the overall evaluation is then described. This may include data on preneoplastic lesions, tumour pathology, genetic and related effects, structure–activity relationships, metabolism and pharmacokinetics, physicochemical parameters and analogous biological agents.

Data relevant to mechanisms of the carcinogenic action are also evaluated. The strength of the evidence that any carcinogenic effect observed is due to a particular mechanism is assessed, using terms such as weak, moderate or strong. Then, the Working Group assesses if that particular mechanism is likely to be operative in humans. The strongest indications that a particular mechanism operates in humans come from data on humans or biological specimens obtained from exposed humans. The data may be considered to be especially relevant if they show that the agent in question has caused changes in exposed humans that are on the causal pathway to carcinogenesis. Such data may, however, never become available, because it is at least conceivable that certain compounds may be kept from human use solely on the basis of evidence of their toxicity and/or carcinogenicity in experimental systems.

For complex exposures, including occupational and industrial exposures, the chemical composition and the potential contribution of carcinogens known to be present are considered by the Working Group in its overall evaluation of human carcinogenicity. The Working Group also determines the extent to which the materials tested in experimental systems are related to those to which humans are exposed.

(c) *Overall evaluation*

Finally, the body of evidence is considered as a whole, in order to reach an overall evaluation of the carcinogenicity to humans of an agent, mixture or circumstance of exposure.

An evaluation may be made for a group of chemical compounds that have been evaluated by the Working Group. In addition, when supporting data indicate that other, related compounds for which there is no direct evidence of capacity to induce cancer in humans or in animals may also be carcinogenic, a statement describing the rationale for this conclusion is added to the evaluation narrative; an additional evaluation may be made for this broader group of compounds if the strength of the evidence warrants it.

The agent, mixture or exposure circumstance is described according to the wording of one of the following categories, and the designated group is given. The categorization of an agent, mixture or exposure circumstance is a matter of scientific judgement, reflecting the strength of the evidence derived from studies in humans and in experimental animals and from other relevant data.

Group 1 — The agent (mixture) is carcinogenic to humans.
The exposure circumstance entails exposures that are carcinogenic to humans.

This category is used when there is *sufficient evidence* of carcinogenicity in humans. Exceptionally, an agent (mixture) may be placed in this category when evidence in humans is less than sufficient but there is *sufficient evidence* of carcinogenicity in experimental animals and strong evidence in exposed humans that the agent (mixture) acts through a relevant mechanism of carcinogenicity.

Group 2

This category includes agents, mixtures and exposure circumstances for which, at one extreme, the degree of evidence of carcinogenicity in humans is almost sufficient, as well as those for which, at the other extreme, there are no human data but for which there is evidence of carcinogenicity in experimental animals. Agents, mixtures and exposure circumstances are assigned to either group 2A (probably carcinogenic to humans) or group 2B (possibly carcinogenic to humans) on the basis of epidemiological and experimental evidence of carcinogenicity and other relevant data.

Group 2A — The agent (mixture) is probably carcinogenic to humans.
The exposure circumstance entails exposures that are probably carcinogenic to humans.

This category is used when there is *limited evidence* of carcinogenicity in humans and sufficient evidence of carcinogenicity in experimental animals. In some cases, an agent (mixture) may be classified in this category when there is inadequate evidence of carcinogenicity in humans and *sufficient evidence* of carcinogenicity in experimental animals and strong evidence that the carcinogenesis is mediated by a mechanism that also operates in humans. Exceptionally, an agent, mixture or exposure circumstance may be classified in this category solely on the basis of limited evidence of carcinogenicity in humans.

Group 2B — The agent (mixture) is possibly carcinogenic to humans.
The exposure circumstance entails exposures that are possibly carcinogenic to humans.

This category is used for agents, mixtures and exposure circumstances for which there is *limited evidence* of carcinogenicity in humans and less than *sufficient evidence* of carcinogenicity in experimental animals. It may also be used when there is *inadequate evidence* of carcinogenicity in humans but there is *sufficient evidence* of carcinogenicity in experimental animals. In some instances, an agent, mixture or exposure circumstance for which there is *inadequate evidence* of carcinogenicity in humans but *limited evidence* of carcinogenicity in experimental animals together with supporting evidence from other relevant data may be placed in this group.

Group 3 — The agent (mixture or exposure circumstance) is not classifiable as to its carcinogenicity to humans.

This category is used most commonly for agents, mixtures and exposure circumstances for which the evidence of carcinogenicity is inadequate in humans and inadequate or limited in experimental animals.

Exceptionally, agents (mixtures) for which the evidence of carcinogenicity is inadequate in humans but sufficient in experimental animals may be placed in this category when there is strong evidence that the mechanism of carcinogenicity in experimental animals does not operate in humans.

Agents, mixtures and exposure circumstances that do not fall into any other group are also placed in this category.

Group 4 — The agent (mixture) is probably not carcinogenic to humans.

This category is used for agents or mixtures for which there is *evidence suggesting lack of carcinogenicity* in humans and in experimental animals. In some instances, agents or mixtures for which there is *inadequate evidence* of carcinogenicity in humans but *evidence suggesting lack of carcinogenicity* in experimental animals, consistently and strongly supported by a broad range of other relevant data, may be classified in this group.

References

Breslow, N.E. & Day, N.E. (1980) *Statistical Methods in Cancer Research*, Vol. 1, *The Analysis of Case–Control Studies* (IARC Scientific Publications No. 32), Lyon, IARC

Breslow, N.E. & Day, N.E. (1987) *Statistical Methods in Cancer Research*, Vol. 2, *The Design and Analysis of Cohort Studies* (IARC Scientific Publications No. 82), Lyon, IARC

Cohen, S.M. & Ellwein, L.B. (1990) Cell proliferation in carcinogenesis. *Science*, **249**, 1007–1011

Gart, J.J., Krewski, D., Lee, P.N., Tarone, R.E. & Wahrendorf, J. (1986) *Statistical Methods in Cancer Research*, Vol. 3, *The Design and Analysis of Long-term Animal Experiments* (IARC Scientific Publications No. 79), Lyon, IARC

Hoel, D.G., Kaplan, N.L. & Anderson, M.W. (1983) Implication of nonlinear kinetics on risk estimation in carcinogenesis. *Science*, **219**, 1032–1037

Huff, J.E., Eustis, S.L. & Haseman, J.K. (1989) Occurrence and relevance of chemically induced benign neoplasms in long-term carcinogenicity studies. *Cancer Metastasis Rev.*, **8**, 1–21

IARC (1973–1996) *Information Bulletin on the Survey of Chemicals Being Tested for Carcinogenicity/Directory of Agents Being Tested for Carcinogenicity*, Numbers 1–17, Lyon

IARC (1976–1996)
Directory of On-going Research in Cancer Epidemiology 1976. Edited by C.S. Muir & G. Wagner, Lyon

Directory of On-going Research in Cancer Epidemiology 1977 (IARC Scientific Publications No. 17). Edited by C.S. Muir & G. Wagner, Lyon

Directory of On-going Research in Cancer Epidemiology 1978 (IARC Scientific Publications No. 26). Edited by C.S. Muir & G. Wagner, Lyon

Directory of On-going Research in Cancer Epidemiology 1979 (IARC Scientific Publications No. 28). Edited by C.S. Muir & G. Wagner, Lyon

Directory of On-going Research in Cancer Epidemiology 1980 (IARC Scientific Publications No. 35). Edited by C.S. Muir & G. Wagner, Lyon

Directory of On-going Research in Cancer Epidemiology 1981 (IARC Scientific Publications No. 38). Edited by C.S. Muir & G. Wagner, Lyon

Directory of On-going Research in Cancer Epidemiology 1982 (IARC Scientific Publications No. 46). Edited by C.S. Muir & G. Wagner, Lyon

Directory of On-going Research in Cancer Epidemiology 1983 (IARC Scientific Publications No. 50). Edited by C.S. Muir & G. Wagner, Lyon

Directory of On-going Research in Cancer Epidemiology 1984 (IARC Scientific Publications No. 62). Edited by C.S. Muir & G. Wagner, Lyon

Directory of On-going Research in Cancer Epidemiology 1985 (IARC Scientific Publications No. 69). Edited by C.S. Muir & G. Wagner, Lyon

Directory of On-going Research in Cancer Epidemiology 1986 (IARC Scientific Publications No. 80). Edited by C.S. Muir & G. Wagner, Lyon

Directory of On-going Research in Cancer Epidemiology 1987 (IARC Scientific Publications No. 86). Edited by D.M. Parkin & J. Wahrendorf, Lyon

Directory of On-going Research in Cancer Epidemiology 1988 (IARC Scientific Publications No. 93). Edited by M. Coleman & J. Wahrendorf, Lyon

Directory of On-going Research in Cancer Epidemiology 1989/90 (IARC Scientific Publications No. 101). Edited by M. Coleman & J. Wahrendorf, Lyon

Directory of On-going Research in Cancer Epidemiology 1991 (IARC Scientific Publications No.110). Edited by M. Coleman & J. Wahrendorf, Lyon

Directory of On-going Research in Cancer Epidemiology 1992 (IARC Scientific Publications No. 117). Edited by M. Coleman, J. Wahrendorf & E. Démaret, Lyon

Directory of On-going Research in Cancer Epidemiology 1994 (IARC Scientific Publications No. 130). Edited by R. Sankaranarayanan, J. Wahrendorf & E. Démaret, Lyon

Directory of On-going Research in Cancer Epidemiology 1996 (IARC Scientific Publications No. 137). Edited by R. Sankaranarayanan, J. Wahrendorf & E. Démaret, Lyon

IARC (1977) *IARC Monographs Programme on the Evaluation of the Carcinogenic Risk of Chemicals to Humans*. Preamble (IARC intern. tech. Rep. No. 77/002), Lyon

IARC (1978) *Chemicals with Sufficient Evidence of Carcinogenicity in Experimental Animals* — IARC Monographs *Volumes 1–17* (IARC intern. tech. Rep. No. 78/003), Lyon

IARC (1978–1993) *Environmental Carcinogens. Methods of Analysis and Exposure Measurement*:

Vol. 1. *Analysis of Volatile Nitrosamines in Food* (IARC Scientific Publications No. 18). Edited by R. Preussmann, M. Castegnaro, E.A. Walker & A.E. Wasserman (1978)

Vol. 2. *Methods for the Measurement of Vinyl Chloride in Poly(vinyl chloride), Air, Water and Foodstuffs* (IARC Scientific Publications No. 22). Edited by D.C.M. Squirrell & W. Thain (1978)

Vol. 3. *Analysis of Polycyclic Aromatic Hydrocarbons in Environmental Samples* (IARC Scientific Publications No. 29). Edited by M. Castegnaro, P. Bogovski, H. Kunte & E.A. Walker (1979)

Vol. 4. *Some Aromatic Amines and Azo Dyes in the General and Industrial Environment* (IARC Scientific Publications No. 40). Edited by L. Fishbein, M. Castegnaro, I.K. O'Neill & H. Bartsch (1981)

Vol. 5. *Some Mycotoxins* (IARC Scientific Publications No. 44). Edited by L. Stoloff, M. Castegnaro, P. Scott, I.K. O'Neill & H. Bartsch (1983)

Vol. 6. *N-Nitroso Compounds* (IARC Scientific Publications No. 45). Edited by R. Preussmann, I.K. O'Neill, G. Eisenbrand, B. Spiegelhalder & H. Bartsch (1983)

Vol. 7. *Some Volatile Halogenated Hydrocarbons* (IARC Scientific Publications No. 68). Edited by L. Fishbein & I.K. O'Neill (1985)

Vol. 8. *Some Metals: As, Be, Cd, Cr, Ni, Pb, Se, Zn* (IARC Scientific Publications No. 71). Edited by I.K. O'Neill, P. Schuller & L. Fishbein (1986)

Vol. 9. *Passive Smoking* (IARC Scientific Publications No. 81). Edited by I.K. O'Neill, K.D. Brunnemann, B. Dodet & D. Hoffmann (1987)

Vol. 10. *Benzene and Alkylated Benzenes* (IARC Scientific Publications No. 85). Edited by L. Fishbein & I.K. O'Neill (1988)

Vol. 11. *Polychlorinated Dioxins and Dibenzofurans* (IARC Scientific Publications No. 108). Edited by C. Rappe, H.R. Buser, B. Dodet & I.K. O'Neill (1991)

Vol. 12. *Indoor Air* (IARC Scientific Publications No. 109). Edited by B. Seifert, H. van de Wiel, B. Dodet & I.K. O'Neill (1993)

IARC (1979) *Criteria to Select Chemicals for* IARC Monographs (IARC intern. tech. Rep. No. 79/003), Lyon

IARC (1982) *IARC Monographs on the Evaluation of the Carcinogenic Risk of Chemicals to Humans*, Supplement 4, *Chemicals, Industrial Processes and Industries Associated with Cancer in Humans* (IARC Monographs, Volumes 1 to 29), Lyon

IARC (1983) *Approaches to Classifying Chemical Carcinogens According to Mechanism of Action* (IARC intern. tech. Rep. No. 83/001), Lyon

IARC (1984) *Chemicals and Exposures to Complex Mixtures Recommended for Evaluation in IARC Monographs and Chemicals and Complex Mixtures Recommended for Long-term Carcinogenicity Testing* (IARC intern. tech. Rep. No. 84/002), Lyon

IARC (1987a) *IARC Monographs on the Evaluation of Carcinogenic Risks to Humans*, Supplement 6, *Genetic and Related Effects: An Updating of Selected* IARC Monographs *from Volumes 1 to 42*, Lyon

IARC (1987b) *IARC Monographs on the Evaluation of Carcinogenic Risks to Humans*, Supplement 7, *Overall Evaluations of Carcinogenicity: An Updating of* IARC Monographs *Volumes 1 to 42*, Lyon

IARC (1988) *Report of an IARC Working Group to Review the Approaches and Processes Used to Evaluate the Carcinogenicity of Mixtures and Groups of Chemicals* (IARC intern. tech. Rep. No. 88/002), Lyon

IARC (1989) *Chemicals, Groups of Chemicals, Mixtures and Exposure Circumstances to be Evaluated in Future IARC Monographs, Report of an ad hoc Working Group* (IARC intern. tech. Rep. No. 89/004), Lyon

IARC (1991a) *A Consensus Report of an IARC Monographs Working Group on the Use of Mechanisms of Carcinogenesis in Risk Identification* (IARC intern. tech. Rep. No. 91/002), Lyon

IARC (1991b) *Report of an Ad-hoc IARC Monographs Advisory Group on Viruses and Other Biological Agents Such as Parasites* (IARC intern. tech. Rep. No. 91/001), Lyon

IARC (1993) *Chemicals, Groups of Chemicals, Complex Mixtures, Physical and Biological Agents and Exposure Circumstances to be Evaluated in Future IARC Monographs, Report of an ad-hoc Working Group* (IARC intern. Rep. No. 93/005), Lyon

Montesano, R., Bartsch, H., Vainio, H., Wilbourn, J. & Yamasaki, H., eds (1986) *Long-term and Short-term Assays for Carcinogenesis — A Critical Appraisal* (IARC Scientific Publications No. 83), Lyon, IARC

Peto, R., Pike, M.C., Day, N.E., Gray, R.G., Lee, P.N., Parish, S., Peto, J., Richards, S. & Wahrendorf, J. (1980) Guidelines for simple, sensitive significance tests for carcinogenic effects in long-term animal experiments. In: *IARC Monographs on the Evaluation of the Carcinogenic Risk of Chemicals to Humans, Supplement 2, Long-term and Short-term Screening Assays for Carcinogens: A Critical Appraisal*, Lyon, pp. 311–426

Tomatis, L., Aitio, A., Wilbourn, J. & Shuker, L. (1989) Human carcinogens so far identified. *Jpn. J. Cancer Res.*, **80**, 795–807

Vainio, H., Magee, P.N., McGregor, D.B. & McMichael, A.J., eds (1992) *Mechanisms of Carcinogenesis in Risk Identification* (IARC Scientific Publications No. 116), Lyon, IARC

Vainio, H., Wilbourn, J.D., Sasco, A.J., Partensky, C., Gaudin, N., Heseltine, E. & Eragne, I. (1995) Identification of human carcinogenic risk in *IARC Monographs*. *Bull. Cancer*, **82**, 339–348 (in French)

Waters, M.D., Stack, H.F., Brady, A.L., Lohman, P.H.M., Haroun, L. & Vainio, H. (1987) Appendix 1. Activity profiles for genetic and related tests. In: *IARC Monographs on the Evaluation of Carcinogenic Risks to Humans*, Suppl. 6, *Genetic and Related Effects: An Updating of Selected IARC Monographs from Volumes 1 to 42*, Lyon, IARC, pp. 687–696

Wilbourn, J., Haroun, L., Heseltine, E., Kaldor, J., Partensky, C. & Vainio, H. (1986) Response of experimental animals to human carcinogens: an analysis based upon the IARC Monographs Programme. *Carcinogenesis*, **7**, 1853–1863

THE MONOGRAPHS

HUMAN IMMUNODEFICIENCY VIRUSES

1. Exposure Data

1.1 Structure, taxonomy and biology

The human immunodeficiency virus type 1 (HIV-1) was discovered in 1983 (Barré-Sinoussi *et al.*, 1983) and firmly associated with the acquired immunodeficiency syndrome (AIDS) in 1984 (Gallo *et al.*, 1984). Later, a second virus was discovered in West Africa (HIV-2) that was sufficiently different from HIV-1 in its serological and molecular characteristics to be considered a separate, but related, virus (Clavel *et al.*, 1986). Initially the virus was referred to as lymphadenopathy-associated virus (LAV) or human T-cell lymphotropic virus type III (HTLV-III); the name human immunodeficiency virus was established in 1986. Between 1985 and 1989, several non-human primates were shown to harbour related retroviruses. All of these retroviruses belong to the lentivirus subfamily, have an RNA genome and replicate via a DNA intermediate (a 'provirus') by means of a viral RNA-directed DNA polymerase, more commonly called reverse transcriptase (RT). It is this 'backward' transfer of genetic information from RNA to DNA which classifies these viruses as retroviruses. HIV-1 and HIV-2 are the only known human lentiviruses.

1.1.1 *Structure*

All retroviruses share a similar overall morphology, but there is variation in detail (Table 1). Lentiviruses contain a diploid, single-stranded RNA genome within a protein core. Each HIV-1 virion measures approximately 120 nm in diameter and has a condensed cylindrical core surrounded by a lipid membrane. The inter-relationship of the genomic RNA, core proteins and surrounding viral envelope is schematically represented in Figure 1. The viral core is a complex made up of RT (p55/66), endonuclease or integrase (IN; p32), protease (PR; p10, p12 or p15[1]), and nucleocapsid proteins (NC; p6 and p7) and two copies of positive strand viral RNA, all of which is surrounded by an icosahedral capsid protein (CA; p24). The myristoylated matrix protein (MA; p17) lies just below the lipid bilayer which surrounds the virion. Embedded within the lipid bilayer are the viral envelope glycoproteins: the external surface glycoprotein (SU; gp120) and the transmembrane glycoprotein (TM; gp41), which are non-covalently associated on the virion surface (Gelderblom, 1991; Barker *et al.*, 1995).

---

[1] According to different researchers

Table 1. Morphological features of retroviruses

Classification	Morphological features	Examples
Oncoviruses		
A-type	Non-infectious, electron-dense, double shell, electron-lucent centre. Intracytoplasmic particles: assembled core particles in B- or D-type infections. Intracisternal particles: unknown function	Precursor of MMTV
B-type	Immature doughnut-shaped cores form prior to budding. Mature cores are located eccentrically within virus particles bearing prominent envelope spikes.	MMTV
C-type	No intracytoplasmic structures, immature cores; electron-lucent centres form simultaneously with budding. A centrally located electron-dense spherical core forms after maturation. Envelope spikes not always visible	MLV, ALV, FeLV, HTLVs, STLVs, BLV, GALV, SSAV, SNV
D-type	Ring-shaped immature cores; electron-lucent centres form prior to budding. Electron-dense, eccentrically located cores form on maturation. Less prominent spikes than MMTV	MPMV (SRV-2) Other SRVs
Lentiviruses	Immature cores form simultaneously with budding. Upon maturation, conical shaped cores are formed.	MVV, HIV-1, HIV-2, SIV, FIV
Spumaviruses	Electron-lucent cores form in the cytoplasm, which bud into extracellular medium or intracytoplasmic vacuoles. Very prominent envelope spikes	HFV, SFVs

MMTV, mouse mammary tumour virus; MLV, murine leukaemia virus; ALV, avian leukosis/sarcoma virus; FeLV, feline leukaemia virus; HTLV, human T-cell lymphotropic virus; STLV, simian T-cell lymphotropic virus; BLV, bovine leukaemia virus; GALV, gibbon ape leukaemia virus; SSAV, simian sarcoma-associated virus; SNV, spleen necrosis virus; MPMV, Mason–Pfizer monkey virus; SRV, simian retrovirus; MVV, maedi-visna virus; HIV, human immunodeficiency virus; SIV, simian immunodeficiency virus; FIV, feline immunodeficiency virus; HFV, human foamy virus; SFV, simian foamy virus
Adapted from Weiss et al. (1985); Coffin (1996)

1.1.2 Taxonomy

Traditionally, retroviruses (family *Retroviridae*) have been classified according to a combination of criteria including disease association, morphology and cytopathic effects *in vitro* (Table 1; Weiss et al., 1985). On this basis three subfamilies were defined. The oncoviruses (Greek, *onkos* = mass, swelling) consist of four morphological subtypes which are associated with tumours in naturally or experimentally infected animals, and non-oncogenic related viruses. The second group, the lentiviruses (Latin, *lentus* = slow), cause a variety of diseases including immunodeficiency and wasting syndromes, usually after a long period of clinical latency. The third subfamily, the spumaviruses (Latin, *spuma* = foam), so called because of the characteristic 'foamy' appearance induced in infected cells *in vitro*, have not been conclusively linked to any disease (Schweizer et al., 1994; Ali et al., 1996).

Figure 1. Schematic representation of a mature retrovirus particle

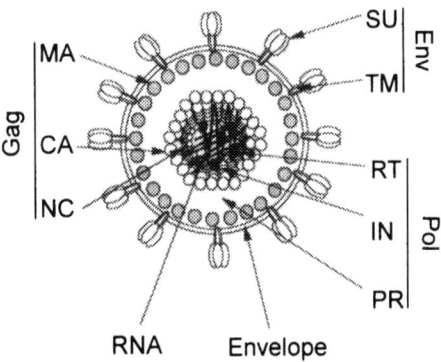

Genomic RNA is contained within a core consisting of NC and CA proteins, along with RT and IN enzymes which are required for the formation of an integrated provirus following infection of a new target cell. MA is thought to be associated with the inner face of the lipid envelope by virtue of N-terminal myristoylation and basic amino acids, although a proportion may be associated with the viral core in some cases (see text). The lipid envelope is traversed by TM oligomers to which are bound SU proteins containing receptor recognition motifs. TM may also contact MA on the inner face of the envelope. The particle is also assumed to contain PR, since Gag and Pol proteins are incorporated into particles as polyprotein precursors, and mature morphology is achieved only after proteolytic processing.

NC, nucleocapsid; CA, capsid; RT, reverse transcriptase; IN, integrase (endonuclease); MA, matrix; TM, transmembrane; PR, protease; SU, surface

More recently, the International Committee on the Taxonomy of Viruses has divided the *Retroviridae* family into seven genera on the basis of genetic structure. The lentiviruses and spumaviruses each constitute a genus; the oncoviruses have been subdivided into five genera.

In addition to their morphological classification, retroviruses have been described as 'simple' or 'complex' according to their genome organization (Cullen, 1993; Figure 2). The defining feature of complex retroviruses is that in addition to *gag*, *pol* and *env* structural genes, they encode genes which regulate expression of structural genes (see Section 1.1.7). Most non-human and human primate lentivirus, oncovirus and spumavirus isolates so far analysed are complex retroviruses (Wilkenson *et al.*, 1994).

1.1.3 *Phylogeny*

(a) *Phylogenetic relationship of HIV-1 and HIV-2 to other retroviruses*

Several lentiviruses have been identified in various species of non-human primates as well as in other mammalian species. Genetically distinct simian immunodeficiency

Figure 2. Genomic organization of human and primate lentiviruses

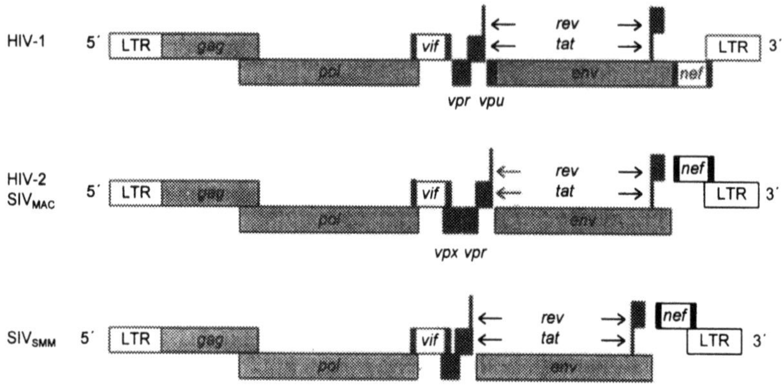

Each genome is between 9 and 10 kb in length and has a similar overall organization of structural genes: *gag, pol, env* (grey), regulatory genes (*tat, rev*) and accessory genes (*nef, vif, vpr, vpx, vpu*) (black). The *vpu* gene is found exclusively in HIV-1, while HIV-2 and the closely related SIVs (SIV_{MAC}, SIV_{SMM}) have an additional gene, *vpx*. The genome is flanked by identical long terminal repeat (LTR) sequences (white).

viruses (SIV) have been isolated from African green monkeys (*Cercopithecus aethiops*; SIV_{AGM}) (Kraus *et al.*, 1989), sooty mangabeys (*Cercocebus atys*; SIV_{SMM}) (Chen *et al.*, 1995; 1996), mandrills (*Mandrillus sphynx*; SIV_{MND}) (Tsujimoto *et al.*, 1988), Sykes' monkeys (*Cercopithecus mitis*; SIV_{SYK}) (Emau *et al.*, 1991) and chimpanzees (*Pan troglodytes*; SIV_{CPZ}) (Peeters *et al.*, 1989). The first primate lentivirus to be identified was SIV_{MAC} at the New England Regional Primate Research Center following an outbreak of lymphoma in rhesus (*Macaca mulatta*) and cynomolgus macaques (*Macaca fascicularis*) (Daniel *et al.*, 1985). SIV_{MAC} is not naturally found in Asian macaques (*Macaca mulatta*) (Lowenstine *et al.*, 1986; Wu *et al.*, 1991), but its close relationship to SIV_{SMM} can be explained by the introduction of SIV_{SMM}-infected mangabeys into primate centres in the United States during the late 1960s and subsequent transfer of SIV into macaques. Each SIV appears to be endemic to the respective monkey species and none has yet been associated with disease in the natural host (Gardner *et al.*, 1994).

Both the human and non-human primate immunodeficiency viruses exist as quasi-species (Wain-Hobson, 1993), i.e., as a population of closely related, yet genetically distinct, viruses which co-exist simultaneously in each infected host. This is a consequence of the sequence diversity generated from the high rates of nucleotide evolution (Coffin, 1986; Hahn *et al.*, 1986). The latter results from a combination of the high error rate associated with RT activity during viral RNA transcription (Ricchetti & Buc, 1990), the extremely high turnover and the ability of retroviruses to undergo recombination (Zhang & Temin, 1994).

Comparison of structural gene sequence data for human and simian lentiviruses has allowed analysis of the evolutionary relationships of these viruses. Basing a phylogenetic analysis on *pol* gene sequences, the primate lentiviruses form five distinct and approximately equidistant lineages: (1) HIV-1 and SIV_{CPZ}, (2) HIV-2, SIV_{SMM} and

SIV_{MAC}, (3) SIV_{AGM}, (4) SIV_{MND} and (5) SIV_{SYK} (Figure 3). Extensive genetic diversity exists within the lineages 1–3. For example, HIV-1 falls into two distinct groups and diverse isolates of HIV-2 constitute another independent group. Diversity within HIV-1 is discussed below. Interestingly, the two HIVs are more closely related to the nearest primate viruses than they are to one another: HIV-1 to SIV_{CPZ} and HIV-2 to SIV_{SMM} (Hirsch et al., 1989; Huet et al., 1990).

Figure 3. Phylogenetic relationships of representative primate lentiviruses, derived from *pol* protein sequences

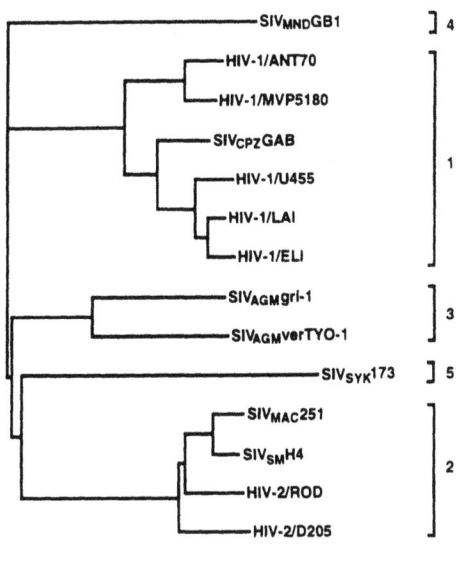

Numbered brackets at the right indicate the five major lineages. Horizontal branch lengths are drawn to scale: the *bar* indicates 0.10 amino acid replacements per site. The approximate position of the root of the tree (at the left) was determined from analyses using nonprimate lentiviruses as outgroups. The precise order of branching of the five major lineages (near the root) is unclear, but bootstrap values for all other nodes (with the exception of the branching order of HIV-2_{D205} and HIV-2_{ROD}) are in the range 99–100%.
From Robertson et al. (1995)

An SIV_{SMM} evolutionary provenance for HIV-2 is supported by their gene sequence relatedness (Gao et al., 1992) and by ecological and social considerations: sooty mangabeys, of which 30% are SIV-infected, are indigenous to West Africa, where HIV-2 is endemic. The human population is frequently exposed to SIV-infected monkey blood, since sooty mangabeys are hunted for food and kept as pets. Genetic characterization of diverse SIV_{SMM} isolates collected from a feral sooty mangabey troop suggests that each HIV-2 subtype found in West Africa originated from widely divergent strains of the simian virus, transmitted by multiple cross-species events in the same geographical region (Chen et al., 1996). Since most chimpanzees in the wild appear to be seronegative for SIV_{CPZ}, there is less evidence for a similar transfer of HIV-1 from chimpanzees.

(b) *Relationship of HIV-1 and HIV-2 isolates to one another*

(i) *Genotypes*

Sequence analysis of the *env*, *gag* and *tat* genes from diverse geographical isolates of HIV-1 has revealed that the sequences cluster into two major groups: M, into which all the earliest known isolates fall, and a genetically distant and more diverse group containing more than 35% nucleotide differences, termed 'O' for outlier (Gürtler et al., 1994; van den Haesevelde et al., 1994). Phylogenetic analyses of Group M sequences have revealed eight subgroups, designated A through H, also called clades (Greek, *klados* = branch) (Myers et al., 1991) or sequence subtypes (Myers, 1993). The term 'genotype' has also been used (Ou et al., 1993) to describe a distinct cluster of genetically related variants within a subtype (McCutchan et al., 1991, 1992; Bobkov et al., 1996) (see Figure 4).

Figure 4. Phylogeny of primate lentiviruses

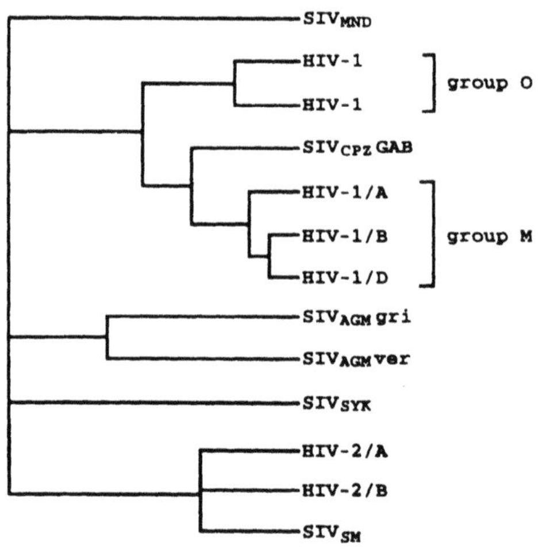

```
┌─────────────── SIV_MND
│               ┌── HIV-1
│           ┌───┤           ] group O
│           │   └── HIV-1
├───────────┤
│           └─────── SIV_CPZ GAB
│               ┌── HIV-1/A
│           ┌───┤
│           │   ├── HIV-1/B   ] group M
│           │   │
│           └───┴── HIV-1/D
│           ┌────── SIV_AGM gri
├───────────┤
│           └────── SIV_AGM ver
├────────────────── SIV_SYK
│               ┌── HIV-2/A
└───────────┬───┤
            │   └── HIV-2/B
            └────── SIV_SM
```

Within the HIV-1 group M there are at least eight different sequence subtypes (A–H), of which just three are shown; within the HIV-2 group there are five known subtypes (A–E) and within the SIV_{AGM} group there are four lineages.
From Sharp et al. (1995)

Clade B is widespread and dominant (almost exclusively) in homosexual men and intravenous drug users throughout North America (Jain et al., 1994) and Europe. With the exception of F, clades A–H have been identified in sub-Saharan Africa (Jain et al., 1994). Clade F has been identified only in Brazil and Romania (Dumitrescu et al., 1994). Clade E is currently being transmitted heterosexually in Thailand (Jain et al., 1994); a clade B variant (B') is circulating in Brazil (Potts et al., 1993) and, besides southern Africa, clade C is found in India (Grez et al., 1994). Moreover, more than one HIV-1 clade is found in some countries: in Uganda, clades A to D predominate over clade G (Kaleebu et al., 1995); in Brazil, clades B, B', C and F have been identified, while in Thailand, clade A circulates among heterosexuals and clade B in intravenous drug users (Ou et al., 1992).

Five clades (A–E) of HIV-2 have been identified (Gao et al., 1994), but currently only clades A and B comprise more than one isolate.

(ii) *Antigenic diversity*

Although there is extensive literature on the genetic diversity of HIV-1 strains, less is known about antigenic diversity. It is clear that sequence data do not translate directly into antigenic information. A principal antigenic determinant of the virus envelope protein which elicits the greatest neutralizing antibody response is an epitope in the third variable domain of gp120, commonly called the V3 loop (Moore & Nara, 1991). A large number of HIV-1 V3 sequences have been reported, but it is still unclear how many distinct antigenic subtypes (also known as serotypes) exist.

HIV-1 neutralization assays were initially carried out using laboratory-adapted viral strains and immortalized T-cell lines (Weiss et al., 1986). Primary isolates may have neutralizing phenotypes which are qualitatively and quantitatively different from T-cell line-adapted viruses. Viral diversity defined in terms of neutralization of field isolates propagated in peripheral blood mononuclear cells (PBMCs) remains to be determined, and may well be an important consideration in the development of a universally effective vaccine.

1.1.4 *Host range*

In addition to humans, HIV-1 and HIV-2 can infect some non-human primates (see Section 3.1).

1.1.5 *Cell tropism*

A distinguishing feature of HIV-1 and HIV-2 is their ability to infect $CD4^+$ T-lymphocytes and macrophages. Indeed, it was this early observation that led to the identification of the cell differentiation antigen CD4 as the receptor for HIV-1 entry into cells (Dalgleish et al., 1984; Klatzmann et al., 1984). All strains of HIV-1 and HIV-2 can infect peripheral blood $CD4^+$ lymphocytes (T-helper cells), but the extent to which immortalized or leukaemic T-cell lines are infected varies from strain to strain (Evans et al., 1987).

Most primary HIV-1 strains (not adapted to propagate in T-cell lines) infect macrophages, although the limited extent of replication of some strains may necessitate co-cultivation of the macrophages with PBMCs to allow detection of the virus (Schrier *et al.*, 1990). Antigen presenting cells such as dendritic and Langerhans' cells may be important in mucosal and sexual transmission of HIV-1 (Pope *et al.*, 1994).

Since the identification of CD4 as the receptor for HIV-1 and HIV-2, it has become apparent that the virus is also capable of limited infection of certain CD4⁺ cells, including fibroblasts, glial cells and rhabdomyosarcoma cells (Clapham *et al.*, 1991). The cellular tropism of HIV-1 appears to be determined primarily by its envelope, although other regions of the virus genome, e.g., *vpr*, may also have an influence. The identification of members of the seven-transmembrane G protein-coupled receptors which act as co-receptors helps to explain the cellular tropisms of HIV-1 (Alkhatib *et al.*, 1996; Deng *et al.*, 1996; Drajic *et al.*, 1996; Feng *et al.*, 1996).

1.1.6 *Target tissues*

(a) *Lymphoid tissue*

HIV-1 localizes in lymphoid tissue early in the course of infection (Biberfeld *et al.*, 1985; Tenner-Rácz *et al.*, 1985; Pantaleo *et al.*, 1993a). The presence of HIV-1 in lymphoid tissues throughout infection has been confirmed by in-situ methods (Embretson *et al.*, 1993). It remains uncertain whether HIV-1 infects other than lymphoid cells (Pantaleo *et al.*, 1993b).

(b) *Central nervous system*

HIV-1 frequently affects the brain. The microglial cells are the main location for viral replication in the central nervous system, although astroglial cells may be abortively infected (Shaw *et al.*, 1985; Epstein *et al.*, 1991; Donaldson *et al.*, 1994). However, there is controversy as to whether the productively infected cells of the brain are the resident microglia or are derived from invading macrophages.

(c) *Gastrointestinal tract*

HIV-1 isolated from the gastrointestinal tract of infected subjects has been reported to be biologically and molecularly different from viruses isolated from the peripheral blood of the same patient (Barnett *et al.*, 1991). In addition to lymphocytes and macrophages of the lamina propria (Smith, 1994), Nelson *et al.* (1988) reported HIV-1 to infect columnar epithelial cells and entero-chromaffin cells. Other investigators have failed to confirm these findings (DuPont & Marshall, 1995).

1.1.7 *The HIV-1 and HIV-2 genome and gene products*

The three major genes of HIV-1 and HIV-2 are the *gag*, *env* and *pol* genes, which initially give rise to polyproteins (respectively Pr55^{gag}, Pr160$^{gag-pol}$ and gp160) that are further processed to yield the structural proteins of the virus and enzymes (see Section 1.1.1 and Figure 1).

The *gag* gene products MA, CA and NC, the *pol* gene products PR, RT and IN and the *env* gene products SU and TM are always present in the same 5'–3' order. In addition, there are regulatory genes (*tat*, *rev*) and four accessory genes (*nef*, *vif*, *vpr*, *vpu*). In the proviral state, open reading frames are flanked by long terminal repeat (LTR) sequences

(Figure 2). These contain promoters of gene expression and specific enhancer elements which control viral gene expression and which are themselves influenced by cellular transcriptional proteins.

(i) *Structural proteins (Gag, Pol, Env)*

The primary product of the *gag* gene is a precursor polypeptide, p55, which undergoes systematic cleavage from its NH_2-terminus to yield the myristoylated MA, p17, and two antigens of the virus core: the CA, p24 and the PR, p15 or p14 (Levy, 1993). The latter is further processed into p7 and p6 (Barker *et al.*, 1995).

Enzymes which catalyse steps in the virus lifecycle are cleaved from the Gag-Pol polyprotein, $Pr160^{gag-pol}$ during virion morphogenesis. These are (i) the mature form of PR, composed of 99 amino acids with a molecular weight of 10 kDa (Katz & Skalka, 1994) and belonging to the category of aspartic proteinases, on the basis of the conserved Asp-Thr/Ser-Gly motif at the active site (Loeb *et al.*, 1989; Luciw, 1996); (ii) RT, which transcribes the viral RNA to DNA, and which has associated RNAse activity to degrade RNA/DNA hybrid molecules (Baltimore, 1970; Temin, 1976); (iii) IN, which results from the COOH-terminal of $Pr160^{gag-pol}$ to yield a 32 kDa protein with DNA cleavage and strand transfer activity, catalysing the covalent linkage of double-stranded DNA into the host genomic DNA (Luciw, 1996).

The initial envelope precursor protein gp160 is cleaved by a cellular protease to produce a mature glycosylated NH_2-terminal protein gp120 and the external spike glycoprotein gp41, which remain non-covalently linked (Figure 1) (reviewed by Moore *et al.*, 1993). The extracellular part of gp120 contains the binding site for the CD4 receptor, as well as the hypervariable region of about 36 amino acids referred to as the V3 loop (Freed *et al.*, 1991) (see Section 1.1.3). The gp 41 TM protein anchors gp120 in the viral lipid membrane and contains a hydrophobic peptide at its amino-terminus that is involved in membrane fusion.

(ii) *Regulatory proteins (Tat, Rev)*

The HIV-1 and HIV-2 genome encodes the major regulatory proteins Tat and Rev (reviewed by Peterlin, 1995; Luciw, 1996). Both are expressed from multiply spliced viral transcripts produced early after infection. Neither are packaged into virions and both are essential for virus replication.

The *tat* gene is bipartite, in that it has two coding exons, one located in the central region of the genome between *vpr* and *env* (Figure 2), the other overlapping the translation frames of *rev* and gp41. The 14 kDa Tat protein is localized in the nucleus by means of an arginine-rich nuclear localization signal within its basic domain. In the nucleus, Tat interacts with a stem-loop RNA structure in the LTR, designated the transactivation response (TAR) element. Tat is essential for viral replication and acts to increase the steady-state levels of viral transcripts (for both structural and regulatory viral proteins) initiated in the LTR.

Viral structural protein expression is additionally regulated by the product of the *rev* gene. Rev is an essential 19 kDa protein which facilitates the appearance of partially spliced and unspliced transcripts in the cytoplasm. In the absence of Rev, only multiply spliced transcripts are translated, so that no structural proteins, enzymes or genomic RNA can be packaged into the virus particle.

Rev, in keeping with its involvement with the splicing machinery, is located in the nucleolus. By binding to viral RNA at the Rev response element (RRE), Rev effectively shifts the balance from multiply spliced transcripts (encoding Tat, Rev, Nef and Vpr in the early stages of the virus replication cycle) to both unspliced and singly spliced transcripts which encode the viral structural proteins at a later stage in infection (Cullen, 1991).

(iii) *Accessory proteins (Nef, Vif, Vpr, Vpu)*

The role of the accessory proteins has been reviewed (Cullen, 1994; Hahn, 1994; Subbramanian & Cohen, 1994; Trono, 1995).

Nef, the first viral protein to be expressed, is a 25–30 kDa protein which is predominantly localized in the cytoplasm and inner surface of the membrane in infected cells (Yu & Felsted, 1992). Nef appears to be multi-functional: it down-regulates expression of the CD4 receptor in infected T-cells (Garcia & Miller, 1991; Aiken *et al.*, 1994), as indeed do Vpu and gp120, although the mechanism is unclear. Since the rate of CD4 endocytosis increases in the presence of Nef, it may be that Nef acts directly or indirectly via a cellular factor, to trigger removal of CD4 by endocytosis (Benichou *et al.*, 1994), thus preventing subsequent re-infection of cells already harbouring virus (Karn, 1991). The effects of Nef *in vivo* and *in vitro* are in sharp contrast. Deletion of *nef* appears to have little effect on infection by HIV-1 in T-cell lines (Cullen, 1994). However, macaques infected with SIV isolates expressing truncated Nef proteins maintain low-level viraemia and remain healthy, but if full-length Nef operates (due to a premature stop codon in SIV_{MAC239}), high-level viraemia and disease develop (Kestler *et al.*, 1991).

The *vpr* gene product is a 15 kDa oligomeric protein expressed from a singly spliced mRNA (Cohen *et al.*, 1990a,b; Zhao *et al.*, 1994). HIV-2 and most SIV strains carry an additional gene, *vpx*, which shares sequence homology with *vpr*, such that it has been suggested that *vpx* arose from *vpr* by gene duplication (Tristem *et al.*, 1992). Both Vpr and Vpx are packaged within the virions and by electron microscopy appear to be located outside the core structure (Wang *et al.*, 1994). Vpr induces differentiation and growth arrest in some tumour cell lines, even in the absence of other viral proteins (Rogel *et al.*, 1995). In terms of its effect on HIV replication, Vpr appears to enhance virus production in primary macrophages and, to a lesser extent in some T-cell lines (Hattori *et al.*, 1990; Connor *et al.*, 1995). Mutation in the nuclear localization signal of both the matrix protein p17 and Vpr of a macrophage tropic clone of HIV-1 led to a lower viral replication rate in macrophages and weakened the localization of uncoated viral complexes in the nucleus. Thus, p17 and Vpr appear to be able to mediate efficient nuclear importation of the pre-integration complex into non-dividing cells (Bukrinsky *et al.*, 1993; Heinzinger *et al.*, 1994). Vpr can also block the proliferation of human rhabdomyosarcoma cells and induce differentiation to muscle cells (Levy *et al.*, 1993a).

Vif, a 23 kDa cytoplasmic protein, is also essential for viral replication (Michaels *et al.*, 1993). In the absence of Vif, HIV-1 virions have abnormal morphology (Borman *et al.*, 1995) and have much reduced capacity to synthesize proviral DNA following infection of new target cells (Sova & Volsky, 1993).

HIV-1 and the related SIV_{CPZ} contain a *vpu* gene (Myers *et al.*, 1994), the 16 kDa phosphorylated product of which is localized in the perinuclear region of infected cells and is thus associated with the endoplasmic reticulum/Golgi system. Vpu-deficient HIV-1 mutants continue to replicate in $CD4^+$ T-cell lines, primary T-lymphocytes and macrophages, but at a reduced titre due to accumulation of virions in intracytoplasmic vesicles (Klimkait *et al.*, 1990). HIV-2 and other SIVs than SIV_{CPZ} lack a *vpu* gene, but its function is probably encoded elsewhere in the genome.

1.1.8 *Replication*

Infection by HIV is initiated when virus binds to the CD4 receptor on a target cell by means of the viral envelope glycoprotein, gp120 (Dalgleish *et al.*, 1984; Klatzmann *et al.*, 1984; Klasse *et al.*, 1993). This binding triggers a conformational change in the Env glycoprotein to expose the TM protein, gp41, resulting in fusion, possibly mediated by the co-receptor, between the virus and the host cell membrane (Weiss, 1993a). HIV-1 and HIV-2 enter the cell via a pH-independent mechanism (McClure *et al.*, 1990). After fusion, the viral core is released into the cell and single-stranded RNA, still associated with capsid protein, is converted to double-stranded proviral DNA through the polymerase and ribonuclease H activities of the viral reverse transcriptase.

The newly formed pre-integration complex enters the nucleus and the viral DNA integrates randomly in the host cellular DNA. This proviral DNA acts as a template for the production of viral RNA progeny. Transcription of the viral genome is driven by a promoter in the 5' LTR of the integrated provirus, resulting in the production of RNA molecules. These in turn serve both as messenger for synthesis of new viral proteins and as genomic RNA. Tat augments levels of viral RNA by increasing transcriptional initiation and/or elongation, and Rev regulates splicing and transport of viral RNA from the nucleus to the cytoplasm (reviewed by Cullen, 1993). Genomic RNA is subsequently packaged into virions which then bud at the surface from the cell membrane. As the virion matures, Gag and Gag–Pol polyproteins are cleaved by the viral protease into subunit proteins, resulting in the mature virion which is directed to the cell surface by the amino-terminal myristoylation of Gag (Smith *et al.*, 1993a). The virion is then released from the cell surface and this completes the life cycle (Figure 5).

1.2 Methods of detection

In this section, HIV refers to both HIV-1 and HIV-2, unless otherwise specified.

1.2.1 *Antibody tests*

The confirmed presence of HIV antibodies is considered to represent current infection because as with other human retroviruses, once acquired, infection is lifelong. An antibody test for HIV-1 was first licensed in 1985, about two years after the virus was

Figure 5. Retrovirus life cycle

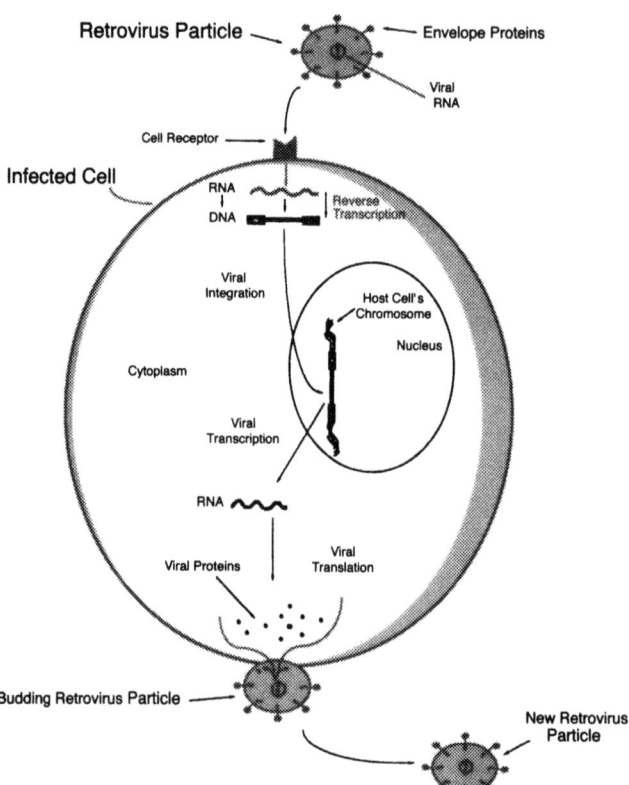

first isolated and identified as the causal agent for AIDS. The most widely used antibody tests for diagnosing HIV infection are enzyme-linked immunosorbent assays (ELISAs), with confirmation by western blot analysis.

(a) ELISA

Disrupted virions, purified from HIV-1-infected T-cells, were used as the antigen source in first-generation ELISAs. These partially purified antigens reacted with antibody to proteins from envelope (gp120 and gp41), core (p24) and reverse transcriptase (p55) regions of the virus. Early antigen preparations were often contaminated with non-viral antigens such as those originating from the major histocompatibility complex (MHC) expressed by the infected T-cells.

Sensitivity and specificity were substantially improved in second-generation ELISAs with the introduction of recombinant viral proteins or synthetic peptides. HIV-1 and HIV-2 are simultaneously detected in more sensitive third-generation ELISAs, also based on synthetic peptides of HIV or recombinant proteins (Simon et al., 1992; Barbé et al., 1994).

(b) Western blot analysis

In the western blot assay, enzyme-conjugated anti-human antibody is then used to detect membrane-bound HIV-specific antibody, observed as bands on the membrane corresponding to an antibody response to HIV proteins. The Centers for Disease Control (CDC; Atlanta, GA; United States of America) recommend that at least two bands corresponding to Gag and Env proteins must be reactive before a specimen can be classified as HIV-1 or HIV-2 antibody-positive (Centers for Disease Control, 1989a).

(c) Indeterminate HIV antibody results

Sera that do not meet the above criteria but exhibit reactivity to one or more bands are classified as 'indeterminate'. The proportion of serum samples that are repeatedly reactive on ELISA testing but interpreted as indeterminate by western blot analysis varies according to geographical region (Centers for Disease Control, 1989a).

HIV-1 indeterminate western blots can be seen in the early stages of HIV-1 infection (Gaines et al., 1987; Ranki et al., 1987; Sloand et al., 1991) and throughout HIV-2 infection (Centers for Disease Control, 1989b). Indeterminate western blot patterns have rarely been found in healthy people with no identifiable risk for HIV infection (Dock et al., 1991; Celum et al., 1991), such as leprosy patients and pregnant women (Kashala et al., 1994).

Further virological and immunological investigations such as HIV culture, quantification of p24 antigen and polymerase chain reaction (PCR) investigations can be used to diagnose HIV infection in individuals with indeterminate western blot results and a relevant exposure history (see Section 1.2.2).

(d) Undetectable HIV antibody

As with other infections, there is a delay between exposure and the development of antibodies (seroconversion), described as a 'window period'. Although antibodies to HIV-1 detectable by current ELISA may develop within weeks after infection, the usual public health practice is to retest 3–6 months after presumed exposure (Petersen et al., 1994). The duration of the window period is variable and may be influenced by the mode of transmission, infectious dose and the host immune response. Improvement of ELISA has greatly reduced the window period.

(e) Diagnosis of HIV infection in infants

The serological diagnosis of HIV infection in children born to mothers with HIV infection is complicated by the passive transfer of maternal anti-HIV IgG antibodies to the baby. These antibodies decline steadily but can be detected for up to 15 months, so that standard serological assays cannot confirm or exclude HIV infection in the infant until then. The detection of IgA antibodies, which can only originate from the child (Livingston et al., 1995), and serial testing to detect a rise in antibody titre after the initial fall during the first six months of life (Palasanthiran et al., 1994), have been used to make an earlier diagnosis. However, where facilities exist, HIV infection is diagnosed in such infants by direct detection of HIV by culture and/or PCR on two occasions (McClure et al., 1996; McMichael et al., 1996).

Tests for HIV-specific antibodies remain useful for large-scale perinatal testing and in developing countries without facilities for viral culture or PCR analysis. To confirm that an infant is infected with HIV, antibody levels should be monitored to see if they persist beyond the first 15 months of life.

(f) Detection of antibodies in saliva

Testing for HIV antibody in saliva specimens has been shown to be a reliable technique for surveillance studies in populations with high prevalence of infection (Behets et al., 1991; van den Akker et al., 1992). The methods of collection of saliva specimens influence the detection of HIV antibody; therefore, these methods have not been recommended for individual diagnostic purposes (WHO, 1993).

1.2.2 Direct detection of HIV

Many of the problems encountered in antibody-based diagnosis of HIV infection, such as long seroconversion periods, the presence of cross-reactive antibody to non-viral proteins and diagnosis of HIV infection in neonates with maternal antibody to HIV, can be overcome by using techniques that detect virus or viral products directly.

HIV diagnosis is influenced by the amount of HIV present in the biological specimen tested. Table 2 shows how HIV load in various body fluids can vary dramatically.

Viral load varies greatly according to the stage of infection. In people recently infected with HIV and in those who have progressed to AIDS, viral load is high. Comparatively low levels of virus are found in asymptomatic individuals.

(a) Viral culture

Isolation of HIV by viral culture involves the co-culture of PBMCs with phytohaemagglutinin (PHA)-stimulated lymphocytes from an uninfected donor or a susceptible uninfected laboratory cell line (Feorino et al., 1987). The presence of virus is then detected by measuring RT activity or p24 antigen.

Viral culture can take between two and four weeks to complete, requires experienced laboratory personnel to handle infectious material and is expensive.

(b) p24 Antigen

A quantitative p24 antigen capture assay has been developed, using a modified ELISA in which specific anti-p24 antibody is fixed to the wells of a microtitre plate so that free p24 antigen in serum is 'captured'. Enzyme-conjugated antibody specific to p24 is then added and the presence of immune complexes is visualized by a standard colour reaction.

The p24 antigen assay can detect HIV infection in some but not all recently exposed people before seroconversion. As antibodies to HIV develop, immune complexes form and p24 levels become low or undetectable. Late in the course of HIV disease, p24 antigen again becomes detectable.

Table 2. Representative data on isolation of HIV-1 from body fluids

Source	No. of specimens with virus isolated/ total specimens	Estimated quantity of HIV[a]
Free virus in fluid		
Plasma	33/33	1–5000[b]
Tears	2/5	< 1
Ear secretions	1/8	5–10
Saliva	3/55	< 1
Sweat	0/2	–[c]
Faeces	0/2	–[c]
Urine	1/5	< 1
Vaginal and cervical fluid	5/16	< 1
Semen	5/15	10–50
Milk	1/5	< 1
Cerebrospinal fluid	21/40	10–10 000
Infected cells in fluid		
Peripheral blood mononuclear cells	89/92	0.001–1%
Saliva	4/11	< 0.01%
Bronchial fluid	3/24	ND[d]
Vaginal and cervical fluid	7/16	ND[d]
Semen	11/28	0.01–5%

From Levy (1993)
[a] For cell-free fluid, quantities are given as infectious particles per millilitre; for infected cells, quantities are the percentage of total cells infected.
[b] High levels associated with symptoms and advanced disease
[c] –, no virus detected
[d] ND, not done

Acid dissociation of immune complexes in serum specimens increases the sensitivity of the p24 assay (Bollinger et al., 1992).

(c) *Detection of viral genomes*

PCR and other nucleic acid amplification methods offer an alternative technique to cell culture for the detection and quantification of HIV in plasma or PBMCs. It is useful for diagnosing HIV infection in people at high risk for infection who remain antibody-negative, in people at low risk with an indeterminate western blot and in infants in whom maternal antibody is still present. Quantitative PCR is increasingly used to guide therapy; PCR is also used to detect mutations, including those which confer drug resistance.

(d) *HIV quantification*

The viral load can be quantified by viral culture and by nucleic acid detection methods (PCR, branched PCR, RT-PCR and nucleic acid sequence–base amplification).

The latter have the advantage of speed (2–3 h) and sensitivity (≤ 50 copies of HIV RNA can be detected per microlitre of plasma) (Holodniy et al., 1991; Piatak et al., 1993). In developed countries, viral load measurements are being introduced into routine patient management (see Section 1.4.2).

1.3 Epidemiology of HIV infection

In this section, HIV refers to HIV-1 unless otherwise specified.

1.3.1 *HIV transmission*

The three primary routes of HIV transmission — sexual intercourse, blood contact and from mother to infant — were proposed on the basis of AIDS case reports, even before the identification of this virus as the causative agent for AIDS. The appearance of AIDS first in homosexual men (Gottlieb et al., 1981) suggested the possibility of sexual transmission, and its occurrence in recipients of blood and blood products (Anon., 1992a) and intravenous drug users (Small et al., 1983) pointed strongly to transmissibility by blood contact. Once tests for detecting HIV antibodies became available in 1984, routes of transmission were established through identification of pairs of individuals with HIV antibody who were linked by a specific form of contact, such as blood donor–recipient, mother–child and members of the same sexual partnership.

(a) Sexual contact

There is extensive documentation of HIV transmission from man to woman and woman to man through vaginal and anal intercourse that is unprotected (i.e., without condom), and from man to man through unprotected anal intercourse. The risk of transmission associated with a single episode of unprotected intercourse appears to be highly variable and dependent on a number of factors (Mastro & de Vincenzi, 1996). Probably most important such factors are the disease stage of the infected partner (de Vincenzi, 1994; Nicolosi et al., 1994a,b), which determines the amount of virus present in body fluids (Anderson et al., 1992), and the presence of genital infection (Plummer et al., 1991; Laga et al, 1993; Telzak et al., 1993), particularly genital ulcerative disease (Cameron et al., 1989). Other factors which have been less conclusively associated with an increased risk of transmission are lack of male circumcision (Cameron et al., 1989; Hunter et al., 1994), cervical ectopy (Moss et al., 1991), intercourse during menstruation and older age for exposed women (European Study Group on Heterosexual Transmission of HIV, 1992). There may be an association between susceptibility to infection and specific HLA subtypes (Rowland-Jones et al., 1995). The likelihood of HIV transmission per episode of sexual contact appears to be somewhat higher from man to woman than from woman to man, and anal intercourse presents a higher risk than vaginal intercourse for the receptive partner (de Vincenzi, 1994).

In the largest prospective study carried out to date (de Vincenzi, 1994), the cumulative risk of sexual transmission over the 20-month follow-up period of the study for couples practising unprotected intercourse was 13% from man to woman and 11% from woman to man. The transmission risks per episode were around 1/1000. A striking feature of this study was that no transmission occurred among the 124 couples who consistently used condoms during sexual intercourse. Transmission risks per unprotected episode have been higher in studies of heterosexual partners from developing countries and in studies of homosexual men (Mastro & de Vincenzi, 1996). [The Working Group noted that some studies using a range of methodologies have found several-fold higher transmission risks than this study.]

A few cases of HIV transmission through penile-oral intercourse to the receptive partner have been reported (Mayer & DeGruttola, 1987; Rozenbaum *et al.*, 1988) but such transmission is thought to occur much less frequently than transmission by vaginal or anal intercourse.

HIV infection can occur through artificial insemination (Stewart *et al.*, 1985).

(b) Blood contact

The most efficient mode of HIV transmission is through direct blood-to-blood contact. In retrospective studies of people transfused with HIV-infected blood, transmission rates were essentially 100% (Donegan *et al.*, 1990). In a number of countries, the prevalence of HIV infection among haemophiliacs reached high levels due to the use of contaminated blood products before the introduction of systematic screening and heat treatment of donations. Transmission in the health care setting has also been documented following minor skin injury with needles and from splash exposure to mucous membranes. Overall, the risk of transmission following percutaneous or mucous membrane exposure to an HIV-infected source via occupational injury has been estimated to be around 0.3% per episode (Henderson *et al.*, 1990). However, the rate of transmission to health care workers who suffer a deep injury from a hollow-bore needle containing HIV-infected blood is much higher (Anon., 1995). HIV infection is also efficiently transmitted by organ transplantation.

Iatrogenic transmission of HIV infection has been minimized in developed countries and many developing countries through the use of procedures to defer (exclude) blood donors at risk of HIV infection and universal screening of blood and tissue donations for HIV antibody (Franceschi *et al.*, 1995a). However, a small number of cases of transmission still occur when a newly infected donor has not yet developed a detectable level of HIV antibody (Ward *et al.*, 1988). In a number of developing countries, the blood supply is not yet universally screened. In South Africa, 80% of HIV-positive donations came from first-time donors, and one approach has been to use only heat-treated blood products from first-time donors (Sitas *et al.*, 1994).

The other major pathway of blood-borne transmission is through the re-use of injecting equipment and related material by intravenous drug users (Friedman & Des Jarlais, 1991). The immediate re-use of a needle and syringe after they have been used by an HIV-infected person is an efficient means of transmitting the virus. Less clear is the extent to which the risk of transmission reduces with the time elapsed between use and re-use of the injecting equipment and by various methods of cleaning the equipment.

(c) Mother-to-child transmission

Between 15% and 35% of babies born to HIV-infected women acquire the infection, the risk depending on a range of factors which vary across population groups (Peckham & Gibb, 1995). As with sexual transmission, a key predictor is the HIV disease stage in the mother (European Collaborative Study, 1992), which is associated with viral load (Roques et al., 1993). Breast-feeding is a strong independent risk factor, as shown by studies of women who became infected post-partum, either by blood transfusion (Ziegler et al., 1985) or sexually (Van de Perre et al., 1991) and of children of women already infected at the time of delivery. The majority of studies have found that delivery by Caesarian section reduces the risk of mother-to-child transmission (reviewed by the European Collaborative Study, 1994), suggesting that most transmission occurs during passage through the birth canal. This is supported by studies of twins in which the first-born twin has the higher risk of HIV infection (Goedert et al., 1991).

(d) Other modes of transmission

There is no evidence that HIV transmission can occur through routes other than those described above (Friedland et al., 1990; Gershon et al., 1990; Anon., 1994). Although it is impossible to prove that a specific form of contact carries a zero likelihood of transmission, studies of the household and casual contacts of people with HIV infection have not revealed any risk of HIV transmission. Similarly, there is no evidence that mosquitoes, bed bugs or other arthropods act as vectors of HIV between humans.

Several well documented pairs or groups of cases of HIV infection are linked both epidemiologically and through molecular typing, but the specific mode of transmission has not been ascertained (Ciesiclski et al., 1992; Chant et al., 1993; Fitzgibbon et al., 1993). It is believed that these cases represent unknowing or unacknowledged blood contact rather than evidence for new modes of transmission.

1.3.2 Geographical distribution

Assessment of the epidemiological pattern of HIV infection was initially based on AIDS case reporting (Buehler et al., 1989). Since 1985, when HIV antibody testing became widely available, case reporting of HIV diagnoses (McDonald et al., 1994) and serological surveys for HIV antibody in population subgroups (Dondero et al., 1988) have complemented AIDS case reporting as mechanisms for monitoring the occurrence of HIV infection. Across geographical and administrative areas, there has been a wide variation in the specific approaches used for epidemiological surveillance of HIV infection, depending on a range of economic, political, cultural and ethical considerations. It is therefore difficult to compile an accurate and current picture of the HIV epidemic as it has spread around the world. Some countries, particularly those of the developed world, have produced national consensus reports on past and predicted patterns of HIV infection, while for other countries, there has been a reliance on estimates made by international bodies, such as WHO.

No single approach to epidemiological monitoring of HIV infection is fully satisfactory. Compilation and analysis of AIDS case reports only provide an indication of past HIV infection patterns, because of the long and variable interval between the acquisition of infection and development of AIDS. AIDS case counts are also prone to substantial under-enumeration, because of reliance on individual medical practitioners to diagnose and report cases centrally. On the other hand, the occurrence of AIDS is generally a severe and life-threatening condition which almost always results in contact with the health system, thereby providing unbiased data in relative, if not absolute, terms within a population and over time. Surveillance based on HIV diagnosis suffers from its dependence on the extent of HIV testing and may be biased by variation in the level of testing across population subgroups. It can nevertheless provide an indication of transmission patterns earlier than would be available from AIDS case reports. Both AIDS and HIV reporting are difficult to implement on a routine basis in countries with limited resources.

Serological surveys for HIV antibody have been carried out in some countries on a routine basis (Gill *et al.*, 1989; Dondero & Gill, 1991; Ministry of Public Health, 1994), while in other countries they are implemented occasionally. Provided sampling frames are carefully chosen, such surveys can provide good estimates of HIV prevalence (and, with more difficulty, incidence) in selected population subgroups. Groups included in serological surveys have generally been either people considered to be at elevated risk of HIV infection, such as homosexual men, sexually transmitted disease clinic attendees, sex workers (prostitutes), intravenous drug users or prisoners. More representative of the general population may be people who are easily accessible within the health system or some other institutional setting, such as pregnant women, hospital in-patients, blood donors (who are now universally tested for HIV antibody in many countries) and military recruits and serving personnel.

(a) Global estimates and projections

At the end of 1995, WHO released a comprehensive set of estimates of HIV prevalence in adults by country (WHO, 1995), along with the Organization's routinely published counts of reported AIDS cases. The prevalence estimates (see Table 3) were provided by national bodies or expert groups in each country or were calculated by WHO if current national estimates were not available. The picture that emerges is one dominated by sub-Saharan Africa, where the HIV epidemic is believed to have started. The proportion of adults estimated to have HIV infection is above 14% in Malawi and Uganda and 17% in Zambia and Zimbabwe. Among the developed countries, the United States and Spain have the highest prevalence rates of HIV infection among adults, above 0.5%, while rates in other developed countries range down to below 0.05%. Apart from Cambodia, Myanmar and Thailand, with prevalence rates of 1.5–2.0%, HIV prevalence remains low in Asia, but India is now estimated to be the single country with the greatest number of people living with HIV infection.

Mathematical models have been used to carry out projections of the future course of the HIV epidemic globally, on the basis of available data and assumptions about future trends in transmission rates. These models predict that in the years up to 2000, there will be a declining annual incidence of AIDS in North America and Europe, a stable or slightly declining incidence in Africa and a sharply rising incidence in Asia (Chin, 1995).

By 2000, it is predicted that Asia will have over 1.3 million new infections per year, compared with 800 000 in Africa and 100 000 in North America and western Europe.

Table 3. Estimated prevalence of HIV infection among adults, in selected countries, at the end of 1994

Country	Number	%	Country	Number	%
North America			Greece	5 000	0.098
Canada	30 000	0.19	Hungary	3 000	0.058
United States	700 000	0.52	Ireland	1 700	0.094
Caribbean			Italy	90 000	0.31
Cuba	1 300	0.021	Netherlands	3 000	0.036
Dominican Republic	40 000	1.0	Norway	1 250	0.057
Haiti	150 000	4.4	Poland	10 000	0.05
Jamaica	12 000	0.91	Portugal	8 000	0.16
Latin America			Romania	500	0.004
Argentina	60 000	0.36	Russian Federation	3 000	0.004
Brazil	550 000	0.65	Spain	120 000	0.58
Chile	10 000	0.13	Sweden	3 000	0.072
Colombia	40 000	0.21	Switzerland	12 000	0.32
Mexico	200 000	0.42	Turkey	500	0.002
Peru	30 000	0.25	United Kingdom	25 000	0.087
Venezuela	35 000	0.32	Ukraine	1 500	0.006
Africa			**Asia**		
Egypt	7 500	0.025	Bangladesh	15 000	0.026
Ethiopia	588 000	2.5	Cambodia	90 000	1.9
Ghana	172 000	2.2	China	10 000	0.002
Kenya	1 000 000	8.3	India	1 750 000	0.38
Malawi	650 000	14	Indonesia	50 000	0.049
Morocco	5 000	0.036	Japan	6 200	0.01
Mozambique	400 000	5.7	Korea, Democratic People's Republic of	100	0.001
Nigeria	1 050 000	2.2			
Rwanda	250 000	7.1	Korea, Republic of	2 000	0.008
Senegal	50 000	1.3	Malaysia	30 000	0.3
South Africa	650 000	3.2	Myanmar	350 000	1.5
Tanzania, United Republic of	840 000	6.4	Pakistan	40 000	0.063
			Philippines	18 000	0.054
Uganda	1 300 000	14	Thailand	700 000	2.1
Zaire	680 000	3.7	Vietnam	25 000	0.069
Zambia	700 000	17	**Oceania**		
Zimbabwe	900 000	17	Australia	11 000	0.12
Europe			New Zealand	1 200	0.065
Denmark	4 000	0.15	Papua/New Guinea	4 000	0.19
Finland	500	0.019	**Middle East**		
France	90 000	0.31	Israel	2 000	0.073
Germany	43 000	0.11	Saudi Arabia	1 000	0.012

From WHO (1995)

More detailed analyses of HIV prevalence and transmission patterns are available for most developed countries and a number of developing countries through national reports or papers published in the scientific literature.

(b) United States and Canada

As the country where AIDS was first recognized (Gottlieb et al., 1981) and the developed country with the highest number of cases of HIV infection in absolute terms (WHO, 1995), the United States has carried out a large number of investigations into HIV infection. It is now apparent that two distinct HIV epidemics have occurred, beginning in the late 1970s and early 1980s. One was focused on the major communities of homosexual men, particularly in San Francisco, Los Angeles and New York. Retrospective tests of stored serum samples from homosexual men taken in the course of longitudinal studies of hepatitis B vaccination revealed a sharp rise in the incidence of HIV infection from the late 1970s (Hessol et al., 1989; van Griensven et al., 1993). These studies, as well as subsequent cohort studies (Winkelstein et al., 1987; Kingsley et al., 1991), showed that the incidence of new infection peaked at around 10% of homosexual men per year in the early 1980s. This finding was confirmed by back-projection (Rosenberg et al., 1992; Rosenberg, 1995), a mathematical method that estimates past incidence of HIV infection based on AIDS case reports combined with knowledge about the rate of progression from HIV infection to the development of AIDS.

The other major epidemic in the United States was among inner-city, largely 'African-American' or 'Hispanic' residents of the major eastern cities, such as New York, Chicago, Philadelphia, Miami, Baltimore and Newark (Centers for Disease Control and Prevention, 1994a). Transmission was associated mainly with the use of illicit drugs, either directly through injection (Schoenbaum et al., 1989) or indirectly through sexual contacts by people seeking money to buy drugs or partners of intravenous drug users (Diaz et al., 1994; Ellerbrock et al., 1995). To the end of 1994, 53% of AIDS cases reported in the United States were men who became infected through homosexual contact, but the proportion of such cases for 1994 alone had fallen to 44%, with corresponding increases in the proportion of AIDS cases attributed to intravenous drug use and heterosexual contact (Centers for Disease Control and Prevention, 1994b; Rosenberg, 1995).

In Canada, the patterns of HIV infection have generally been similar to those in the United States, but the overall rates of infection have been lower, and a higher proportion of cases have been transmitted through homosexual contacts between men (Remis & Sutherland, 1993).

(c) Caribbean

Early case reports of AIDS in the United States documented an association with Haitian origin (Anon., 1992b), and subsequent serological surveys confirmed high rates of HIV infection in Haiti and some other Caribbean countries (WHO, 1995; Cáceres & Hearst, 1996). The predominant mode of transmission in the Caribbean is heterosexual contact (Cáceres & Hearst, 1996). An apparent exception to the pattern of high HIV infection rates in the Caribbean is Cuba, where the adult prevalence has been estimated to be 0.02% (WHO, 1995).

(d) Latin America

In the early 1980s, the pattern of HIV transmission in Latin American countries closely resembled those in the United States and Europe, being largely through sexual contact between men and among intravenous drug users (Cáceres & Hearst, 1996). More recently, some Latin American countries have experienced substantial increases in the extent of heterosexual transmission. In Brazil, the most populous country of the region, 23% of AIDS cases reported in 1992 were attributed to heterosexual transmission of HIV infection, compared with 7% in 1987 (Ministério da Saúde, 1993). There remains considerable variation between countries in the extent to which HIV transmission has extended beyond the population subgroups initially affected (Cáceres & Hearst, 1996).

(e) Sub-Saharan Africa

From retrospective testing of stored sera and tissue, HIV infection is known to have existed in Africa since before 1963 (Quinn et al., 1986). Numerous serological surveys have documented the rapid spread of HIV infection through sub-Saharan Africa over the past decade. The most affected countries have been in central and southern Africa, including Kenya, Malawi, Rwanda, Tanzania, Uganda, Zambia and Zimbabwe (Nkowane, 1991; WHO, 1995). Within these countries, HIV prevalence has generally been substantially higher in cities than in rural communities (Berkley et al., 1989) and epidemic spread has been associated with major transport routes (Grosskurth et al., 1995), but is not strongly associated with social class, as measured by characteristics such as educational level attained (Malamba et al., 1994). Transmission to adults has been mainly through heterosexual contact, with roughly equal numbers of men and women infected (Rwandan HIV Seroprevalence Study Group, 1989). Medical procedures such as injections and blood transfusion have also played a role.

Studies of women engaged in commercial sex work (prostitution) had already found HIV prevalence as high as 80% by the late 1980s in several African countries (Padian, 1988). The prevalence of infection in pregnant women has reached 30% in some urban surveys, resulting in high numbers of babies being born with HIV infection (Allen et al., 1991).

In west Africa, HIV-2 was the predominant form in the mid-1980s, but in some urban areas, HIV-1 is now becoming more prevalent (Kanki et al., 1994).

(f) Europe

In most European countries, HIV infection and AIDS were first reported among homosexual men in the early to mid-1980s (Downs et al., 1987), but three distinct epidemiological patterns have emerged subsequently. In Germany, the Netherlands, the Nordic countries and the United Kingdom, sexual transmission between men has remained by far the most important route of transmission. In these countries, the cumulative proportions of AIDS cases attributed to male homosexual contact exceeded 60% in 1994 (European Centre for the Epidemiological Monitoring of AIDS, 1995a) and the prevalence of HIV infection in pregnant women has generally been below 0.1% (European Centre for the Epidemiological Monitoring of AIDS, 1994). There are exceptions, such as parts of inner London, where large sections of the population are ethnic minority groups, in which the prevalence in pregnant women has been estimated at 0.4% (PHLS (Public Health Laboratory Service) Communicable Diseases Surveillance Centre, 1993).

In other European countries, the pattern of HIV infection became dominated by transmission related to intravenous drug use during the 1980s. Particularly affected were Italy, Spain and Switzerland, where HIV prevalence among people who inject drugs exceeded 50% in several cities (Friedman & Des Jarlais, 1991; European Centre for the Epidemiological Monitoring of AIDS, 1995a). As a consequence, these countries have experienced increasing rates of HIV infection and AIDS among women, acquired either through the sharing of injecting equipment or by sexual contact with male intravenous drug users, and of mother-to-child transmission of HIV infection (Franceschi et al., 1994; European Centre for the Epidemiological Monitoring of AIDS, 1995b).

In a third group of European countries, primarily those of eastern Europe, HIV transmission appears to have been very limited so far (European Centre for the Epidemiological Monitoring of AIDS, 1995b). There are notable exceptions, such as a major outbreak of nosocomially-acquired HIV infection among children in Romania in the mid-1980s (Patrascu & Dumitrescu, 1993). In Poland, nearly half of the reported AIDS cases have been among intravenous drug users (European Centre for the Epidemiological Monitoring of AIDS, 1995a).

(g) *Asia*

There has been considerable variation between Asian countries in the extent to which rates of HIV infection have been monitored. However, there appears to be substantial heterogeneity, both within and across countries, in the patterns of HIV transmission (Kaldor et al., 1994). As in Europe, the first Asian cases of HIV infection and AIDS were reported in homosexual men (Weniger et al., 1991), but other routes of transmission later became predominant in a number of countries. In Myanmar (Htoon et al., 1994) and Thailand (Brown et al., 1994a), the prevalence of HIV infection among intravenous drug users increased rapidly during the mid- to late 1980s, reaching levels of 40–50% within a few years. High prevalences were reported among intravenous drug users in Yunnan Province, China (Xinhua et al., 1994), the north-east Indian state of Manipur (Sarkar et al., 1993) and, more recently (and to a lesser extent so far), in Malaysia (Singh et al., 1994) and Vietnam (Kaldor et al., 1994).

A separate HIV epidemic in Thailand initially arose through transmission between sex workers and their clients. Some surveys of prostitutes have found up to 70% having HIV infection, with a strong inverse association between prevalence of infection and the price charged per client, presumably through association with frequency of contact and prevalence in client groups (Brown et al., 1994a).

A high prevalence of HIV infection has also been found among female prostitutes in a number of Indian cities (Jain et al., 1994).

In several Asian countries, monitoring of population subgroups more representative of the general population, such as pregnant women and military recruits, has revealed a steady increase in HIV prevalence, presumably as a consequence of heterosexual transmission. By 1993, the prevalence of HIV infection in pregnant women had reached 2% in Thailand overall and 8% in the northern province of ChiangMai. The prevalence among military recruits in northern Thailand (men aged around 20) was of the order of 10% (Brown *et al.*, 1994a). In several other countries, including Cambodia and India, the reported HIV prevalence among volunteer blood donors has already exceeded 1% (Jain *et al.*, 1994; Kaldor *et al.*, 1994).

Nevertheless, a large part of the Asian population so far appears to be relatively untouched by the global spread of the HIV epidemic. The small numbers of cases reported from China (mostly from Yunnan province), Pakistan, Bangladesh and Indonesia (WHO, 1995) may to some extent be attributable to limited surveillance systems, but probably also reflect very low rates of HIV transmission in these countries.

(h) Oceania

In Australia and New Zealand, HIV transmission has overwhelmingly been through sexual contact between men (Crofts *et al.*, 1994). Transmission via this route occurred at high levels in the early 1980s but declined sharply in the second half of the decade.

In Papua New Guinea, heterosexual contact has emerged as the most important route of transmission (Malau *et al.*, 1994).

(i) Middle East

Few cases of HIV infection or AIDS have been reported from Middle Eastern countries (WHO, 1995), and distinct transmission patterns have not been discerned.

1.4 Clinical description of non-neoplastic disorders

1.4.1 *Seroconversion syndrome*

The 'seroconversion syndrome', also known as 'primary HIV infection' or 'acute retroviral syndrome', refers to a complex of symptoms that occur in the first one to six weeks after HIV-1 infection in many adult patients (Tindall *et al.*, 1988a,b) during the 'window period' before HIV antibody is detectable (see Section 1.2.1). Early observations on a few patients (Cooper *et al.*, 1985; Ho *et al.*, 1985a) indicated that these included truncal maculopapular rash, fever, arthralgia, myalgia, sore throat, lymphadenopathy, abdominal cramps, diarrhoea and headache (Ho *et al.*, 1985a). Subsequent studies of series of patients in the United States (Fox *et al.*, 1987), Australia (Tindall *et al.*, 1988a,b), Italy (Sinicco *et al.*, 1990) and Switzerland (Kinloch-de Loës *et al.*, 1993) have confirmed this constellation of signs and symptoms (see Table 4), although the frequency varies somewhat depending on the definitions used, the means of determination (e.g., self-reported versus observed) and the severity or persistence of symptoms. Additional signs and symptoms in persons with primary HIV infection include lethargy and malaise, anorexia and weight loss, retro-orbital pain and, more rarely, rhinorrhoea, dark urine and irritability (Cooper *et al.*, 1985; Tindall *et al.*, 1988a,b).

Table 4. Selected common symptoms in series of patients with seroconversion syndrome

Reference	No.[a]	Percentage with						
		Fever	Skin rash	Sore throat	Myalgia/ arthralgia	Headache	Diarrhoea	Enlarged[b] nodes
Kinloch-de Loës et al. (1993)	31	87	68	48	42	39	32	57
Sinicco et al. (1990)	12	100	58	75	75	NR	17	92
Tindall et al. (1988a)	39	77	23	56	56	49	28	43
Fox et al. (1987)	22	23	14	23	14	23	14	36

[a] Number of patients in series
[b] Enlarged nodes, polyadenomegaly; enlarged lymph nodes/lymphadenopathy
NR, not reported

In the first weeks of HIV-1 infection, there are very high levels of circulating virus (Clark et al., 1991; Daar et al., 1991) and 'antigen excess' as determined by p24 antigen assays (Kessler et al., 1987; Henrard et al., 1995). Numbers of peripheral CD4⁺ T-lymphocytes decrease markedly and CD8⁺ T-lymphocytes increase (Roos et al., 1992; Weiss et al., 1992; Zaunders et al., 1995). Leukopenia and thrombocytopenia may be seen (Cooper et al., 1985; Ho et al., 1985a; Scully et al., 1989; Kinloch-de Loës et al., 1993) (Figure 6).

The occurrence of the seroconversion syndrome and its clinical severity may be prognostic of a rapid rate of progression to AIDS (Sinicco et al., 1993; Henrard et al., 1995).

1.4.2 Immunological decline

Following infection, there is a variable period during which most patients are asymptomatic but undergo progressive immunological decline. This may be measured by various parameters such as CD4⁺ T-cell counts and percentages of total lymphocytes, the ratio of CD4⁺ to CD8⁺ T-cells and serum levels of β_2-microglobulin and neopterin (Fahey et al., 1990; Gruters et al., 1991). Immunological decline is not smooth or consistent over the prolonged course of infection. As a general rule, some parameters, such as CD4⁺ T-cell count, percentage and CD4⁺ to CD8⁺ ratio, decline with duration of HIV infection and appearance of symptomatic disease, whereas markers of lymphocyte activation, such as serum levels of β_2-microglobulin and neopterin, increase (see Figure 6).

Peripheral blood measurements, particularly the absolute CD4⁺ T-cell count (or CD4⁺ T-cell percentage), are used clinically to indicate the stage of HIV disease. CD4⁺ T-cell decline and rate of decline have proven to be useful, if imperfect, markers of the development of the disease (Fahey et al., 1990; Phillips et al., 1991). During primary HIV infection, CD4⁺ T-cells and their percentage typically fall rapidly, rise again with the appearance of HIV antibody, then gradually decline during a long 'latent' (asymptomatic) period of several years (Margolick et al., 1993, 1994; Holmberg et al., 1995a). Subsequently, a more rapid drop in CD4⁺ T-cell count or percentage presages the onset of AIDS-defining conditions and opportunistic infections (Krämer et al., 1992; Galai et al., 1993; Phillips et al., 1994a). The prognostic value of rapidly declining or low CD4⁺ T-cell counts as predictors of AIDS onset has been amply demonstrated in populations at risk for HIV infection, including homosexual and bisexual men (Schechter et al., 1989; Veugelers et al., 1993), intravenous drug users (Zangerle et al., 1991; Margolick et al., 1992; Muñoz et al., 1992; Alcabes et al., 1993a), heterosexual women (Flanigan et al., 1992) and haemophilic men (Eyster et al., 1987; Phillips et al., 1989).

Figure 6. Schematic model of the natural history of HIV-1 infection

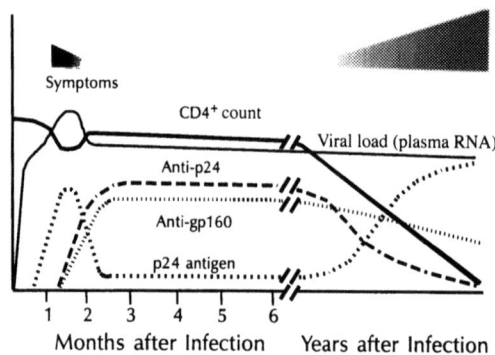

Markers of immunological decline other than CD4⁺ T-cells have been investigated for prognostic purposes. In particular, serum levels of β_2-microglobulin and neopterin, non-specific markers of inflammation, correlate with declining immunity and the onset of AIDS-related conditions (Krämer et al., 1992; Lifson et al., 1992; Muñoz et al., 1992; Galai et al., 1993). Some investigators have found that addition of serum β_2-microglobulin or neopterin determinations to CD4⁺ T-cell counts improves prognostic ability, but in general, the clinical role of these markers is diminishing (Melmed et al., 1989; Fahey et al., 1990; Krämer et al., 1992; Muñoz et al., 1992; Galai et al., 1993).

The various immunological markers do not reflect accurately the total body burden of HIV (Pantaleo et al., 1993a). HIV is actively replicating throughout the long asymptomatic period of infection. Although the decline in CD4⁺ T-cells is gradual (Figure 6), up to 30% of the PBMCs may be infected by HIV and lost each day. The total viral load varies, but 10^{10} or more new virions may be generated per day and viral load measurements have been shown to have prognostic value beyond the CD4⁺ count (Ho et al., 1995; Wei et al., 1995; Mellors et al., 1996; O'Brien et al., 1996).

During HIV-1 and HIV-2 infection, cellular immunity is compromised more than humoral immunity (Fauci et al., 1991; Pantaleo & Fauci, 1995). Not only the number but also the function of CD4⁺ and CD8⁺ cytotoxic T-lymphocytes decrease, particularly in the initial stages of HIV infection (Gruters *et al.*, 1991; Mackewicz *et al.*, 1991; Margolick *et al.*, 1993; Torpey *et al.*, 1993; Koup *et al.*, 1994). Anergy to delayed-type hypersensitivity skin tests is also more likely to occur as the disease progresses (Blatt *et al.*, 1993; Gordin *et al.*, 1994).

1.4.3 *Non-AIDS-defining manifestations of HIV infection*

(a) *Classification of HIV disease*

The use of the term 'AIDS' has been complicated by changes in its definition and the need to apply somewhat different definitions depending upon local situations. The initial definition of AIDS was developed in 1982 by the CDC and subsequently accepted by WHO in 1985. There were major revisions of the classification system in 1987 (WHO, 1988); cervical cancer, recurrent pneumonia, pulmonary tuberculosis and, for persons in the United States, a CD4$^+$ T-cell count of less than 200 cells/mm^3 (or percentage less than 14%) in HIV-positive individuals were added to the definition at the beginning of 1993 (Centers for Disease Control and Prevention, 1992a). Each of these revisions resulted in a large increase in reported numbers of AIDS cases in subsequent years, as AIDS was diagnosed earlier by including a broader range of conditions and, particularly in the United States, by including CD4$^+$ T-cell counts in patients who had not developed an AIDS-defining opportunistic infection or malignancy.

Because of the different spectrum of AIDS-related diseases in developing countries, and the shortage of sophisticated diagnostic equipment there, a WHO workshop in 1985 adopted a provisional clinical case definition of AIDS for use in such regions of the world (WHO, 1986).

Some non-malignant, non-AIDS-defining conditions have been described in the past as 'persistent generalized lymphadenopathy' and 'AIDS-related complex'. The former term was used to describe the lymphadenopathies often seen in HIV-infected persons before AIDS was recognized as an entity (Centers for Disease Control, 1982). In 1983, the Extramural AIDS Working Group of the US National Cancer Institute and National Institutes of Allergy and Infectious Diseases first defined the term 'AIDS-related complex' to cover the status of persons whose clinical condition did not meet the AIDS surveillance definition but who exhibited clinical and laboratory abnormalities that appeared to be related to AIDS (Abrams, 1988). This definition was never widely adopted. AIDS-related complex originally referred to persistent lymphadenopathy (Kaplan *et al.*, 1988), fever, weight loss, diarrhoea, fatigue and night sweats and, in standard laboratory tests, leukopenia, thrombocytopenia (Abrams, 1988; Sloand *et al.*, 1992) and anaemia. Later, other non-fatal conditions such as oral candidiasis, oral hairy leukoplakia and herpes zoster (Buchbinder *et al.*, 1992; Holmberg *et al.*, 1995b) were included, as well as some major manifestations that later became part of the most recent CDC definition of AIDS (Centers for Disease Control and Prevention, 1992a; see Table 5).

Table 5. Conditions included in the 1993 AIDS surveillance case definition[a]

Candidiasis of bronchi, trachea or lungs
Candidiasis, oesophageal
Cervical cancer, invasive[b]
Coccidiomycosis, disseminated or extrapulmonary
Cryptococcosis, extrapulmonary
Cryptosporidiosis, chronic intestinal (> 1 month's duration)
Cytomegalovirus disease (other than liver, spleen or nodes)
Cytomegalovirus retinitis (with loss of vision)
Encephalopathy, HIV-related
Herpes simplex; chronic ulcer(s) (> 1 month's duration); or bronchitis, pneumonitis or oesophagitis
Histoplasmosis, disseminated or extrapulmonary
Isosporiasis, chronic intestinal (> 1 month's duration)
Kaposi's sarcoma
Lymphoma, Burkitt's (or equivalent term)
Lymphoma, immunoblastic (or equivalent term)
Lymphoma, primary, of brain
Mycobacterium avium complex or *M. kansasii*, disseminated or extrapulmonary
Mycobacterium tuberculosis, any site (pulmonary[b] or extrapulmonary)
Mycobacterium, other species or unidentified species, disseminated or extrapulmonary
Pneumocystis carinii pneumonia
Pneumonia, recurrent[b]
Progressive multifocal leukencephalopathy
Salmonella septicaemia, recurrent
Toxoplasmosis of brain
Wasting syndrome due to HIV
Immunodeficiency as measured by a $CD4^+$ T-cell count less than 200 cells/mm^3 or $CD4^+$ T-cell percentage less than 14%[b,c]

[a] From Centers for Disease Control and Prevention (1992a) [Appendix B]
[b] Added in the 1993 expansion of the AIDS surveillance case definition
[c] United States only

(b) Non-AIDS illness

To summarize a large body of research and clinical observations, it is clear that there are many pre-AIDS conditions, signs and symptoms of HIV infection. In persons with immunological impairment, many of these conditions reflect opportunistic or reactivated infection. Generally, these include 'constitutional' symptoms, namely persistent weight loss, diarrhoea, sweating and headaches (independent of intracranial causes) (Greenberg *et al.*, 1992; Hoover *et al.*, 1993; Holmberg *et al.*, 1995b); oral and sinus problems, including oral candidiasis, oral hairy leukoplakia and sinusitis (Farizo *et al.*, 1992;

Holmberg et al., 1995b); skin manifestations, such as herpes zoster, seborrhoeic dermatitis and eczema; and anogenital problems, such as ulcers, fissures, warts and vaginal candidiasis (Renzullo et al., 1991; Holmberg et al., 1995b). Finally, several early neurological manifestations can be added to the spectrum of morbidity suffered by persons before they develop AIDS (Janssen et al., 1989; Holmberg et al., 1995b).

(c) *Time to AIDS*

The incubation time between HIV infection and the appearance of clinical AIDS conditions is of obvious importance to clinicians caring for HIV-infected patients, to epidemiologists and statisticians trying to model the size and direction of the HIV epidemic, to health care planners and administrators attempting to anticipate future health care needs of the HIV-infected population and last but not least to the patients themselves. This incubation period has been examined in populations in which dates of HIV-1 infection could be ascertained or interpolated, including homosexual and bisexual men (Lui et al., 1988; Bacchetti & Moss, 1989; Biggar et al., 1990; Giesecke et al., 1990; Rutherford et al., 1990; Kuo et al., 1991) and transfusion recipients (Ward et al., 1989). Almost all studies indicate that the median incubation period is 7–11 years (Alcabes et al., 1993b). Many studies have attempted to discern host factors that may shorten or lengthen the incubation period of HIV infection, but only one 'cofactor', age, has been found consistently. In adults, the older the HIV-infected patient is, the shorter is the incubation period (Biggar & International Registry of Seroconverters, 1990; Mariotto et al., 1992; Darby et al., 1996). Antiretroviral therapies against HIV and prophylactic therapies against diseases associated with it, such as *Pneumocystis carinii* infection, have been shown to delay the onset of AIDS (Collier et al., 1996).

1.4.4 *AIDS manifestations*

Table 5 lists the 26 AIDS-defining conditions recognized by CDC. Apart from the recognized HIV-associated malignancies, almost all are opportunistic infections. However, there is geographical variation, probably related to the varying prevalence of relevant pathogens. In Thailand, *Penicillium marneffei*, not included in CDC's definition of AIDS, is a very common fungal pathogen in AIDS patients (Sirisanthana & Sirisanthana, 1995).

The most frequently reported opportunistic infection of HIV-infected adults and children in the United States and most other developed countries is *Pneumocystis carinii* pneumonia (PCP) (Hughes, 1995). However, as treatment recommendations and guidelines have been published and promulgated (Centers for Disease Control and Prevention, 1992b), the incidence of cases of AIDS-defining PCP has declined (Muñoz et al., 1993; Katz et al., 1994; Centers for Disease Control and Prevention, 1995a; see Section 1.5.3).

Tuberculosis and non-tuberculous mycobacterial infections, particularly *Mycobacterium avium* complex (*M. avium* and *M. intracellulare*) (Horsburgh, 1991) are common. These have received much attention, because many multi-drug-resistant strains of *M. tuberculosis* have become epidemic in HIV-1-infected persons, especially in New York City in recent years (Frieden et al., 1993). The continuing high rates of tuberculosis in

HIV-infected persons in developing countries present great problems for prevention, diagnosis and treatment (Pitchenik, 1990).

Candidiasis of the oesophagus, bronchi, trachea and lungs are all AIDS-defining conditions in HIV-infected persons.

Other fungal infections, such as cryptococcosis, coccidioidomycosis and histoplasmosis, are AIDS-defining opportunistic infections (Galgiani & Ampel, 1990; Currie & Casadevall, 1994; Stevens, 1995; Rinaldi, 1996) and have been included in several comprehensive clinical guidelines and preventive efforts for persons with HIV infection (Centers for Disease Control and Prevention, 1995b).

Parasitic infections of the central nervous system, notably with *Toxoplasma gondii*, are life-threatening complications in the HIV-immunocompromised host and require early diagnosis to optimize treatment (Wang *et al.*, 1995). The protozoans *Cryptosporidium* and *Isospora* have long been recognized as important causes of chronic diarrhoea in AIDS patients (DeHovitz *et al.*, 1986; Lopez & Gorbach, 1988).

Cytomegalovirus infections of the retina and intestines are often seen late in the course of HIV infection. Cytomegalovirus retinitis and colitis are much more difficult to prevent or treat than PCP and some other parasitic and bacterial infections. Therefore, as a proportion of AIDS diagnoses, their frequency has increased in developed countries, while that of PCP has decreased (Katz *et al.*, 1994).

Bacterial infections are frequent in HIV-infected persons, especially community-acquired pneumonia (Caiaffa *et al.*, 1993; Holmberg *et al.*, 1995b) and septicaemia (Whimbey *et al.*, 1986). Recurrent salmonellosis, an AIDS-defining condition, is an important, if less frequent, enteric infection (Lopez & Gorbach, 1988).

Progressive multifocal leukoencephalopathy is caused by the JC virus (Fong *et al.*, 1995). Focal neurological manifestations can be caused by opportunistic infections, such as toxoplasmosis, or by lymphoma. HIV can also directly cause peripheral nervous system abnormalities, such as sensory neuropathy, and AIDS-related dementia in late HIV infection (Simpson & Tagliati, 1994).

Wasting syndrome (DuPont & Marshall, 1995; Grunfeld, 1995), originally referred to as 'Slim disease' in Africa (Serwadda *et al.*, 1985), has long been recognized as a major cause of HIV-related morbidity and mortality. Reduced calorific intake is the prime determinant of this weight loss (Macallan *et al.*, 1995).

Paediatric AIDS has a somewhat different clinical profile, with an increased incidence of lymphocyte intestinal pneumonia in HIV-infected children (Horowitz & Pizzo, 1990; Chintu *et al.*, 1993).

1.4.5 *Long-term non-progressors*

'Long-term non-progressors', 'healthy long-term survivors' and other such terms describe persons known to be infected for several years but who have no or minor symptoms of HIV infection and who have $CD4^+$ T-cell counts that are normal or near normal (e.g., more than 500 $CD4^+$ T-cells/mm^3). About 5–10% of HIV-infected persons remain asymptomatic and maintain $CD4^+$ T-lymphocyte counts above 500 cells/mm^3 for 10 or more years (Buchbinder *et al.*, 1994). With time after infection, the percentage of long-term non-progressors declines (Baltimore, 1995). While few in number, these persons have become the focus of much current research from two broad points of view: the host and the virus.

Most research into host factors has focused on factors associated with preserved immune function, and indicates that non-progressors, compared with other HIV-infected persons, have higher $CD8^+$ T-lymphocyte counts and lower antigenaemia and viral load (Lifson *et al.*, 1991; Buchbinder *et al.*, 1994; Cao *et al.*, 1995; Hogervorst *et al.*, 1995; Pantaleo *et al.*, 1995). $CD8^+$ T-cell function appears to be important in the control of viral replication (Lifson *et al.*, 1991; Landay *et al.*, 1993), while the role of neutralizing antibodies is unclear (Hogervorst *et al.*, 1995).

Viral variants may have different pathogenicity. Evidence of at least one less virulent strain of HIV-1 with a variant form of *nef* gene has come from a cluster of long-term healthy survivors infected from a single blood donor (Deacon *et al.*, 1995).

1.4.6 *Human immunodeficiency virus type 2 (HIV-2)*

HIV-2 has been recovered mainly from patients in west Africa. A seroconversion syndrome has also been described in relation to HIV-2 infection (Besnier *et al.*, 1990). Symptomatic patients usually have been described as having chronic diarrhoea, weight loss, lymphadenopathy and tuberculosis. However, HIV-2-infected persons can have the same immunological and clinical spectrum of disease as HIV-1 (Clavel *et al.*, 1987; Marlink *et al.*, 1988; Nauclér *et al.*, 1989; Odehouri *et al.*, 1989). Sexual and mother–child transmission seem to be less efficient (Matheron *et al.*, 1990; Markowitz, 1993; Kanki *et al.*, 1994). There is evidence that HIV-2 is less pathogenic than HIV-1. HIV-2-infected patients may have longer incubation periods between infection and AIDS-defining conditions than do HIV-1-infected patients (Burin Des Roziers *et al.*, 1987; Pepin *et al.*, 1991; Markowitz, 1993; Whittle *et al.*, 1994).

1.5 Control and prevention

1.5.1 *Behavioural prevention*

In the absence of a vaccine, behavioural change remains necessary to stem the worldwide HIV epidemic. To prevent sexual transmission, two general categories of preventive activity are usually urged: reducing the number of sexual partners and modifying the types of sexual contact; and the use of condoms.

Protection of sex partners from exposure to semen, blood and vaginal fluid during intercourse can be accomplished by the consistent and correct use of condoms, and this recommendation has been promulgated worldwide (Choi & Coates, 1994; Johnson, 1994; Stryker *et al.*, 1995). Other strategies to minimize risk of infection may be useful, such as penile withdrawal prior to ejaculation (de Vicenzi *et al.*, 1994) and the use of the vaginal pouch (or 'female condom') (Farr *et al.*, 1994).

Various programmes to change behaviour — such as increasing the use of condoms — have been effective to varying extents (Choi & Coates, 1994; Kelly *et al.*, 1994; Moore *et al.*, 1994; Stryker *et al.*, 1995). The greatest change has occurred among older

European and American homosexual men, who dramatically decreased their sexual exposures and HIV infection rates as early as the mid-1980s (Winkelstein *et al.*, 1987; Centers for Disease Control and Prevention, 1992c). The change in sexual behaviour and use of condoms among heterosexual men and women has been more modest (Catania *et al.*, 1992; Diaz *et al.*, 1994).

Empirical evidence indicates that behaviourally based HIV prevention programmes have had a favourable impact in specific populations, especially when delivered with sufficient resources, intensity and cultural sensitivity (Holtgrave *et al.*, 1995; Office of Technology Assessment, 1995). However, outcomes of prevention programmes, such as partner notification (Potterat *et al.*, 1989), have not been well evaluated. Some programmes or measures have been evaluated, and found to be ineffective, for example, programmes for counselling and testing (Higgins *et al.*, 1991a) and mandatory premarital testing for HIV (Turnock & Kelly, 1989).

Behavioural interventions are thought to have reduced the spread of HIV among intravenous drug users who share needles, syringes and other blood-tainted effects (Booth & Watters, 1994; Chitwood, 1994; Watters, 1994). Firstly, treatment for drug dependence can reduce the number of intravenous drug users in a community and so, presumably, decrease HIV transmission (Sisk *et al.*, 1990). Secondly, previously used needles may be disinfected, usually with bleach, but the contact times with bleach that are necessary to reduce or eliminate HIV in injection equipment are considerably longer than those generally applied by intravenous drug users (Centers for Disease Control and Prevention, 1994b; Garza *et al.*, 1994; Gleghorn *et al.*, 1994). Thus, it is not clear that bleach disinfection has reduced the risk of HIV infection among intravenous drug users (Booth & Watters, 1994; Titus *et al.*, 1994).

Recent attention has focused on the effectiveness of needle and syringe exchange and distribution programmes. There is accumulating evidence that providing sterile needles reduces the transmission of HIV among intravenous drug users (Donoghoe *et al.*, 1989; Hart *et al.*, 1989; Hartgers *et al.*, 1989; Stimson, 1989; van Ameijden *et al.*, 1994; Heimer *et al.*, 1994; Watters *et al.*, 1994; Centers for Disease Control and Prevention, 1995c; Hagan *et al.*, 1995). A recent international comparison of cities with and without needle exchange programmes supports the effectiveness of such measures (Feachem *et al.*, 1995). To provide sterile needles for injection, the deregulation of the sale and possession of needles and syringes has been advocated (Des Jarlais *et al.*, 1994; Vlahov, 1995). However, some countries in which disposable syringes are commercially available and cheap, such as Italy, have nevertheless experienced a high prevalence of HIV among intravenous drug users.

1.5.2 *Screening*

Antibody-test screening of all blood or plasma donors has been universal in developed countries since the mid-1980s and has resulted in a marked reduction in HIV transmission by blood transfusion or use of clotting factor concentrates. For example, it has been estimated that among 12 million blood donations collected in the United States, only 18–27 are now infectious (Lackritz *et al.*, 1995) because the donors were in the 'window period'. Blood transfusion has remained a major mode of HIV transmission in some developing countries, where screening of blood donors is not universal (N'tita et al., 1991; Vos et al., 1994).

Several countries recommend the counselling and voluntary screening of pregnant women for HIV infection (Centers for Disease Control and Prevention, 1995d) to allow them to take informed decisions about continuation of pregnancy, and enable suitable medical care and interventions to reduce the risk of vertical transmission to be applied. The rationale for screening mothers antenatally has received additional impetus from the finding that zidovudine (also called azidothymidine, AZT) taken by infected pregnant women and their newborns substantially reduces the probability of mother-to-child transmission (Connor et al., 1994; Centers for Disease Control and Prevention, 1995e). Studies of simplified treatment protocols, particularly for use in developing countries, are being conducted (Dabis et al., 1995).

1.5.3 Treatment

Zidovudine may reduce the levels of HIV in the semen of HIV-infected men (Anderson et al., 1992) and hence its infectiousness; similarly, women taking zidovudine may be less likely to transmit HIV to their HIV-uninfected regular male partners (Nicolosi et al., 1994b). However, the evidence that use of zidovudine prevents the sexual transmission of HIV should be considered as tentative and zidovudine-resistant strains of HIV are now being identified in newly acquired infections.

The literature on the efficacy of zidovudine and other reverse transcriptase inhibitors (e.g., didanosine (also called dideoxyinosine, ddI); dideoxycytidine (also called zalcitabine, ddC); stavudine) in prolonging survival of patients with HIV infection and AIDS is extensive. Briefly, improvements in survival time after AIDS diagnosis have been observed in America and Europe (Fischl et al., 1987; Lafferty et al., 1991; Jacobson et al., 1993; Whitmore-Overton et al., 1993; Blum et al., 1994; Lundgren et al., 1994). However, most recent reports indicate that zidovudine monotherapy is of modest benefit in the prolongation of this incubation time (Holmberg & Byers, 1993; Concorde Coordinating Committee, 1994; Volberding et al., 1994, 1995). It has been suggested that improved incubation and survival times may be more attributable to improved prophylaxis and treatment of *Pneumocystis carinii* pneumonia than to use of zidovudine and other antiretroviral drugs (Lundgren et al., 1994).

Antiretroviral therapy is in constant evolution. Chemotherapeutic agents have been evaluated on the basis of their ability to reduce viral load, as measured by the level of HIV-1 RNA in plasma (O'Brien et al., 1996). A number of promising new agents may retard the development of HIV disease and prolong survival (Hirsch & D'Aquila, 1993; Saag et al., 1993; Sande et al., 1993). At present, interest has centred on the so-called 'protease inhibitors' (Danner et al., 1995; Kitchen et al., 1995), on combination therapy with two or more antiretroviral drugs used together or in rotation (Fauci, 1992; Kahn et al., 1992; Abrams et al., 1994; Yarchoan et al., 1994; Collier et al., 1996) and on the use of ILs (Schnittman et al., 1994).

1.5.4 *Prospects for vaccines*

The development of a safe, effective and cheap preventive vaccine for HIV-1 or HIV-2 faces many obstacles: the considerable antigenic variability of the virus; the integration of proviral DNA in the host gene; the viability of the virus both inside and outside cells; the mucosal (sexual) and blood-borne modes of transmission; and the persistent nature of the infection even in the presence of host immunity (Girard, 1995; Graham & Wright, 1995; Hilleman, 1995). Nevertheless, more than 20 candidate vaccines have undergone preclinical evaluation for safety and immunogenicity in about 2000 volunteers. Several have entered phase I clinical testing in uninfected volunteers, and a few vaccines are now being evaluated in phase II studies in larger numbers of persons at risk for HIV infection. Candidate vaccines have been of various types, including whole killed virus and recombinant live vectors (e.g., canary pox) expressing antigens. Most of those still under consideration rely on immunization with recombinant or synthetic HIV peptides or envelope proteins such as gp120 or gp160 (see Section 1.1.7). These may induce neutralizing antibodies or lymphoproliferative responses (e.g., cytotoxic T-cell activity), but only variably and, even then, only to laboratory-adapted HIV-1 strains (not primary or wild-type isolates) (Johnston *et al.*, 1993; Dolin, 1995). Furthermore, several 'breakthrough' HIV infections have been documented in volunteers who received partial or complete series of vaccinations (Kahn *et al.*, 1995). In addition to immunization with antigenic peptides or proteins, another direction of research has been the use of live, attenuated mutant virus, which has provided immunological protection in some simian models. However, serious concerns about the use of live, attenuated virus vaccines in humans remain because viruses with deleted *nef* gene have been shown to cause disease in neonatal macaques (Baba *et al.*, 1995).

1.5.5 *Other approaches*

There is considerable interest in the safety and efficacy of agents such as Nonoxyl 9 (Elias & Meise, 1993) and dextrin sulfate (Stafford *et al.*, 1995) as vaginal virucides to protect against heterosexual transmission of HIV-1 and HIV-2. A perceived advantage of such agents over condoms is that they may be used unobtrusively by women in situations where condom usage is not acceptable to either or both partners.

Recent data from Tanzania show that HIV transmission can be reduced by effective, syndromic treatment of other sexually transmitted diseases (Grosskurth *et al.*, 1995; Hayes *et al.*, 1995; Dik *et al.*, 1995; Foulkes *et al.*, 1995; O'Reilly *et al.*, 1995; Rygnestad *et al.*, 1995; Whitaker & Renton, 1995).

2. Studies of Cancer in Humans

Most epidemiological studies of HIV have not differentiated between HIV-1 and the rarely seen HIV-2, which occurs almost exclusively in West Africa. In this section, unless specifically designated as HIV-2, the term HIV should be assumed to refer to HIV-1.

As described in Section 1.1.3, several different clades of both HIV-1 and HIV-2 have been defined. To date, there are no conclusive epidemiological data on the association between infection with specific clades and the occurrence of cancer in humans.

2.1 Kaposi's sarcoma

Kaposi's sarcoma is an AIDS-defining condition (see Section 1.4.4).

2.1.1 *Pathology and clinical disease*

In 1872, Dr Moriz Kaposi, a Hungarian dermatologist, first described an idiopathic, multiple, pigmented sarcoma, now called 'classic' Kaposi's sarcoma (Kaposi, 1872; Breimer, 1994). For many years, Kaposi's sarcoma was thought to be a lesion predominantly affecting elderly men of Mediterranean and eastern European origin (Dörffel, 1932; Landman *et al.*, 1984; Franceschi & Geddes, 1995). However, in the 1950s, as cancer registries became established in Africa, it was found that Kaposi's sarcoma comprised up to 8% of malignancies in some sub-Saharan regions, with an unusual endemic focus in parts of central Africa (Oettlé, 1962; Hutt & Burkitt, 1965). This 'endemic' Kaposi's sarcoma, like classic Kaposi's sarcoma, predominated in elderly men, but also occasionally affected children. In the 1960s and 1970s, Kaposi's sarcoma constituted up to 5% of cancers among immunosuppressed patients who had organ transplants (Penn, 1983, 1988a,b). In the early 1980s, a fourth variant of Kaposi's sarcoma, the so-called 'epidemic' Kaposi's sarcoma, heralded the onset of the AIDS epidemic in the United States (Hymes *et al.*, 1981).

The main pathological features of Kaposi's sarcoma are described in Section 4.2.1. The histopathology is identical in all variants (Templeton, 1981; Cockerell, 1991).

(a) *Clinical disease in HIV-seronegative individuals*

Classic or endemic Kaposi's sarcoma predominantly affects the skin of the lower limbs, and internal organs are rarely involved. The disease typically follows an indolent course, with patients surviving for an average of 10–15 years (Tappero *et al.*, 1993). Young children tend to have more severe disease than adults, often affecting the lymphatic system and internal organs rather than the skin, and shorter survival (Oettlé, 1962; Ziegler & Katongole-Mbidde, 1996). Adults develop plaques or nodules that may progress to sarcomatous or deeply infiltrative lesions (Taylor, 1971; Templeton, 1981). Kaposi's sarcoma in immunocompromised individuals (mainly transplant recipients and long-term users of steroids and cytotoxic drugs) often involves internal organs, lymph nodes and the face, mimicking the 'epidemic' type (Tappero *et al.*, 1993). In transplant recipients, Kaposi's sarcoma appears before most other tumours and may regress completely when immunosuppressive therapy is terminated (Penn, 1988a,b).

(b) *Clinical disease in HIV-seropositive individuals*

Kaposi's sarcoma may occur at milder levels of immunosuppression than other AIDS-defining illnesses. Lesions are usually multiple, progress rapidly, and may affect any area of the skin as well as internal organs. The tumours frequently begin as dusky-red or violet macules, progressing over weeks or months to raised, painless, firm nodules and plaques. Although the tumour may affect the legs, as seen with classic Kaposi's sarcoma, lesions on the trunk, arms, genitalia and face are also common (Smith & Spittle, 1987). Lymph nodes and the oral cavity, most notably the palate, may be extensively involved. Oral Kaposi's sarcoma is often associated with involvement elsewhere in the gastrointestinal tract (Levine, 1993; Regezi et al., 1993). Pulmonary Kaposi's sarcoma generally presents with shortness of breath and cough and is clinically difficult to distinguish from other pulmonary complications of AIDS (Levine, 1993).

Median survival following diagnosis of AIDS-related Kaposi's sarcoma is 14–18 months, a relatively long survival compared with other AIDS-defining illnesses (Casabona et al., 1993; Jacobson et al., 1993; Lundgren et al., 1994; 1995; Luo et al., 1995).

2.1.2 Descriptive epidemiology of Kaposi's sarcoma

(a) Demographic variations: age and sex

Formerly a tumour predominantly affecting the elderly (Oettlé, 1962; Templeton, 1981; Hutt, 1984; Geddes et al., 1994; Hjalgrim et al., 1996), Kaposi's sarcoma has shown a substantial alteration in age distribution in recent years, both in Africa and in Europe and the United States. In developed countries, the median age is now in the late thirties.

Age-specific incidence rates of Kaposi's sarcoma in Uganda and Zimbabwe in the early 1990s show a modest peak in children aged 0–4 years, a decline until age 15, and then the main peak at age 35–39 in men and age 25–29 in women (Wabinga et al., 1993; Bassett et al., 1995). In Europe and the United States, childhood Kaposi's sarcoma is very rare, only 32 cases having being recorded up to 1993 (Serraino & Franceschi, 1996a). Many of the European cases were in Romania, where intravenously acquired HIV infection had previously been documented (Hersh et al., 1991; Orlow et al., 1993).

Before the advent of AIDS, Kaposi's sarcoma was generally more frequent in men than in women, except among transplant recipients and children (Qunibi et al., 1993; Serraino & Franceschi, 1996a,b), with a male : female ratio in developed countries as high as 15 : 1, although later studies found ratios of 2–3 : 1 in persons thought to be HIV-seronegative, possibly reflecting improved case ascertainment in women (Biggar et al., 1984a; Franceschi & Geddes, 1995; Hjalgrim et al., 1996). In Africa, male : female ratios above 10 from earlier surveys (Wahman et al., 1991), have declined to about 3 : 1 more recently (Wabinga et al., 1993; Bassett et al., 1995; Newton et al., 1996).

(b) Geographical variations

The incidence of Kaposi's sarcoma exhibits wide geographical variation.

In the 1960s, it represented up to 8% of all malignancies in some parts of sub-Saharan Africa (Table 6; Oettlé, 1962; Templeton, 1981; Hutt, 1984). Elsewhere, relatively high incidence rates were recorded in Israel (1970–79, 1.5/100 000 in both sexes combined; Landman et al., 1984) and Italy (1976–84, 1.05/100 000 in men, 0.27/100 000 in women;

Geddes et al., 1994), particularly in the south. The rates were lower in the United States (1973–79, 0.29/100 000 in men and 0.07/100 000 in women; Biggar et al., 1984a) than in Europe (Grulich et al., 1992; Hjalgrim et al., 1996).

Table 6. Relative frequencies of Kaposi's sarcoma among all cancers in various areas of Africa

Reference	Location	Year(s) of study or report	Percentage of all cancers		
			Men	Women	Both
Oettlé (1962)	Belgian Congo	1956–57	–	–	9–13
	French Equatorial Africa	1953	–	–	5
	French West Africa	1954	–	–	1
	Gold Coast	1956	–	–	1
	Kenya	1948–61	–	–	2–4
	Mozambique	1958	–	–	2
	Natal	1957	–	–	1
	Nigeria	1934–44	–	–	2
	Rhodesia	1949	–	–	1
	South Africa	1960, 51	–	–	1–3
	Tanganyika	1960	–	–	3
	Tunisia	1960	–	–	< 1
Hutt & Burkitt (1965)	Uganda	1964	–	–	4
Bayley (1984)	Zaire	1983	–	–	9
Melbye et al. (1987)	Zaire	1984	16	–	–
Otu (1986)	Nigeria	1986	–	–	15–20
Ngendahayo et al. (1989)	Rwanda	1979–86	–	–	6
Wabinga et al. (1993)	Uganda	1989–91	49	18	–
Bassett et al. (1995)	Zimbabwe	1990–92	23	10	–
Newton et al. (1996)	Rwanda	1991–93	10	3	–
Patil et al. (1995)	Zaire	1980–89	–	–	7.0
Sitas et al. (1996)	South Africa				
	Black	1990–91	0.54	0.14	0.3
	White	1990–91	0.12	0.03	0.1

Since the advent of the AIDS epidemic, Kaposi's sarcoma has become even more common in parts of Africa (Table 6; Ziegler, 1993; Patil et al., 1995). The prevalence of Kaposi's sarcoma in different areas of the world reflects both the proportion of homosexual and bisexual men and the proportion of people from high-risk countries such as Africa (see Section 2.1.5(a)).

Although widespread in parts of Africa before the AIDS epidemic, endemic Kaposi's sarcoma was not associated with HIV infection (Biggar et al., 1984b). In some countries, modest increases in the incidence of Kaposi's sarcoma were already occurring before the onset of the AIDS epidemic (Dictor & Attewell, 1988; Hjalgrim et al., 1996).

Volcanic dust has been proposed to contribute to the etiology of Kaposi's sarcoma. The evidence supporting this hypothesis came largely from the ecological observation that, for endemic Kaposi's sarcoma, the areas of highest incidence are located in seismically active regions around the Rift Valley of east Africa and (to a lesser extent) parts of Italy and Greece (Ziegler, 1993). One report described a two-fold increase (of borderline significance) in the risk for endemic Kaposi's sarcoma in a volcanic area of Italy (Montella *et al.*, 1996). However, many areas of endemic Kaposi's sarcoma are not volcanic regions. In a study of the distribution of endemic Kaposi's sarcoma in Italy, residence in flat lands and former malaria areas was a risk factor (Geddes *et al.*, 1995). [The Working Group noted that these hypotheses cannot explain the higher risk among homosexual men than other HIV-infected persons.]

(c) Temporal changes

The incidence of Kaposi's sarcoma increased dramatically with the arrival of the HIV epidemic. This increase is still being observed in some developing countries (Wabinga *et al.*, 1993; Bassett *et al.*, 1995) and some southern European countries, but the incidence appears to have reached a plateau in other developed countries, such as the United States (Dal Maso *et al.*, 1995).

2.1.3 *Descriptive epidemiological studies*

(a) Studies in men in relation to marital status

Studies of various types have attempted to quantify the incidence of Kaposi's sarcoma in groups affected by the HIV epidemic. Never-married young men were used as a surrogate representing homosexual men, who had the highest incidence of HIV infection in the populations studied (Table 7).

From 1973–80 to 1981–82, a significant increase in the odds ratio (OR) for Kaposi's sarcoma among never-married men compared to ever-married men was observed in San Francisco, CA, United States: 51.8 (95% confidence interval (CI)), 18.6–143.6), and in other areas covered by the Surveillance, Epidemiology and End Results (SEER) Program: 18.6 (95% CI, 2.2–154.5) (Biggar *et al.*, 1985). In San Francisco County, an OR of approximately 2000 was estimated in young single men when comparing data from 1973–79 and 1982. No similar increase was recorded among ever-married men. By 1984, Kaposi's sarcoma represented 56% of all malignancies among young never-married men in San Francisco city. In single men, the relative risk for Kaposi's sarcoma in 1984 compared with 1973–78 approached 2500 (Biggar *et al.*, 1987). In Los Angeles County, CA, United States, for never-married men, the proportionate OR for Kaposi's sarcoma in 1983–85 was nearly 100 times greater than that of 1972–79 (Bernstein *et al.*, 1989).

In 1985–87 in San Francisco County, compared with 1973–78, the incidence of Kaposi's sarcoma had increased over 5000-fold in single men under 50 years old and 200-fold in young married men. In the nine SEER areas combined (including low AIDS-incidence areas), the corresponding increase in young single men was 733-fold (Rabkin *et al.*, 1991).

Table 7. Increase in risk for Kaposi's sarcoma among never-married men since the beginning of the AIDS epidemic in the United States

Reference	Study area	Control group	Time period	Risk measure		95% CI[a] or χ^2_1 for trend
Biggar et al. (1985)	San Francisco County	Never-married men aged 20–49, 1973–79	1982	OR	2043	$p < 0.001$
	San Francisco area	Never-married men aged 20–49, 1973–80	1981–82	OR	52	19–144
	Other SEER areas	Never-married men aged 20–49, 1973–80	1981–82	OR	19	2–155
Biggar et al. (1987)	San Francisco City	Never-married men aged 20–49, 1973–78	1984	OR	2479	$p < 0.0001$
	San Francisco area	Never-married men aged 20–49, 1973–78	1984	OR	182	$p = 0.0001$
Rabkin et al. (1991)	San Francisco County	Never-married men aged 20–49, 1973–78	1985–87	RIR	5060	$p < 0.001$
	Total SEER areas	Never-married men aged 20–49, 1973–78	1985–87	RIR	733	$p < 0.002$
Bernstein et al. (1989)	Los Angeles County	Never-married men aged 18–54, 1972–79	1983–85	POR	96	$p < 0.0001$
Biggar et al. (1989)	Manhattan	Never-married men aged 20–49, 1973–76	1985	OR	1851	$p < 0.0001$
	Rest of New York City	Never-married men aged 20–49, 1973–76	1985	OR	484	$p < 0.0001$
	New York State	Never-married men aged 20–49, 1973–76	1985	OR	109	$p < 0.0001$

CI, confidence interval; OR, odds ratio; RIR, relative incidence ratio; SEER, Surveillance, Epidemiology and End Results; POR, proportionate OR
[a] In the absence of 95% CI, p value or χ^2_1 for trend is given

Rabkin and Yellin (1994) examined the incidence of Kaposi's sarcoma in a population-based study of never-married men, aged 25–54 years, in San Francisco, of whom an estimated 20 000 (24%) were HIV-seropositive in late 1984. In 1988–90, the estimated standardized incidence was 540/100 000, over 20 times higher than the concurrent rate in ever-married men (25/100 000; $p < 0.001$).

In 1985, the OR for Kaposi's sarcoma in single men in Manhattan, NY, United States, compared with the pre-AIDS period (1973–76), was 1851 (Biggar et al., 1989). ORs were somewhat lower for the rest of New York City (484) and rest of New York State (109).

In New York City, small but consistent increases in the numbers of cases of Kaposi's sarcoma were seen also among married men and women of the same age group (Biggar et al., 1989). Between 1976–78 (baseline period) and 1987–88, the annual incidence of Kaposi's sarcoma in women aged 20–49 years increased from 0 to 1.8/100 000 in black women and 0 to 0.8/100 000 in white women in New York City, but did not change in the remainder of New York State (Rabkin *et al.*, 1993a).

(b) Linkage studies between AIDS and cancer registries

Record linkage between AIDS and cancer registration databases is an alternative methodology for examining associations between HIV infection and cancer in a population (Coté *et al.*, 1995). Such studies are facilitated by the relative completeness of AIDS and cancer registries with respect to Kaposi's sarcoma (Reynolds *et al.*, 1990; Barchielli *et al.*, 1995; Coté *et al.*, 1995). By matching 2528 AIDS registry cases with 62 500 cancer registry cases from the State of Illinois, United States, Coté *et al.* (1991) found a standardized incidence ratio (SIR) of Kaposi's sarcoma in AIDS patients of 972 compared with the general population of Illinois, an area of low risk for AIDS. This ratio was based on 137 linked cases of Kaposi's sarcoma.

Reynolds *et al.* (1993) linked 1454 cases of Kaposi's sarcoma in the California Tumor Registry (active since 1969) with all AIDS cases diagnosed in San Francisco since 1980. Before 1980, Kaposi's sarcoma was very rare. In 1980–87, the relative risk in AIDS patients was 716 compared with the general population.

Similar results have been reported from Italy and Switzerland (Franceschi *et al.*, 1992; Barchielli *et al.*, 1995; Serraino *et al.*, 1995a). Data for children are shown in Table 8 (Serraino & Franceschi, 1996a,b).

2.1.4 *Analytical studies*

(a) Cohort studies

Veugelers *et al.* (1994) from the Tricontinental Seroconverter Study studied 407 homosexual men with known date of HIV seroconversion, among whom 37 developed Kaposi's sarcoma.

Lundgren *et al.* (1995) studied 687 AIDS patients diagnosed in Denmark up to the end of 1990. Among these, 437 were homosexual or bisexual men who had died at the end of follow-up and 138 had developed Kaposi's sarcoma either at the time of AIDS diagnosis or during follow-up.

Dore *et al.* (1996) carried out a retrospective cohort study of 2580 people diagnosed with AIDS in Australia in 1983–94, among whom Kaposi's sarcoma was the AIDS-defining illness for 451, and among the remaining 2129 patients, Kaposi's sarcoma developed subsequently in 265.

[The Working Group noted that, although none of these studies reported the number of expected cases based on the incidence in the corresponding general population, the high proportions of persons in these cohorts who developed Kaposi's sarcoma must reflect a very high relative risk.]

Table 8. Odds ratio (OR) and 95% confidence interval (CI) for Kaposi's sarcoma (KS) according to selected characteristics and geographical area in children with AIDS, 1981–93

Characteristic	Europe			United States		
	KS/AIDS[a]	OR[b]	95% CI	KS/AIDS[a]	OR[c]	95% CI
Age (years)						
≤ 4[d]	5/3875	1		15/3796	1	
5–12	5/525	12.0	2.22–52.4	7/914	1.95	0.7–5.1
Gender						
Females[d]	3/1920	1		12/2224	1	
Males	7/2480	[1.5]	0.3–7.2]	10/2486	0.8	0.3–1.9
Ethnic group						
White[d]		–		5/2136	1	
Black		–		17/2574	2.8	1.0–8.6
Transmission category						
Mother to child[d]	2/1802	1		20/4121	1	
Haemophiliacs and transfused	7/1671	3.13	0.4–162.1	2/523	0.9	0.1–4.2
Period of diagnosis						
≤ 1990[d]	[3/2440]	1		[20/3283]	1	
1991–93	[7/1788]	[2.3]	[0.5–12.5]	[2/1427]	[0.2]	[0.04–1.01]

Modified from Serraino & Franceschi (1996a,b)
[a] Some numbers do not add up to the same total because of missing values.
[b] Adjusted for age and European country
[c] Adjusted for age
[d] Reference category
[ ] calculated by the Working Group

(b) Case–control studies

Early studies measured the prevalence of antibodies to HIV in AIDS patients, including those with Kaposi's sarcoma, compared with various control groups. These studies established that antibodies to HIV were strongly associated with the development of Kaposi's sarcoma.

HIV infection was found in 11/18 Kaposi's sarcoma patients and in 8/200 control persons with other cancers in Rwanda (relative risk, 35.0; 95% CI, 8.2–206.7) (Newton *et al.*, 1995).

(c) Analytical studies of the relationship between degree of immunosuppression and Kaposi's sarcoma among HIV-infected persons

Muñoz *et al.* (1993) followed a cohort of HIV-infected homosexual and bisexual men during 1985–91. Among the 873 AIDS cases observed in the cohort, 194 had Kaposi's sarcoma as AIDS-defining illness. A diagnosis of Kaposi's sarcoma was strongly associated with $CD4^+$ T-cell count, with an incidence of 15/100 person-years for those with

CD4+ count below 100 cells/mm³ to 0.3/100 person-years for those with CD4+ count above 500. Only 7.8% (12/153) of all initial AIDS-defining diagnoses of Kaposi's sarcoma were made in men with a CD4+ count above 500 cells/mm³. These data clearly show that the risk for Kaposi's sarcoma among AIDS patients is associated with the degree of immunosuppression.

In the early period of the AIDS epidemic, Kaposi's sarcoma was considered to be a relatively early manifestation of AIDS compared with, for example, lymphomas and many opportunistic infections. In recent years, Kaposi's sarcoma has been reported to occur later in the course of HIV disease than in the past. Lundgren et al. (1995) documented a significant decline in median CD4+ count among AIDS patients from Denmark with Kaposi's sarcoma as initial AIDS diagnosis from 96 cells/mm³ before 1987 to 28 cells/mm³ in 1989–90.

Very similar results were obtained by Dore et al. (1996), who found a significant decline in median CD4+ count for Kaposi's sarcoma patients as initial AIDS diagnosis from 92 cell/mm³ in 1983–87 to 40 cells/mm³ in 1991–94 ($p < 0.0005$).

Veugelers et al. (1995) studied the AIDS outcomes among 407 homosexual men. Their data showed that HIV-infected men who seroconverted before 1985 did not progress faster to Kaposi's sarcoma than men who seroconverted later.

2.1.5 Factors influencing the occurrence of Kaposi's sarcoma in HIV-1-infected individuals

(a) Behavioural cofactors

(i) *Descriptive studies*

The risk for Kaposi's sarcoma varies greatly with HIV transmission risk group, being particularly high in homosexual and bisexual men (see Tables 9–12, which were produced on the basis of AIDS surveillance data (Dal Maso et al., 1995)). Figure 7 shows that even in young homosexual and bisexual men (aged 13–24 years), there is already an elevated proportion with Kaposi's sarcoma compared with other HIV-transmission groups. Since first homosexual intercourse must have been recent, this finding implies a rapid increase in risk following sexual transmission of the putative Kaposi's sarcoma agent (Franceschi & Serraino, 1995).

Beral et al. (1990) found that, among 88 739 AIDS patients in the United States, 13 616 (15%) developed Kaposi's sarcoma. The proportion varied from 21% in homosexual or bisexual men to 3% in heterosexuals, 2% in intravenous drug users, 3% in transfusion recipients, 1% in haemophiliacs and 1% in children infected by perinatal transmission.

In Spain, Casabona et al. (1990) found that, among 1074 AIDS patients, 124 presented with Kaposi's sarcoma: 36% in homosexual or bisexual men, 2% in intravenous drug users and none in 35 heterosexuals, 5 transfusion recipients, 23 haemophiliacs and 33 children infected by perinatal transmission.

Table 9. Numbers and proportions of male AIDS cases with Kaposi's sarcoma as AIDS-defining condition, by country and HIV transmission group, in Europe and United States, 1981–94

Country[a]	Homo/bisexual men		Intravenous drug users		Heterosexuals				Haemophiliac and transfused		Other/ unknown		All	
					Pattern II countries[b]		Natives							
	KS cases	(%)[d]	KS cases	(%)[d]	KS	(%)[d]	KS	(%)[d]	KS cases	(%)[d]	KS cases	(%)[d]	KS cases	(%)[d]
Austria	106	(20)	2	(1)	0	(0)	3	(4)	0	(0)	9	(6)	120	(11)
Belgium	209	(28)	2	(2)	40	(14)	9	(5)	4	(7)	1	(2)	265	(19)
Denmark	217	(18)	0	(0)	1	(6)	2	(2)	1	(2)	1	(2)	222	(15)
France	5 396	(31)	122	(2)	94	(6)	157	(9)	34	(3)	188	(11)	5 991	(20)
Germany	2 151	(24)	35	(3)	10	(10)	22	(7)	5	(1)	88	(14)	2 311	(20)
Greece	107	(19)	2	(7)	2	(25)	8	(14)	2	(2)	18	(11)	139	(15)
Italy	934	(21)	300	(2)	10	(6)	96	(7)	21	(5)	100	(9)	1 461	(7)
Netherlands	493	(19)	0	(0)	1	(2)	8	(5)	0	(0)	4	(9)	506	(16)
Portugal	216	(28)	15	(2)	0	(0)	55	(12)	3	(3)	13	(14)	302	(15)
Spain	1 333	(26)	217	(1)	0	(0)	85	(5)	10	(1)	91	(5)	1 736	(7)
Sweden	134	(18)	0	(0)	4	(8)	5	(7)	1	(2)	0	(0)	144	(14)
Switzerland	480	(26)	28	(2)	6	(12)	38	(11)	2	(3)	9	(11)	563	(16)
UK	1 569	(20)	5	(1)	59	(12)	11	(5)	0	(0)	10	(6)	1 654	(17)
USA White	30 255	(21)	548	(4)	–[c]	–[c]	93	(5)	109	(2)	382	(8)	31 387	(19)
Black	4 198	(10)	711	(2)	–[c]	–[c]	101	(2)	30	(3)	331	(4)	5 371	(6)
Other	5 583	(19)	560	(3)	–[c]	–[c]	67	(4)	30	(4)	204	(6)	6 444	(12)

KS, Kaposi's sarcoma

[a] Only countries with > 100 cases of Kaposi's sarcoma over the period 1981–94 are included.
[b] Individuals originating from Pattern II countries (countries in which extensive spread of HIV began in the mid-to-late 1970s or early 1980s and in which heterosexual transmission has predominated and continues to)
[c] Data not available
[d] Number of Kaposi's sarcoma cases as percentage of total AIDS cases in the respective risk group

Data derived from the European Non-aggregate AIDS Data Set (ENAADS) updated to June 1995, prepared by the European Centre for the Epidemiological Monitoring of AIDS, Paris, and from the AIDS Public Information Data Set (PIDS) updated to December 1994, prepared by the National Center for Infectious Diseases, Centers for Disease Control and Prevention (CDC), Atlanta, GA, United States

Table 10. Numbers and proportions of female AIDS cases with Kaposi's sarcoma as AIDS-defining condition, by country and HIV transmission group, in Europe and United States, 1981–94

Country[a]	Intravenous drug users		Heterosexuals		Haemophiliacs and transfused		Other/ unknown		All	
	KS cases	(%)[b]	KS cases	(%)[b]	KS cases	(%)[b]	KS cases	(%)[b]	KS cases	(%)[b]
Belgium	1	(3)	22	(7)	2	(4)			25	(5)
France	33	(1)	83	(3)	16	(2)	6	(1)	138	(2)
Italy	55	(2)	33	(2)	3	(2)	13	(4)	104	(2)
Spain	55	(1)	16	(7)	2	(1)			74	(1)
UK			42	(7)	1	(1)			43	(5)
US White	60	(1)	42	(1)	18	(1)	14	(2)	134	(1)
Black	136	(1)	48	(1)	9	(1)	46	(1)	250	(1)
Other	56	(1)	37	(1)	5	(1)	4	(1)	103	(1)

KS, Kaposi's sarcoma
[a] Only countries with > 25 cases over the period 1981–94 are included.
[b] Number of Kaposi's sarcoma cases as percentage of total AIDS cases in the respective risk group
[c] Data derived from the European Non-aggregate AIDS Data Set (ENAADS) updated to June 1995, prepared by the European Centre for the Epidemiological Monitoring of AIDS, Paris, and from the AIDS Public Information Data Set (PIDS) updated to December 1994, prepared by the National Center for Infectious Diseases, Centers for Disease Control and Prevention (CDC), Atlanta, GA, United States

In the United Kingdom, Beral et al. (1991a) found that, among 2830 AIDS patients, 566 developed Kaposi's sarcoma. The proportion varied from 23% in homosexual or bisexual men and 10% in heterosexuals to 0% in 83 intravenous drug users, 47 transfusion recipients, 163 haemophiliacs and 23 children infected by perinatal transmission.

European (Serraino et al., 1992a; Franceschi et al., 1995b; Serraino et al., 1995b) and Australian (Elford et al., 1993) surveillance data have confirmed that Kaposi's sarcoma is more common among homosexual and bisexual men and women who reported sexual rather than parenteral exposure to HIV. This finding is particularly notable since a high proportion of transfusion-associated AIDs cases have received blood from homosexual or bisexual men, so that even massive blood contact does not appear to increase the risk as much as sexual contact (Busch et al., 1991).

Among people who acquired HIV by heterosexual contact, the risk for developing Kaposi's sarcoma varies according to country of origin: Kaposi's sarcoma occurred in 18% of AIDS cases in Rwanda (Van de Perre et al., 1984), 16% in Zaire (Piot et al., 1984), 13% of infected Africans resident in Belgium (Clumeck et al., 1984), 8% of infected Africans resident in the United States, 6% of AIDS cases in Haitians resident in the United States and 14% of infected Africans resident in the United Kingdom, as compared to 2–5% of AIDS patients in the United States or Europe (Beral et al., 1990, 1991a) [Data calculated by Beral (1991a) from the original papers.]

Table 11. Numbers and proportions of AIDS cases with Kaposi's sarcoma as AIDS-defining condition, by country and year of AIDS diagnosis, among homosexual and bisexual men in Europe and the United States, 1981–94

Country[a]	Year of diagnosis											
	Pre-1985		1985–86		1987–88		1989–90		1991–92		1993–94	
	KS cases	%[c]	KS cases	%[c]	KS cases	%[c]	KS cases	%[c]	KS cases	%[c]	KS cases	%[c]
Austria	6	50	5	22	18	20	17	14	35	24	25	18
Belgium	4	29	15	35	30	29	41	23	64	29	55	28
Denmark	11	31	22	24	34	19	47	17	54	19	49	16[b]
France	107	45	485	41	968	33	1274	31	1353	30	1209	28[b]
Germany	53	39	227	36	420	26	538	25	547	24	366	17[b]
Greece			4	17	12	17	16	14	40	24	35	21
Italy	8	38	39	22	126	26	202	21	263	21	296	19[b]
Netherlands	17	35	44	24	97	21	115	18	135	19	85	15[b]
Portugal	3	100	13	36	29	30	46	24	77	32	48	24
Spain	12	60	54	33	181	29	313	25	429	27	344	22[b]
Sweden	4	25	22	30	25	21	31	17	33	21	19	10[b]
Switzerland	14	44	63	40	102	31	106	24	107	22	88	22[b]
UK	54	39	169	28	276	21	315	19	374	18	381	19[b]
USA												
White	2525	44	4603	29	6485	22	7260	21	7043	18	2339	15[b]
Black	249	20	460	13	741	10	1091	10	1112	8	545	8[b]
Other	292	32	678	26	1080	21	1370	19	1522	17	641	14[b]

KS, Kaposi's sarcoma

[a] Only countries with > 100 cases of Kaposi's sarcoma over the period 1981–94 are included.

[b] χ^2_1 for trend, > 3.84; $p < 0.05$

[c] Number of Kaposi's sarcoma cases as percentage of total AIDS cases in the respective calendar period

Data derived from the European Non-aggregate AIDS Data Set (ENAADS) updated to June 1995, prepared by the European Centre for the Epidemiological Monitoring of AIDS, Paris, and from the AIDS Public Information Data Set (PIDS) updated to December 1994, prepared by the National Center for Infectious Diseases, Centers for Disease Control and Prevention (CDC), Atlanta, GA, United States

Table 12. Numbers and proportions of AIDS cases with Kaposi's sarcoma as AIDS-defining condition, by country and year of AIDS diagnosis, among men (other than homosexual and bisexual) and women in Europe and the United States, 1981–94

Country[a]	Year of diagnosis											
	Pre 1985		1985–86		1987–88		1989–90		1991–92		1993–94	
	KS cases	%[c]	KS cases	%[c]	KS cases	%[c]	KS cases	%[c]	KS cases	%[c]	KS cases	%[c]
Men												
Belgium	8	12	8	14	13	14	9	8	10	6	8	5[b]
France	12	12	34	9	94	6	119	4	171	5	165	4[b]
Germany	6	16	13	9	37	8	28	4	44	6	32	5[b]
Italy	2	10	20	6	69	4	113	3	149	3	174	3[b]
Portugal			2	8	7	8	17	9	14	4	46	7
Spain	4	9	8	2	44	2	81	2	130	2	136	2
UK			2	2	8	4	15	4	31	6	29	5
USA												
White	40	7	83	5	165	4	272	5	349	5	223	5
Black	76	6	104	4	174	3	274	3	327	2	218	2[b]
Other	29	6	65	4	143	3	200		283	4	141	3[b]
Women												
France	3	8	12	5	22	3	28	2	36	2	37	2[b]
Italy			6	5	12	2	22	2	19	1	45	2
Spain	1	14	4	4	10	2	15	1	17	1	27	1
UK	3	43	1	5			5	3	18	6	15	4
USA												
White	17	9	24	3	26	1	39	1	48	1	21	1[b]
Black	23	5	28	2	56	2	83	1	107	1	65	1[b]
Other	1	1	17	3	29	2	41	2	52	2	30	1

KS, Kaposi's sarcoma
[a] Only countries with > 40 cases of Kaposi's sarcoma in each group over the period 1981–94
[b] χ^2_1 for trend, > 3.84; $p < 0.05$
[c] Number of Kaposi's sarcoma cases as percentage of total AIDS cases in the respective calendar period
Data derived from the European Non-aggregate AIDS Data Set (ENAADS) updated to June 1995, prepared by the European Centre for the Epidemiological Monitoring of AIDS, Paris, and from the AIDS Public Information Data Set (PIDS) updated to December 1994, prepared by the National Center for Infectious Diseases, Centers for Disease Control and Prevention (CDC), Atlanta, GA, United States

In addition, the proportion of sexually infected female AIDS patients presenting with Kaposi's sarcoma was highest in those whose reported sexual partners were bisexual men (2.6% in the United States, Peterman *et al.*, 1993; 6.9% in Europe, Serraino *et al.*, 1995b) (Figure 8).

Figure 7. Percentage of Kaposi's sarcoma as AIDS-defining illness by age in homosexual and non-homosexual males and females in selected European countries and the United States (whites and blacks), 1981–94

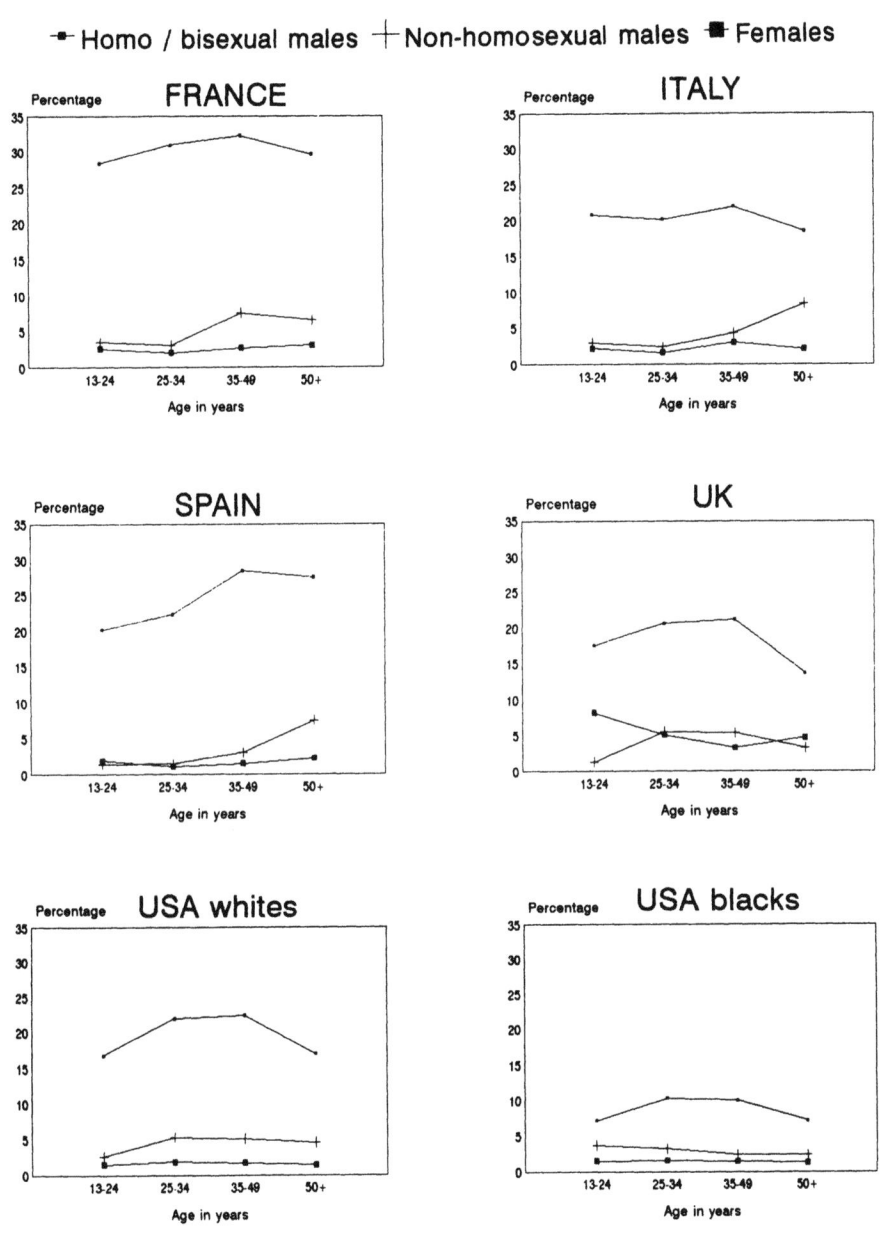

Data derived from the European Non-aggregate AIDS Data Set (ENAADS) updated to June 1995, prepared by the European Centre for the Epidemiological Monitoring of AIDS, Paris, and from the AIDS Public Information Data Set (PIDS) updated to December 1994, prepared by the National Center for Infectious Diseases, Centers for Disease Control and Prevention (CDC), Atlanta, GA, United States

Figure 8. Percentage of Kaposi's sarcoma in women who acquired AIDS via heterosexual contact by their sexual partner's reported HIV-transmission group, Europe, 1981-93 and United States, [1981-91]

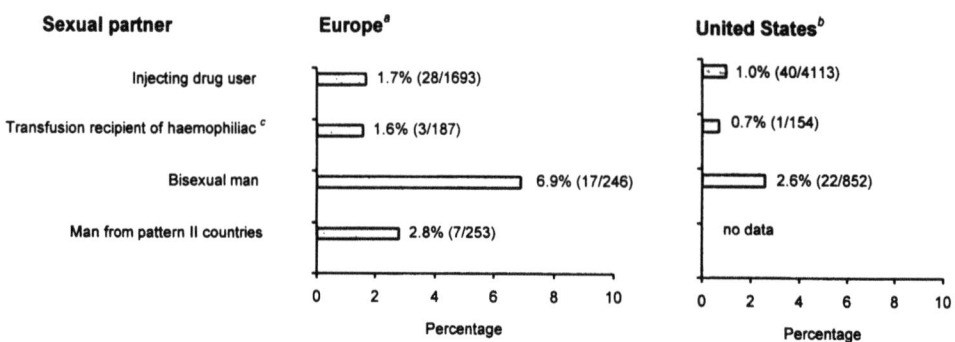

Pattern II countries: Extensive spread of HIV began in the mid-to-late 1970s or early 1980s. Heterosexual transmission has predominated and continues to.
[a] Modified from Serraino et al. (1995b)
[b] Modified from Peterman et al. (1993)
[c] In United States, transfusion recipient of haemophiliac. In Europe, blood recipient

(ii) *Analytical studies*

A number of studies have contrasted the sexual practices of homosexual men with Kaposi's sarcoma with those of men with opportunistic infections or other manifestations of AIDS (Tables 13 and 14).

Several studies have reported on the number of sexual partners among homosexual and bisexual men with Kaposi's sarcoma compared with homosexual and bisexual men with other AIDS manifestations (Table 13). Most of these studies (Haverkos et al., 1985; Goedert et al., 1987; Archibald et al., 1990; Armenian et al., 1993), but not all (Lifson et al., 1990a,b), found that the Kaposi's sarcoma patients had a higher number of sexual partners. Goedert et al. (1987) also reported that Kaposi's sarcoma patients had more sexually transmitted diseases.

Similar studies have been undertaken of insertive oral–anal contact among Kaposi's sarcoma patients compared with men with other AIDS manifestations. Some studies (Archibald et al., 1990; Beral et al., 1992; Darrow et al., 1992), but not all (Lifson et al., 1990b; Elford et al., 1992; Kaldor et al., 1993; Page-Bodkin et al., 1992; Armenian et al., 1993) have found this sexual practice to be more common among Kaposi's sarcoma patients than among other AIDS patients (Table 14).

In conclusion, men who developed Kaposi's sarcoma have tended to be more sexually active, have had more sexually transmitted diseases and had more sexual partners from areas where Kaposi's sarcoma is common. In conjunction with the much higher risk for

Kaposi's sarcoma in homosexual men than in other HIV transmission groups, the data have led some authors to suggest that an infectious and sexually transmitted agent (independent of HIV) is associated with Kaposi's sarcoma. It should be noted that very few data on risk factors for Kaposi's sarcoma are available from Africa.

Table 13. Studies of the association between risk factors and Kaposi's sarcoma in homosexual men

Reference	Risk behaviour	AIDS manifestations	Proportion of cases No.	%
Haverkos et al. (1985)	≥ 100 male sexual partners in year before illness	KS PCP	29/47 6/20	61 30
Goedert et al. (1987)	≥ 100 homosexual partners during the previous year	KS PCP	3/8 3/10	38 30
	≥ 3 STDs	KS PCP	1/8 0/10	13
Archibald et al. (1990)[a]	> 20 male sexual partners in prior year	KS Other infections	19/25 25/48	76 52
	> 20 sexual partners from areas of high risk for KS[b]	KS Other infections	14/25 10/48	56 21
Lifson et al. (1990a,b)	Median no. of sexual partners: 300	KS	71 cases	
	Median no. of sexual partners: 278	Other	107 cases	
Armenian et al. (1993)[c]	≥ 49 male partners in the last 2 years	KS Non-cancerous AIDS controls	159/314 194/508	51 38
	Having partners from high risk areas[d]	KS Non-cancerous AIDS controls	65/314 61/508	21 12

KS, Kaposi's sarcoma; PCP, *Pneumocystis carinii* pneumonia; STD, sexually transmitted disease
[a] A reanalysis of the same cohort in 1992 found very similar results (Archibald et al., 1992)
[b] San Francisco, Los Angeles, New York
[c] This cohort was first studied by Jacobson et al. (1990)
[d] From San Francisco for participants from other than Los Angeles

(b) *Infectious cofactors*

(i) *Human herpesvirus 8*

For a more detailed description of human herpesvirus 8 (HHV-8), see Section 4.2.4.

Chang et al. (1994) announced the discovery of a previously unknown human herpesvirus in Kaposi's sarcoma tissue of AIDS patients from the United States. The

Table 14. Studies of insertive oro-anal contact as a risk factor for Kaposi's sarcoma among AIDS patients

Reference	Location	Period of interview	Period of sexual behaviour assessed	KS post-AIDS included in cases	Index of IOAC	Proportion reporting IOAC[a] Numbers (%)	
						AIDS patients with KS	AIDS patients without KS
Armenian et al. (1993)	4 US cities	1984–85, 1987–91	2 years before enrolment	No	Being rimmed	240/314 (76%)	357/508 (70%)
Beral et al. (1992)	London, UK	1984–85	Previous five years	Yes	Insertive rimming, less than once a month and at least once a month but less than once a week	[14/30 (47%)]	[5/35 (14%)]
Darrow et al. (1992)	4 US cities	1981	Previous one year	No	> 10% of sexual contacts	22/49 (45%)	0/8
Archibald et al. (1990)	Vancouver, Canada	1982–84	At enrolment	Yes	Insertive fists	18/25 (72%)	23/48 (48%)
Lifson et al. (1990b)	San Francisco, USA	1983–86	1978–80 to 1983–84	Yes	Proportion of steady sexual partners with whom practised	4/71 (5%)	5/107 (5%)
Elford et al. (1992)	Sydney, Australia	1984, then 6-monthly[b]	1984 to diagnosis of AIDS	No	Any	29/55 (53%)	65/116 (56%)
Page-Bodkin et al. (1992)	San Francisco, USA	1984–91	2 years before interview	Yes	With some or most of sexual partners	43/87 (49%)	51/100 (51%)
Kaldor et al. (1993)	Sydney, Australia	1984–85	3 months before enrolment	No	[Insertive rimming]	[22/45 (49%)]	[34/88 (39%)][c]

KS, Kaposi's sarcoma; IOAC, insertive oro-anal contact
[a] Except where specified
[b] Self-administered questionnaire
[c] Numbers recalculated by the Working Group

virus, described as 'Kaposi's sarcoma-associated herpesvirus' (KSHV) or as human herpesvirus 8 (HHV-8), was identified by the use of representational difference analysis to discern DNA sequences in tumour tissue that were absent from normal DNA. The sequences, which showed similarity to a number of gammaherpesviruses (including Epstein–Barr virus (EBV)), were found in 21/27 (78%) people with AIDS-related Kaposi's sarcoma, 6/39 (15%) AIDS patients without Kaposi's sarcoma and 0/103 non-AIDS controls ($p < 10^{-7}$ using non-Kaposi's sarcoma controls).

A number of laboratories have since reported the detection of HHV-8 in biopsies of all epidemiological forms of Kaposi's sarcoma and/or in PBMCs from Kaposi's sarcoma patients (see Table 15). Overall, HHV-8 has been detected in more than 98% of Kaposi's sarcoma biopsies, but much less frequently and in lower amounts in skin of Kaposi's sarcoma patients. Using PCR, HHV-8 has been detected in PBMCs from about 50% of Kaposi's sarcoma patients (Ambroziak et al., 1995 (in 100%); Howard et al., 1995; Whitby et al., 1995), but not at all (Ambroziak et al., 1995; Whitby et al., 1995) or in only 9% (Bigoni et al., 1996) in those of healthy blood donors. In asymptomatic HIV-infected individuals, detection of HHV-8 in peripheral blood strongly predicts progression to Kaposi's sarcoma (Collandre et al., 1995; Howard et al., 1995; Whitby et al., 1995). These findings suggest that HHV-8 has only a limited distribution in developed countries, but is an independent risk factor for classic (Mediterranean), African endemic and AIDS-associated Kaposi's sarcoma. However, the distribution of HHV-8 in the general population is not yet fully clear. Two groups have found HHV-8 in semen samples and prostate of healthy HIV-seronegative individuals (Lin et al., 1995; Monini et al., 1996), whereas others have not confirmed this observation (Ambroziak et al., 1995; Li et al., 1995).

Preliminary serological data also support the view that HHV-8 is infrequent in the general populations of developed countries. Antibodies to several proteins of HHV-8 can be detected in the majority of Kaposi's sarcoma patients, but only infrequently in HIV-infected individuals without Kaposi's sarcoma (Miller et al., 1996; Moore et al., 1996) and in the general population. These findings underline the strong association between detection of HHV-8 and the presence of Kaposi's sarcoma. However, in view of the conflicting PCR-based evidence, it needs to be established whether the presence of antibodies to HHV-8 reflects infection with, rather than reactivation of, HHV-8.

The advent of serological tests for HHV-8 should allow larger and more thorough epidemiological studies to be conducted, looking at the prevalence of the agent in populations at differing risk of developing Kaposi's sarcoma. If the virus is ubiquitous, it throws into question the issue of causality for Kaposi's sarcoma. Using an immunoblot assay for two latent nuclear antigens specific for HHV-8, Gao et al. (1996a) showed that the seroprevalence of HHV-8 did vary between groups with differing risk of Kaposi's sarcoma, being most prevalent in those at highest risk. Of 40 patients with Kaposi's sarcoma (recruited from the Multicentre AIDS cohort study (MACS)), 32 (80%) were positive for antibodies to HHV-8, compared to 7/40 (18%) homosexual men without the disease (just before the onset of AIDS). Of 122 HIV-seronegative blood donors and

Table 15. Proportion of patients with HHV-8 in relation to Kaposi's sarcoma and HIV/AIDS status

Reference	HHV-8-positive proportion of patients				Comments
	AIDS/HIV+ KS+	AIDS/HIV− KS+	AIDS/HIV+ KS−	AIDS/HIV− KS−	
Chang et al. (1994)	21/27		6/39[a]	0/103[b]	[a] Lymphomas, lymph nodes biopsies [b] Non-AIDS lymphomas, lymph nodes, cancers, other biopsies
Su et al. (1995)	4/4	2/3	0/5[a]	0/32[b]	[a] AIDS lymph nodes [b] Benign and malignant lymphoid tissue
Dupin et al. (1995)	4/4[a]	5/5[b]		0/6[c]	[a] Homosexual [b] Mediterranean KS [c] Other patients
Boshoff et al. (1995a)	14/14[a]	16/17[b] 8/8[d] 1/1[e]		0/11[c]	[a] 12 males, 2 females [b] Mediterranean patients [c] Various skin lesions (9 M, 2 F) [d] Organ transplant recipients [e] Homosexual
Ambroziak et al. (1995)	12/12[a] 7/7[b]	1/1[a] 3/3[b]	0/6[b]	0/14[b,c]	[a] Homosexual patients [b] HHV-8 detected in PBMCs [c] Healthy lab volunteers
Moore & Chang (1995)	10/11[a]	6/6[b] 4/4[a]		1/11 0/10[c]	[a] 10/11 Homosexual [b] Mediterranean 'classic' [c] PBMCs
Howard et al. (1995)	11/14[a,c] 0/6[b,c] 11/17[d]		1/19[c,e] 0/6[a]		All homosexual [a] Pulmonary and cutaneous KS [b] Cutaneous KS only [c] Bronchoalveolar lavage fluid [d] HHV-8 detected in PBMCs [e] The patient re-presented with [a] 3 months later

Table 15 (contd)

Reference	HHV-8-positive proportion of patients				Comments
	AIDS/HIV+ KS+	AIDS/HIV+ KS−	AIDS/HIV− KS+	AIDS/HIV− KS−	
Whitby et al. (1995)	24/46[a]		11/143[a]	0/160[a,b]	[a] HHV-8 detected in PBMCs [b] 134 blood donors, 26 cancer patients
Buonaguro et al. (1996)	19/19[a] 0/5[c]	42/42[b] 9/13[c]	0/15[c]	0/17[d]	[a] 5 Italian, 5 North American, 3 Ugandan, 3 Kenyan origin, KS tissues [b] 28 classic KS (5 Greek, 6 North American, 17 Italian), 2 iatrogenic (Greek), 12 African endemic KS (Ugandan) [c] PBMCs [d] Human biopsies from healthy individuals or affected by other pathologies [e] Autologous uninvolved skin of a and b
Chang et al. (1996)[a]	22/24	17/20	1/7	2/15	[a] Ugandan patients
Huang et al. (1995)	12/12[a]	14/18[b]			[a] US origin [b] Mediterranean (classic) and African origin
Lebbé et al. (1995)	2/2	14/14[a] 0/5[b]			[a] Immunosuppressed (1), classic (10), endemic (3) KS [b] PBMCs
Schalling et al. (1995)	17/17[a] 8/8[b]	18/18[a] 3/3[b]			[a] KS biopsies, Ugandan origin [b] KS biopsies, Swedish origin

Table 15 (contd)

Reference	HHV-8-positive proportion of patients				Comments
	AIDS/HIV+ KS+	AIDS/HIV− KS+	AIDS/HIV+ KS−	AIDS/HIV− KS−	
Bigoni et al. (1996)			0/10[b] — 4/58[d]	7/80[b] 1/11[c] 5/56[d]	[a] Italian patients [b] Non-Hodgkin's lymphoma patients [c] Reactive lymphadenopathy [d] HHV-8 detected in PBMCs
Prospective studies:	No. developing KS[a] HIV+				[a] AIDS patients KS-free at recruitment; average 30 months follow-up
	HHV-8+[b]	HHV-8−[b]			[b] HHV-8 detected in PBMCs
Whitby et al. (1995)	6/11 55% ($p < 0.00005$)	12/132 (9%)			

KS, Kaposi's sarcoma; PBMC, peripheral blood mononuclear cell; M, male; F, female

20 HIV-infected haemophiliacs, none were seropositive. The 40 patients with HIV-associated Kaposi's sarcoma had each been followed for a period of between 13 and 103 months before diagnosis of the disease (all were HIV-seropositive on entry). In that time, 11/40 (28%) were seropositive for HHV-8 throughout, 21 (52%) became positive between 6 and 75 months prior to diagnosis, 6/40 (15%) remained seronegative throughout and 2/40 (5%) changed from seropositive to seronegative during the course of the study. These data support the hypothesis that HHV-8 is causal for Kaposi's sarcoma and suggest that many of those who get the disease seroconvert to antibodies against the virus relatively soon before its onset. Further studies in these patients (using a different serological assay: an immunofluorescent assay) showed that they had an antigen profile suggestive of primary infection with HHV-8 rather that reactivation of a chronic existing infection (high titres of IgC and absence of IgA and IgM).

A second study by Gao *et al.* (1996b) compared the prevalence of HHV-8 in those with and without Kaposi's sarcoma from Uganda, Italy and the USA. There is a very strong association between seropositivity for HHV-8 and Kaposi's sarcoma, both in HIV-seropositive and in HIV-seronegative patients. However, the prevalence of HHV-8 in HIV-seronegative blood donors or patients with cancers other than Kaposi's sarcoma (for which there is no evidence of an association with HHV-8), varied dramatically between countries, being highest in Uganda (51%), followed by Italy (4%) and then the USA (0%). Kaposi's sarcoma remains virtually unknown outside of HIV-seropositive homosexual men in the USA (and some immigrant groups), but has existed at a low incidence in Italy and a considerably higher incidence in Uganda since well before the early 1980s (Templeton, 1973). Therefore, these results might be expected if HHV-8 were causal for Kaposi's sarcoma.

(ii) *Cytomegalovirus*

Even before the HIV epidemic, there were reports that cytomegalovirus antibody was more commonly present in persons with endemic forms of Kaposi's sarcoma (Giraldo *et al.*, 1975, 1978); cytomegalovirus genome was detected in Kaposi's sarcoma tissue from endemic cases (Giraldo *et al.*, 1980). Early in the AIDS epidemic, it was observed that the great majority of homosexual men had cytomegalovirus antibodies, compared with only half of the general population of the same age (Drew *et al.*, 1982; Melbye *et al.*, 1983; Rogers *et al.*, 1983), leading some investigators to suggest that it was a plausible candidate for the causal agent of AIDS itself (Urmacher *et al.*, 1982; Mintz *et al.*, 1983). However, other studies failed to confirm the consistent presence of the cytomegalovirus genome within Kaposi's sarcoma tissue (Ambinder *et al.*, 1987; Kempf *et al.*, 1995).

In retrospect, the reported associations between AIDS, immunosuppression or Kaposi's sarcoma and cytomegalovirus antibody prevalence or titre were probably due to failure to obtain controls adequately matched by sexual habits (Johnston *et al.*, 1990).

(iii) *Other infectious agents*

There is little evidence to support a relationship between human herpesvirus 6 (HHV-6) and Kaposi's sarcoma. One study failed to detect an elevated HHV-6 prevalence in

Kaposi's sarcoma tissue compared with normal skin; when detected, it was the more common B variant (Kempf et al., 1995). However, another study reported that the less common A variant of HHV-6 was present in nearly a third of both endemic and HIV-related cases (Bovenzi et al., 1993). Infection with HHV-6 occurs early in life and antibodies are common in adults (Krueger et al., 1988; Dolcetti et al., 1994).

Two studies have found human papillomaviruses (see IARC, 1995) in Kaposi's sarcoma tissue from AIDS cases, detected by PCR (Huang et al., 1992) and by immunohistochemistry (Nickoloff et al., 1992), but other investigations have failed to confirm these findings (Biggar et al., 1992; Kaaya et al., 1993a).

Rochalimaea henselae is a bacterium associated with angiomatoses that might be confused with Kaposi's sarcoma. It has been considered as a causal agent for Kaposi's sarcoma (Bignall, 1993) but is thought unlikely to be related to this disease (Taylor et al., 1993).

Mycoplasma fermentans has been isolated from cells transformed with human DNA from Kaposi's sarcoma tissue (Lo et al., 1989). However, there are no epidemiological data to support an association with Kaposi's sarcoma. Katseni et al. (1993) found HIV-positive and HIV-negative subjects to have comparable frequencies of *M. fermentans*. Another mycoplasma, *M. penetrans* (Lo et al., 1991), seems to be more common in HIV-infected than in HIV-negative individuals, as shown by the prevalence of antibodies to this organism (Wang et al., 1992). Serological evidence suggests that *M. penetrans* might be more common in HIV-infected homosexuals, but not in intravenous drug users or haemophiliacs, suggesting a link to those patient groups known to be at an increased risk for Kaposi's sarcoma (Wang et al., 1993).

(c) Genetic susceptibility

In 1983, early in the AIDS epidemic, the HLA-DR5 haplotype was reported to be associated with the occurrence of Kaposi's sarcoma in homosexual men from New York City (Pollack et al., 1983a; Prince et al., 1984), an association also reported among cases of endemic Kaposi's sarcoma (Pollack et al., 1983b; Contu et al., 1984; Papasteriades et al., 1984). Subsequent studies have failed to confirm such an association in either AIDS-related or endemic Kaposi's sarcoma (Melbye et al., 1987; Brunson et al., 1990; Mann et al., 1990; Ioannidis et al., 1995; Strichman-Almashanu et al., 1995).

One suggestion to explain this discrepancy was that HIV-infected persons with elevated genetic susceptibility (in this case, DR5-positive) developed Kaposi's sarcoma sooner after infection and hence were not seen in later studies. However, large numbers of newly infected persons continue to enter the pool of persons at risk and exhaustion of the susceptible subgroups seems an unlikely explanation. Another explanation is that this marker is more common in some subgroups, particularly in Mediterranean and Jewish populations, and that control for this factor was inadequate. Reported associations with other HLA markers have not been confirmed (summarized by Ioannidis et al., 1995), and the relationship between HLA and Kaposi's sarcoma is still controversial. [The Working Group noted that the multiple comparisons made in the analysis of the HLA data make it difficult to interpret the findings.]

(d) Miscellaneous factors

The use of amyl nitrite inhalants has been considered as a factor increasing risk for Kaposi's sarcoma in homosexual men. Use of these drugs was especially popular among very sexually active homosexual men at the time when the AIDS epidemic was emerging in the late 1970s and early 1980s (Jaffe *et al.*, 1983; Melbye *et al.*, 1983). They act as smooth muscle relaxants and potent vasodilators (Newell *et al.*, 1984) and are thought to be potentially carcinogenic (Jørgensen & Lawesson, 1982). Therefore, they seemed plausible candidate etiological agents for a tumour prominently involving blood vessels. Early studies found their use to be associated with both immunosuppression and with development of Kaposi's sarcoma (Goedert *et al.*, 1982; Marmor *et al.*, 1982; Haverkos *et al.*, 1985).

However, since nitrite inhalants were often used to facilitate anal intercourse, their use was correlated with the frequency of receptive anal intercourse with multiple partners. In one study, adjusting for anal intercourse eliminated the relationship between Kaposi's sarcoma and nitrite inhalant use (Darrow *et al.*, 1992), although in another study (Archibald *et al.*, 1990), a residual 'independent' effect remained. [The Working Group noted that, among homosexual men in developed countries, nitrite inhalant users also became HIV-infected early in the epidemic and thus manifested AIDS symptoms (including Kaposi's sarcoma) earlier. Thus, the evidence of the association between nitrite inhalants and Kaposi's sarcoma is not convincing.]

Data about androgen levels is conflicting. Klauke *et al.* (1995) report higher testosterone levels in 17 HIV-infected men with Kaposi's sarcoma than other HIV-infected men who had no symptoms (11), mild symptoms (12) or non-Kaposi's sarcoma AIDS (29). In contrast, Christeff *et al.* (1995) found higher levels of testosterone and dehydroepiandrosterone in 28 men with Kaposi's sarcoma compared to 34 HIV-infected men without Kaposi's sarcoma, after stratifying for $CD4^+$ T-cell count. Further studies are needed to clarify this issue.

Lunardi-Iskandar *et al.* (1995a) reported that Kaposi's sarcoma Y1 cells could not be grown in pregnant mice and that human chorionic gonadotropin (HCG) appeared to induce apoptosis in Kaposi's sarcoma derived cells in culture (see Section 4.2.1). The incidence of Kaposi's sarcoma in HIV-infected pregnant women (who would have high HCG levels soon after conception) in Africa was similar to that in post-pregnant women or women not recently pregnant, arguing against a role for HCG at physiological doses. Similarly, there was no difference between pregnant and non-pregnant women in the frequency of disseminated Kaposi's sarcoma lesions (Rabkin *et al.*, 1995a).

2.1.6 *Human immunodeficiency virus type 2*

Because of a paucity of data, it is unclear whether the clinical spectrum of diseases in HIV-2-infected individuals differs from that of HIV-1, particularly with respect to Kaposi's sarcoma (De Cock & Brun-Vézinet, 1989).

Kaposi's sarcoma in people with HIV-2 infection was reported in two patients from Senegal (Le Guenno *et al.*, 1987), one from France (Brücker *et al.*, 1987), four of 17 HIV-2-associated AIDS cases from western Africa (Clavel *et al.*, 1987), but not in two follow-up studies, namely a one-year follow-up of 62 HIV-2-seropositive individuals (Poulsen *et al.*, 1989) and a two-year follow-up of 133 similar subjects from Guinea Bissau, a few of whom had an AIDS diagnosis (Ricard *et al.*, 1994).

No Kaposi's sarcoma was observed in a few case reports and small case series of HIV-2-seropositive individuals (Clavel *et al.*, 1986; Mølbak *et al.*, 1986; Ancelle *et al.*, 1987; Brun-Vézinet *et al.*, 1987; Burin Des Roziers *et al.*, 1987; Kroegel *et al.*, 1987; Saimot *et al.*, 1987; Veronesi *et al.*, 1987; Vittecoq *et al.*, 1987; Agut *et al.*, 1988; Centers for Disease Control, 1988; Hugon *et al.*, 1988)

2.2 Non-Hodgkin's lymphoma

In this monograph, Hodgkin's disease is covered under other cancers (Section 2.3.3).

2.2.1 *Description of the clinical disease and pathology*

Lymphomas have been classified on the basis of pathological appearance in various classification schemes. The use of different schemes and changes in these over time have complicated comparisons of the occurrence of non-Hodgkin's lymphoma between places and between time periods.

Non-Hodgkin's lymphoma is a recognized complication of other immunosuppressed conditions. Both primary and iatrogenic immunosuppression are associated with increased risk for non-Hodgkin's lymphoma (see Section 4.3.1). In particular, Burkitt's lymphoma incidence is increased in X-linked lymphoproliferative disease and ataxia telangiectasia, but not in relation to iatrogenic immunosuppression (Filipovich *et al.*, 1994).

Non-Hodgkin's lymphoma accounts for approximately 4% of cancer cases and 4% of cancer deaths in the general population not infected with HIV (Parkin *et al.*, 1992). Incidence rates for non-Hodgkin's lymphoma rise exponentially with age, and there is a male predominance (ratio 3 : 2), which is more marked at younger than older ages. The incidence has been rising steadily for several decades, since long before the advent of HIV. Among United States men aged 0–64 years, the increase over the past 40 years has been estimated to be above 40%. Even after accounting for the effect of HIV, the incidence of non-Hodgkin's lymphoma has continued to increase more rapidly than that of most other tumours (Devesa *et al.* 1987; Coleman *et al.*, 1993). The incidence of high histological grades of disease has increased more than that of low-grade ones, and extranodal disease has increased more rapidly than nodal disease (Rabkin *et al.*, 1993b). The reasons for these increases are not understood. Even after accounting for the impact of changes in diagnosis and well established risk factors on the trends, there remains an unexplained increase in the incidence of non-Hodgkin's lymphoma in the United States (Hartge & Devesa, 1992).

(*a*) *Classification of AIDS-related lymphomas*

Most types of non-Hodgkin's lymphoma are AIDS-defining conditions.

Non-Hodgkin's lymphoma can arise either in the lymph nodes or in extranodal lymphoid tissue. In the absence of HIV infection, approximately three quarters of the cases have a nodal primary site and one quarter originate extranodally. The central nervous system is an unusual site of non-Hodgkin's lymphoma in the absence of HIV infection. In 2687 HIV-negative cases reported to a Danish Lymphoma Registry, the central nervous system was the primary site in 4.2% of extranodal non-Hodgkin's lymphomas and in 1.6% of all non-Hodgkin's lymphomas (Krogh-Jensen et al., 1994).

HIV-associated lymphomas are distinctive in their site distribution. Nearly half of the cases of HIV-associated lymphoma have an extranodal primary site. The central nervous system is a particularly favoured primary site, accounting for about 20% of all AIDS-related non-Hodgkin's lymphoma in the United States (Beral et al., 1991b).

As shown in Table 16, the spectrum of HIV-related lymphoproliferative disorders includes: (i) systemic non-Hodgkin's lymphomas; (ii) body cavity-based lymphoma; (iii) primary lymphoma of the brain; and (iv) multicentric Castleman's disease.

(i) *Systemic non-Hodgkin's lymphomas*

Systemic AIDS-related non-Hodgkin's lymphomas are a heterogeneous group of malignancies, usually of the B-cell phenotype. The overwhelming majority fall within three Working Formulation histological categories: large non-cleaved-cell lymphoma; large-cell immunoblastic lymphoma; and small non-cleaved-cell lymphoma, which includes Burkitt's tumour. It has been proposed that large non-cleaved-cell lymphoma and large-cell immunoblastic lymphoma be classified as a single category under the term 'diffuse large-cell lymphoma'. This latter definition has been further expanded to include also $CD30^+$ anaplastic large-cell lymphoma of B-cell origin (Harris et al., 1994). $CD30^+$ anaplastic large-cell lymphomas constitute a heterogeneous group of high-grade lymphomas at the borderline between Hodgkin's disease and non-Hodgkin's lymphomas, and have been described in association with AIDS (Carbone et al., 1991; Chadburn et al., 1993; Tirelli et al., 1995a).

An interesting feature of systemic lymphomas in HIV patients is the frequency of pleomorphic features, with overlap between established histological subtypes (Raphael et al., 1991). An atypical variant made up mainly of blastic cells exhibiting features intermediate between small non-cleaved-cell lymphoma with plasma-cell differentiation and immunoblastic plasmacytoid cells has also been observed in HIV patients (Lennert & Feller, 1990; Carbone et al., 1995a). These atypical morphological features may bias a correct discrimination of small non-cleaved-cell lymphoma from large-cell immunoblastic lymphoma. This intermediate variant also includes Burkitt-like tumours (Harris et al., 1994).

Whether extramedullary plasmacytoma should be included among AIDS-related lymphomas is still debated (reviewed by Levine, 1993).

(ii) *Body cavity-based lymphoma*

Body cavity-based lymphoma, growing in the pleural, pericardial and peritoneal cavities as primary lymphomatous effusions, represents an additional rare AIDS-related non-Hodgkin's lymphoma variant (Knowles et al., 1989; Cesarman et al., 1995). This lymphoma has morphological features between those of large-cell immunoblastic lymphoma and anaplastic large-cell lymphoma (Ansari *et al.*, 1996; Carbone *et al.*, 1996a; Cesarman *et al.*, 1996). Its identification is based on pathology, clinical features, phenotype, genotype and etiology (Jaffe, 1996).

Table 16. Pathological features of AIDS-related non-Hodgkin's lymphomas and other lymphoproliferative disorders

Non-Hodgkin's lymphomas
  Systemic lymphomas
    (a) *'Blastic'[a] cell lymphomas*
      Large non-cleaved cell (G - WF)
      Immunoblastic (H - WF) with or without plasma cell differentiation
      Small non-cleaved cell (J - WF) with or without plasma cell differentiation
      Extramedullary (plasmacytoma)[b]
      Blastic cells with 'intermediate' features
    (b) *'Anaplastic'[c] cell lymphomas*
      Anaplastic large cell (CD30/Ki-1')
    (c) *Others (rare types)*
  Body cavity-based lymphoma
  Primary brain lymphoma (immunoblastic)

Multicentric Castleman's disease

Updated and adapted from Gaidano & Carbone (1995)
WF, International Working Formulation for non-Hodgkin's lymphomas
[a] The term 'blastic' is used in analogy with the suffix 'blastic' used in the Kiel Classification (Stansfeld *et al.*, 1988).
[b] Whether extramedullary plasmacytomas should be included among HIV-related lymphomas is still debated.
[c] The term 'anaplastic' is used in analogy with the term used in the definition of CD30' anaplastic large-cell lymphomas; it indicates blastic large cells which display marked pleomorphism, with giant cells possessing bizarre and irregular nuclei and large nucleoli (Harris *et al.*, 1994).

(iii) *Primary lymphoma of the brain*

Unlike the heterogeneous systemic AIDS-related non-Hodgkin's lymphomas, non-Hodgkin's lymphomas arising in the central nervous system represent a more uniform group and, in the majority of cases, tend to display histological features consistent with immunoblastic–plasmacytoid lymphomas (Remick *et al.*, 1990; Camilleri-Broët *et al.*, 1995).

(iv) *Multicentric Castleman's disease*

Multicentric Castleman's disease, also called multicentric angiofollicular lymphoid hyperplasia, is an atypical, usually polyclonal lymphoproliferative disorder which involves multiple lymphoid organs. Multicentric Castleman's disease in HIV-infected individuals is a distinct clinicopathological entity (Oksenhendler *et al.*, 1996). It is characteristically associated with Kaposi's sarcoma, which occurs during the clinical course of most HIV-associated cases of multicentric Castleman's disease (Soulier *et al.*, 1995).

(*b*) *Phenotypic and genotypic features*

The vast majority of AIDS-related non-Hodgkin's lymphomas are B-cell neoplasms (reviewed by Levine, 1993). Most of them, especially systemic and primary brain lymphomas, express monotypic surface immunoglobulin or B-cell antigens (CD19, CD20, and CD22), but lack T-cell-associated antigens (reviewed by Knowles, 1993). The remaining AIDS-related B-cell non-Hodgkin's lymphomas, particularly $CD30^+$ anaplastic large-cell lymphomas (Carbone *et al.*, 1993a, 1996b) and those preferentially involving body cavities (Knowles, 1993; Cesarman *et al.*, 1995), usually exhibit an indeterminate immunophenotype. Both lymphoma types lack surface immunoglobulin and B-cell-associated antigens, but express the leukocyte common antigen and various antigens associated with activation (Cesarman *et al.*, 1995; Carbone *et al.*, 1996b).

Almost all AIDS-related non-Hodgkin's lymphomas, including those displaying B-cell phenotypes as well as those displaying indeterminate phenotypes, exhibit clonal immunoglobulin heavy-chain and light-chain gene rearrangements and lack clonal T-cell receptor β-chain gene rearrangements (reviewed by Knowles, 1993). A higher proportion of anomalously matured B-cell neoplasms has been observed in HIV-infected individuals than among non-Hodgkin's lymphomas in the general population (Boiocchi *et al.*, 1990).

Polyclonality has been reported in rare instances, based on absence of immunoglobulin heavy chain gene rearrangements in three B-cell tumours (McGrath *et al.*, 1991). However, Raphael *et al.* (1994) reported that two cases without rearrangement did have clonal EBV termini. Similarly, Boiocchi *et al.* (1993a) noted clonal light chain rearrangement in all of three cases of AIDS-associated non-Hodgkin's lymphoma without heavy chain rearrangement.

2.2.2 *Descriptive epidemiology of non-Hodgkin's lymphoma*

As a primary AIDS-defining illness, non-Hodgkin's lymphoma accounts for 2.9% of AIDS cases in United States (Beral *et al.*, 1991b; Biggar & Rabkin, 1992) and 3% in European (Serraino *et al.*, 1992b) surveillance data. However, at least as many non-Hodgkin's lymphomas occur as a clinically recognized secondary diagnosis after another AIDS-defining illness. In the United States death certification data for 1992, 5.7% of persons dying of HIV infection had non-Hodgkin's lymphoma recorded (Selik *et al.*, 1995).

(a) *Cancer registry data*

Population-based cancer registration data yield indirect estimates of HIV-associated risk for non-Hodgkin's lymphoma based on surrogate indicators of groups at risk for HIV infection, such as never-married marital status as a surrogate indicator of homosexuality among men (see Table 17).

Table 17. Increase in risk for non-Hodgkin's lymphoma among US never-married men since beginning of the AIDS epidemic

Reference	Study area	Age group	Time period Before	Time period After	Relative risk	p value
Kristal et al. (1988)	New York City, high AIDS mortality neighbourhood	25–54	1980	1984	[2.6	<0.01]
Biggar et al. (1989)	Manhattan	20–49	1973–76	1985	6.2	<0.01
Harnly et al. (1988)	San Francisco	25–44	1975	1985	5.3	<0.01
Ross et al. (1985)	Los Angeles	18–54	1972–79	1983	1.6	<0.05
Rabkin & Yellin (1994)	San Francisco	25–54	1973–79	1988–90	20	<0.01

Ross *et al.* (1985) studied the incidence of non-Hodgkin's lymphoma in never-married men aged 18–54 years in Los Angeles, CA, United States, from 1972 to 1983. Starting in 1982, there was a 60% increase in incidence; increases were especially marked for Burkitt-like lymphoma and immunoblastic sarcoma (lymphoma). During 1980–83, these high-grade tumours accounted for 20% of all cases of non-Hodgkin's lymphoma.

Kristal *et al.* (1988) examined cancer surveillance data and mortality statistics for residents of New York City, NY, United States, aged 25–54 years for the period 1980–85. They detected a three-fold increase in the incidence of non-Hodgkin's lymphoma up to 1984 among never-married men living in neighbourhoods with high AIDS mortality.

Biggar *et al.* (1989) examined lymphoma incidence among never-married men aged 20–49 years in Manhattan, NY, United States, from 1973 through to 1985. They detected a six-fold increase from baseline rates by the end of their study period. Increases were greatest for Burkitt-like lymphoma and immunoblastic lymphoma.

Harnly *et al.* (1988) examined cancer incidence in never-married men aged 25–44 years in San Francisco, CA, United States, for the period 1975–85. In census tracts with a high incidence of AIDS, the incidence of non-Hodgkin's lymphoma was increased five-fold by 1985.

Rabkin and Yellin (1994) found that the incidence of non-Hodgkin's lymphoma in never-married men aged 25–54 years in San Francisco increased 20-fold between 1973–79 and 1988–90. However, the increases were not uniform for all sub-types of non-Hodgkin's lymphoma. Burkitt-like tumours peaked in incidence in 1985–87, then decreased in 1988–90, whereas incidence of immunoblastic lymphomas increased continuously through to 1990. The incidence of extranodal (especially central nervous system) lymphoma increased more rapidly than that of nodal disease, accounting for half of the incidence in the most recent period. [On the basis of the estimated 25% prevalence of HIV in this population, the incidence of non-Hodgkin's lymphoma in HIV-infected San Francisco men was 0.7% per year in 1988–90.]

Rabkin *et al.* (1993a) examined cancer registration data for New York women at high risk for HIV infection. Between 1976–78 and 1987–88, the incidence of non-Hodgkin's lymphoma doubled in black women, but not in white women, consistent with the distribution of AIDS, which was also primarily concentrated among black women.

Another set of studies has relied on linkage between cancer registry and AIDS registry data.

Coté *et al.* (1991) used linkage of AIDS and cancer registries in Illinois, United States, to detect cases of non-Hodgkin's lymphoma in patients diagnosed with AIDS between 1 January 1981 and 15 February 1989. Compared with general population rates, they found a 140-fold increase in incidence of non-Hodgkin's lymphoma among AIDS patients.

Reynolds *et al.* (1993) linked AIDS and cancer registry data in San Francisco for the period 1980–87. Risk for non-Hodgkin's lymphoma was increased 71-fold over concurrent general population incidence rates and 97-fold over the 1973–77 rates in the same geographical area. [The Working Group noted that the former risk estimate may be biased downwards by HIV-associated non-Hodgkin's lymphoma not being recognized as AIDS, whereas the latter may be biased upwards by the temporal trend in non-Hodgkin's lymphoma independent of HIV infection.]

(b) Cohort data

Lyter *et al.* (1995) examined the incidence of non-Hodgkin's lymphoma in 430 HIV-seropositive homosexual men in Pittsburgh, PA, United States, between 1984 and 1993. The annual incidence was [0.6%], which was 83 times that of contemporaneous population rates.

Ragni *et al.* (1993) followed a cohort of 1295 HIV-positive haemophiliacs in a collaborative study. The overall incidence of non-Hodgkin's lymphoma was 0.16 case/100 person-years, which constituted a 36.5-fold increase over expected rates.

Peters *et al.* (1991) reported a case-series of 347 AIDS patients treated at a hospital in London, United Kingdom, between October 1982 and December 1989. They found that the proportion of AIDS deaths due to lymphoma increased from 0 to 16% between 1984 and 1989. [The Working Group noted that these figures may be confounded by the introduction of *Pneumocystis carinii* pneumonia prophylaxis.]

2.2.3 Role of immunosuppression

Non-Hodgkin's lymphoma is considered to be a relatively late manifestation of AIDS, compared with Kaposi's sarcoma and some opportunistic infections.

Muñoz et al. (1993) analysed the incidence of non-Hodgkin's lymphoma in 2627 HIV-infected homosexual men in four United States cities between 1985 and 1991. They noted a nonsignificant increase with decreasing $CD4^+$ T-cell count: the relative risk for non-Hodgkin's lymphoma as an initial AIDS-defining illness was 0.38 (95% CI, 0.14–1.09) with 101–200 $CD4^+$ cells/mm^3 versus ≤ 100 cells/mm^3.

Rabkin et al. (1992) followed a cohort of 1701 haemophiliacs, of whom 1065 (63%) were HIV-seropositive. The incidence of non-Hodgkin's lymphoma after HIV seroconversion averaged 0.15 cases/100 person-years and rose exponentially with increasing duration of HIV infection. However, $CD4^+$ T-cell counts of cases of non-Hodgkin's lymphoma were similar to those in AIDS-free subjects after the same duration of HIV infection. Haemophiliac patients without HIV infection showed no increased risk for non-Hodgkin's lymphoma.

In clinical trials of zidovudine and dideoxyinosine in AIDS and AIDS-related complex patients, the three-year cumulative incidence of non-Hodgkin's lymphoma among 116 patients was 19%. There was no significant difference between subjects receiving the two antiretroviral treatments (Pluda et al., 1990, 1993). Patients with less than 50 $CD4^+$ T-cells/mm^3 were at significantly higher risk for primary central nervous system lymphoma, but not for systemic lymphoma (Pluda et al., 1993).

Moore et al. (1991) followed 1030 patients with AIDS or advanced AIDS-related complex receiving zidovudine at 12 sites in the United States between 1987 and 1990. The incidence of non-Hodgkin's lymphoma was 1.6 cases/100 person-years. Kaposi's sarcoma, oral hairy leukoplakia and cytomegalovirus disease, markers of immune dysfunction, were each independently associated with increased risk for non-Hodgkin's lymphoma.

The association between immune decline and non-Hodgkin's lymphoma appears to differ with the subtype of the disease. Roithmann et al. (1991) reported 131 HIV-associated non-Hodgkin's lymphomas recorded at a French registry during 1987–89. The median $CD4^+$ T-cell count was significantly higher in cases of small non-cleaved-cell lymphoma (266/mm^3) than in those of large-cell (125/mm^3, $p < 0.05$) or immunoblastic (80/mm^3, $p < 0.01$) lymphoma.

These studies have consistently found increasing risk of non-Hodgkin's lymphoma with increasing duration of HIV infection and with progression in immune dysregulation. It is not clear what aspect of immune dysfunction corresponds directly to this risk.

The potential role of HIV as a direct cause of non-Hodgkin's lymphoma is addressed in Section 4.3.

2.2.4 Co-factors

(a) Demographic

The proportion of AIDS patients presenting with non-Hodgkin's lymphoma is greater in adults than in children. In United States surveillance data, 0.5% of AIDS cases under one year and 1.9% of cases one to nine years of age had non-Hodgkin's lymphoma (Beral et al., 1991b). Children were somewhat more likely to have Burkitt-like lymphoma, and older adults were more likely to have immunoblastic or large-cell lymphoma. In this series, women were one third to one half less likely than men to have non-Hodgkin's lymphoma as an AIDS-defining illness.

Biggar and Rabkin (1992) reviewed United States AIDS surveillance data for AIDS-defining lymphomas. The proportion of AIDS cases presenting with non-Hodgkin's lymphoma was higher in older persons, men and whites. As the authors noted, these same characteristics are associated with increased risk for non-Hodgkin's lymphoma in non-HIV-infected individuals, suggesting that an environmental cofactor(s) for AIDS lymphoma is unlikely to be important.

In European surveillance data, the proportion of AIDS patients presenting with non-Hodgkin's lymphoma is also greater in adults than in children (Serraino et al., 1992c). In cases reported up to the end of June 1991, among intravenous drug users, females had a relative risk for non-Hodgkin's lymphomas of 0.7 (95% CI, 0.6–0.9) compared with males in the same risk group, whereas among AIDS patients with heterosexually acquired HIV infection, females had a relative risk of 1.2 (95% CI, 0.8–1.8).

(b) Geographic

Non-Hodgkin's lymphoma accounts for a similar proportion of AIDS cases in various locations. In surveillance data, non-Hodgkin's lymphoma accounted for 2.9% of United States AIDS cases recorded up to June 1989 and 3.0% of European cases up to June 1991 (Beral et al., 1991b; Serraino et al., 1992c). In European surveillance data, there was little difference between four regions (northern, central, southern and eastern) in the fraction of AIDS with non-Hodgkin's lymphoma as the initial diagnosis (Serraino et al., 1992c).

Casabona et al. (1991) analysed national surveillance data from 15 European countries up to March 1989. They found similar proportions of AIDS-related non-Hodgkin's lymphoma in three regions (northern, central, southern) for homosexual men and for other risk groups, and there was no consistent variation in the geographic pattern with time for either transmission category.

Data from Africa are less complete and it is unclear whether the risk for non-Hodgkin's lymphoma is the same as that observed in developed countries. In South African AIDS surveillance data, seven (5.6%) of the first 126 cases reported between 1982 and 1988 had non-Hodgkin's lymphoma (Sitas et al., 1993). However, most of these patients were of Caucasian origin.

Lucas et al. (1994) reported an autopsy study of HIV-positive adults and children admitted in 1991 and 1992 to the largest hospital in Abidjan, Côte d'Ivoire. In this series, 7/247 (2.8%) adult (> 14 years) decedents had non-Hodgkin's lymphoma at autopsy versus 0/78 paediatric decedents. The proportion was similar in patients seropositive for HIV-1 and HIV-2.

Bassett et al. (1995) examined cancer incidence rates in the African population of Harare, Zimbabwe, for 1990–92 and compared them with rates in Bulawayo, Zimbabwe, 20–30 years earlier. With the advent of the AIDS epidemic, annual age-standardized (world standard) Kaposi's sarcoma incidence increased by [22 and 88/100 000] in men and women, respectively. In contrast, the respective increases in non-Hodgkin's lymphoma incidence were only [2 and 3/100 000], similar to increases over this period in populations without HIV infection.

Wabinga et al. (1993) examined cancer surveillance data for Kampala, Uganda, for the period between September 1989 and December 1991. They noted a marked increase in Kaposi's sarcoma compared with baseline data from 1954–1960. In contrast, there was no detectable increase in the incidence of non-Hodgkin's lymphoma. Annual age-standardized (world standard) rates of non-Hodgkin's lymphoma actually decreased slightly between these two periods, from 3.9 to 3.2/100 000 for men and from 2.9 to 2.6/100 000 for women.

Newton et al. (1995) reported 245 cancer cases registered in Butare, Rwanda, between October 1992 and April 1994. Seven (37%) of 19 patients with non-Hodgkin's lymphoma were HIV-seropositive compared with 4% of control cancer cases, corresponding to an odds ratio of 12.6 (95% CI, 2.2–54.4).

[The Working Group noted that the apparent deficit of AIDS-associated non-Hodgkin's lymphoma in Africa cannot be explained by underdiagnosis only. It is possible that patients with severe immunodeficiency in this part of the world tend to die from infectious diseases before manifesting non-Hodgkin's lymphoma.]

(c) *Behavioural*

In contrast to the variation in risk for Kaposi's sarcoma, there are relatively small differences in risk for non-Hodgkin's lymphoma between HIV exposure groups in developed countries.

As seen in Tables 18 and 19, the proportion of AIDS cases presenting with non-Hodgkin's lymphoma is consistently between 2 and 5% in western European countries and the United States, and varies little between HIV-exposure categories.

In United States surveillance data up to 30 June 1989, 5.2% of haemophilic AIDS cases, 3.4% of homosexual or bisexual male cases and 1.6% of intravenous drug user cases were reported with non-Hodgkin's lymphoma (Beral et al., 1991b).

Reynolds et al. (1993) linked AIDS and cancer registries in San Francisco, CA, United States, for an analysis of cancers diagnosed during 1980–87. Intravenous drug users comprised 2% of 3826 AIDS cases without cancer versus 1% of 234 AIDS-associated non-Hodgkin's lymphoma, but this difference was not statistically significant.

Serraino et al. (1992c) analysed data on 53 042 AIDS cases reported from the World Health Organization European Region as of June 1991. Non-Hodgkin's lymphoma accounted for 1% of initial AIDS diagnoses among HIV-infected children and 4% among

Table 18. Numbers and proportions of male AIDS cases with non-Hodgkin's lymphoma as the AIDS-defining condition, by country and HIV transmission group in Europe and the United States, 1981–94

Country	Homo/bisexual men		Intravenous drug users		Heterosexuals (Pattern II countries)[b]		Heterosexuals (other)		Haemophiliacs and transfused		Others/unknown		Total NHL	
	NHL cases	%[c]	NHL cases	%	NHL cases	%	NHL cases	%	NHL cases	%	NHL cases	%	NHL cases	%
Austria	14	3	8	3	0	0	5	7	2	3	7	5	36	3
Belgium	26	3	3	3	7	3	15	9	0	0	3	10	54	4
Denmark	45	4	2	3	1	6	6	5	4	4	2	5	60	4
France	642	4	204	3	25	2	84	5	61	5	50	5	1096	4
Germany	372	4	37	3	1	1	11	3	31	5	52	9	504	4
Greece	16	3	0	0	1	12	3	5	5	5	6	4	31	3
Italy	168	4	386	3	6	4	54	4	16	4	50	5	682	3
Netherlands	105	4	5	2	1	2	6	4	1	2	1	2	119	4
Portugal	19	2	6	1	0	0	8	2	1	1	2	3	36	2
Spain	160	3	265	2	0	0	36	2	25	4	49	3	535	2
Sweden	38	5	4	5	0	0	1	1	2	3	0	0	45	4
Switzerland	68	4	23	2	0	0	14	4	1	2	1	2	107	3
United Kingdom	246	3	15	4	14	3	12	5	28	5	5	3	320	3
United States White	3821	3	301	2	—[d]	—[d]	53	3	137	3	146	3	4518	3
United States Black	549	1	315	1	—[d]	—[d]	57	1	19	2	103	1	1043	1
Other	581	2	284	1	—[d]	—[d]	26	1	20	2	69	2	980	2

NHL, non-Hodgkin's lymphoma
[a] Only countries with > 30 cases of NHL over the period 1981–94 are included.
[b] Individuals not originating from Pattern II countries (countries in which extensive spread of HIV began in the mid-to-late 1970s or early 1980s and in which heterosexual transmission has predominated and continues to) which include Africa and the Caribbean.
[c] Number of NHL cases as percentage of total AIDS cases in the respective risk group
[d] Data not available

Data derived from the European Non-aggregate AIDS Data Set (ENAADS) updated to June 1995, prepared by the European Centre for the Epidemiological Monitoring of AIDS, Paris, and from the AIDS Public Information Data Set (PIDS) updated to December 1994, prepared by the National Center for Infectious Diseases, Centers for Disease Control and Prevention (CDC), Atlanta, GA. United States

Table 19. Numbers and proportions of female AIDS cases with non-Hodgkin's lymphoma as the AIDS-defining condition, by country and HIV transmission group in women in Europe and the United States, 1981–94

Country[a]	Intravenous drug users		Heterosexual (Pattern II countries)[b]		Heterosexual (other)		Haemophiliacs and transfused		Other/ unknown		Total NHL	
	NHL cases	%[c]	NHL cases	%	NHL cases	%	NHL cases	%	NHL cases	%	NHL cases	%
France	55	3	17	2	50	3	18	2	21	4	161	3
Germany	14	2	1	1	8	2	3	2	6	5	32	2
Italy	79	2	2	3	32	2	5	4	9	2	127	2
Spain	36	1	0	0	24	2	2	1	9	3	71	1
Switzerland	13	2	0	0	8	3	0	0	0	0	21	2
United Kingdom	5	3	6	2	7	3	5	7	1	1	24	3
United States White	43	1	—[d]	—[d]	80	2	32	2	24	2	179	2
Black	60	0	—[d]	—[d]	80	1	10	1	38	1	188	1
Other	38	1	—[d]	—[d]	42	1	8	2	13	1	101	1

[a] Countries with > 30 cases of NHL over the period 1981–94 are included.
[b] Individuals not originating from Pattern II countries (countries in which extensive spread of HIV began in the mid-to-late 1970s or early 1980s and in which transmission has predominated and continues to), which include Africa and the Caribbean.
[c] Number of NHL cases as percentage of total AIDS cases in the respective risk group
[d] Data not available

Data derived from the European Non-aggregate AIDS Data Set (ENAADS) updated to June 1995, prepared by the European Centre for the Epidemiological Monitoring of AIDS, Paris, and from the AIDS Public Information Data Set (PIDS) updated to December 1994, prepared by the National Center for Infectious Diseases, Centers for Disease Control and Prevention (CDC), Atlanta, GA, United States

haemophiliacs; homosexual men were significantly more likely to have non-Hodgkin's lymphoma than intravenous drug users.

Pedersen *et al.* (1995) investigated 6550 European patients with AIDS followed at 52 centres, diagnosed with AIDS from 1979 up to the end of 1989. In this study, non-Hodgkin's lymphoma constituted a higher fraction of AIDS-defining illnesses in intravenous drug users (4.1%) than in homosexual men (3.0%); however, lymphoma incidence after AIDS diagnosis was significantly lower among intravenous drug users than among homosexual men. The authors suggested that their results indicate that national surveillance data may underreport AIDS-related non-Hodgkin's lymphoma in drug users.

Similarly, the Italian Cooperative Group for AIDS-Related Tumours (GICAT) (1988) reported that intravenous drug users accounted for a slightly higher proportion of AIDS-associated non-Hodgkin's lymphoma than of total AIDS cases in Italy. They identified 93 AIDS-associated non-Hodgkin's lymphomas diagnosed between January 1980 and November 1987, of which 63 (68%) were in intravenous drug users as compared with 59% of all AIDS cases in the United States.

(d) Infections

AIDS-associated non-Hodgkin's lymphoma is a heterogeneous entity, and subsets of cases have been associated with various viruses, particularly two herpes viruses, EBV and HHV-8.

(i) *Epstein–Barr virus*

Monoclonal Epstein–Barr virus (EBV) infection is found in AIDS-related non-Hodgkin's lymphomas, especially those in the central nervous system, which are almost always EBV-positive (MacMahon *et al.*, 1991). Table 20 lists studies in which central nervous system lymphomas have been tested for EBV. MacMahon *et al.* (1991) found EBV in all of 21 cases of AIDS-related central nervous system lymphoma, and this high prevalence is consistent with results of most other studies (DeAngelis *et al.*, 1992; Cinque *et al.*, 1993; Arribas *et al.*, 1995). An exception is the study by Morgello (1992), which reported only 50% of cases to be EBV-positive, perhaps because of a less sensitive method of detection. Cinque *et al.* (1993) found EBV in cerebrospinal fluid to be highly predictive of central nervous system lymphoma at subsequent necropsy. These data suggest that EBV is necessary for lymphomagenesis in the central nervous system in patients with AIDS.

In AIDS-related systemic non-Hodgkin's lymphoma, EBV is less frequently detected (Table 21). It is found preferentially in tumours with immunoblastic histology. The prevalence of EBV-positivity reported has varied from 28% (Ernberg & Altiok, 1989) to 66% (Shibata *et al.*, 1993). No single histological type was uniformly positive for EBV, which suggests that the systemic AIDS-related lymphomas have a more complex etiology than primary central nervous system disease. However, where EBV clonality has been examined, EBV-positive tumours have been uniformly monoclonal (Ballerini *et al.*, 1993; Shibata *et al.*, 1993). Thus, EBV infection precedes clonal outgrowth of

Table 20. Prevalence of Epstein–Barr virus in central nervous system non-Hodgkin's lymphoma and control tissue in relation to HIV status

Reference	Study area	Lymphoma site	EBV detection method	EBV+ non-Hodgkin's lymphoma cases		EBV+ controls		Comments
				HIV+	HIV−	HIV+	HIV−	
MacMahon et al. (1991)	Baltimore, USA	CNS	EBER1 ISH	21/21	2/15	0/13	0/6	1/1 HIV–transplant patient EBV-positive
DeAngelis et al. (1992)	New York, USA	CNS	BamHI-W PCR	11/13	7/13			
Morgello (1992)	New York, USA	CNS	EBNA-1 PCR	6/12				
Cinque et al. (1993)	Stockholm and Milan	CNS	EBER ISH	16/16 0/2				
		CSF	EBNA-1 PCR	17/17 0/2	1/66		0/10	
Arribas et al. (1995)	St Louis, MO, USA	CNS	LMP PCR	6/6 1/1				
		CSF	EBNA-1 PCR	4/7[a] 1/1		0/16		Systemic lymphoma
			BamHI-W PCR	6/7[b] 1/1		1/16		Systemic lymphoma

Abbreviations: CNS, central nervous system; EBER, Epstein–Barr encoded RNA; ISH, in-situ hybridization; EBNA, Epstein–Barr nuclear antigen; PCR, polymerase chain reaction; CSF, cerebrospinal fluid; BamHI-W, first internal repeat sequence; LMP, latent membrane protein

[a] Including 3/6 patients with CNS lymphoma
[b] Including 5/6 patients with CNS lymphoma

Table 21. Prevalence of Epstein–Barr virus in systemic lymphoma tissue in relation to HIV status

Reference	Study area	Histology	EBV detection method	EBV+ non-Hodgkin's lymphoma cases		Comments
				HIV+	HIV–	
Ernberg & Althiok (1989)	Sweden		Southern blot	7/25		1/7 PGL nodes also positive
MacMahon et al. (1991)	Baltimore, USA		EBER1 ISH	3/7	0/2	
Shibata et al. (1993)	Los Angeles, USA	Diffuse large-cell	EBNA-1 PCR + (EBER-1 ISH or Southern blot)	6/11	0/12	EBV clonal in 12/12 cases
		Immunoblastic		17/20	1/13	
		Small non-cleaved-cell		16/28	1/12	
Carbone et al. (1993b)	Aviano, Italy	Diffuse large-cell	EBER1/2 ISH	1/6		
		Immunoblastic		1/1		
		Small non-cleaved-cell		2/4		
		Anaplastic large-cell		3/4		
		Immunoblastic	BamHI-W PCR	2/6		
		Small non-cleaved-cell		4/11		
		Anaplastic large-cell		10/12		
		Diffuse large-cell	LMP PCR	0/6		
		Immunoblastic		3/7		
		Small non-cleaved-cell		0/15		
		Anaplastic large-cell		9/12		
Ballerini et al. (1993)	New York, USA	Diffuse large cell	Southern blot	1/4		EBV clonal in all positive cases
		Immunoblastic		4/4		
		Small non-cleaved cell		5/16		
Finn (1995)	New York, USA		Immunohistochemistry	8/17	9/23	Head and neck lymphomas

Abbreviations: PGL, persistent generalized lymphadenopathy; EBER, Epstein–Barr encoded RNA; ISH, in-situ hybridization; EBNA, Epstein–Barr nuclear antigen; PCR, polymerase chain reaction; BamHI-W, first internal repeat sequence; LMP, latent membrane protein these tumours, which is consistent with an etiological role of this virus. The specific role of EBV in lymphomagenesis is uncertain.

Detection of EBV in lymph nodes from patients with persistent generalized lymphadenopathy has been associated with subsequent non-Hodgkin's lymphoma. Shibata *et al.* (1991) studied 32 patients with persistent generalized lymphadenopathy who were non-Hodgkin's lymphoma-free. Two of 10 patients with EBV-positive lymph nodes versus one of 22 patients with EBV-negative lymph nodes developed non-Hodgkin's lymphoma over a median follow-up of 12 months ($p > 0.1$). [The Working Group noted that insufficient data were presented to allow analysis by survival methods accounting for duration of follow-up.]

(ii) *HHV-8*

HHV-8 is a recently identified human herpes virus that is a nearly universal infection in Kaposi's sarcoma tissues (see Section 2.1.5). In the first report of this virus, Chang *et al.* (1994) examined 27 AIDS lymphomas and 29 non-AIDS lymphomas by PCR. Three (11%) of the AIDS lymphomas and none of the non-AIDS lymphomas had HHV-8 sequences in the tumour tissue.

In a follow-up to this study, Cesarman *et al.* (1995) reported on an examination of 193 AIDS-associated lymphomas in 42 patients from New York, United States, which included the 27 from the report by Chang *et al.* (1994). HHV-8 was detected in all eight tumors associated with lymphomatous effusions (body-cavity based), but not in 185 others without effusions. Furthermore, there were on average 40–80 copies of the HHV-8 sequence per cell, whereas Kaposi's sarcoma tissue contained 1–2 copies per cell. Significantly, all eight tumors also contained EBV detected by PCR, which was clonal by Southern blot in 6/6 cases.

Pastore *et al.* (1995) tested 180 lymphoid malignancies in Italy and Spain. HHV-8 was present in all of three cavity-based lymphomas, but was not found in 177 other non-Hodgkin's lymphomas.

(iii) *HHV-6*

In a French study, the presence of HHV-6 DNA was determined by PCR in HIV-positive and HIV-negative patients with non-Hodgkin's lymphoma or lymph node follicular hyperplasia. Twelve (44%) of the 27 AIDS-associated lymphomas versus seven (35%) of the 20 lymphomas from HIV-seronegative patients contained HHV-6 DNA ($p = 0.51$) (Fillet *et al.*, 1995). HHV-6 prevalence was similar in the hyperplastic lymph nodes from both HIV-positive (2/4, 50%) and HIV-negative patients (5/9, 55%).

In an Italian study, HHV-6 DNA was detected by PCR in DNA extracted from paraffin-embedded tissue from 16 (89%) of 18 HIV-infected individuals. However, nine (64%) of 14 non-lymphoma tissue samples from the same patients also contained detectable HHV-6 (Trovato *et al.* 1995).

In summary, EBV and HHV-8 are almost always found in AIDS-related lymphoma of the brain and body cavity-based lymphomas, respectively, and may be found in other AIDS lymphomas (HHV-8 has been detected in all (14/14) cases of HIV-associated lymphomas). Their role in the etiology of these malignancies will be examined in Section 4.3. HHV-6 has not been specifically related to non-Hodgkin's lymphoma.

(e) Zidovudine and other therapy

As non-Hodgkin's lymphoma occurs more frequently in advanced-stage HIV infection, concern has been raised regarding a potential role of antiretroviral therapy in lymphomagenesis. An exceptionally high risk of non-Hodgkin's lymphoma was found in Phase I trials of nucleoside analogues in patients with advanced HIV infection at the National Institutes of Health in the United States (Pluda *et al.*, 1990, 1993). Patients treated with either zidovudine or dideoxyinosine had a 19% risk of non-Hodgkin's lymphoma three years after starting therapy, with no significant difference between these two antiretroviral agents.

Levine *et al.* (1995) performed a case–control study of AIDS-related non-Hodgkin's lymphoma compared with other AIDS diagnoses. The matched odds ratio for prior use of zidovudine was 0.43 (95% CI, 0.17–1.12).

Muñoz *et al.* (1993) examined antiretroviral therapy as a risk factor for non-Hodgkin's lymphoma in a cohort study of homosexual men. They found a protective effect of treatment, with a relative risk of 0.47, which was not statistically significant.

Coté and Biggar (1995) linked AIDS and cancer registries to compare risk for non-Hodgkin's lymphoma before and after zidovudine therapy became available in 1987. The observed : expected ratios for non-Hodgkin's lymphoma incidence were 222 pre-zidovudine (1981–86) and 193 post-zidovudine (1988–90).

Rabkin *et al.* (1993c) examined the incidence of non-Hodgkin's lymphoma in relation to $CD4^+$ count in a cohort of HIV-infected homosexual men. They compared incidence in the periods before and after January 1988 to assess changes after zidovudine was introduced. The cumulative risk for non-Hodgkin's lymphoma at 50 $CD4^+$ cells/mm^3 was $25 \pm 12\%$ before January 1988 and $10 \pm 5\%$ after that date ($p = 0.4$).

In summary, there is no consistent evidence from these studies that antiretroviral therapies increase the risk for non-Hodgkin's lymphomas in AIDS patients.

2.2.5 *HIV-2 and non-Hodgkin's lymphoma*

When they occur, HIV-2-associated non-Hodgkin's lymphomas appear to have clinical features similar to those of HIV-1-associated non-Hodgkin's lymphomas. In a report of three cases of non-Hodgkin's lymphomas associated with HIV-2 infection, all were high-grade malignancies with B-cell immunophenotype (Forjaz Lacerda *et al.*, 1990).

In the study from the Côte d'Ivoire by Lucas *et al.* (1994) (see Section 2.2.4), 7/247 HIV-positive adult decedents had non-Hodgkin's lymphoma. The proportion was similar in patients who were seropositive for HIV-1 (5/154), HIV-2 (1/40) and both (1/53).

2.3 Cervical, anal and other cancers

Cancers other than Kaposi's sarcoma and non-Hodgkin's lymphoma have been studied considerably less often and reported in far fewer HIV-positive patients. Some positive findings may have been inflated by publication bias, surveillance bias or misclassification with Kaposi's sarcoma and non-Hodgkin's lymphoma; confounding is also possible on account of the existence of several risk factors shared by HIV infection and some neoplasms. Data on cancer occurrence in HIV-infected individuals are particularly inadequate in developing countries, where the largest numbers of AIDS cases occur.

Research attempting to clarify the potential relationship between HIV and anogenital cancers has so far been based primarily on small cross-sectional and case–control studies of populations at particular risk for HIV infection and with the outcome variable being precancerous lesions rather than invasive cancer. The short existence of the HIV epidemic, the initial male predominance, and the young populations at risk have in particular limited the possibilities for studying large numbers of HIV-infected female cases — especially HIV-infected cases with cervical cancer.

Specific genital types of human papillomavirus (HPV) are involved in the etiology of invasive cervical cancer and in some of its precursor lesions. There is also preliminary evidence for an association with anal cancer and anal intraepithelial lesions (IARC, 1995). Both HIV and most known oncogenic types of HPV are sexually transmitted. Therefore, the ability to control for confounding is particularly essential in studying the influence of HIV on anogenital malignancies. The small sample size in many of the studies undertaken so far has limited their ability to control adequately for behavioural covariates and risk factors associated with HIV infection.

2.3.1 *Cervical intraepithelial neoplasia and invasive cancer*

The influence of HIV on invasive cervical cancer and its precursor lesions has been reviewed (Palefsky, 1991; Rabkin & Blattner, 1991; Sillman & Sedlis, 1991; Northfelt & Palefsky, 1992; Braun, 1994; Stratton & Ciacco, 1994).

(*a*) *Precancerous lesions*

(i) *Association with HIV*

In the late 1980s, the first case reports and case series were published which suggested an association between HIV infection and cervical intraepithelial neoplasia (CIN) (Bradbeer, 1987; Byrne *et al.*, 1989; Henry *et al.*, 1989). In a review by Mandelblatt *et al.* (1992), 21 of the earliest case reports and series were described in more detail. Table 22 summarizes relevant data.

In a blind cytological analysis of cervicovaginal smears, a significantly higher percentage of cytological squamous atypia was documented in HIV-positive (11/35; 31%) than HIV-negative women (1/23; 4%) (Schrager *et al.*, 1989). Furthermore, cytological or histopathological findings suggestive of HPV infection were observed in 26% of HIV-positive women compared with 4% of HIV-negative women. [The Working Group noted that the controls in this study were not comparable with HIV-positive cases in terms of sexual behaviour, history of sexually transmitted diseases or frequency of barrier methods used.]

Fruchter *et al.* (1994) estimated that approximately 13% of 482 women referred to a public colposcopy clinic in Brooklyn, NY, United States, with abnormal Papanicolaou

Table 22. Studies of precancerous lesions of the uterine cervix in HIV-infected persons

Reference, study area	No. and type of HIV+ cases	No. and type of HIV– controls	HPV prevalence Percentage	HPV prevalence Odds ratio (95% CI)	Cervical abnormality Percentage	Cervical abnormality Odds ratio (95% CI)	HPV test	Pathology reading	Comments
Schrager et al. (1989) USA	35	23	HIV+ 26% HIV– 4%		Squamous atypia HIV+ 31% HIV– 4%		Cytological or histopathological findings	Pap smear	HIV-infected: fewer barrier methods, more STD
Feingold et al. (1990) USA	35	32	HIV+ 49% HIV– 25%		SIL HIV+ 40% HIV– 9%		Southern blot (cervico-vaginal lavage)	Pap smear	48 IVDU 18 heterosexual partners of IVDU
Vermund et al. (1991a) USA	51 (18 asymptomatic 33 symptomatic)	45	HIV+ symptomatic 53% asymptomatic 70% HIV– 22% 22%		SIL HIV+ symptomatic 42% asymptomatic 17% HIV– 13%	12 (1.3–108) [2.0 (0.1–30)] 4.6 (0.8–28)	Southern blot (lavage)	Pap smear	IVDU, heterosexual contacts with IVDU
Byrne et al. (1989) UK	19 recruited from HIV+ STD clinic attenders				3 CIN III 1 CIN II 1 Atypia 1 SPI 1 HPV		Colposcopy	Pap smear and biopsy	
ter Meulen et al. (1992) Tanzania	313 gynaecological in-patients		Any type HIV+ 78% HIV– 56% HPV 16/18 HIV+ 30% HIV– 14%	HPV (total)* 2.5 (p = 0.02) HPV-16/18* 2.4 (p = 0.02)	HIV+ 2.4% HIV– 2.8%		PCR	Pap smear	*Adjusted for age
Kreiss et al. (1992) Nairobi, Kenya	147 prostitutes	51 prostitutes	HIV+ 37% HIV– 24%	1.7 (0.8–3.6)*	CIN HIV+ 26% HIV– 24% HPV+ HIV+ 47% HIV– 57% HPV– HIV+ 9% HIV– 7%	0.9 (0.2–3.5) 9.4 (1.7–52.1) 17.3 (1.4–217)		Cytology	*Adjusted for age and years of prostitution

Table 22 (contd)

Reference, study area	No. and type of HIV+ cases	No. and type of HIV− controls	HPV prevalence Percentage	Odds ratio (95% CI)	Cervical abnormality Percentage		Odds ratio (95% CI)	HPV test	Pathology reading	Comments
Laga et al. (1992) Kinshasa, Zaire	47 prostitutes	48 prostitutes	HIV+ 38% HIV− 8% HIV+/CIN+ 73% HIV+/CIN− 30%	6.8 (1.9–26.8) 6.2 (p = 0.02)	CIN HIV+ HIV−	27% 3%	14.7 (1.8–95.3)	ViraType™ Southern blot	Cytology	13 Pap smears inadequate for interpretation
Conti et al. (1993) Italy	273 former IVDU	161 former IVDU			HIV+ HIV−	42% 8%	4.2 (2.1–8.4) HPV−/HIV+ 1.2 (0.2–0.6) HPV+/HIV− 10.8 (2.8–41.6) HPV+/HIV+ 64.0 (19.2–214)	Cytological diagnosis	Cytology confirmed by biopsy	Cross-sectional study, potential selection bias (inflated), odds ratios CIN II,III/HIV+ CD4+ ≥ 500 1.0 CD4+ < 500 5.4 (2.6–11)
Maggwa et al. (1993) Nairobi, Kenya	205 attenders, family planning clinic	3853 attenders, family planning clinic			HIV+ HIV−	4.9% 1.9%	2.8 (1.3–5.9) adj. sexual behaviour, demographic variables		Cytology	
Van Doorrum et al. (1993) The Netherlands	25 IVDU and prostitutes	44 IVDU and prostitutes	HIV+ 32% HIV− 7%	6.4 (1.3–40.1)	HIV+ HIV−	0% 4.6%		PCR	Cytology	HIV−: More clients per month than HIV+ women
Smith et al. (1993b) UK	43 mostly IVDU	43 matched to HIV+ cases	HPV-6/11 HIV+ 11.6% HIV− 2.3% HPV-16 HIV+ 11.6% HIV− 4.7%		HIV+ HIV−	14% 9%		Southern blot	Histology	Tendency to increased CIN prevalence in HIV+ women with increasing immunosuppression
Ho et al. (1994) New York, USA	97 IVDU, HIV-related disease, IVDU partner	110 same	All HPV types HIV+ 49.5% HIV− 22.7% CD4+ > 20% 45.0% CD4+ ≤ 20% 60.7% Oncogenic types HIV+ 14.4% HIV− 6.4%	3.3 (1.8–6.1) 2.8 (1.3–6.0) 5.3 (2.2–12.7) 3.5 (1.3–9.2)				Southern blot hybridization		*Strong HPV signal,* odds ratios: HIV− 1.0 HIV+ CD4+ > 20% 2.6 CD4+ ≤ 20% 5.9

Table 22 (contd)

Reference, study area	No. and type of HIV+ cases	No. and type of HIV− controls	HPV prevalence Percentage	Odds ratio (95% CI)	Cervical abnormality Percentage	Odds ratio (95% CI)	HPV test	Pathology reading	Comments
Klein et al. (1994) New York, USA	114 IVDU, HIV-related disease, sex partner IVDU	139 same			HIV+ 21.9% HIV− 10.1% CD4 > 20% 16.7% CD4 ≤ 20% 35% Multivariate analysis HPV infection high-risk HPV Strong HPV signal Low CD4+ count	2.5 (1.2–5.1) 1.8 (0.7–4.6) 4.8 (2.0–11.6) 6.8 (2.9–15.7) 11.8 (4.1–34.1) 10.8 (3.5–33.7) 3.1 (1.0–9.5)	Southern blot hybridization	Cytology	No demographic or behavioural variables associated with SIL
Williams et al. (1994) San Francisco, USA	55 IVDU	59 IVDU	Dot blot HIV+ 19% HIV− 5% PCR HIV+ 57% HIV− 13%		9 out of 11 abnormal smears in HIV+	6.1 (1.2–60.5)	ViraType™ and PCR	Cytology	Recruited from larger cohort, see also Table 23
Sun et al. (1995) New York, USA	344 cross-sectional	325	All HPV types HIV+ 60% HIV− 36% HPV-16 HIV+ 27% HIV− 17% HPV-18 HIV+ 24% HIV− 9%	< 0.001	All HPV types HIV+/CIN II/III 53% HIV−/CIN II/III 50% HPV-16 HIV+/CIN II/III 35% HIV−/CIN II/III 0 HPV-18 HIV+/CIN II/III 35% HIV−/CIN II/III 50%		PCR	Cervico-vaginal lavage, colposcopy and sometimes biopsy	HIV+ HPV+ women had more CIN irrespective of CD4+ level than HIV− HPV+ women
Langley et al. (1996) Senegal	HIV-1 68 HIV-2 58 both 14 commercial sex workers	619 commercial sex workers	HIV-1+ 57% HIV-2+ 50.0% both 75.0% HIV− 40.1%	2.3 (1.4–3.7) 1.7 (1.0–3.0) 3.9 (1.9–8.1) 1.0	HIV-1 7.5 HIV-2 11.1 both 16.7 HIV− 6.8	1.8 (0.7–4.7) 2.9 (1.2–7.2) 5.2 (1.4–19.6) 1.0 Adjusted for no. of sexual partners and study site	PCR	Cytology	No analysis of the independent effect of HIV and HPV on CIN development was presented

STD, sexually transmitted disease; SIL, squamous intraepithelial lesions; CIN, cervical intraepithelial neoplasia; SPI, subclinical papillomavirus infection; PCR, polymerase chain reaction; IVDU, intravenous drug user; | | calculated by the Working Group smears were HIV-seropositive. A more detailed characterization of 208 of these women showed the 47 HIV-positive women had more advanced CIN, larger cervical lesions and more associated vulvo-vaginal lesions than the 161 HIV-seronegative women.

Johnstone et al. (1994) conducted a retrospective case–control study in Edinburgh, United Kingdom, which included IVDU women or women having a seropositive IVDU partner and computer-matched neighbourhood controls. Cytological smears were retrieved subsequently for both cases and controls. There were more abnormal smears from the HIV-seropositive group than from the drug-related seronegative ($p < 0.01$) group or the neighbourhood control group ($p < 0.001$). [The Working Group noted that no information on HPV was presented.]

(ii) *Association with HIV and HPV*

Vermund et al. (1991) extended a study by Feingold et al. (1990) on HPV-associated disease in women taking intravenous drugs in the United States. In this study of 96 women, non-white subjects were disproportionately represented among HIV-infected women but other behavioural and sociodemographic characteristics were similar. Symptomatic HIV-positive women had more HPV DNA (70%), measured by Southern blot hybridization, compared with asymptomatic (22%) and seronegative women (22%). Among symptomatic HIV-positive women, a strong association between HPV and squamous intraepithelial lesions was documented (odds ratio, 12; 95% CI, 1.3–108), whereas the association was nonsignificant for the other two groups. These and other studies conducted in the late 1980s and early 1990s suggest that more severe HIV disease might exacerbate HPV-mediated cervical cytological abnormalities (Maiman et al., 1991; Schäfer et al., 1991; Johnson et al., 1992; Conti et al., 1993).

In a cross-sectional study of 359 gynaecological in-patients without cancer in Tanzania (ter Meulen et al., 1992), 1/42 (2.4%) HIV-positive women compared with 8/285 (2.8%) HIV-negative women had an abnormal Pap smear. However, none of the HIV-positive women was suspected to be severely immunosuppressed, in view of the lack of severe HIV-related symptoms. HIV-positive women were 3.3 times more likely to be positive for HPV types 16 or 18, as detected by PCR, after adjusting for differences in sexual behaviour, history of sexually transmitted diseases and other factors. [The Working Group noted that no analysis of the association between HPV and smear abnormality by HIV status was presented.]

Kreiss et al. (1992) performed a nested case–control study of 147 HIV-positive and 51 HIV-negative women within a large cohort of prostitutes in Nairobi, but did not observe a significant difference with respect to the prevalence of HPV DNA between the two groups (adjusted odds ratio, 1.7; 95% CI, 0.8–3.6). A strength of this study is that the populations studied were relatively homogeneous with respect to sexual behaviour and condom use. Papanicolaou smears were available only for the most recently enrolled 63 women in the study. Among women with cervical HPV DNA, HIV infection was not associated with an increased prevalence of CIN (47% in HIV-positive versus 57% in HIV-negative women).

In contrast, in a somewhat smaller but otherwise similarly designed study conducted in Kinshasa, Zaire, Laga et al. (1992) found a significantly higher prevalence of HPV

DNA in HIV-positive cases (18/47; 38%) than in HIV-negative controls (4/48; 8%; odds ratio, 6.8; 95% CI, 1.9–26.8). HPV was detected both by ViraType™ and Southern blot. Eight (73%) of 11 HIV-positive women who had CIN also had HPV DNA detected compared with nine (30%) of 30 with no CIN (Fisher's exact test $p = 0.02$). Cases and controls in this study did not differ in terms of important demographic or sexual behavioural characteristics, but clinical AIDS was more frequent (7% of HIV-positive cases) than in the population studied by Kreiss *et al.* (0.7%).

In a large study of 4058 women attending two semi-urban family planning clinics in Nairobi, Kenya, Maggwa *et al.* (1993) observed CIN on Pap smears of 10/205 (4.9%) HIV-positive women compared with 72/3853 (1.9%) HIV-seronegative women (odds ratio, 2.8; 95% CI, 1.3–5.9) controlled for sexual behaviour and other risk factors. [The Working Group noted that the association with HPV was not evaluated in this study.]

Langley *et al.* (1996) studied the effect of both HIV-1 and HIV-2 on the development of CIN lesions in a cross-sectional analysis of 759 female commercial sex workers in Senegal. After adjustment for number of sexual partners per week and study site, HIV-2 seropositivity was associated with a 2.9-fold increased risk for CIN (95% CI, 1.2–7.2) compared with a 1.8-fold (0.7–4.7) risk in HIV-1 infected women. Women infected with both HIV types had a 5.2-fold increased risk (1.4–19.6). [The Working Group noted that the authors did not report HPV status or $CD4^+$ T-cell counts in these analyses.]

(iii) *HIV, HPV and $CD4^+$ T-cell counts*

Whereas most studies reviewed above have used either HIV-positivity *per se* or degree of severity of HIV-associated disease as a surrogate marker for level of immune status, recent studies have often included an evaluation by $CD4^+$ T-cell count. Ho *et al.* (1994) found that among 207 primarily intravenous drug-using women, young age (less than 35 years) (odds ratio, 2.5; 95% CI, 1.3–4.8) and HIV-positivity (3.0; 1.5–5.7) were the only independent covariates associated with HPV DNA positivity. The association with HIV changed only marginally between the univariate and the multivariate analysis, indicating little influence of confounding. Prevalence of HPV increased with decreasing $CD4^+$ count, from 23% among immunocompetent HIV-negative subjects to 45% in mild or moderate immunosuppressive conditions (HIV-positive and $CD4^+$ percentage > 20%) and to 61% in severe immunosuppression ($CD4^+$ percentage < 20%). Oncogenic HPV types (16, 18, 31, 33 and 35) were not particularly strongly associated with HIV-positivity. A general increase in the quantity of viral copies of HPV detected was indirectly supported by the finding of a significant association between strong Southern blot hybridization signal strength and increasing HIV-induced immunosuppression (see Table 22). Among 29 study subjects who had no sexual exposure in the previous year, 1/16 (6.3%) HIV-seronegative women were HPV-positive compared to 8/13 HIV-positive women (61.5%). [The Working Group noted that this observation supports the conclusion that individuals with HIV-induced immunosuppression are prone to persistent HPV infection rather than self-limiting infection].

The influence of immunosuppression was also evaluated in a cross-sectional study by Williams *et al.* (1994) of 114 intravenous drug users in San Francisco. A close association between HIV, HPV and abnormal cervical cytology was observed (see Table 23).

In a multivariate model of risk factors for cervical epithelial abnormalities which excluded those showing only atypia with inflammation, both cervical HPV detected by dot blot (odds ratio, 32.1; 95% CI, 2.9–354) and HIV-seropositivity with $CD4^+$ T-cell count below 250 cells/mm³ (odds ratio, 126.8; 95% CI, 7.5–2133) were independent predictors.

Table 23. Relation between human immunodeficiency virus serostatus, presence of cervical human papillomavirus, and cervical cytology (from Williams et al., 1994)

HPV/HIV status	Cervical cytology		Odds ratio	95% CI	p value[a]
	Abnormal	Normal			
Dot blot					
HPV–/HIV–	0	47	1		
HPV–/HIV+	5	31	7.3	0.7–354	0.08
HPV+/HIV–	1	2	15.7	0.2–1254	0.2
HPV+/HIV+	4	4	37.6	2.7–1888	0.001
PCR					
HPV–/HIV–	0	41	1		
HPV–/HIV+	3	17	6.8	0.5–367	0.1
HPV+/HIV–	1	6	5.8	0.07–471	0.3
HPV+/HIV+	6	18	12.9	1.4–610	0.009

[a] p values compared with referent values (negative/negative)

In a population-based study of HIV-positive women exposed by intravenous drug use or from partners using intravenous drugs in Edinburgh, United Kingdom, Johnstone et al. (1994) found an association between prevalence of abnormal smears and reduced $CD4^+$ count ($p < 0.0005$), but there was no clear relation between $CD4^+$ count and the severity of the lesions.

Sun et al. (1995) conducted a large cross-sectional study in New York including 325 HIV-seronegative and 344 HIV-seropositive women. The two groups had similar age distribution, income and education. HPV of any type was detected in 60% of HIV-positive women and 36% of seronegative women. HPV-positive women who were also HIV-positive were significantly more likely to have CIN than were HPV-infected HIV-seronegative women. This difference was observed at all levels of immunosuppression. [The Working Group noted that these epidemiological data suggest that the association between HIV and CIN lesions cannot be explained exclusively by activation of a latent HPV infection mediated by HIV-induced immunosuppression. Thus, HIV could have an effect on the development of CIN which is independent of systemic immunosuppression. Such an effect could reflect a direct biological action but could also be a result of confounding by factors for which no adjustment was made, e.g., a behavioural variable linked with HIV seropositivity and often associated with CIN lesions.]

(iv) *Progression of disease and treatment of CIN lesions*

Adachi *et al.* (1993) conducted a prospective study among 48 women with abnormal Papanicolaou smear out of an original cohort of 232 women at high risk for HIV infection in the Bronx, New York. Subsequent colposcopic or histological findings in 36/38 were no more severe than those observed by cytology, indicating that abnormal cytological smears accurately reflect the severity of cervical and vaginal disease in HIV-positive women. Similar results were obtained by Korn *et al.* (1994) and Johnstone *et al.* (1994). A follow-up of between 3 and 37 months, based on small numbers, showed that all three HIV-negative and five out of ten HIV-positive women had normal examinations, whereas three HIV-positive women had persistent disease and two had progression to condyloma (Adachi *et al.*, 1993).

Sha *et al.* (1995) followed 82 HIV-positive women who were seen between 1986 and 1992 at a hospital in Chicago, IL, United States. Among 10 who presented with CIN confirmed by Papanicolaou smears, none developed invasive cervical cancer during a median follow-up time of 13 months (range, 3–61 months).

Maiman *et al.* (1993a) in Brooklyn, NY, found an equal distribution of CIN severity and lesion size among 44 HIV-positive and 125 HIV-negative women. However, more HIV-positive women (39%) developed biopsy-proven recurrent CIN after treatment than HIV-negative women (9%), and, among HIV-positive women, recurrent disease was clearly associated with degree of immunosuppression as measured by $CD4^+$ T-cell count.

Wright *et al.* (1994) performed a retrospective chart review of patients treated by electrosurgical excision for CIN at a hospital in Manhattan, NY, United States, during 1991–92. All patients had at least six months of follow-up or had documented recurrent and/or persistent disease during less than six months of follow-up. Age-distribution and grading of disease stage were similar in HIV-positive and -negative patients, but recurrent and/or persistent CIN occurred significantly more frequently in HIV-positive women (56%, 19/34) than in HIV-negative women (13%, 10/80; $p < 0.001$). In HIV-positive women, the occurrence of recurrent and/or persistent CIN was associated with degree of immunosuppression (> 500 $CD4^+$ cells/mm^3: 20%; ≤ 500 $CD4^+$ cells/mm^3: 61%).

These studies suggest that HIV infection and/or HIV-related immunosuppression accelerate the progression of CIN.

(b) *Invasive cervical cancer*

Since January 1993, CDC included invasive cervical cancer as an AIDS-defining illness in HIV-positive women (Centers for Disease Control and Prevention, 1992a) (see Table 5).

(i) *Case series*

Maiman *et al.* (1993b) studied 16 HIV-positive women (19%) out of 84 women below 50 years of age with invasive cervical cancer, at a hospital in Brooklyn. Three were known to be HIV-positive before enrolment whereas 81 were subsequently tested for HIV. Almost 70% of the HIV-positive patients were at clinical stage III or IV disease, compared with 28% in the HIV-negative group ($p = 0.01$).

Zanetta et al. (1995) made a retrospective evaluation of all patients referred during 1991–94 to a hospital in Milan, Italy, with a diagnosis of invasive cervical carcinoma. Six (1.8%) out of 340 women with invasive cervical carcinoma were HIV-positive. The mean age at diagnosis was 30 years (range, 27–36) for the HIV-seropositive women, but 49 for the remaining population. Furthermore, HIV-seropositive women had more advanced disease ($p = 0.04$). [The Working Group noted that four out of the six seropositive women were intravenous drug addicts ($p < 0.0001$).]

(ii) *Prognosis*

Maiman et al. (1990, 1993b) reported a poorer response to therapy and a poorer prognosis among HIV-infected patients with invasive cervical cancer in Brooklyn, with higher recurrence and death rates compared with HIV-uninfected patients. The patient's immune status had a significant impact on subsequent disease. Thus, only seropositive patients with $CD4^+$ counts greater than 500 cells/mm^3 had prolonged or disease-free follow-up.

(iii) *Descriptive epidemiology*

Rabkin et al. (1993a) used cancer registry incidence data from New York and northern New Jersey in the United States to study time trends in cervical cancer rates. The annual incidence of AIDS among women in upstate New York is low among white women and also significantly lower in black women compared to women from New York City and northern New Jersey. Nevertheless, cervical cancer in New York and northern New Jersey blacks declined during the study period (1976–88) by approximately 40% for invasive tumors and 50% for in-situ lesions (Figure 9). Because the incidence in whites remained rather stable, the ratio of incidence of invasive cervical carcinoma in blacks to incidence in whites decreased in all three regions.

Data from a pathological review of cervical cancer series from Lusaka, Zambia (Rabkin & Blattner, 1991; Patil et al., 1995) indicated that both the total incidence and the age-distribution of cervical cancer remained stable during the period between 1980 and 1989 when HIV was rapidly spreading to large segments of the population. Nearly 10% of pregnant women and 18% of normal blood donors were already HIV-infected by 1985 (Melbye et al., 1986).

Wabinga et al. (1993) compared cervical cancer incidence data for different time periods based on the cancer registry in Kyadondo County in Uganda. Invasive cervical cancer almost doubled from 22.2/100 000 in 1954–60 to 43.6 in 1989–91. The overall increase in cancer incidence during the same period was nearly 50%. [The Working Group noted that the quality of the data is uncertain and the incidence of cervical cancer appears to have been increasing in this population before the advent of HIV.]

In a large linkage study between AIDS and cancer registries in seven health departments in the United States, published as an abstract, Coté et al. (1993) found invasive cervical carcinoma in AIDS patients to be only marginally increased over background.

Figure 9. Incidence per 100 000 of AIDS and selected cancers in black New York City women aged 20–49, 1976–1988. Data smoothed by 3-point moving means

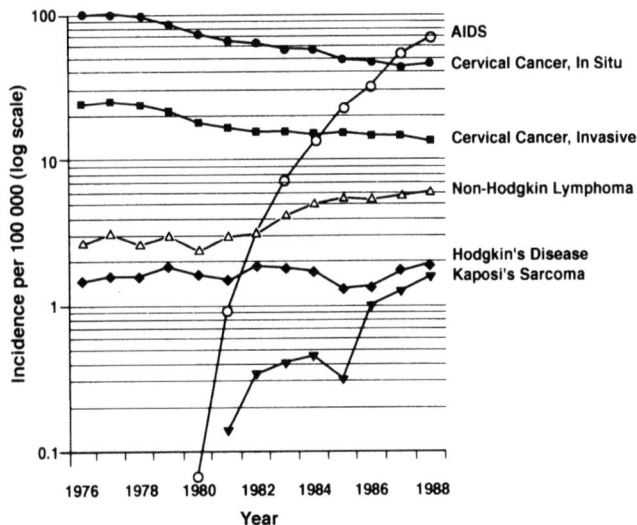

From Rabkin *et al.* (1993a)

(iv) *Case–control studies*

In Tanzania, ter Meulen *et al.* (1992) found that 8/270 (3%) cases of invasive cervical cancer were HIV-seropositive compared with 46/359 (13%) controls. [The Working Group noted that many of the controls were gynaecological patients and may have had conditions associated with other sexually transmitted diseases.]

In a study of cancer patients in Rwanda (Newton *et al.*, 1995), 0/23 cases of cervical cancer were HIV-seropositive compared to 8/200 (4%) in controls comprising other cancers.

In summary, the above studies are generally consistent in demonstrating an association between late-stage HIV infection and increased prevalence of CIN. However, there is at present no evidence of a significantly increasing incidence of invasive cervical carcinoma as a consequence of the HIV epidemic. This lack of increased risk of invasive disease may be partly explained by the late spread of HIV infection in the female population. In addition, active screening programmes among HIV-infected women may reduce the likelihood of progression to invasive cervical carcinoma. One result could be that HIV-infected women die from other causes before CIN progresses to invasive cervical carcinoma. HIV-infected women have in general higher rates of sexually transmitted diseases than women in the general population and are therefore more likely to be in close contact with the health care system both before and after their HIV infection.

2.3.2 Anorectal intraepithelial neoplasia and invasive cancer

A comprehensive and detailed review of anal cancer in HIV-infected individuals has been presented by Palefsky (1994).

The assessment of anorectal epithelial cytology poses special problems because of variable quality of sample collection and faecal contamination. Furthermore, biopsy materials have only rarely been obtained for confirmation of cytological results. A significant association between cytological and histopathological findings was observed in one study (Palefsky et al., 1990), whereas Surawicz (1993) reported a three-fold greater prevalence of dysplasia for biopsy evaluation than by cytology in 90 homosexual men referred for internal lesions from a cross-sectional community-based study (see Table 24).

Table 24. Correlation of anal abnormalities with histological diagnosis

Anoscopic abnormalities	Negative	Low grade (AIN I)	High grade (AIN II-III)	Total
Discrete warts	3	26	8	37[a]
Circumferential ring of warts	2	14	7	23
Flat white epithelium	1	11	6	18
Normal or non-HPV-associated findings	7	0	1	8[a]
Total	13	51	22	86[a]

From Surawicz et al. (1993)
AIN, anal intraepithelial neoplasia
[a] Biopsies from two HIV-seronegative men in each of these categories were unsatisfactory.

(a) Precancerous lesions

(i) Association with HIV

Denis et al. (1992) studied 190 patients diagnosed with advanced HIV-associated disease (Group IV, CDC). Thirty-five patients had anal abnormalities, including one case of non-Hodgkin's lymphoma, but there was no case of anal carcinoma.

(ii) Association with HIV and HPV

The main features and results of published studies are summarized in Table 25.

Frazer et al. (1986) reported, from a prospective study of 61 homosexual men in Australia, cytological evidence of dysplasia with concomitant features of HPV infection in 24 men and of HPV without dysplasia in a further 26 men. HIV infection was associated with dysplasia in a univariate analysis, but the small sample size hindered more sophisticated analyses.

HUMAN IMMUNODEFICIENCY VIRUSES

Table 25. Studies of precancerous lesions of the anorectal region in HIV-infected persons

Reference, study area	No. and type of HIV+ cases	No. and type of HIV− cases	HPV prevalence		Anal abnormality			HPV test	Pathology reading	Comments
			Percentage	Odds ratio (95% CI)	% HIV+/HIV−		Odds ratio (95% CI)			
Frazer et al. (1986) Australia	20 homosexual men	41 homosexual men			HIV+ HIV−	[45%] [15%]		Cytological reading	Cytology	
Palefsky et al. (1990) San Francisco, USA	97 homosexual men with CDC group IV disease	None	HPV, all types 54% HPV-6/11* 23% HPV-16/18* 29% HPV-31,33,35* 20%		HIV+ condyloma atypia AIN I AIN II	39% 4 19 11 4		ViraType™	Cytology + histology	*Alone or in combination
Melbye et al. (1990) Denmark	33 homosexual men	87 homosexual men	HIV+ 61.1%				ASIL+HPV CD4/CD8 ratio ≥ 1.0 5.9 < 1.0 30.0	ViraType™	Cytology (ASIL)	
Caussy et al. (1990) USA	43 homosexual men	62 homosexual men	HIV+ 53% HIV− 29%	p = 0.01	HIV+ HIV−	24% 7%	p = 0.03	ViraType™ and PCR	Cytology (ASIL)	
Kiviat et al. (1990) USA	49 homosexual men	47 homosexual men	HIV+ 26% HIV− 6%					ViraType™		
Critchlow et al. (1992) USA	26 consecutive homosexual men for HIV testing	119 same	HIV+ 31% HIV− 8%	5.8 (1.1–30.1) adj. for STD history, age, anorectal symptoms				Dot filter hybridization		HIV positivity did not influence type of HPV. HPV prevalence up with severity of HIV-disease
Bernard et al. (1992) France	54 homosexual and IVDU men	54 partners of women with genital HPV or cervical dysplasia	HIV+ Any type [66%] HPV-6/11 17% HPV-16/18 and/or 83% 31/35/51 HIV− Any type [54%] HPV-6/11 62% HPV-16/18 and 38% 1/35/51					In situ hybridization		Link between CMV and high-risk HPV observed irrespective of HIV status

Table 25 (contd)

Reference, study area	No. and type of HIV+ cases	No. and type of HIV− cases	HPV prevalence		Anal abnormality			HPV test	Pathology reading	Comments
			Percentage	Odds ratio (95% CI)	% HIV+/HIV−	Odds ratio (95% CI)				
Kiviat et al. (1993) USA	285 homosexual men seeking HIV testing	204 same	*Southern blot* HIV+ 55% HIV− 23% *PCR* HIV+ 92% HIV− 78%	4.0 (2.7–6.2) 3.1 (1.6–5.8)	HIV+ 26% HIV− 8% *HIV+ only* Atypia: CD4⁻ <200 28% 200–500 25% 501–800 25% >800 30% ASIL: CD4⁻ <200 36% 200–500 35% 501–800 25% >800 8%	5.6 (3.0–10.5) *HIV+* Atypia: 4.2 3.3 2.7 2.6 ASIL: 9.9 8.7 5.1 1.3		Southern transfer hybridization and PCR	Cytology Bethesda recommendation	*Southern transfer hybridization* CD4⁻ ≤500 2.6 (1.2–5.7) CD4⁻ >500 1.0 *PCR alone* CD4⁻ ≤500 6.3 (0.8–72.2) CD4⁻ >500 1.0
Breese et al. (1995) Denver, USA	93 homosexual men	116 homosexual men	*HIV+* HPV, any type 61% HPV-6/11 8% HPV-16/18 12% HPV-31/35/35 18% Mixed HPV-16/18+ 19% Mixed HPV-16/18− 4% *HIV−* HPV, any type 17% HPV-6/11 4% HPV-16/18 7% HPV-31/33/35 0.8% Mixed HPV-16/18+ 4% Mixed HPV-16/18− 0.8%					ViraPap[19]/ ViraType[15]	None	HPV prevalence associated with increasing immunodeficiency

ASIL, anal squamous intraepithelial lesions; PCR, polymerase chain reaction; IVDU, intravenous drug users; STD, sexually transmitted disease; CMV, cytomegalovirus

Kiviat et al. (1990) reported that 13/49 (26.5%) HIV-infected homosexual men compared with 3/47 (6.4%) HIV-negative homosexual men had detectable anal HPV by dot-blot hybridization ($p = 0.002$). No data on anal cytology or histology were available.

Critchlow et al. (1992) reported a significant association between HIV infection and HPV DNA as measured by dot filter hybridization, after adjustment for sexually transmissible disease history, age and current anorectal disease (odds ratio, 5.8; 95% CI, 1.1–30.1). HIV infection was not associated with the type of HPV detected but the severity of HIV-related disease was positively related to HPV prevalence.

In anal swabs or biopsies from homosexual men, Critchlow et al. (1995) reported a progressive increase in the detection of HPV-16 or HPV-18 DNA with declining $CD4^+$ T-cell count.

Bernard et al. (1992) studied 54 HIV-positive and 54 HIV-negative men, all presenting with anogenital lesions such as flat condyloma or condyloma acuminata. HIV-positive subjects were homosexual men (71%) or intravenous drug users (24%). HIV-negative subjects were partners of women with genital HPV infection or cervical dysplasia. High-risk types of HPV (16, 18, 31, 35, 51) were more prevalent (83.4%) in HIV-positive persons and the low-risk HPV types (6, 11) were more common in HIV-negative subjects (62.1%). Anal intraepithelial neoplasia (AIN) II/III was highly associated with high-risk HPV types (15/16, 94%) compared with low-risk HPV (1/24, 6%).

(iii) *HIV, HPV, and $CD4^+$ T-cell count*

Palefsky et al. (1990), in their study of 97 homosexual men with advanced HIV infection in San Francisco, CA, United States, found HPV DNA (detected by ViraPap™/ViraType™) in 54% and abnormal anal cytology in 39% (for details see Table 25). AIN was diagnosed in 15 specimens (15%). Abnormal cytology was significantly associated with anal HPV infection (odds ratio, 4.6; $p = 0.003$) and, among those infected with two or more HPV types, 10/12 had abnormal anal cytology (odds ratio, 39.0). $CD4^+$ counts obtained from medical records were inversely associated with cytological abnormality but did not contribute significantly in a multiple regression model which also included HPV.

Caussy et al. (1990) found that 41 (39%) of 105 homosexual men from Washington DC, and New York, United States, had infection with HPV-6/11, -16/18, or -31,33,35. The corresponding figures were 53% in 43 HIV-infected subjects and 29% in 64 HIV-negative subjects ($p = 0.01$). In HIV-infected subjects, low $CD4^+$ count was independently associated with anal HPV detection, whereas the number of partners and the frequency of receptive anal intercourse were unimportant. Abnormal cytology was seen in 9/37 (24%) HIV-infected men and in 4/55 (7%) HIV-negative men ($p = 0.03$) and was strongly associated with the detection of any HPV genotype. None of 15 subjects with HPV detected only by PCR had anal epithelial abnormality.

In a sample of 112 Australian homosexual men consecutively presented for routine screening for sexually transmitted diseases and HIV infection, 19% showed evidence of mild to moderate dysplastic changes (AIN I or AIN II). HPV DNA (types 6/11, 16/18) by dot blot hybridization was detected in 40% (6/11 in 18%; 16/18 in 11%; both groups in

12%). There was a significant association between presence of HPV-16/18 and anal dysplasia, but not between HPV infection or anal dysplasia and HIV-positivity, immune status, sexual practices or other sexually transmitted diseases (Law et al., 1991).

In a larger study (Kiviat et al., 1993), a random sample of 285 HIV-positive and 204 HIV-negative homosexual men was surveyed. HPV DNA was found by Southern blot hybridization in 55% and 23% (odds ratio, 4.0; 95% CI, 2.7–6.2) of HIV-positive and -negative men and by PCR in 92% and 78% (odds ratio, 3.1; 95% CI, 1.6–5.8), respectively. Each specific group of HPV DNA types surveyed was most common in HIV-infected men (Table 26). Detection of HPV by both Southern blot hybridization and PCR (high-level HPV infection) was significantly associated with anal intraepithelial lesions. However, after adjustment for level of HPV DNA, severely immunosuppressed HIV-positive men (CD4$^+$ count < 500 cells/mm^3) were at higher risk for anal intraepithelial lesions than men with a CD4$^+$ count of more than 500 cells/mm^3 (odds ratio, 2.9; 95% CI, 1.4–6.2). [The Working Group noted that this finding indicates a possible independent role of immunosuppression in addition to that of HPV].

Table 26. Prevalence of anal HPV DNA in HIV-positive and HIV-negative homosexual men as detected by dot-filter hybridization, low- and high-stringency Southern transfer hybridization, and PCR

	HIV+	HIV–	OR	95% CI
Dot blot	(n = 304)	(n = 211)		
Any HPV	52%	18%	5.1	3.3–7.9
Southern	(n = 285)	(n = 204)		
Any HPV	55%	23%	4.0	2.7–6.2
HPV-16,18[a]	21%	7%	5.0	2.6–9.6
HPV-31,33,35[a]	15%	3%	8.7	3.5–25.7
HPV-6,11[a]	21%	7%	5.0	2.6–9.6
Unclassified	16%	8%	3.7	1.7–6.3
Multiple	15%	3%	8.5	3.4–25.2
PCR	(n = 241)	(n = 152)		
Any HPV	92%	78%	3.1	1.6–5.8
HPV-16,18	53%	38%	3.6	1.8–7.2
HPV-31,33,35	43%	15%	7.4	3.4–16.2
HPV-6,11	47%	39%	3.1	1.6–6.2
Unclassified	19%	22%	2.2	1.0–4.9
Multiple	44%	23%	4.9	2.4–10.1

From Kiviat et al. (1993)
[a] Alone or in combination

Sixty-six (22%) HIV-positive and 24 (11%) HIV-negative men from the above-mentioned study were referred for biopsies of internal anorectal lesions (Surawicz et al., 1993). Whereas only 31 (36%) had dysplasia diagnosed by cytology, 73/86 (85%) had dysplasia evident on biopsy (26% high-grade). The correlations of anal abnormalities with histological diagnosis are presented in Table 24. HIV status did not influence the prevalence of high-grade lesions. Both high- and low-risk HPV types were common in many of the biopsy specimens.

In a study of 37 HIV-positive and 28 HIV-negative homosexual men, Palefsky *et al.* (1994) found both anal intraepithelial lesions and the presence of HPV to be closely associated with HIV-positivity in men with CD4$^+$ T-cell counts below 200 cells/mm^3. Furthermore, multivariate analysis indicated a possible influence of current smoking.

Several studies among women are in progress, but the results of only one have been published (Williams *et al.*, 1994). Among 114 intravenous drug users, anal infection with HPV was twice as frequent as cervical infection and was associated with HIV-positivity by both dot blot (odds ratio, 2.5; 95% CI, 0.9–7) and PCR (2.6; 1.03–6.8). Anal intraepithelial lesions were seen in 14% (15/109) of the women, of whom 11 were HIV-infected (odds ratio, 3.4; 95% CI, 0.9–15.5). The presence of anal squamous intraepithelial lesions (ASIL) was closely associated with a simultaneous high level (dot blot positive) of HPV DNA and HIV-positivity (odds ratio, 9.2; 95% CI, 1.6–63.6), whereas no association was found with CD4$^+$ count.

Breese *et al.* (1995) studied the expression of HPV in a cross-sectional, follow-up study of 116 HIV-seronegative and 93 HIV-seropositive homosexual men. HPV was significantly more common among HIV-positive persons and HPV types 16/18 accounted for more than 50% of the infections. HPV prevalence increased significantly with decreasing CD4$^+$ count; persistence of HPV during a six-month follow-up was also more common among men with clinical signs of severe immunosuppression (AIDS/ARC (AIDS-related complex)) (95%) compared with asymptomatic HIV-seropositive men (62%) and HIV-seronegative men (61%).

(iv) *Progression of disease*

Irrespective of HIV status, there are few data available relevant to the association between the different intraepithelial lesions and invasive anal cancer.

In San Francisco, Palefsky *et al.* (1992) followed 37 homosexual men with advanced HIV disease prospectively for an average of 17 months and found an increase in anal epithelial abnormality from 27% to 65%. The percentage of men with AIN increased from 8 to 32% and that of men with high-grade AIN from 0 to 16%. Presence of HPV DNA (detected by Virapap™/Viratype™) increased from 60 to 89%.

Morgan *et al.* (1994) identified all patients who had undergone excision biopsy of anal condylomata during 1984–88 at a hospital in London, United Kingdom. Overall, 27 had evidence of AIN and for these patients, results of HIV testing were traced. Five of six patients having carcinoma *in situ* (AIN III) were found to be HIV-seropositive and were followed for between four and six years without any evidence of progression of disease.

(b) *Invasive anal cancer*

(i) *Case reports and series*

Only a few case reports and series describe invasive anal cancer in HIV-infected persons (Rüdlinger & Buchmann, 1989; Lorenz *et al.*, 1991; Chadha *et al.*, 1994; Jebakumar *et al.*, 1994; Nasti *et al.*, 1994). Most cancers occurring in the anal region are of the (transitional) epidermoid type. Other anal cancers associated with HIV include small-cell carcinoma (Read *et al.*, 1985; Smitherman *et al.*, 1990; Nakahara *et al.*, 1993), non-Hodgkin's lymphoma and Kaposi's sarcoma.

(ii) *Prognosis*

Very little information is available on the possible influence of HIV infection on the prognosis of anal cancer. Some cases have shown an aggressive clinical course with low response to treatment (Lorenz *et al.*, 1991; Jebakumar *et al.*, 1994), whereas others have not (Chadha *et al.*, 1994; Nasti *et al.*, 1994).

(iii) *Descriptive epidemiology*

Reports from Sweden, Denmark and the United States have shown significant increases in the incidence of epidermoid anal cancer over the last 30 years, not only during the period of the AIDS epidemic (Goldman *et al.*, 1989; Frisch *et al.*, 1993; Melbye *et al.*, 1994a). The increase has been more pronounced in women than in men and more in urban than in rural areas. Furthermore, black people are at higher risk than whites and never-married men are at higher risk than ever-married men. The increased risk of anal cancer in never-married men has been documented as early as the 1940s and 1950s (Frisch *et al.*, 1993). These trends suggest that important behavioural and environmental changes were taking place before the beginning of the AIDS epidemic.

Melbye *et al.* (1994a) compared the proportion of men who were never-married (as a surrogate for homosexuality) among anal cancer patients with that in colon cancer patients (controls) in four metropolitan areas (San Francisco–Oakland, CA; Detroit, MI; Seattle, WA; Atlanta, GA) included in the SEER Programme in the United States. The relative risk for anal cancer patients rose from 5.8 (95% CI, 3.9–8.7) in 1973–78 to 6.7 (4.7–9.5) in 1979–84 and 10.3 (7.5–14.1) in 1985–89 (p_{trend} = 0.02). Among white men from the San Francisco Bay area, the incidence of anal cancer increased from 0.5/100 000 in 1973–75 to 1.2/100 000 in 1988–89 (p_{trend} < 0.001).

Biggar *et al.* (1987) and later Rabkin and Yellin (1994) used data from the SEER programme to study the evolution in anal cancer incidence in single, young (25–54 years) men within the city of San Francisco. The incidence of anal cancer in 1973–79 was 9.9 (95% CI, 4.5–18.7) times that expected from general population rate and in 1988–90 was 10.1 (95% CI, 5.0–18.0) times that expected.

Biggar *et al.* (1989) used a proportional incidence method to study cancers (period 1973–85) occurring among single young men and married young men in New York. A significant increase in anal/anorectal cancers was recorded for single but not for married men. However, the increase appeared to have already occurred by 1979–80, without a clear increasing trend thereafter.

Reynolds et al. (1993) linked AIDS registry files (San Francisco residents only) with the California Tumor Registry (period 1980–87) and compared the incidence of cancer in the AIDS population with that of the general population of the San Francisco Bay Area. Six cases of anal or rectal cancer were seen among the AIDS patients, which were more than expected (standardized incidence ratio [SIR], 3.5; 95% CI, 1.3–7.5). In-situ cancer of the anorectal area was also significantly elevated among persons with AIDS (7 cases; SIR, 65; 95% CI, 26.1–134). The SIR analysis included cancers that occurred before, concurrently with and subsequent to the diagnosis of AIDS.

Melbye et al. (1994b) used a linkage between AIDS (50 050 reports) and cancer (859 398 reports) registries in seven health departments in the United States to investigate the association between HIV infection and epidermoid anal cancer. Compared with general population rates, the relative risk for anal cancer at and after AIDS diagnosis was 84.1 (95% CI, 46.4–152) among homosexual men and 37.7 (9.4–151) among non-homosexual men. The relative risk was 13.9 (6.6–29.2) for occurrence of anal cancer in the period two to five years before AIDS diagnosis and 27.4 (15.9–47.2) during the two years before AIDS diagnosis (p for trend = 0.004) (Table 27).

Table 27. Relative risk (observed/expected ratio) of epidermoid anal and anorectal cancer among AIDS patients compared with population controls matched for age, sex, and race

Time from AIDS diagnosis	No. of cases		Relative risk (95% CI)
	Observed	Expected	
2–5 years before	7	0.502	13.9 (6.6–29.2)
0.25–2 years before	13	0.475	27.4 (15.9–47.2)
0.25 years before or after	9	0.113	79.6 (41.4–153)
0.25–0.75 years after	3	0.072	41.7 (13.4–129)
> 0.75–2.25 years after	4	0.082	48.7 (18.3–130)

From Melbye et al. (1994b)

In summary, the above studies are generally consistent in demonstrating an association between HIV infection (and the associated immunodeficiency) and anal dysplasias. However, even in the absence of HIV infection, anal cancer is more common in AIDS risk groups. Thus, a specific association of HIV infection with invasive cancer has not been convincingly demonstrated.

2.3.3 *Hodgkin's disease*

Misclassification of non-Hodgkin's lymphoma cases as cases of Hodgkin's disease occurs (Herndier & Friedman, 1992; Reynolds et al. 1993; Rabkin & Yellin, 1994; Knopf & Locker, 1995) and may at least partly explain the reported increased rates of Hodgkin's disease in HIV-positive persons. Non-Hodgkin's lymphoma incidence is greatly increased in HIV-positive persons and only a small misclassification rate of these cases would cause a false impression of an elevation in rates of Hodgkin's disease (Glaser & Swartz, 1990). Assignment to a specific type is particularly difficult for those cases of Hodgkin's disease that have been reported in HIV-positive persons with an atypical lymphoid background. Sometimes even unusual atypical reactive processes make a firm diagnosis rather difficult (Herndier & Friedman, 1992).

(a) *Distribution of histological types*

(i) *Hodgkin's disease in HIV-uninfected persons*

Hodgkin's disease is a heterogeneous entity which is often described as two different diseases. In developed countries, it has a bimodal age–incidence curve with a first peak at 15–34 years and another among persons older than 55 years of age. Histologically, nodular sclerosis is primarily diagnosed in young Hodgkin's disease patients, whereas mixed cellularity predominates in the older age groups. Population-based data from the SEER programme show a significant increase in the incidence of nodular sclerosis, particularly in adolescents and young adults, whereas the mixed cellularity type has remained stable over time. A decrease in incidence in recent years among older age groups was explained by earlier misclassification of non-Hodgkin's lymphoma as Hodgkin's disease. Among 9418 microscopically confirmed cases of Hodgkin's disease reported to the SEER programme between 1973 and 1987, 51.0% were of the nodular sclerosis type, 23.8% of mixed cellularity, 6.7% with lymphocytic predominance, 5.7% with lymphocytic depletion and 12.8% were miscellaneous Hodgkin's disease (Medeiros & Greiner, 1995).

(ii) *Hodgkin's disease in HIV-infected persons*

Since the mid-1980s, a large number of case reports and small case series of Hodgkin's disease in HIV-infected persons have appeared (see Rubio, 1994) which, together with larger and more recent case series (Table 28), describe a particular natural history and histological distribution of Hodgkin's disease which are different from those of Hodgkin's disease in HIV-uninfected persons. Despite a young median age of the patients, mixed cellularity and lymphocyte depletion are the predominant histological features. The majority of cases have B symptoms and approximately 80% have advanced disease (stages III or IV). Extranodal dissemination and, in particular, bone marrow involvement are common, whereas mediastinal involvement is less frequent than is observed in HIV-uninfected persons (Rabkin & Blattner, 1991; Tirelli *et al.*, 1995b).

The Italian Cooperative Group on AIDS-related Tumors (GICAT) in 1988 and subsequently Monfardini *et al.* (1991), Tirelli *et al.* (1992), Serraino *et al.* (1993), Errante *et al.* (1994) and Tirelli *et al.* (1995b) have described cases of Hodgkin's disease in HIV-infected persons. Among 63 cases in intravenous drug users (median age, 27 years), reported to the organization during 1980–89, 74% were histologically characterized as showing mixed cellularity or lymphocyte depletion. Overall, 83% were in advanced stage, but atypical presentations (central nervous system, skin, endobronchial site or lung involvement with lack of mediastinal adenopathy) were uncommon (Monfardini *et al.*, 1991).

Table 28. Characteristics of Hodgkin's disease in HIV-infected persons (only studies with more than 20 cases)

Reference	Period	N	Age median (range)	Male no.	Female no.	Histopathology					Advanced stage (III, IV)	B symptoms	Extra nodal	Bone marrow involvement
						Mixed cellularity	Lymphocyte depletion	Nodular sclerosis	Lymphocytic predominance					
Rubio (1994) Spain	1984–91	46	27 (mean) (18–55)	43	3	41%	22%	22%	4%		89%	83%	50%	41% at diagnosis
Andrieu et al. (1993) France	1987–89	45[a]	30	39	6	49%	4%	40%	0		75%	80%	in all stage IV	[24%]
Monfardini et al. (1991) Italy	1980–89	63	27 (20–44)	59	4	48%[b]	23%	23%	0		83%	NR		
Tirelli et al. (1995b) Italy	1986–94	114[c]	29 (19–57)	103	11	45%	21%	30%	4%		81%	77%	63%	
Ree et al. (1991) USA	1983–90	24	34 (24–51)	23	1	100%	0	0	0		92%	100%		50% at presentation, confirmed in 25% by biopsy

[a] Three cases had undetermined histological subtype.
[b] 3% had lymphocyte depletion and mixed cellularity
[c] Seven cases not classified histopathologically

Tirelli et al. (1995b) compared 114 HIV-positive cases reported to GICAT during 1986–94 with 104 HIV-negative cases of Hodgkin's disease from a single institution. HIV-positive cases included a higher percentage of stage IV disease despite a lower median age.

Andrieu et al. (1993) compared all 45 cases of Hodgkin's disease collected by the French registry of HIV-associated tumours between 1987 and 1989 with a cohort of 407 HIV-negative Hodgkin's disease patients for whom similar diagnostic criteria had been used. The groups had a similar median age (30 and 31 years) but differed significantly with respect to advanced clinical stage (75% versus 33%), proportion of mixed cellularity (49% versus 20%) and absence of mediastinal disease (87% versus 29%).

In a series of 46 patients with Hodgkin's disease and HIV infection diagnosed in 1984–91 in nine hospitals in Madrid, Spain, 41% were classified as being of mixed cellularity, 22% with lymphocytic depletion, 22% with nodular sclerosis and 4% with lymphocytic predominance. Advanced disease (stages III or IV) was found in 89%; 83% had B symptoms and 41% had bone marrow involvement (Serrano et al., 1990; Rubio, 1994).

(iii) *Prognosis*

Hodgkin's lymphoma in the immunocompromised host is particularly aggressive and difficult to treat (Carbone et al., 1991).

Errante et al. (1994) studied treatment response and survival in 84 Italian HIV-negative and 92 HIV-positive patients. Remission was achieved in 51% of HIV-infected patients and in more than 90% of the HIV-negative patients. When HIV-infected patients were compared with only the older HIV-negative patients, who were primarily diagnosed with the mixed cellularity type of Hodgkin's disease, similar differences were observed. The estimated four-year survival was 33% in HIV-positive patients compared with 88–100% in HIV-negative patients, depending upon the age group.

In the French study, Roitmann et al. (1992), Andrieu et al. (1993) and Lévy et al. (1995) found a high rate (79%) of complete remission after standard therapy in 45 HIV-positive Hodgkin's disease patients, but haematological and infectious complications were very frequent. Overall, two-year survival was 41%.

Other authors have found full remission in HIV-positive persons to range between 47% and 58% (Serrano et al., 1990; Monfardini et al., 1991; Tirelli et al., 1995b).

(b) *Descriptive epidemiology*

Already in the early 1980s, analyses of data from the SEER programme detected marked increases in the incidence of Kaposi's sarcoma and non-Hodgkin's lymphoma among never-married young men, but no similar increase in Hodgkin's disease was observed (Biggar et al., 1985; Bernstein et al., 1989). Among never-married young men from San Francisco, CA, United States, Biggar et al. (1987) found a small but non-significant increase while Rabkin and Yellin (1994) observed an increase which predated the AIDS epidemic and which was not restricted to the mixed cellularity subtype most often associated with HIV-positive cases of Hodgkin's disease. Analyses of data from a cancer registry in New York State, not part of the SEER programme, revealed an abrupt increase in Hodgkin's disease among never-married men in 1985 (Biggar et al., 1989), whereas a study of women based on cancer registry data from New York and New Jersey did not detect an increase in the incidence of Hodgkin's disease during 1976–88 (Rabkin et al., 1993a).

Medeiros and Greiner (1995) studied trends in Hodgkin's disease over three time periods (1973–77, 1978–82 and 1983–87), using data from the SEER programme. In San Francisco County, where young men are known to have a high prevalence of HIV infection, the age-specific incidence rates for Hodgkin's disease of mixed cellularity increased for men and was the most common subtype by the age of 50. This was in contrast to an unchanged age-adjusted rate among men based on the entire SEER database.

In another study based on SEER data, the risk was evaluated of developing another primary cancer after a diagnosis of Kaposi's sarcoma. Because of the more than 40 000-fold increase in risk for Kaposi's sarcoma among never-married men since the beginning of the HIV epidemic, this tumour was used as a surrogate for HIV-positivity. No indication of an increased risk for Hodgkin's disease was found among never-married men with Kaposi's sarcoma (Biggar et al., 1994).

(c) Cohort studies

Reynolds et al. (1993) linked data from AIDS and cancer registries in San Francisco between 1980 and 1987. Compared with concurrent population rates for the same geographical area, the SIR for Hodgkin's disease in men with AIDS increased from 1.9 in 1980–81 to 18.3 in 1986–87. This observation was based on only 16 cases and the standardized intervals overlapped for each of the four periods studied. [The Working Group noted that the SIR analysis included 14 cases in which Hodgkin's disease was diagnosed before the AIDS diagnosis. This would tend to overestimate the risk in AIDS patients when comparing with population rates, because these cases entered the analysis only if they survived until AIDS diagnosis.]

Hessol et al. (1992) compared the risk for Hodgkin's disease in a cohort of 6704 homosexual men from the San Francisco City Clinic Cohort study with population-based rates from the SEER programme. Information on cancer events in the cohort was obtained by computer-matched identification of participants with the records of the Northern California Cancer Center registry. Among HIV-infected men, the age-adjusted standardized relative risk for Hodgkin's disease was 5.0 (95% CI, 2.0–10.3).

Ragni et al. (1993) found no increased incidence of Hodgkin's disease among 3041 haemophiliacs from the United States during 1978 and 1989. In fact, no case of Hodgkin's disease was reported among the 1295 HIV-positive patients.

In the NCI Multicenter Haemophilia Cohort Study, there were two cases of Hodgkin's disease among 1065 HIV-seropositive subjects and one case among 636 HIV-seronegative subjects (Rabkin et al., 1992). These cases were 6.6 and 8.2 times the expected frequencies in HIV-seropositive and HIV-seronegative subjects, respectively, although neither excess was statistically significant.

Lyter *et al.* (1995) studied cancer events occurring during 1984–93 in a cohort of 769 HIV-seronegative and 430 HIV-seropositive homosexual men in Pittsburgh, PA, United States. Cancer information was collected through semiannual visits, medical records and death certificates. There was no difference in Hodgkin's disease rates between the seronegative homosexual men and the general male population of Pennsylvania, whereas two cases observed in the HIV-seropositive group were more than expected (SIR, 19.8; 95% CI, 2.4–71.5).

(d) Cofactors

Little is known about potential cofactors for Hodgkin's disease occurring in HIV-positive persons. HIV-positive persons express a higher proportion of EBV-positive B-lymphocytes that are capable of spontaneous outgrowth *in vitro* than HIV-uninfected persons (Birx *et al.*, 1986).

Moran *et al.* (1992) used PCR to detect the presence of EBV DNA sequences in 10 HIV-positive patients with Hodgkin's disease. Eight (80%) were positive for EBV, compared with 23 (40%) of 57 specimens from HIV-negative patients with Hodgkin's disease.

Tirelli *et al.* (1995b) observed the expression of the EBV-encoded latent membrane protein-1 (LMP-1) in the diagnostic Reed–Sternberg cells (Mueller, 1996) in 14/18 (78%) HIV-positive and 27/104 (25%) HIV-negative Hodgkin's disease patients ($p < 0.001$). Monoclonal expression of EBV genomes was found in 8/10 (80%) tumours from HIV-infected persons compared with 12/44 (38%) tumours from HIV-negative individuals. Using PCR-based amplification of EBNA-2-specific sequences, the authors showed 6/11 EBV-positive tumours in HIV-positive persons to contain type 2 EBV compared with 1/26 such tumours from HIV-negative persons. The great majority of tumour biopsies from HIV-1-positive patients with Hodgkin's disease have been consistently found to be positive for the EBV genome or viral proteins (Mueller, 1996).

In summary, the above studies indicate that Hodgkin's disease in the presence of HIV infection is more likely to have mixed cellularity or lymphocyte-depleted histology and is clinically more aggressive. Absolute Hodgkin's disease incidence may also be elevated in HIV-infected persons, particularly injecting drug users, but an association is not proven because of the modest magnitude of the observed increases and the diagnostic overlap with non-Hodgkin's lymphoma.

2.3.4 *Testicular cancer*

The incidence of both testicular germ-cell tumours and infection with HIV is highest in young men aged 20–40 years. It is to be expected that a proportion of testicular cancer patients will be HIV-positive by chance.

(a) Case reports and series

A number of case reports and small case series of testicular cancer in HIV-infected men have been published. Some of these have been summarized by Csiszar and Zimmern (1993) and Buzelin *et al.* (1994) and together with other series (Moyle *et al.*, 1991;

Bernardi et al., 1995; Timmerman et al., 1995) constitute a total of at least 120 cases. Of these, five were reported as being lymphomas, often with accompanying extensive systemic disease. The remaining cases were testicular germ-cell tumours. Seminomas were the most frequently observed histological type of germ-cell tumour (49–67%). Non-seminomatous tumours comprised a proportion similar to that reported in uninfected individuals with testicular germ-cell tumours (Einhorn et al., 1993).

Moyle et al. (1991) reported three testicular seminomas among 2205 known HIV-seropositive patients attending a hospital clinic in London, United Kingdom. They calculated the risk among HIV-infected persons to be increased 68-fold compared with expected rates.

Timmerman et al. (1995) reviewed 294 cases of testicular germ-cell tumours diagnosed between 1980 and 1993 at four hospitals in San Francisco, CA, United States, using cancer registry files and pathology reports. Overall, 11 HIV-seropositive cases (4%) were identified. These were further evaluated together with four additional seropositive cases diagnosed at private medical centres in San Francisco and compared with the remaining 279 cases without evidence of HIV infection. There was no difference in tumour stage at presentation (low-stage (I and IIA) tumours in HIV-positive persons, 67%; those in HIV-negative persons, 63%). Standard therapy including orchiectomy, retroperitoneal lymph node dissection, radiation therapy and chemotherapy was well tolerated. In these HIV-positive patients, there was no indication of a more aggressive course of disease compared with that seen in HIV-negative patients.

Bernardi et al. (1995) performed a retrospective analysis of 26 cases of testicular germ-cell tumours diagnosed between 1986 and 1994 in HIV-positive men in Italy. Of these patients, 61% had low-stage tumours (stages I to IIb) and only 35% had advanced disease, a proportion similar to that observed among HIV-seronegative patients. The complete response rate of 95% and overall three-year survival of 65% in this series did not differ substantially from those in HIV-uninfected persons (Kaplan, 1995). The median $CD4^+$ T-cell count at presentation was 261 cells/mm^3 (range, 2–1229) and only six had a $CD4^+$ count below 200 cells/mm^3, which suggests that the clinical behaviour of testicular cancer in HIV-positive persons is not directly related to level of immunosuppression.

(b) Descriptive and cohort studies

Descriptive studies based on cancer incidence data from various parts of the United States have unanimously failed to show a link between cancer of the testis and the HIV epidemic. Biggar et al. (1987) used never-married men as a surrogate for homosexuality in their study of cancer incidence trends in San Francisco from 1973 to 1984. Neither this study nor that of Rabkin and Yellin (1994), with the same data series updated to 1990, showed any indication of an increasing trend in the 1980s for cancer of the testis. In an analysis of cancer incidence data from New York City based on the period 1973–85, Biggar et al. (1989) similarly found no increasing trend for cancer of the testis.

Reynolds et al. (1993), using data from population-based registries for AIDS and cancer for San Francisco residents for the period 1980–87, found no indication of an increased risk for testis cancer in AIDS patients (1973–77: SIR, 1.0; 95% CI, 0.2–2.8); 1980–87: SIR, 0.7; 95% CI, 0.2–2.2).

Lyter et al. (1995) found two cases of testicular seminoma in a prospective cohort study of 430 HIV-infected men (SIR, 8.2 (95% CI, 1.0–30)). When a third case of extragonadal seminoma was included and the age-adjusted population rates for all seminomas were compared, a 21-fold increase ($p < 0.001$) in the HIV-infected cohort was observed.

In summary, there is some suggestion of an association of testicular cancers with HIV infection, but the studies are not yet conclusive.

2.3.5 Non-melanoma cancers of the skin

Skin cancers and, in particular, squamous-cell carcinomas have been associated with a wide variety of immunodeficiency conditions (Hintner & Fritsch, 1989). Transplant patients who are immunocompromised have a disproportionately high incidence of squamous-cell carcinomas as compared to basal-cell carcinomas, in a ratio of 15 : 1 according to one study (Barr et al., 1989) (see Section 4.1).

(a) Case reports and series

A number of case reports on skin cancers other than Kaposi's sarcoma in HIV-infected persons have been published (for references see Smith et al., 1993c). However, only one large series has been described.

Lobo et al. (1992) identified all HIV-infected male patients with a non-melanoma skin cancer diagnosed in the dermatology clinic at the University of California, San Francisco, United States, and performed a retrospective case–control study with age-matched controls. Overall, 116 non-melanoma skin cancers were identified in 48 patients, 101 occurring in 47 patients were basal-cell carcinomas and 15 in 10 patients were squamous-cell carcinomas. The basal-cell : squamous-cell carcinoma ratio (6.7 : 1) was similar to that observed in HIV-uninfected persons in the same area but different from that observed among transplant patients, as discussed above. The major risk factors associated with non-melanoma skin cancer in this group of men were the same as those in the normal population: fair skin, a family history of skin cancer and sun exposure.

(b) Descriptive and cohort studies

Reynolds et al. (1993) found, in their linkage study of AIDS and cancer cases among San Francisco residents, three non-melanoma skin cancers (one dermatofibroma, one haemangiosarcoma, one sarcoma unspecified), a significantly higher number than expected (SIR, 10.0). Because the study was purely registry-based, it was impossible to confirm that these cases were not misclassified Kaposi's sarcoma cases.

Non-melanoma skin cancers are not registered in the SEER programme. The incidence of melanoma of the skin has been found to be marginally increased among never-married men from New York City and from San Francisco (Biggar et al., 1989; Rabkin & Yellin, 1994), but these findings are possibly related to the specific behaviour of single men in terms of recreational sun exposure, rather than to the HIV epidemic. No increase incidence with time was observed in any of the studies.

Smith et al. (1993c) followed 724 HIV-infected military employees in the United States for a period of 36 months and diagnosed 13 cases of basal-cell carcinoma (1.8%), two cases of squamous-cell carcinoma (0.3%) of the face, 2 cases of squamous-cell carcinoma (0.3%) in the anus and three malignant melanomas (0.6%). The basal-cell : squamous-cell carcinoma ratio was more similar to that of the general population than to that observed among transplant recipients. Most of the patients studied were at an early stage of their HIV disease and not severely immunosuppressed, and had lightly pigmented skin.

In their cohort study of 1701 haemophiliacs (see Section 2.2.3), Rabkin et al. (1992) observed five cases of basal-cell carcinoma (2 in HIV+, 3 in HIV− persons), corresponding to rates of [0.2 and 0.8 per 1000 person-years] in HIV-infected and HIV-uninfected subjects, respectively. No comparison was made with rates in the general population.

Ragni et al. (1993) performed a retrospective cohort study of 3041 haemophiliacs (56.6% HIV-infected) from 18 haemophilia centres in the United States during the period 1978–89. The incidence of basal-cell carcinoma in HIV-infected patients was 18.3 times greater than that in HIV-uninfected patients ($p < 0.0001$) but 11.4 times greater than that in the general population, a finding which remains unexplained. Among HIV-infected patients, the observed-to-expected ratio was 2.0 ($p < 0.001$).

In a large cohort study of 1199 homosexual men (period 1984–1993) (Lyter et al., 1995) found three cases of basal-cell carcinoma in HIV-infected persons and seven cases of basal-cell carcinoma and two of squamous-cell carcinoma in seronegative men. No more cases were found in either HIV-infected or -uninfected men than expected from general population rates.

In a study of 1073 homosexual and bisexual men (434 HIV+) in three United States cities, followed for over 10 000 person-years, the relative risk for incidence of skin cancers —25/35 basal-cell carcinomas — was 2.2 in HIV-infected compared with uninfected men (Holmberg et al., 1995b).

In summary, there is conflicting evidence regarding an association between non-melanoma skin cancers and HIV infection. [The Working Group noted that the diagnosis and reporting of these tumours are highly variable and this possible association may be particularly difficult to investigate.]

2.3.6 *Conjunctival tumours*

Although rare in Europe and North America, squamous-cell carcinoma of the conjunctiva was already more common in Africa before the advent of AIDS (Templeton, 1973; Newton et al., 1996). Strong associations have been reported between dysplasia and invasive carcinoma of the conjunctiva and HPV (IARC, 1995).

(a) *Case reports*

Two case reports of squamous-cell carcinoma of the conjunctiva in HIV-seropositive men in the United States (Winward & Curtin, 1989; Kim et al., 1990), coupled with a dramatic increase in the number of tumours being seen by ophthalmologists in at least two African centres, led to the suggestion of an association with HIV infection (Kestelyn *et al.*, 1990; Ateenyi-Agaba, 1995). Several studies from Africa and one from the United States have investigated this association.

(b) *Descriptive study*

In an analysis based on the Multistate AIDS-Cancer Match Registry in the United States, Goedert and Coté (1995) found four AIDS patients with a diagnosis of conjunctival squamous-cell carcinoma, a significantly higher number than expected (observed : expected, 13 [95% CI, 4–34]).

(c) *Case–control studies*

In Rwanda, Kestelyn *et al.* (1990) found that 9/11 cases of conjunctival squamous-cell carcinoma were HIV-seropositive, compared with 6/22 controls (odds ratio, 13.0; 95% CI, 2.2–76.9).

In Uganda, Ateenyi-Agaba (1995) found that 36/48 cases of conjunctival squamous-cell carcinoma were HIV-seropositive, compared with 9/48 controls (odds ratio, 13.0; 95% CI, 4.5–39.4).

In Rwanda, Newton *et al.* (1995) examined the association of HIV infection with all ocular tumours, excluding retinoblastoma and melanoma. The proportion of HIV-positive cases was 2/8 versus 8/200 controls (odds ratio, 8.4; 95% CI, 0.8–96.9).

In summary, HIV infection has been consistently associated with conjunctival carcinoma in case–control studies in several African locations. The association has been inconsistent in western countries and the discrepancy between these regions may be due to the lower background rates of this tumour in developed countries.

2.3.7 *Leiomyosarcoma*

Leiomyosarcoma is an extremely rare tumour in childhood, with an annual incidence of less than two cases per 10 million children (Lack, 1986). It has been reported in immunocompromised children following liver and renal transplantation (Ha *et al.*, 1993).

(a) *Case reports and series*

Spindle-cell tumours (leiomyoma and leiomyosarcoma) in HIV-infected children have been described relatively frequently, at sites such as the gastrointestinal tract (Chadwick *et al.*, 1990; McLoughlin *et al.*, 1991; Mueller *et al.*, 1992), liver (Mueller *et al.*, 1992; Ross *et al.*, 1992; Levin *et al.*, 1994), tracheobronchial tree (Martinez *et al.*, 1990; Balsam & Segal, 1992), lung (Chadwick *et al.*, 1990) and subcutaneous tissue (Orlow *et al.*, 1992). Several of the cases were discovered only at autopsy as solitary small spherical tumour masses.

DiCarlo *et al.* (1990) described eight cancers in 102 HIV-infected children followed at the Children's Hospital AIDS programme of New Jersey, NY, during 1984–88, of which one was an unusually aggressive case of leiomyosarcoma.

The above reports and a further one by McClain *et al.* (1995, 6 cases in 5 children) document at least 14 spindle-cell tumours in HIV-infected children, a much higher number than expected considering that less than 10 000 children are infected with HIV in developed countries.

A few cases of spindle-cell tumours of the liver, colon, adrenal glands and spinal cord in HIV-infected adults have also been reported (Radin & Kiyabu, 1992; Steel *et al.*, 1993; Prévot *et al.*, 1994; McClain *et al.*, 1995).

(b) Descriptive studies

Rabkin and Yellin (1994) found, using cancer incidence data from the SEER programme, an increasing although nonsignificant trend in the observed-to-expected ratio of leiomyosarcomas among never-married men resident in San Francisco, CA, United States.

(c) Cofactors

McClain *et al.* (1995) suggested that EBV may contribute to the pathogenesis of leiomyomas and leiomyosarcomas in HIV-infected patients but not in HIV-uninfected persons. Using in-situ hybridization, they detected EBV genomes in all muscle cells of five leiomyosarcomas and two leiomyomas from six HIV-infected persons but not in three leiomyosarcomas or four leiomyomas from HIV-uninfected persons. Quantitative PCR showed high levels of EBV in the tumour tissues. Furthermore, separate tumours in the same patients contained different episomal EBV clones, signifying the presence of distinct monoclonal EBV-related tumours.

Lee *et al.* (1995) studied three children who developed smooth muscle tumours following organ transplantation. In each case, clonal EBV genome was detected in tumour tissue. In the two cases studied, the tumours were positive for EBNA-2 and the tumours from each of the patients were positive for EBERs. Both viral protein products expressed in latent infection.

In summary, leiomyomas and leiomyosarcomas appear to be associated with HIV infection in children. EBV appears to be an important etiological co-factor. The association is not apparent in HIV-infected adults.

2.3.8 *Other cancers*

There have been a large number of case reports and small case series of tumours other than those described above in HIV-infected persons.

Apart from effects on specific tumours, HIV infection and associated immunosuppression have been suspected of causing a global increase in the incidence of cancers of all types. This hypothesis has been examined in cohort studies (Rabkin & Yellin, 1994; Lyter *et al.*, 1995) and in analyses of registry data (Coté *et al.*, 1991; Reynolds *et al.*, 1993; Biggar *et al.*, 1994). Excluding cases of Kaposi's sarcoma and non-Hodgkin's lymphoma, total incidence of other cancers was either not increased or minimally increased. Since HIV-infected persons may have increased exposure to other cancer risk factors (e.g., cigarette smoking), the significance of the elevations seen in some of these studies is uncertain.

A small increase in the number of registered hepatomas at the SEER cancer registry in San Francisco, CA, United States, was observed among single white men between 1973–78 (baseline) and 1984 (Biggar *et al.*, 1987). However, there was no obvious further increase in incidence when the data were followed through to 1990 (Rabkin & Yellin, 1994). No case of liver cancer was recorded in a cohort of San Francisco AIDS patients followed from 1980 to 1987 (Reynolds *et al.*, 1993). Similarly, no case of liver cancer was found among 1065 HIV-infected haemophiliacs in the United States followed over 12 years (Rabkin *et al.*, 1992). In another study of United States haemophiliacs (Ragni *et al.*, 1993), no significant difference in liver cancer was seen in HIV+ and HIV– patients. In a study of 1227 HIV-infected haemophiliacs in the United Kingdom between 1985 and 1992, the risk of death from liver cancer (compared with the United Kingdom population) was similar in the HIV-infected (observed : expected, 15.1) and HIV-uninfected cohorts (observed : expected, 18.7) (Darby *et al.*, 1995). No association between HIV infection and liver cancer was found in Rwanda (Newton *et al.*, 1995); 1 person out of 35 (3%) with liver cancer was HIV-positive versus 7/165 (4%) controls.

In a large linkage analysis based on AIDS and cancer records from different regions within the United States, no association between EBV-associated nasopharyngeal carcinoma and AIDS was found (Melbye *et al.*, 1996).

Oral squamous-cell carcinomas have been hypothetically linked to infection with HPV. A small number of case reports have described these tumours, primarily located on the tongue, in HIV-infected persons (Salas-Buzon & Saez-Eligido, 1992). However, there are no data to support an association with HIV-infection (Ficarra & Eversole, 1994). *Nasal cavity tumours* were in excess ($n = 2$) in a linkage study of AIDS and cancer registry data from San Francisco (Reynolds *et al.*, 1993) but the authors ascribed this finding to possibly misclassified Kaposi's sarcoma cases.

Plasma-cell tumours that have been hypothetically linked with EBV infection have been described at unusual sites with widespread dissemination and a clinically aggressive course in HIV-infected persons (Israel *et al.*, 1983; Vandermolen *et al.*, 1985; Kaplan *et al.*, 1987; Monfardini *et al.*, 1989; Voelkerding *et al.*, 1989; Kumar *et al.*, 1994). *Lymphomatoid granulomatosis* (Mittal *et al.*, 1990) and a number of typical and more atypical cases of *acute myeloblastic leukaemia* have been reported (Al-Bahar *et al.*, 1994; Rabaud *et al.*, 1995). However, there has been no indication from either registry studies or cohort studies of an increased risk for leukaemia associated with the HIV epidemic (Biggar *et al.*, 1989; Rabkin & Yellin, 1994; Ragni *et al.*, 1993; Reynolds *et al.*, 1993; Lyter *et al.*, 1995).

Reports on *lung cancer* in HIV-infected persons have reflected differences in the clinical course in comparison with HIV-uninfected persons. Survival is short and appears to be worse than that seen in HIV-uninfected lung cancer patients (Flores *et al.*, 1995). However, these data probably reflect the dismal course of infection with HIV. Rabkin and Yellin (1994) reported a small relative increase in lung cancer among never-married men in San Francisco, but unrelated behavioural risk factors such as cigarette smoking may be responsible.

Other tumours that have been reported in HIV-positive persons but for which an association with the infection is not convincing include *mesothelioma* (Behling *et al.*, 1993), *cerebral glial tumours* (Chamberlain, 1994; Moulignier *et al.*, 1994) and *cancer of the colon* (Kaplan *et al.*, 1987; Cappell *et al.*, 1988), *pancreas* (Kaplan *et al.*, 1987; Monfardini *et al.*, 1989) and *kidney* (Monfardini *et al.*, 1989).

In summary, the available data do not support an association of these other tumours with HIV infection.

3. Studies of Cancer in Animals

3.1 HIV-1 and HIV-2

There have been many unsuccessful attempts to infect a variety of laboratory animal species (rats, hamsters, guinea-pigs) with HIV-1 and HIV-2 (Morrow *et al.*, 1987). In some studies, rabbits have been infected successfully (Filice *et al.*, 1988; Kulaga *et al.*, 1989), but the most reliable models involve HIV infection of nonhuman primates.

Chimpanzees (*Pan troglodytes*) (Morrow *et al.*, 1989), gibbons (*Hylobates lar*) (Lusso *et al.*, 1988) and pigtailed macaques (*Macaca nemestrina*) (Frumkin *et al.*, 1993; Gartner *et al.*, 1994) can be infected with HIV-1, whereas HIV-2 infection has been reported in rhesus monkeys (*M. mulatta*), cynomolgus monkeys (*M. fascicularis*) and baboons (*Papio papio sp.*) (Stahl-Hennig *et al.*, 1990; Castro *et al.*, 1991; Barnett *et al.*, 1994).

Despite persistent infection and immunological disorders such as lymphopenia and a decrease in $CD4^+$ T-cell counts, clinical signs are rare in HIV-1- and HIV-2- infected non-human primates. Chimpanzees show definite serological and haematological features of HIV infection (Morrow *et al.*, 1989). No clinical disease was seen in HIV-1-infected pigtailed macaques with persistent HIV-1 infection more than one year after first incubation (Gartner *et al.*, 1994).

Transient lymphadenopathy and/or splenomegaly have been observed in HIV-2-infected rhesus and cynomolgus monkeys (Stahl-Hennig *et al.*, 1990; Livartowski *et al.*, 1992), but in most cases they remained clinically healthy (Putkonen *et al.*, 1989). Diarrhoea and weight loss were reported in one of eight infected rhesus macaques (Castro *et al.*, 1991). A case of central nervous system and lung lesions due to actinomycetes was reported by Livartowski *et al.* (1992).

One rapidly growing mammary adenocarcinoma has been observed in an HTLV-I/-HIV-1-infected rabbit (Kulaga *et al.*, 1989). [The Working Group considered that the occurrence of this tumour was probably unrelated to the retroviral infection.]

Among six HIV-2 infected baboons (*Papio cynocephalus*), five animals became persistently infected. After 28 months, one baboon developed an AIDS-like condition with fibromatosis involving lymph nodes, skin, thyroid and pancreas. Another animal was reported to follow a similar clinical course (Barnett *et al.*, 1994).

3.2 Lymphomas in nonhuman primates

Prior to the first documented lymphoma outbreak in colonies of rhesus monkeys, malignant lymphomas in nonhuman primates had been reported only rarely (Stowell et al., 1971). However, lymphomas have been reported to develop in various species of monkeys treated with immunosuppressive agents (Reitz et al., 1980) and in newborn tamarins experimentally infected with Epstein-Barr virus (EBV) (Young et al., 1989). Lymphomas have also been found in various nonhuman primates naturally or experimentally infected with herpesvirus saimiri (HVS) (Adamson et al., 1975), or with STLV-I (see Section 3.2.1 of the monograph on HTLV in this volume, p. 308).

3.2.1 Occurrence of lymphomas in nonhuman primates infected with simian immunodeficiency virus

Lymphomas in simian immunodeficiency virus (SIV)-infected nonhuman primates have been documented in rhesus, cynomolgus and pigtailed macaques, but the incidence of these lymphomas is not well defined. In a study of cynomolgus macaques, an incidence of 38% (9/24) was reported (Feichtinger et al., 1990). In a retrospective necropsy study in the USA, King et al. (1983) observed nodular lymphoproliferative infiltrates of well differentiated lymphocytes in liver, kidney and bone marrow tissues in 3/16 macaques (M. mulatta and M. fascicularis) and, in addition, a clear malignant lymphoma was found in one macaque (M. mulatta). All four animals were immunodeficient. Letvin et al. (1983) also reported three lymphoma cases in the same colony. [The Working Group noted that it was unclear whether these were the same animals as previously reported.] It was subsequently recognized that this colony was infected with SIV (Letvin & King, 1990).

The likely transfer of nonpathogenic SIV from its natural host (the sooty mangabey monkey: Cercocebus atys) to the highly sensitive macaques, as manifested by the development of lymphoma, was demonstrated by Baskin et al. (1986). These studies involved the inoculation of a rhesus macaque (M. mulatta) with a homogenate of a cutaneous leprosy lesion from a sooty mangabey monkey. Subsequently, the rhesus monkey developed a lymphoma, and cells from this lymphoma induced a further lymphoma when injected into another rhesus macaque. Lymphoblastoid cell lines from the second rhesus macaque were established in vitro from tumour cell suspensions and shown to produce a herpesvirus related to EBV and a retrovirus morphologically similar to SIV (Baskin et al., 1986). Baskin et al. (1988) also observed one case of lymphoma in a study of 24 rhesus monkeys experimentally infected with this virus designated SIV_{SMM}. SIV_{MNE} was also isolated from a pigtailed macaque (M. nemestina) with lymphoma (Benveniste et al., 1986; Henderson et al., 1988). SIV_{MNE} was shown to be related to HIV-2.

Five lymphoma cases out of 49 necropsied stump-tailed macaques (M. arctoides) were observed by Lowenstine et al. (1992). Among these 49 animals, 75% had pathological lesions compatible with a diagnosis of SIV infection and the SIV-related mortality was 68%. SIV_{STM} was pathogenic for rhesus macaques.

In the UK, Ramsay et al. (1991) observed B-cell lymphomas in 2/26 rhesus monkeys infected with SIV_{MAC} over a two-year period. These lymphomas occurred 11.5 and 20 months after infection. In a study of 7 rhesus and 3 cynomolgus monkeys infected with SIV_{MAC} or SIV_{SMM}, one animal developed a lymphoma involving the lumbar spinal cord 11.5 months after the onset of SIV infection (Baskerville *et al.*, 1990).

In a Swedish study, malignant lymphoma was observed in 10/33 wild-caught cynomolgus monkeys 5 to 15 months after intravenous inoculation with SIV_{SMM} (Feichtinger *et al.*, 1990, 1992a,b).

3.2.2 *Pathological and molecular features of lymphoma*

The SIV_{SMM}-associated lymphomas in cynomolgus monkeys were clinically malignant, with visceral metastasis, and were in some cases also observed to develop in testis, brain and spinal cord (Feichtinger *et al.*, 1990; Ramsay *et al.*, 1991; Feichtinger *et al.*, 1992a,b). By histology, the lymphomas were mostly high grade and all those tested were phenotypically B-cell derived. Most showed clonal heavy- and light-chain immunoglobulin restrictions and immunoglobulin gene rearrangements (Feichtinger *et al.*, 1990; Ramsay *et al.*, 1991; Feichtinger *et al.*, 1992a,b; Rezikyan *et al.*, 1995).

No integrated viral genomes were found in lymphoma cells (Feichtinger *et al.*, 1990, 1992a,b). In another study, an SIV-like virus was identified in a lymphoblastoid cell line established from a transmissible lymphoma associated with SIV infection (Baskin *et al.*, 1986).

In a monkey cohort in Sweden, the time to lymphoma development varied from five to 46 months after SIV infection. The lymphomas were all of B-cell origin. DNA analysis of VDJ immunoglobulin genes showed both monoclonal and oligoclonal rearrangements. In some instances, the lymphoma clone was already detectable in lymph nodes soon after SIV infection and before manifestation of clinically apparent lymphoma (Rezikyan *et al.*, 1995). All the lymphomas were associated with an EBV-like B-lymphotropic herpesvirus (HVMF-1) (Feichtinger *et al.*, 1990, 1992a,b; Rezikyan *et al.*, 1995; Li *et al.*, 1993a, 1994), which had 65% DNA homology in exonic regions with EBV (Li *et al.*, 1994).

The SIV_{SMM}-related lymphomas have features very similar to those of the AIDS-related lymphomas in man which are associated with EBV, supporting the hypothesis of an important role of EBV-type viruses in the pathogenesis of such lymphomas.

3.2.3 *Other neoplastic conditions*

Neoplastic conditions other than lymphomas have not been documented as being related to SIV infection, with the possible exception of occasional cases of retroperitoneal fibromatosis. However, retroperitoneal fibromatosis has been seen mostly in macaques infected with the simian immunosuppressive type D retrovirus (SRV-2) (Giddens *et al.*, 1985; Tsai *et al.*, 1995) and in one case of SIV-induced AIDS (Baskerville *et al.*, 1990) (see also Section 4.2.3).

3.2.4 *Cofactors in SIV oncogenesis*

As discussed for AIDS-related malignant lymphoma in humans (Section 2.2.4), the interaction of several oncogenic cofactors at various stages of the lymphomagenic process has to be considered. These factors can be classified into those inducing: (a) activation, (b) deregulated proliferation and (c) genomic abnormalities in B-cells.

Marked B-cell follicular hyperplasia, seen in early stages of SIV as well as HIV infection (Biberfeld et al., 1985; Chalifoux et al., 1986; Kaaya et al., 1993b), could predispose to B-cell lymphomagenesis. In both SIV and HIV infections, viral antigens appear after infection in hyperplastic follicles on the follicular dendritic cells (FDC). These cells have the foremost antigen-presenting effect on follicular B-cells and are therefore related to the development of the characteristic follicular hyperplasia (Biberfeld et al., 1985; Tenner-Rácz et al., 1986; Kaaya et al., 1993b). With progression of infection, the FDC-antigen-presenting cell-reticulum is destroyed, probably by immunopathological mechanisms and/or viral cytopathic effects (Biberfeld et al., 1985; Stahmer et al., 1996). This leads to the breakdown 'lysis' of follicles, which probably is reflected functionally by the development of impaired immune responses to neoantigens. This follicle 'lysis' may promote the selection of FDC-independent, deregulated autocrine B-cells which during migration through extranodal tissues settle and develop into malignant lymphomas. This extranodal homing is probably promoted by the capacity of AIDS-related malignant lymphomas in humans to produce growth factors (IL-6, IL-10) with possible autocrine functions (Emilie et al., 1992).

A highly deregulated cytokine growth factor homeostasis and the disruption of the antigen-presenting FDC network are thus likely also to play an important role in B-cell activation and proliferation with an increased risk for genomic changes and lymphomagenesis in SIV-infected monkeys (Kaaya et al., 1993b).

Despite the clear association of SIV infection with lymphomagenesis, no evidence yet indicates a direct oncogenic effect of the SIV or HIV genome. However, in-vitro experiments have suggested a transforming effect on 3T3 cells transfected with the SIV PBj_{14} nef gene (Du et al., 1995).

The well recognized oncogenic effects of EBV in certain human lymphomas appear to be mirrored in SIV-infected nonhuman primates. Thus studies have shown a direct transforming/immortalizing effect of the EBV-like HVMF-1 in cynomolgus monkeys associated with SIV-related lymphomas (Li et al., 1994).

3.3 Feline immunodeficiency virus infection in cats

Lentiviral infections of animals other than non-human primates include infections with feline immunodeficiency virus (FIV), bovine immunodeficiency virus, maedi-visna virus, caprine arthritis-encephalitis virus and equine infectious anaemia virus (Coffin, 1992). An association between viral infection and the development of neoplasia, in particular B-cell lymphomas, has been documented only for FIV infections.

FIV was first isolated in 1986 and has become recognized as a common infection in pet cats worldwide (Pedersen et al., 1987). Initial epidemiological studies of a representative sample of the pet cat population in the United Kingdom reported a 19% prevalence of FIV in sick cats, a 6% prevalence in healthy cats and a 21% prevalence among cats in households with more than one cat (Hosie et al., 1989). In studies in the United States, 10–14% of sick cats and 1–4% of healthy cats were FIV-positive (Grindem et al., 1989;

Shelton et al., 1989; Yamamoto et al., 1989; O'Connor et al., 1991). In Japan, infection rates as high as 44% in sick cats and 12% in healthy cats have been recorded (Ishida et al., 1989).

High-grade B-cell neoplasms in association with both naturally acquired and experimentally induced infections have been described. The term 'lymphosarcoma' is used throughout the text to designate tumours of lymphoid lineage. Five cases of lymphosarcoma and one case of a poorly differentiated myeloproliferative disorder are the only tumours that have been documented in association with experimental FIV infections (Yamamoto et al., 1988; English et al., 1994; Poli et al., 1994; Callanan et al., 1996). A broader range of tumours in cats with naturally acquired infections has been described and case reports include lymphosarcomas (Shelton et al., 1990; Hutson et al., 1991; Barr et al., 1993; Callanan et al., 1996), fibrosarcomas (Ishida et al., 1989), myeloproliferative diseases (Ishida et al., 1989; Shelton et al., 1990; Hutson et al., 1991), mast-cell tumours (Shelton et al., 1990; Barr et al., 1993; Terry et al., 1995), cutaneous squamous-cell carcinomas (Hutson et al., 1991; Pedersen & Barlough, 1991), miscellaneous adenomas and carcinomas (Gruffydd-Jones et al., 1988; Hopper et al., 1989) and oligodendrogliomas (Hurtrel et al., 1992).

3.3.1 Occurrence of lymphosarcomas in FIV infection

In natural FIV infection, the majority of clinical and epidemiological studies demonstrate that lymphosarcomas occur in less than 10% of FIV-infected cats (Hopper et al., 1989; Hosie et al., 1989; Ishida et al., 1989; Yamamoto et al., 1989; Shelton et al., 1990). Evaluation of the association between FIV infection and lymphoid malignancies is confounded by concurrent infection with the C-type feline leukaemia virus (FeLV), the most common cause of lymphosarcoma in cats (Hardy, 1981). In a study of 161 cats with leukaemia and/or lymphoma, Shelton et al. (1990) performed a stratified analysis controlling for FeLV infection using the Mantel–Haenszel test, which revealed a significant association between FIV infection and leukaemia/lymphoma. The estimated relative risk for developing leukaemia/lymphoma was 5.0 for cats infected with FIV only, compared with uninfected cats. In the same study, a relative risk of 62.1 was found for FeLV-infected animals and, when animals were co-infected with both viruses, the risk was 77.3.

Two reports have described lymphosarcomas in two of seven experimentally infected cats at 9 and 21 months after infection (English et al., 1994) and in two of 20 experimentally infected cats at 30 and 42 months after infection (Callanan et al., 1996); the specific pathogen-free cats were infected intravenously or intraperitoneally with the North Carolina State University (NCSU1) or Glasgow (Gla-8) strains of FIV, respectively. Lymphosarcoma associated with experimental infection has also been documented in a cat intravenously infected with FIV (Pisa M2 strain), 18 months after infection (Poli et al., 1994) and a myeloproliferative disorder was reported 8.5 weeks after inoculation with FIV (Petaluma strain) (Yamamoto et al., 1988).

3.3.2 *Pathological and molecular features of lymphosarcoma*

In FIV-associated lymphosarcomas, as with HIV and SIV, sites of tumour distribution are predominantly extranodal, with involvement of the heart, eyes, brain, spinal cord, pancreas and urinary bladder (Hutson *et al.*, 1991; Callanan *et al.*, 1996).

Limited information is available on the immune function of FIV-infected cats with lymphosarcomas. Callanan *et al.* (1992) found normal responses of lymphocytes to mitogens in one case, and Poli *et al.* (1994) detected a marked reduction in circulating $CD4^+$ T-lymphocytes in another case.

In a series of eight FIV-infected cats (two experimental and six natural) with lymphosarcoma, seven of the tumours were high-grade B-cell lymphomas of the centroblastic or immunoblastic subtypes. The remaining case was a T-cell tumour associated with concurrent FeLV infection (Callanan *et al.*, 1996). Lymphosarcomas in experimental infection described by English *et al.* (1994) and Poli *et al.* (1994) were also of B-cell origin, based on immunoglobulin expression. However, the single neoplasm described by Poli *et al.* (1994) was low-grade.

Four of the tumours reported by Callanan *et al.* (1996) were examined with molecular probes to establish tumour cell lineage and to screen for integrated viral sequences (Terry *et al.*, 1995). Confirmation of a B-cell origin was supported by the identification of monoclonal or oligoclonal immunoglobulin heavy-chain gene rearrangements and the lack of rearrangements of T-cell receptor β-chain genes in all four cases. Rearrangement of the *c-myc* locus, which occurs in many FeLV lymphosarcomas, was not found in any of the FIV-associated tumours and none of the tumours showed evidence of integrated FIV sequences by Southern blot hybridization. Poli *et al.* (1994) identified DNA of the FIV *gag* gene in many tissues including tumour tissue of an experimentally FIV-infected cat. However, in this tumour tissue, it could not be determined whether the infection was of neoplastic cells.

Thus lymphosarcomas in FIV-infected cats share similar morphological, immunophenotypic and molecular qualities to those associated with HIV and SIV infections. The evidence available supports an indirect role for FIV in tumour development. FIV induces activation of lymphoid tissue, polyclonal B-cell activation and increased serum cytokine levels, all of which may facilitate malignant transformation of B cells (Lawrence *et al.*, 1992; Rideout *et al.*, 1992; Callanan *et al.*, 1993; Flynn *et al.*, 1994).

4. Other Data Relevant to an Evaluation of Carcinogenesis and its Mechanisms

4.1 Immunity and cancer

In mice and humans with inherited or acquired immunodeficiency, only certain types of malignancy are significantly increased in incidence (Weiss, 1993b). Many of these tumours are associated with viruses that have established persistent infections, and others are tumours arising within the immune system. Consideration of malignancies developing in cases of immunodeficiency caused by factors other than HIV is restricted in this monograph to humans. The highest relative risks in human non-AIDS immunodeficiency are for non-Hodgkin's lymphoma, Kaposi's sarcoma and non-melanoma skin cancer (Beral, 1991b).

4.1.1 *Types of cancer seen in non-HIV-associated human immunodeficiency*

The vast majority of data concerning the incidence of malignancies occurring in persons with an acquired immunodeficiency other than those with HIV infection comes from patient populations undergoing organ transplantation. In addition to immunosuppressive therapy and the foreign graft, such patients are exposed to incidental infections of donor origin. Birkeland *et al.* (1995) reported on the subsequent risk of malignancy in all 5692 renal transplant patients during 1964–86 within the Nordic countries, using the national population-based cancer registries for long-term follow-up. The data were analysed by standardized incidence ratios (SIR), using the population rates as the reference. Overall, there was a significant increase in overall cancer rates of 4.5 for women and 4.6 for men. Very highly increased risks (SIR, ≥ 10-fold) were seen for cancers of the lip, kidney, cervix and vulva–vagina and non-melanoma cancer of the skin and for non-Hodgkin's lymphoma. In addition, there were significantly increased SIRs (2–5-fold) for a range of common malignancies including cancers of the colon, larynx, lung, bladder, prostate and testis. However, only two cases of Kaposi's sarcoma were reported.

Penn (1993) analysed data on a series of 7192 organ transplant patients followed by the Cincinnati Transplant Tumor Registry in the United States up to 1993. [The institutional sources of these patients were not specified.] Only the numbers of subsequent cancer cases were reported; these were compared with the proportional distribution of site-specific malignancy in the 'general population' without statistical analysis. [It is not clear whether the referent distribution was corrected for age and sex.] The most common tumours in the transplant patients were cancers of the skin (predominantly squamous-cell carcinoma) and lip and non-Hodgkin's lymphoma. There were 307 cases (2.4%) of Kaposi's sarcoma. Other common sites included vulva/peritoneum and kidney. The proportion of cervix cancer cases [3.5%] was reported to be the same as that in the general population. Subsequently, Penn and Porat (1995) reported on cases of central nervous system non-Hodgkin's lymphoma in this registry. Of a total of 1332 non-Hodgkin's lymphoma cases recorded, 289 (22%) involved the central nervous system. Penn (1994) similarly reported on the 326 paediatric patients recorded in the Cincinnati Registry. [These patients appear to be also included in the report above.] Compared with the distribution of cancer sites in adult transplant patients, paediatric patients had a higher frequency of lymphoma (50% versus 15%) and a lower proportion of cancers of the skin and lip (20% versus 38%).

Kinlen *et al.* (1979) reported on the follow-up of 3823 renal transplant patients in Australia, New Zealand and the United Kingdom. Compared with age- and sex-specific national mortality rates, the relative risk for any malignancy was 3.5 and that for non-Hodgkin's lymphoma was almost 60, with an excess evident for squamous skin cancer and mesenchymal tumours including one Kaposi's sarcoma.

In a hospital-based series from London, United Kingdom, Gaya et al. (1995) reported on 274 renal transplant patients whose graft survived three years or more, using survival analysis and comparison with national rates. Skin cancers were most common, particularly among men, followed by lymphomas and renal, urinary bladder and bronchial cancer. The actuarial risk of development of any tumour was 18.4% at 10 years and 49.6% at 20 years. There was a higher risk among males than among females, which was attributable to a higher incidence of skin cancer.

Schmidt et al. (1995) reported on the occurrence of genito-urinary malignancies among 868 renal transplant patients in a hospital-based series in Germany. Twelve cases were noted, of which one was transplanted in the graft. The 11 de-novo cases included four kidney, three cervical and one each of testicular, vulvar, urinary bladder and renal duct carcinomas.

Levy et al. (1993b) reported on 556 liver transplant patients followed between 1985 and 1991 at Baylor University in Dallas, TX, United States. Of these, 25 developed new malignancies, including 10 with lymphoma and 9 with at least one skin cancer. Other malignancies seen included lung, breast, prostate, pancreas, hepatocellular and colon cancers and Kaposi's sarcoma.

Dresdale et al. (1993) reported on 112 cardiac transplant patients seen at a hospital in Detroit, MI, United States, between 1985 and 1991. Of these, nine developed a new malignancy, including four cancers of the skin, two of the colon, and one each of the bone and bladder and one Kaposi's sarcoma. Guettier et al. (1992) reported on 174 cardiac transplant patients from a hospital in Paris between 1984 and 1990. The only malignancies reported were four gastrointestinal non-Hodgkin's lymphomas. Zahger et al. (1993) reported two cases of Kaposi's sarcoma occurring among 18 cardiac transplant patients in Jerusalem; both patients were Mediterranean Jews.

Table 29 summarizes the data from more than 15 000 organ (mostly kidney) transplant patients. The most common findings are the substantial excesses of squamous-cell carcinoma of the skin and non-Hodgkin's lymphoma. In addition, risks for cancers of the kidney and urinary bladder, cervix and vulva, and head and neck were commonly increased. Less frequently seen are unusual tumours including Kaposi's sarcoma and testicular cancer.

Table 30 summarizes the experience of more than 11 000 patients receiving bone marrow transplants, primarily for haematopoietic malignancies and disorders. The findings in this patient population were similar to those in the organ transplant patients, with the additional common finding of leukaemia. Kolb et al. (1992) reported only the number of new malignancies occurring among the 9732 bone marrow transplant patients reported to the International Bone Marrow Registry and among the 226 patients reported to the European Bone Marrow–European Late Effects Project. Of the former, 116 had a subsequent cancer: 58 were lymphoma, 15 leukaemias including myelodysplasia, 14 cancers of the skin including 5 melanomas, 4 cervical including dysplasia, 3 vulvar/-vaginal, 2 oropharyngeal, 2 breast and 2 thyroid cancers, among others. Among the latter group of patients, there were 11 new cancers including 6 skin cancers.

Table 29. Cancer risks following organ transplants: cohort studies

Reference	Population, number	Time period	Case identification	Comparison group	Sites	Results SIR M	(Σ)	F	Notes
Birkeland et al. (1995)	Nordic countries: kidney transplant only 5692 (32 392 person-years) Follow-up for life	1964–86	Population registries	Population rate	Lip	14.0		117.0	SIR increase seen within first 5 years, peaking in the next decade with some decrease after 15 years. Risk higher in younger patients (< 45) and if the donor was a family member. Cyclosporin and OKT3 not used. (All SIRs listed are statistically significant.)
					Colon	3.2		3.9	
					Rectum	4.5		–	
					Larynx	3.8		15.0	
					Lung	1.8		4.9	
					Cervix	–		8.6	
					Vulva/vagina	–		31.0	
					Prostate	2.1		–	
					Testis	3.9		–	
					Ureter/kidney	4.6		19.0	
					Urinary bladder	3.1		17.0	
					Non-melanoma skin	29.0		18.0	
					Brain, etc.	3.0		–	
					Thyroid	16.0		5.1	
					Connective tissue	7.3		–	
					NHL	10.0		11.0	
					Hodgkin's lymphoma	–		11.0	
Gaya et al. (1995)	Hammersmith Hospital, London — Graft survived 3 years: kidney transplant only 274 (2622 person-years) 29-year follow-up	1961–90	Hospital follow-up	Population rates	Skin	23.3	(45.0)	12.0	4-fold RR increase for non-skin cancers seen within first 5 years and stabilized 2–3 thereafter. RR for skin cancer increased with time. Greater risk in younger patients (< 40 years). No effect seen for cyclosporin. Median time to diagnosis, 7.7 years.
					NHL	34.0	25.0		
					Kidney				
					Urinary bladder	9.5	(7.6)		

Table 29 (contd)

Reference	Population, number	Time period	Case identification	Comparison group	Sites	Results	Notes
Schmidt et al. (1995)	University of Cologne: kidney transplant only 868 (1209 person-years) Follow-up 42 ± 45 months	1968–94	Hospital follow-up	Population rates	Genito-urinary cancer only: sites 6 Kidney, renal duct 3 Cervical 1 Testis 1 Bladder 1 Vulva		RR for males, 7.3; females, 11.2. All but one cancer developed in the 324 patients aged 20–40 years [$p = 0.001$]
Penn (1993)	Cincinnati Transplant Tumor Registry 6798	[1968]–93	Special registry	General population	Skin Lymphoma Lip KS Kidney Vulva/perineum Cervix Hepatobiliary Other sarcomas	Proportional incidence 52% vs 32%[a] 23% vs 5% 7% vs 0.3% 6% vs < 0.1% 5% vs 2% 4% vs 0.5% 3% vs 3% 2.6% vs 1.4% 1.7% vs 0.5%	Mean time to diagnosis: KS, 22 months (2–226); lymphomas, 32 months (1–254); epithelial excl. vulva and perineum, 69 months (1–299); vulva, perineum, 113 months (3–286); 94% lymphomas were NHL. In heart or heart–lung transplant cases, 42% were cardiac lymphomas. Large increase in SCC.
Penn (1994)	Cincinnati Transplant Tumor Registry: paediatric patients 326	1968–93	Special registry	Adult transplant patients	Lymphoma Skin and lip Malignant melanoma Vulva/perineum KS[c] Other sarcoma Liver Thyroid Cervix	50% vs 15% 20% vs 38% 15% vs 5%[b] 4% vs 3% 2% vs 4% 3% vs 1% 3% vs 2% 3% vs 1% 2% vs 4%	Mean time to diagnosis: KS, 46 months (4–197); lymphoma, 20 months (1–177); skin and lip, 118 months (10–282); vulva/perineum, 140 months (43–262), 98% lymphomas were NHL — these were much more frequent in non-renal transplants. There were six cases of cervix cancer (including in situ) among the 158 females: mean age at diagnosis, 25 years.

Table 29 (contd)

Reference	Population, number	Time period	Case identification	Comparison group	Sites	Results		Notes
Kinlen et al. (1979)	United Kingdom Australasian Transplant Study 3823	1970–77/8	Special registry	Population rates	NHL Skin[a] Other	RR 58.6 4.5 1.7	No. 34 5 30	(Other: Kidney/bladder, 6; colon, 4; lung, 3; genital, 3; leukaemia, 3; other, 11)
Levy et al. (1993b)	Baylor University Medical Center: liver transplant only 556	1985–91	Hospital follow-up	NG	Lymphomas Skin	CI 1.7% 1.6%		Mean time to diagnosis: lymphomas, 7 months; skin, 18 months. For skin, ratio of BCC to SCC, 1:4.
Dresdale et al. (1993)	Henry Ford Hospital, Detroit: cardiac transplant treated with antilymphocyte globulin 112	1985–91	Hospital follow-up	None	SCC Colon Other	[3%] [2%] [4%]		
Guettier et al. (1992)	Hôpital Broussais, Paris: cardiac transplant 174	1984–90	Hospital follow-up	None	NHL	3%[c]		All were gastrointestinal

SIR, standardized incidence rate; OKT3, orthotopic kidney transplantation therapy; NHL, non-Hodgkin's lymphoma; KS, Kaposi's sarcoma; RR, relative risk; NG, not given; CI, cumulative incidence; BCC, basal cell carcinoma of the skin; SCC, squamous cell carcinoma of skin
[a] Proportion of all malignancies
[b] Proportion of all skin cancers
[c] Two of these KS patients were HIV-positive
[d] United Kingdom only

Table 30. Cancer risks following bone marrow transplants: cohort studies

Reference	Population number	Time period	Case identification	Comparison group	Results	Notes
Lowsky et al. (1994)	Princess Margaret Hospital, Toronto 557 (1608 person-years)	1970–93	Hospital follow-up	Population rates	Any cancer, relative risk = 4.2 (10 malignancies in 9 patients) 2 oral cavity, 1 malignant melanoma, 2 skin, 1 endometrium, 1 breast, 1 NHL, 1 AML (donor cells), 1 lung. 7 patients developed in situ cancer: 5 cervical, 1 vulvar, 1 rectal Addendum: 1 endometrium, 1 NHL	Risk associated with total body irradiation and development of acute GVHD
Socié et al. (1993)	European Bone Marrow Transplantation–Severe Anaplastic Anemia Working Group 748	1971–92	Hospital follow-up	Population rates	Any cancer, relative risk = 28.6 (9 malignancies) 2 acute leukaemia, 5 head and neck, 1 stomach, 1 liver	Rish higher among males, increased with age, and with use of radiation-based conditioning regimen
Socié et al. (1991)	Hôpital Saint-Louis, Paris; Fanconi anaemia patients 40	1976–90	Hospital follow-up	Population rates	1 tongue cancer	

Table 30 (contd)

Reference	Population number	Time period	Case identification	Comparison group	Results	Notes
Kolb et al. (1992)	International Bone Marrow Transplant Registry: cancer patients 9732				(116 malignancies) 58 lymphoma, 15 leukaemia including myelodysplasia, 14 skin including 5 melanoma, 4 cervical including dysplasia, 3 vulva/vaginal, 12 other solid, 10 unspecified	
	Late Effect Study Group 226				(11 malignancies) 4 within 6 years: 2 squamous cell of skin, 1 breast, 1 chloroma; 7 > 10 years: 4 basal cell of skin, 1 'spinalioma', 1 parotid, 1 uterus	

GVHD, graft versus hot disease; AML, acute myeloid leukaemia; NHL, non-Hodgkin's lymphoma

Lowsky et al. (1994) reported on 557 consecutive bone marrow transplant patients from a hospital in Toronto, Canada between 1970 and 1993. The actuarial probability of having a new malignancy was 12% at 11 years after the transplant for the first nine cancers reported. Of the total of 11 patients who developed cancer, three had developed cancer of the skin, two of the oral cavity, two of the endometrium (of whom one also had breast cancer), two had myelogenous leukaemias (one of donor origin), and one each had non-Hodgkin's lymphoma and cancer of the lung.

Socié et al. (1993) reported on the experience of 748 patients followed by the European Bone Marrow Transplantation–Severe Aplastic Anemia Working group from 1971 to 1991. [The Working Group noted that these patients may overlap with those of Kolb et al. (1992) noted above.] Of these, 748 were treated by bone marrow transplantation. Of the latter, all but 20 (3%) received short-term immunosuppression (primary cyclophosphamide) as a conditioning regimen before transplantation. Nine patients developed a new malignancy, including five cancers of the head and neck, two acute leukaemias, one stomach and one liver cancer. In the group receiving only immunosuppression, 28 myelodysplasias and 15 acute leukaemias were diagnosed, plus 3 liver, 2 breast, and 1 each of stomach and head/neck cancer and non-Hodgkin's lymphoma. The cumulative incidence at 10 years for any secondary malignancy was much higher in the immunosuppressed group (18.8%) than in the bone marrow transplant group (3.1%). In another report, Socié et al. (1991) reported on 40 patients who received a bone marrow transplant to treat Fanconi anaemia. [The Working Group noted that these patients may also overlap with those reported by Kolb et al. (1992) noted above.] Of these, one boy developed a cancer of the tongue 74 months after the transplantation.

Mueller and Pizzo (1995) reviewed reports on cancers in children with primary immunodeficiencies (Table 31). In these conditions, the occurrence of malignancy is substantial (5–25%) over a variable number of years and is mostly lymphoma, followed by leukaemia. An earlier review by Kinlen (1992) noted that about half of these malignancies were non-Hodgkin's lymphoma, 13% leukaemia and 9% Hodgkin's disease.

4.1.2 *Time of onset of cancers in non-HIV-associated immunodeficiency*

Among the 5692 renal transplant recipients followed on average for 5.7 years reported by Birkeland et al. (1995) (see Section 4.1.1), the risk for cancer at all sites was increased nearly four-fold in the first five years, over five-fold in the next decade and four-fold in the subsequent period. The risk for skin cancers increased continuously with time since receiving the transplant. In the registry-based series of 7668 tumours in 7192 patients reported by Penn (1993), the 307 Kaposi's sarcomas appeared on average at 22 (range, 1–226) months after organ transplantation; the 1252 lymphomas at 32 (1–254) months and other tumours at 67 (1–299) months. The average time of onset of non-Hodgkin's lymphoma involving the central nervous system was the same as that seen for all non-Hodgkin's lymphoma: 33 (0.1–249) months (Penn & Porat, 1995). In the paediatric patients from this cohort, the range of time intervals for any malignancy was the same as that for adults. However, the average time of onset of the 8 Kaposi's

Table 31. Cancers arising in children with primary immunodeficiency

Syndrome	Malignancy	Cumulative incidence (%)	Estimated latency in years
X-linked gamma globulinaemia	Leukaemia, NHL	6	10
Wiskott–Aldrich	NHL, leukaemia, Hodgkin's disease	>10	6
Bloom's syndrome	Leukaemia, NHL, Hodgkin's disease, adenocarcinoma	25	During first 40 years
Ataxia telangiectasia	Leukaemia, NHL, Hodgkin's disease, other	>12	9
Common variable immunodeficiency	NHL, stomach	8–10	16
Severe combined immunodeficiency	NHL	5	< 1
X-linked lympho-proliferative	NHL	4	(following EBV infection)
Selective IgA deficiency	NHL, gastric, thymoma	NG	NG

Modified from Mueller & Pizzo (1995)
NHL, non-Hodgkin lymphoma; EBV, Epstein-Barr virus; NG, not given

sarcomas was only 13 months (0–34) and that for the 167 lymphomas was 22 (0.2–217) months (Penn, 1994). In the United Kingdom–Australasian study of 3823 renal transplant patients, the authors noted that the risk for any malignancy was elevated within the first two years, and remained so through ≥ 4 years of follow-up. In the series of 274 renal transplant patients followed on average for 9.6 years reported by Gaya et al. (1995), the relative risk was also about four-fold within the first five years, and remained within the same range thereafter. Among non-skin tumours, there did not appear to be a time trend. However, the appearance of skin cancer increased significantly with time. Among the 868 renal transplant patients followed on average for 41.8 months for genito-urinary system malignancies, the 11 cancers (excluding the transplanted kidney adenocarcinoma) occurred on average at 66 (24–131) months (Schmidt et al., 1995).

Fewer follow-up data are available for other organ transplants. In patients who generally receive more immunosuppression, malignancies occur earlier. Among the 556 liver transplant patients followed on average for 35 months by Levy et al. (1993b), the 10 lymphomas occurred on average at 8 (1–29) months after transplantation, 1 Kaposi's sarcoma at 16 months, 6 other solid tumours at 34 (12–66) months and 9 skin cancers at 17 (2–66) months. Among the 112 cardiac transplant recipients followed on average for 41.5 months by Dresdale et al. (1993), there were one patient with Kaposi's sarcoma at 47 months, four with skin cancer at an average of 43 (8–70) months and four others at 23 (6–60) months. Guettier et al. (1992) reported that the four gastrointestinal tract non-

Hodgkin's lymphomas occurring in a cohort of 174 cardiac transplant patients had an average time of onset of 22 (15–29) months. The two cases of Kaposi's sarcoma in cardiac transplant patients in Israel occurred two months after transplantation (Zahger et al., 1993). Among 9732 bone marrow recipients, who generally receive both radiation and chemotherapy, Kolb et al. (1992) reported that most of the new malignancies found occurred 'in the first few months', although 9% of 79 patients developed malignancies after more than 10 years of follow-up.

In 1608 patients treated with either immunosuppression or bone marrow transplantation for aplastic anaemia reported by Socié et al. (1993) after mean follow-up times of 30 and 47 months, respectively, the median time to development of myelodysplasia syndrome was 52 (2–122) months, that for acute leukaemia was 47 (7–115) months, that for non-Hodgkin's lymphoma was 33 months (one case) and that for other tumours was 52 (1–94) months.

Of 557 bone marrow transplant patients followed by Lowsky et al. (1994), a non-Hodgkin's lymphoma developed at 7 months, a leukaemia at 46 months, three skin cancers at an average of 47 (30–64) months and five other cancers at 84 (31–127) months.

Among the cases of congenital immunodeficiency reviewed by Mueller and Pizzo (1995), the length of time to cancer diagnosis ranged from an average of less than one year in severe combined immunodeficiency syndrome to over 40 years in Bloom's syndrome.

4.1.3 *Similarities and differences between AIDS- and transplantation-associated tumours*

(a) *In immunity*

HIV-associated immunodeficiency shares with the other acquired or inherited immunodeficiencies reviewed above a diminution of host cellular immunity, the primary control mechanism of latent viral infections. The effect of cyclosporin A, which has been causally associated with an increased incidence of both non-Hodgkin's lymphoma and Kaposi's sarcoma in organ transplant patients, is quite similar to that seen in HIV-infection, with the selective inhibition of T-helper function (IARC, 1990). The populations reviewed above were immunosuppressed by a variety of means, either by inborn genetic defect, by cytotoxic chemotherapy or, in the vast majority of cases, by exposure to a range of therapeutic agents designed to create tolerance to a foreign organ or tissue. In the latter case, the level of immunosuppression can be modulated or withdrawn in response to clinical status, and there is regression of a lymphoma and of Kaposi's sarcoma with reduction or cessation of the treatment (IARC, 1990; Penn, 1993). Further, the impact on the immune system is generally immediate, unlike the apparently cumulative effect that is seen in the natural history of HIV infection. A general characteristic of malignancy occurring in non-HIV/AIDS-related immunosuppression is that the risk and rapidity of onset are directly related to the severity of the immunosuppression (Brusamolino et al. 1989; IARC, 1990; Kinlen, 1992; Gaya et al., 1995).

(b) *In cancer types*

The types of malignancy which develop excessively in non-HIV-infected patients are generally similar to those seen in AIDS, with a predominance of non-Hodgkin's lymphomas, of which a high proportion involves the central nervous system, and Kaposi's sarcoma. A much higher proportion of non-Hodgkin's lymphomas (> 90%) in transplant recipients are EBV-positive than in AIDS-related non-Hodgkin's lymphoma (~ 50%). Among non-Hodgkin's lymphomas, Burkitt's lymphoma is relatively frequent in AIDS patients and in inherited ataxia telangiectasia and X-linked lymphoproliferative disease (Duncan's syndrome), but rare in adult transplant recipients. Further, in both AIDS and transplant patients, the malignancies tend to be more aggressive and include sites other than those usually seen in the general population (Bayley *et al.*, 1985; Kinlen, 1992; Barrett *et al.*, 1993). In regions where Kaposi's sarcoma in non-immunocompromised patients is relatively frequent, it occurs in transplant recipients at a higher frequency than non-Hodgkin's lymphoma (Qunibi *et al.*, 1988).

Transplant patients also differ from those with AIDS in their excessive development of cancers of the skin, primarily squamous-cell but also basal-cell — particularly with long-term follow-up. In renal transplant patients, there is commonly an excess of cancers of the urinary tract; however, an excess of these cancers has been seen in patients with chronic renal failure without transplantation. In patients treated for haematopoietic diseases, there is an excess of leukaemias; however, this is part of the spectrum of disease seen in many of these conditions. It used to be supposed that the excess cancer risk in transplant patients did not include those fatal malignancies which are common in older non-immunocompromised populations in the developed countries (Kinlen, 1992), and Prehn (1994) postulated that immune reactions may exert a stimulatory effect on such tumours. However, a report from the Nordic countries (Birkeland *et al.*, 1995), consolidating population-based registry data for 5692 renal transplant patients linked to the generally mutually standardized population cancer registries, found, in contrast to other studies, significantly increased risks for the incidence of cancers of the colon, lung, testis, thyroid and prostate.

(c) *In onset*

New malignancies in non-HIV-infected immunosuppressed individuals can occur within a very short period. A substantially increased relative risk is consistently seen in the first five years. This is in contrast to the extended latent period preceding the diagnosis of the malignancies seen in HIV-1 infection. The time from start of immunosuppressive therapy to tumour development is shorter in patient groups with more severe immunosuppression. In general, the relative risk for the associated tumours remains fairly constant over time since initiation of treatment, although Kaposi's sarcoma tends to occur earlier than non-Hodgkin's lymphoma; however, the relative risk for skin cancer shows a marked increase with time. In those studies in which both Kaposi's sarcoma and non-Hodgkin's lymphoma were seen, the former generally occurred earlier than the latter, as is seen in AIDS.

4.1.4 *Occurrence of other viruses in malignancies associated with non-HIV immunosuppression*

HHV-8 has been detected in 11/11 biopsies of Kaposi's sarcoma in transplant patients (Boshoff *et al.*, 1995a; Lebbé *et al.*, 1995; Buonaguro *et al.*, 1996). EBV was detected in 28/29 non-Hodgkin's lymphomas from transplant patients (Ho *et al.*, 1985b; Shapiro *et al.*, 1988; Nakhlen *et al.*, 1991). Transplantation of PBMCs from EBV-positive healthy humans into severe combined immunodeficient (SCID) mice frequently results in the development of immunoblastic lymphoma in the immunodeficient mouse.

IARC (1995) reviewed the data on the role of HPV in malignancies among transplant patients. In the case–control studies, the prevalence of cervical infections with HPV detected in women with organ transplants ranged from 22 to 45%, which was significantly higher than that in controls (3–6%). [The Working Group noted that these studies preceded the introduction of more sensitive primers for PCR detection of the high-risk HPV types and probably underestimated HPV prevalence.]

IARC (1995) also reviewed the prevalence of detectable HPV in skin cancers occurring in transplant patients. For 539 squamous-cell carcinoma specimens tested using the more sensitive methods, the positivity rate ranged between studies from zero to 100%, with half of the 16 studies having case positivity rates of at least 50%. Similarly, in eight published studies, among a total of 40 basal-cell carcinomas in transplant patients, nine cases (23%) were scored HPV-positive. A study using new PCR primers detected a high frequency of HPV-5, HPV-8 and other strains related to those occurring in epidermodysplasia verruciformis in skin cancer of renal transplant recipients (Berkhout *et al.*, 1995).

4.1.5 *Mechanisms by which immune dysfunction may contribute to the genesis of cancer*

(*a*) *Activation of oncogenic viruses with immunosuppression*

In immunocompetent persons, cell-mediated immunity may act to limit viral oncogenesis at two levels: first by controlling the overall viral burden by eliminating cells productively infected by the virus; second by recognizing viral antigen expressed on latently preneoplastic and neoplastic cells.

(*b*) *Stimulation and hyperreactivity of remaining cells in immunosuppressed persons*

The presence of the graft itself may modulate the immune system as a source of chronic antigenic stimulation. Lowsky *et al.* (1994) reported that the risk for new malignancies in bone marrow transplant patients was significantly associated with the presence of acute graft versus host disease, but not with the treatment modality itself. Bouwes Bavinck *et al.* (1991) observed that HLA-B mismatching (as well as homozygosity for HLA-DR) was significantly associated with the risk for squamous-cell carcinoma of the skin in renal transplant patients. This association appeared to be independent of the amount and type of treatment. However, B-cell hyperplasia is not a feature of iatrogenic immunosuppression as it is in HIV infection, which may explain why a larger proportion of non-Hodgkin's lymphomas in AIDS are EBV-negative (see Section 4.3.2).

4.2 Kaposi's sarcoma

Epidemiological and clinical studies (summarized in Section 2.1) have yielded the following conclusions regarding the etiology of Kaposi's sarcoma in HIV-infected individuals:

(i) the immunosuppressive effect of HIV is a major factor;

(ii) HIV component(s) may directly promote the development of Kaposi's sarcoma lesions, as the disease is often more aggressive in HIV-infected patients;

(iii) an infectious agent distinct from HIV and mainly transmitted sexually may have an important role.

This section reviews the virological and cell biological evidence which is relevant to these observations.

4.2.1 *Cell biology of Kaposi's sarcoma lesions*

(a) *Origins of Kaposi's sarcoma spindle cells*

The hallmark of the advanced Kaposi's sarcoma lesion is the spindle cell surrounding slit-like spaces. Endothelial cells (either vascular or lymphatic endothelium), cells from venous lymphatic junctions, fibroblasts, smooth muscle cells and dermal dendrocytes have all been proposed as possible progenitors of Kaposi's sarcoma spindle cells (reviewed by Roth *et al.*, 1992; Stürzl *et al.*, 1992a; Kaaya *et al.*, 1995). Rappersberger *et al.* (1991) reported that spindle cells stain with the monoclonal antibody EN-4 (which detects both vascular and lymphatic endothelium) but lack reactivity with the monoclonal antibody Pal-E (which reacts with blood-vessel but not lymphatic endothelial cells). This observation is compatible with spindle cells originating from lymphatic endothelium. However, other markers for blood vessel endothelium (but not lymphatic endothelium; OKM-5 and anti-factor VIII-related antigen; von Willebrand factor; vWF) stain Kaposi's sarcoma endothelial or spindle cells, although slightly varying results have been reported by different laboratories (Nadji *et al.*, 1981; Modlin *et al.*, 1983a; Little *et al.*, 1986; Rappersberger *et al.*, 1991; further references in Roth *et al.*, 1992).

Ultrastructural examination has failed to show the presence of Weibel–Palade bodies, the storage vesicles for vWF and therefore a characteristic feature of vascular endothelium, in spindle cells from Kaposi's sarcoma lesions (Rappersberger *et al.*, 1991). Staining with monoclonal antibody BMA 120, that detects an antigen specific to endothelial cells, lends support to an endothelial origin of Kaposi's sarcoma cells (Roth *et al.*, 1988). Kaposi's sarcoma spindle cells and endothelia lining vascular spaces in lesions express leukocyte adhesion molecule-1 (LAM-1) and thrombomodulin, which are markers of lymphokine-activated endothelial cells (Zhang *et al.*, 1994). This observation supports the notion that Kaposi's sarcoma spindle cells are of endothelial origin and are activated by growth factors (see below).

The staining (observed by some laboratories but not by others) of spindle cells with antibodies to CD14, CD68 and factor XIIIa has been interpreted to reflect a possible link between Kaposi's sarcoma spindle cells and cells of the monocyte/macrophage lineage, possibly dermal dendrocytes (Nickoloff et al., 1989; Rappersberger et al., 1991; Kaaya et al., 1995). These cells are distinct from Langerhans' cells (Nickoloff et al., 1989). The staining of cultured Kaposi's sarcoma spindle cells with an antibody to smooth muscle α-actin (Weich et al., 1991) and other similar histochemical data have been interpreted to suggest a relationship with smooth muscle cells or myofibroblasts (reviewed by Roth et al., 1992). These discrepant results suggest either that cells of different lineages can adopt a spindle-like morphology or that these markers are common to different cells of mesenchymal origin. [The Working Group considered that the weight of evidence pointed to the spindle cells being most closely related to vascular endothelial cells.]

A number of laboratories have cultured cells from Kaposi's sarcoma that express markers characteristic for vascular or lymphatic endothelium (Delli-Bovi et al., 1986; Nakamura et al., 1988; Roth et al., 1988; Siegal et al., 1990; Corbeil et al., 1991; Herndier et al., 1994a), but cultures expressing smooth muscle α-actin (Albini et al., 1988; Wittek et al., 1991) as well as mixed populations (Siegal et al., 1990; further references in Roth et al., 1992) have also been reported. The lineage identity of cultured cells has been defined by staining for the same markers as in the in-situ studies, notably vimentin and cytokeratin (for discrimination of mesenchymal and epithelial cells respectively), the endothelial markers vWF, Pal-E, OKM-5, BMA 120 (specific for blood-vessel endothelium), and EN-4 and UEA-I lectin (reactive with blood-vessel and lymphatic endothelium), CD14, CD68 and factor XIIIa (for the monocyte/macrophage lineage), SMC α-actin (smooth muscle and myofibroblast) and others (reviewed by Roth et al., 1992; Stürzl et al., 1992a; Kaaya et al., 1995). Spindle-shaped cells showing a moderate expression of endothelial antigens have been cultured from peripheral blood of Kaposi's sarcoma patients (Browning et al., 1994).

(b)   Vascular lesions induced by Kaposi's sarcoma cell cultures in nude mice

The various cell cultures established from Kaposi's sarcoma lesions differ in their ability to induce the growth of Kaposi's sarcoma-like vascular lesions in nude mice. A cell line expressing endothelial markers induced Kaposi's sarcoma-like tumours of human origin in nude mice (Siegal et al., 1990; Herndier et al., 1994a). This cell line had a normal diploid karyotype and expressed the endothelial markers factor VIII, EN-4 and UEA-I lectin. In addition, it produced high levels of urokinase plasminogen activator (uPA) and plasminogen activator inhibitor (PAI-1; Herndier et al., 1994a). Plasminogen activator has been shown to be involved in the development of endothelial tumours in mice transgenic for the polyoma middle T protein (Montesano et al., 1990). More recently, a second cell line capable of causing tumours of human origin in nude mice has been described and these lesions could be inhibited by β-human chorionic gonadotropin (β-HCG) (Lunardi-Iskander et al., 1995a). These cell lines meet the criteria for a tumorigenic cell line.

In contrast, a few other Kaposi's sarcoma cell cultures, also of an endothelial phenotype, are angiogenic *in vivo*, and induce transient Kaposi's sarcoma-like vascular lesions of *murine* origin, when inoculated into nude mice (Nakamura *et al.*, 1988; Salahuddin *et al.*, 1988). Spindle-shaped cells grown from the peripheral blood of Kaposi's sarcoma patients have also been reported to induce murine angiogenesis in nude mice (Browning *et al.*, 1994). This angiogenic property, together with other in-vitro findings (see below), suggests that growth factors produced by the cultured cells could induce murine cells to produce lesions resembling early Kaposi's sarcoma.

However, most other cell cultures established from Kaposi's sarcoma lesions, including some which are capable of acidic low-density lipoprotein uptake and expressing the endothelial marker BMA 120 (Roth *et al.*, 1988), did not induce tumour formation in nude mice, were not capable of growing in soft agar and showed only a slightly reduced serum dependence. Similarly, cultures expressing the endothelial marker OKM-5 were not tumorigenic in nude mice (Delli-Bovi *et al.*, 1986).

Cell cultures of smooth muscle origin do not induce Kaposi's sarcoma-like lesions *in vivo* but are capable of local invasion in muscle organ cultures and through artificial basal membranes (Albini *et al.*, 1988; Wittek *et al.*, 1991). The reason for these differences is not clear but may be linked to differences in the cytokine profile secreted by these different cultures (see below).

(c) *Growth factors involved in the proliferation of spindle cells*

Extensive work by several laboratories has examined the role that lymphokines might play during the development of Kaposi's sarcoma. However, probably because of the different cell types grown by different laboratories, the findings reported are inconsistent. Fibroblast growth factors (FGFs) and platelet-derived growth factors (PDGFs) have been found to be expressed in Kaposi's sarcomas, or to be present in short-term cultures from Kaposi's sarcoma biopsies.

(i) *Fibroblast growth factors*

Basic fibroblast growth factor (bFGF) has been reported to be secreted by Kaposi's sarcoma cultures expressing endothelial cell markers and may promote the growth of these cells *in vitro* (Ensoli *et al.*, 1989). Other groups, working with Kaposi's sarcoma cultures of either an endothelial phenotype (Corbeil *et al.*, 1991) or mixed fibroblastoid/-endothelial appearance (Werner *et al.*, 1989) also found an FGF-like activity in supernatants of their Kaposi's sarcoma cultures which stimulated the growth of normal fibroblasts and endothelial cells.

Members of the FGF family, including bFGF and endothelial cell growth factor (ECFG), are known to stimulate the growth of normal endothelial cells, and cultured Kaposi's sarcoma cells with endothelial characteristics have been shown to induce transient neoangiogenesis in nude mice (Nakamura *et al.*, 1988). The FGF family of cytokines may thus play a crucial role during the development of Kaposi's sarcoma. In Kaposi's sarcoma, the expression of bFGF and FGF5 in spindle cells has been shown by in situ hybridization (Xerri *et al.*, 1991). Acidic FGF and FGF6 are also expressed in Kaposi's sarcoma (Li *et al.*, 1993b), but the technique employed in this study (RT-PCR) does not permit the identification of the cell type(s) secreting these two members of the FGF family. The importance of bFGF in the development of experimental Kaposi's sarcoma-like lesions is further supported by the report that a bFGF-specific antisense oligonucleotide can inhibit the angiogenic effect of cultured Kaposi's sarcoma cells in nude mice (Ensoli *et al.*, 1994a).

(ii) *Platelet-derived growth factor*

Normal endothelial cells (Ensoli *et al.*, 1989; Roth *et al.*, 1989) as well as short-term cultures of endothelial cells with endothelial characteristics (Ensoli *et al.*, 1989) produce PDGF. Kaposi's sarcoma cell cultures that produce PDGF thus do not require exogenous PDGF to promote proliferation (Ensoli *et al.*, 1989; Corbeil *et al.*, 1991). However, PDGF has been found to be essential for the propagation *in vitro* of Kaposi's sarcoma cells expressing the endothelial cell marker BMA 120 and capable of acidic low-density lipoprotein uptake but exhibiting fibroblast-like growth properties. These cultures were also shown to express mRNA for the receptors for PDGF-A and PDGF-B (Roth *et al.*, 1989; Werner *et al.*, 1990). Kaposi's sarcoma spindle cells express *in vivo* mRNA for PDGF-B receptor, whereas mRNAs for PDGF-A and PDGF-B were expressed on some tumour cells located in the vicinity of slit-like spaces (Stürzl *et al.*, 1992b). Taken together, these findings suggest that Kaposi's sarcoma cells related to endothelial cells produce PDGF which is required for the growth of spindle cells exhibiting at least some fibroblastoid characteristics, thus highlighting the interdependence of the different cell lineages found in Kaposi's sarcomas.

(d) *Clonality of Kaposi's sarcoma and chromosomal abnormalities*

Individual nodules of HIV-associated Kaposi's sarcoma may contain predominant clonal populations (Rabkin *et al.*, 1995b). It is unknown whether different Kaposi's sarcomas from the same patient contain the same or different clonal populations. Therefore, whether individual lesions are derived from the same (as in a metastatic lesion) or different clones is also unknown. A tumorigenic cell line established from a Kaposi's sarcoma was reported to contain a marker chromosome (Lunardi-Iskandar *et al.*, 1995b). [The Working Group noted that evidence for chromosomal anomalies in primary Kaposi's sarcoma tissue is lacking.] Some short-term cultures of Kaposi's sarcoma biopsies have been noted to contain chromosomal rearrangements, but no consistent pattern has been confirmed either in primary sporadic tumours (Ottolenghi *et al.*, 1974; Scappaticci *et al.*, 1986) or in AIDS-associated tumours (Delli-Bovi *et al.*, 1986; Alonso *et al.*, 1987; Saikevych *et al.*, 1988).

Thus, clonal populations may develop in Kaposi's sarcoma and give rise to monoclonal tumorigenic cell lines.

4.2.2 *The role of HIV-1 Tat in the development of Kaposi's sarcoma lesions*

Experimental evidence suggests that the Tat protein of HIV-1 can enhance the growth of cultured 'endothelial' Kaposi's sarcoma cells (Ensoli *et al.*, 1990; Barillari *et al.*, 1993). In this in-vitro model, Tat is thought to cooperate with bFGF to enhance Kaposi's sarcoma cell proliferation. The effect of Tat seems to be mediated by its binding to a5 a1 and aV a3 integrins via an RGD (i.e. arginine-glycine-aspartic acid) sequence element in a manner similar to, and replaceable by, their physiological ligands fibronectin and vitronectin (Barillari et al., 1993; Ensoli et al., 1994b).

Several cytokines, including tumour necrosis factor (TNF), interleukin (IL)-1 and γ-interferon, can render normal endothelial and smooth muscle cells susceptible to the growth-promoting effect of Tat (Barillari et al., 1992), possibly by increasing the expression of integrin receptors which interact with Tat (Barillari et al., 1993; Ensoli et al., 1994b). Injection of Tat into nude mice (Ensoli et al., 1994b) or immunocompetent C57/Bl mice (after incorporation into Matrigel; Albini et al., 1994) induces angiogenesis and this effect is potentiated by bFGF (Ensoli et al., 1994b) or heparin (Albini et al., 1994). The formation of Kaposi's sarcoma-like lesions induced by Tat and heparin can be inhibited by the matrix metalloproteinase inhibitor TIMP-2 (Albini et al., 1994) and Tat and bFGF act synergistically to increase the expression of collagenase IV in nude mice (Ensoli et al., 1994b). These studies suggest the involvement of tissue proteinases in the development of Kaposi's sarcoma.

Several groups have investigated the role of HIV-1 *tat* in Kaposi's sarcoma pathogenesis using transgenic mice. Vogel et al. (1988) reported the emergence of Kaposi's sarcoma-like lesions in mice transgenic for HIV-1 *tat*. Transgenic mice carrying the early region of BK virus, included in an LTR-*tat* construct, also develop Kaposi's sarcoma-like lesions in addition to other malignancies (Corallini et al., 1993) and extracellular Tat protein released by tumour cell lines derived from these animals protects them from apoptosis under conditions of serum starvation (Campioni et al., 1995). The growth-promoting effect of extracellular Tat on cultured Kaposi's sarcoma cells and endothelial cells (Ensoli et al., 1990; Barillari et al., 1992) suggests that infection by HIV-1 of cells not directly involved in the Kaposi's sarcoma lesion may be sufficient for triggering the sequence of events leading to the development of Kaposi's sarcoma. In keeping with this interpretation, in *tat*-transgenic mice which did develop Kaposi's sarcoma-like lesions, the expression of *tat* was found not in spindle cells but in neighbouring keratinocytes (Vogel et al., 1988). However, other lines of transgenic mice, carrying the complete HIV-1 genome, failed to develop similar lesions (Leonard et al., 1988).

With regard to the question of whether sufficient levels of HIV-1 Tat are present in AIDS-related Kaposi's sarcoma lesions to achieve an angiogenic effect, Ensoli et al. (1994b) claimed that HIV-1 Tat could be detected on spindle cells by histochemical techniques. They suggested that Tat originated from a few HIV-1-infected mononuclear cells infiltrating these lesions.

Thus, the ability of Tat, in concert with other growth factors, to induce vascular lesions resembling Kaposi's sarcoma has been documented in a variety of experimental systems. However, this property may not be unique to HIV-1 infection, as supernatants from T-cell lines infected with HTLV-II have been shown to induce the propagation of Kaposi's sarcoma-derived cells *in vitro*. The lymphokine responsible for this growth-enhancing effect has been identified as oncostatin M (Nakamura et al., 1988; Miles et al., 1992; Nair et al., 1992). This suggests that infection by other human retroviruses can lead to the production of lymphokines which promote the growth of cells found in Kaposi's sarcomas. Since some non-human retroviruses have been shown to induce

Kaposi's sarcoma-like lesions in several animal models (see Section 4.2.3), and since mice transgenic for the middle T gene of polyomavirus develop endothelial cell tumours (Bautch et al., 1987), it is conceivable that various microorganisms could initiate such a cascade of events.

4.2.3 *An infectious agent as a cause of Kaposi's sarcoma*

Extensive epidemiological studies, reviewed in Section 2.1, suggest the involvement in the pathogenesis of Kaposi's sarcoma of an agent which can be transmitted sexually, although not exclusively so.

There is no convincing evidence to associate cytomegalovirus, HHV-6, papillomaviruses, hepatitis B virus (IARC, 1994), *Mycoplasma fermentans* or *M. penetrans* with Kaposi's sarcoma.

In the last two decades, several laboratories have either observed or tried to isolate viruses from Kaposi's sarcomas. Giraldo et al. (1972) reported the presence of herpes-like viruses in short-term cultures from Kaposi's sarcoma biopsies. The identity of these particles has never been satisfactorily established. Occasional herpes viral particles have also been seen in Kaposi's sarcoma tissue sections (Walter et al., 1984).

C-Type retroviruses were detected in Kaposi's sarcoma biopsies from a group of HIV-negative Kaposi's sarcoma patients from a distinct region of the southern Peloponnese in Greece (Rappersberger et al., 1991). Some of the clinical features of the disease in this group of patients (involvement of oral and genital mucosa and gastrointestinal tract; extensive involvement of facial skin) were reminiscent of African or AIDS-associated Kaposi's sarcoma rather than 'classical' Kaposi's sarcoma. Retroviral particles have also been found in Kaposi's sarcoma biopsies from patients with AIDS (Gyorkey et al., 1984; Schenk, 1986). It is possible that these particles represented HIV-1.

As discussed in Section 3.2.3, there is no really good animal model for Kaposi's sarcoma. However, several animal models have provided indirect evidence supporting a possible role of retroviruses in the pathogenesis of Kaposi's sarcoma. Macaque monkeys infected with the D-type simian retrovirus type 2 (SRV-2) develop retroperitoneal and subcutaneous fibrosis with progressive fibrovascular proliferation, reminiscent of Kaposi's sarcoma lesions (Tsai et al., 1995). Cell cultures established from these lesions induced self-limited, transient spindle cell proliferation, accompanied by pronounced vascularization, when inoculated into nude mice. In fowl, some strains of avian leukosis virus can induce, in addition to lymphoma, disseminated haemangiomatosis characterized by a progression from early patch-like lesions with predominant endothelial cell proliferation to haemangiosarcoma (Victor & Jarplid, 1988). In BALB/c mice, a strain of Moloney murine sarcoma virus (MMSV 349), containing the *mos* oncogene, induces lesions that resemble human Kaposi's sarcoma on the basis of both histopathology and electron microscopy. The *mos* oncogene does not seem to be sufficient to induce these lesions, as another strain of MMSV, also containing the *mos* oncogene, does not induce similar lesions (Stoica et al., 1990).

In addition to some HIV-1 *tat* transgenic mice which develop Kaposi's sarcoma-like lesions (see Section 4.2.2), mice transgenic for the middle T antigen of polyomavirus develop endothelial tumours (Bautch *et al.*, 1987). These reports indicate that a variety of infectious agents or their proteins can induce vascular proliferation which bears some resemblance to Kaposi's sarcoma lesions. Yet it is difficult to extrapolate from these animal models to a candidate for an infectious agent involved in the pathogenesis of human Kaposi's sarcoma.

4.2.4 *The role of human herpesvirus 8*

A new human γ-herpesvirus (HHV-8), also termed Kaposi's sarcoma herpesvirus (KSHV), has been discovered in AIDS-associated Kaposi's sarcoma biopsies (Chang *et al.*, 1994) and is a strong candidate for the 'Kaposi's sarcoma agent' (see Section 2.1.5).

(*a*) *Genomic organization and relationship to other primate herpesviruses*

HHV-8 belongs to the γ_2 subgroup of herpesviruses and is most closely related to herpesvirus saimiri, a T-lymphotropic herpesvirus with transforming potential, found in squirrel monkeys (*Saimiri sciureus*) (Moore *et al.*, 1996). Several of the HHV-8 structural genes show significant levels of sequence homology to the corresponding genes of herpesvirus saimiri, but also to those of the slightly more distantly related EBV, and the organization of a 20 kb central segment of the HHV-8 genome is highly similar to that of these other two γ-herpesviruses (Moore *et al.*, 1996). In addition, HHV-8 contains a homologue of the human *cyclin D* gene and a member of the family of six-protein coupled receptors (Cesarman *et al.*, 1995). The HHV-8 cyclin homologue has been shown to be active in abrogating the function of the retinoblastoma tumour-suppressor protein and could thus be involved in dysregulating cellular proliferation or differentiation.

(*b*) *In-vivo tropism and association with Kaposi's sarcoma*

As described in Section 2.1.5, HHV-8 is consistently found in the vast majority (> 95%) of biopsies from all epidemiological forms of Kaposi's sarcoma, i.e. AIDS-associated Kaposi's sarcoma, classical Mediterranean Kaposi's sarcoma, post-transplant Kaposi's sarcoma and African endemic Kaposi's sarcoma (see Table 15).

HHV-8 has been found by PCR in-situ hybridization in the flat endothelial cells lining ectatic vascular spaces, as well as in spindle cells of Kaposi's sarcoma lesions (Boshoff *et al.*, 1995b). These two cell types represent the bulk of the lesion and this observation is therefore compatible with an important etiopathological role of HHV-8 in the development of Kaposi's sarcoma.

However, primary cultures established from fresh Kaposi's sarcoma biopsies lose HHV-8 after a few passages, and established Kaposi's sarcoma cell cultures, including permanent cell lines (see above) are negative for this virus (Ambroziak *et al.*, 1995; Lebbé *et al.*, 1995). The implications of this observation are unclear.

Therefore, it is possible that the murine angioproliferative lesions induced by Kaposi's sarcoma cell cultures in nude mice are not an adequate model for Kaposi's sarcoma. However, it is also possible that HHV-8 is not required for the development of Kaposi's sarcoma *in vivo* and may only infect and/or replicate preferentially in already established Kaposi's sarcoma endothelial or spindle cells.

In peripheral blood of HIV-infected individuals, HHV-8 is present in B-cells (Ambroziak *et al.*, 1995) and its detection correlates inversely with the number of $CD4^+$ T-cells, suggesting that its replication is under immunological control (Whitby *et al.*, 1995).

Thus, the available evidence suggests that HHV-8 is a strong candidate for the long-sought 'Kaposi's sarcoma agent', but its precise role and epidemiology remain to be established.

4.3 Non-Hodgkin's lymphomas and other lymphoproliferative disorders

As discussed in Sections 2.2 and 2.3.3 and listed in Table 16, the incidence of several types of lymphoproliferative disease is increased in HIV-infected patients.

4.3.1 *Pathological models of lymphomagenesis*

The biological basis and molecular genetics underlying the pathogenesis of AIDS-related non-Hodgkin's lymphomas and other lymphoproliferative disorders (Hodgkin's disease and multicentric Castleman's disease) are not well understood. Several pathological conditions seem to contribute to AIDS-related lymphomagenesis: immunosuppression, dysregulation of cytokine loops, accumulation of genetic lesions within the proliferating clones and infection by viruses (reviewed by Knowles, 1993; Gaidano & Carbone, 1995). These contributory factors may act at different stages of a proposed multistage model of lymphomagenesis (Pelicci *et al.*, 1986; Feichtinger *et al.*, 1992a; Gaidano & Dalla-Favera, 1992; Knowles, 1993; Gaidano *et al.*, 1994a; Herndier *et al.*, 1994b).

The development of AIDS-related non-Hodgkin's lymphoma is often preceded by polyclonal hypergammaglobulinaemia and persistent generalized lymphadenopathy (PGL) (Carbone *et al.*, 1991; Raphael *et al.*, 1991); furthermore, chromosomal abnormalities (Alonso *et al.*, 1987) and oligoclonal immunoglobulin gene rearrangements are detectable in a fraction of these HIV-associated lymphadenopathies (Pelicci *et al.*, 1986; Carbone *et al.*, 1989). Unlike PGL, AIDS-related non-Hodgkin's lymphoma is usually monoclonal and is characterized by a number of molecular alterations of dominantly-acting oncogenes and of tumour-suppressor genes (Ballerini *et al.*, 1993; Gaidano *et al.*, 1993). According to this model of lymphomagenesis, the emergence of oligoclonal B-cell expansions representing a pre-malignant condition is at first driven by several factors including immune dysregulation and viral infections. This phase clinically and pathologically corresponds to PGL. In subsequent phases, the neoplastic transformation of a B-cell clone is due to the accumulation of genetic lesions which eventually transform the clone developing the non-Hodgkin's lymphoma (Figures 10–12). The

Figure 10. Schematic representation of follicle disruption during the course of HIV infection, showing the progression from follicular hyperplasia to follicular involution

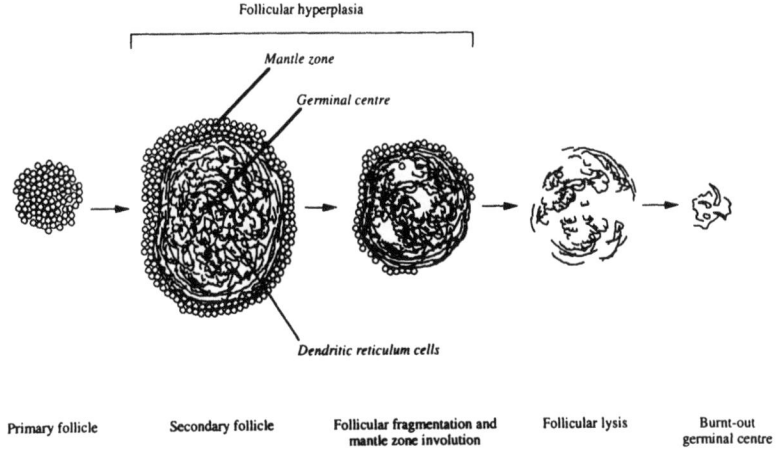

Figure 11. Genetic lesions contributing to pathogenesis of AIDS-related small non-cleaved-cell lymphoma

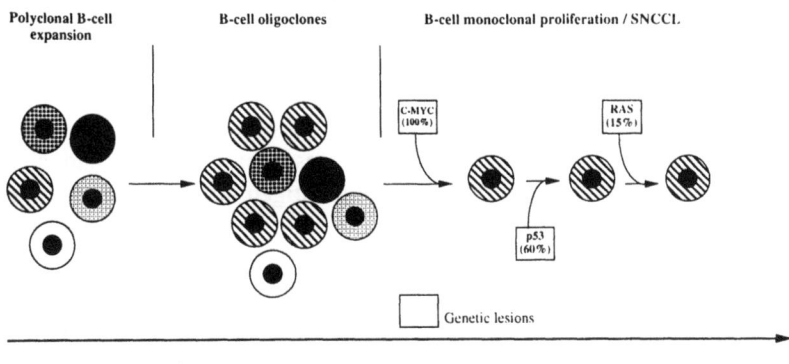

Adapted from Gaidano et al. (1994a)
SNCCL, small non-cleaved cell lymphoma

complex pathophysiological milieu of HIV infection is obviously of importance in the pathogenesis of AIDS-related lymphomas. Morphological, immunopathological, molecular and cytogenetic analyses of the pathological changes in lymphoid tissues during HIV infection have improved the understanding of the mechanisms leading to lymphoma onset and progression.

Figure 12. Genetic lesions contributing to the pathogenesis of AIDS-related diffuse large-cell lymphoma

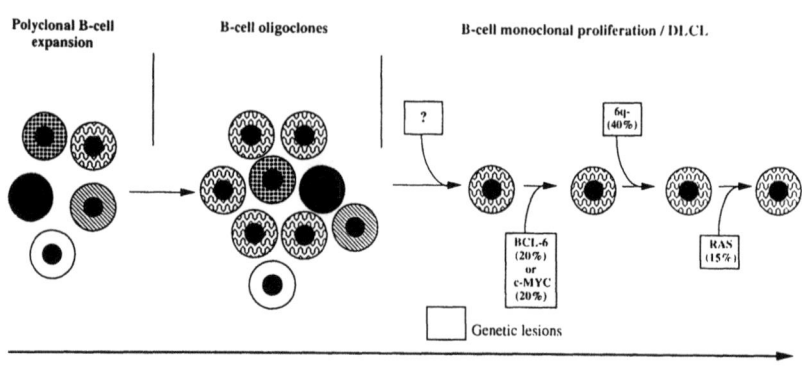

Adapted from Gaidano et al. (1994a)
DLCL, diffuse large-cell lymphoma

As depicted in Figures 11 and 12, three biological stages in the development of B-cell lymphoma can be distinguished: (a) polyclonal B-cell hyperplasia; (b) oligoclonal expansion and (c) genetic changes. Combination of these factors leads to the eventual emergence of monoclonal lymphoma.

(a) *HIV infection of lymphoid tissue and polyclonal B-cell hyperplasia*

A critical event in initiating and establishing HIV infection is the localization of HIV in lymphoid organs which become the major reservoirs of HIV and sites of viral replication (Fox et al., 1991). Viral particles and antigen become trapped on the surface of the web-like processes of the follicular dendritic cells which permeate the germinal centres. These cells then expand to form the core of the lymphoid tissue (Biberfeld et al., 1985; Tenner-Rácz et al., 1985; Pantaleo et al., 1993a,b). Persistence of virus in lymphoid organs causes chronic stimulation of the immune system which ultimately leads to degeneration of the follicles (reviewed by Pantaleo & Fauci, 1995). Morphological analyses at different stages of HIV infection have demonstrated that lymphoid tissues undergo progressive destruction and depletion of B-cell areas as the disease advances (Biberfeld et al., 1985, 1987; Ioachim et al., 1990; Fox et al., 1991). The severe immunosuppression at advanced stages of disease is one of the functional consequences of this process (reviewed by Pantaleo & Fauci, 1995). In contrast, lymph-node architecture and immune function appear to be intact in some HIV-infected individuals who remain free of disease for many years (Pantaleo et al., 1995).

(i) *Pathological changes in HIV-infected lymphoid follicles*

The lymph nodes in HIV-infected patients with PGL have been extensively studied both histologically and immunophenotypically (Ioachim *et al.*, 1983; Baroni *et al.*, 1985; Janossy *et al.*, 1985; Wood *et al.*, 1985; Carbone *et al.*, 1986; Wood *et al.*, 1986). The first lymphadenopathic change is follicular hyperplasia (Biberfeld *et al.*, 1985), which is the expansion of the germinal centre by recruitment, proliferation and differentiation of antigen-reactive B-cells (follicular hyperplasia). Morphologically, follicles appear to be increased in size and number and show a marked variation in shape and irregular marginal zones. By immunohistochemical methods, a colocalization of HIV p24 antigen with follicular dendritic cells is clearly visible in the secondary germinal centres (Biberfeld *et al.*, 1985; Baroni *et al.*, 1986). Follicular fragmentation, which may represent an early degenerative change, can be perceived as a disruption of the dendritic reticulum of the germinal centre (Biberfeld *et al.*, 1985). Also, the follicular mantle zones become progressively reduced (Wood *et al.*, 1985). Such follicular changes in lymph nodes have also been detected in mucosal, 'hypertrophic' nasopharyngeal lymphoid tissue (Barzan *et al.*, 1989; Shahab *et al.*, 1994). Nasopharyngeal lymphoid tissue 'hypertrophy', often associated with PGL (Barzan *et al.*, 1990), is apparently linked to the early phase of HIV infection in the same way as follicular hyperplasia is in PGL (Carbone *et al.*, 1995b).

As HIV disease progresses, germinal centres show a reduction in the number of $CD4^+$ T-lymphocytes and an increase in the percentage of $CD8^+$ T-cells (Modlin *et al.*, 1983b; Said *et al.*, 1984; Carbone *et al.*, 1985; Biberfeld *et al.*, 1986), reflecting the decrease in $CD4^+ : CD8^+$ lymphocyte ratio of peripheral blood. The destruction of the follicular dendritic cell network and the collapse of the germinal centres become increasingly evident (the so-called burning-out phenomenon) (Biberfeld *et al.*, 1985). Follicular involution is characterized by hypervascularity, with small follicles resembling those seen in multicentric Castleman's disease. Germinal centres are small and show hyalinization and fibrosis (Figure 10).

These pathological changes, ranging from follicular hyperplasia to follicular involution, usually involve most lymphoid tissue, including tonsils, abdominal lymph nodes and spleen (Burke *et al.*, 1993).

(ii) *Destruction of follicular centres and B-cell hyperplasia*

It has been suggested that abnormal B-cell proliferation takes place when follicular architecture is disrupted by HIV (Armstrong & Horne, 1984; Tenner-Rácz *et al.*, 1985; Feichtinger *et al.*, 1992a). According to one version of this hypothesis, the destruction of follicular dendritic cells interferes with apoptosis and allows the proliferation of B-cell clones expressing low-avidity cell surface immunoglobulin (Herndier *et al.*, 1994b). Another aspect is the dissemination of follicular dendritic cells outside of lymphoid tissue, which could permit the formation of germinal centres in non-lymphoid tissue from which a polyclonal B-cell proliferation and B-cell lymphoma would emerge (Feichtinger *et al.*, 1992a; Herndier *et al.*, 1994b).

(iii) *Chronic antigen stimulation*

Chronic antigen stimulation, pathologically observed as florid B-cell hyperplasia, has been postulated to be a key factor in Burkitt's lymphoma pathogenesis in patients with AIDS (reviewed by Karp & Broder, 1992). Evidence for this is the finding that AIDS-related Burkitt's lymphomas frequently produce antibodies directed against self antigens; furthermore, the hypervariable regions of the immunoglobulin genes utilized by AIDS-related Burkitt's lymphoma carry somatic mutations, which may have been selected by antigen stimulation (Ng *et al.*, 1994; Riboldi *et al.*, 1994). Together, these data suggest that a process of B-cell clonal selection is involved in AIDS lymphomagenesis.

(iv) *Presence of HIV in tumour cells*

Tumours from AIDS-related non-Hodgkin's lymphoma are almost all of B-cell origin. In these tumours, HIV has not been detected in the B-lymphocytes. For example, Morgello (1992) reported a series of 12 primary central nervous system lymphomas from New York, United States. None was positive for HIV *gag* sequences by the sensitive technique of PCR. Similarly, Cornford *et al.* (1991) studied the immunohistochemical localization of HIV in seven cases of central nervous system lymphoma in Los Angeles, CA, United States. While they detected HIV near the mass lesions in five (70%) of the cases, in no instance was HIV detected within the neoplastic lymphoid cells themselves.

Insertional mutagenesis with a direct role of HIV has been proposed to explain some cases of AIDS-related non-Hodgkin's lymphoma. Shiramizu *et al.* (1994) reported four cases that had HIV clonally integrated in the tumour. In one case of T-cell immunophenotype, HIV was detectable in T-cells by anti-p24 immunostaining. The other three cases having a B-, T- or null phenotype contained a large histiocytic reactive component; HIV was localized to these reactive cells. All four cases were reported to have a common integration site of HIV upstream from the c-*fes/fps* proto-oncogene, which suggested an insertional mutagenesis role for HIV in a subset of AIDS-related lymphomas.

In another study, it was also suggested that HIV could play a direct role in B-cell transformation. This was based on the increased proliferation *in vitro* of B-lymphocytes dually infected with HIV and EBV (Laurence & Astrin, 1991). In addition, Astrin *et al.* (1992) reported detection by PCR of, on average, one HIV proviral DNA copy per cell in B-lymphoma tissue, but did not observe monoclonal integration of HIV DNA in B-lymphoma cells. These results therefore fall short of confirming a direct oncogenic effect of HIV in B-cells.

Indeed, consistent failure to detect HIV sequences unequivocally within the tumour clone has suggested that HIV is not directly involved in the development of malignancy (reviewed by Knowles, 1993).

(b) *Oligoclonal B-cell proliferation*

Three main groups of cofactors, cytokines, lymphotropic viruses and genetic changes, are thought to be involved during the transition from polyclonal B-cell proliferation to the expansion of oligoclonal B-cell populations.

(i) *Immunosuppression*

As for some other cancers in AIDS, immunosuppression also predisposes to the frequent development of B-cell lymphoma (reviewed by Gaidano & Dalla Favera, 1992; Karp & Broder, 1992).

The relation between immunosuppression and the development of lymphoma is recognized in several clinical conditions other than AIDS, including congenital and iatrogenic immunodeficiencies (Frizzera, 1994) (see Sections 2.2.1 and 4.1.3). The relative risk for AIDS-related non-Hodgkin's lymphoma increases with progressive immune dysfunction (Section 2.2.1) (Pluda et al., 1993). Immunosurveillance is known to play an important role in controlling the replication of EBV-infected B-lymphocytes in humans (Rickinson et al., 1992). The specific importance of cytotoxic T-lymphocytes (CTLs) in the control of virus-associated lymphoproliferative disease in immunosuppression has been demonstrated in animal studies by Boyle et al. (1993). They showed that EBV-specific CTLs adaptively transferred into SCID mice engrafted with EBV-transformed and immortalized B-lymphoblastoid cell lines delayed or prevented the development of B-cell lymphomas. In another study, five patients who developed EBV-associated lymphoproliferative disease following bone marrow transplantation were given infusions of leukocytes from the original donors. The proliferating cells were of donor cell origin and contained EBV DNA which was clonally integrated in two out of the three cases adequate for study. Since the lymphoproliferation derived from donor cells, the leukocytes included EBV-sensitized CTLs. Complete responses, pathological or clinical, were sustained in the three surviving patients (Papadopoulos et al., 1994). EBV-specific CTLs are now generated in some clinical centres for the prevention and treatment of EBV-associated lymphoproliferative disease or treatment of organ transplant recipients (Smith et al., 1995). The impaired immunosurveillance in AIDS patients may give rise to the oligoclonal B-cell expansion seen in PGL (Birx et al., 1986). Consistently, one third of hyperplastic lymph nodes from HIV-infected individuals with PGL contain EBV-positive clones (Shibata et al., 1991). The presence of EBV-containing B-cell clones in PGL correlates with the simultaneous occurrence or subsequent development of EBV-containing non-Hodgkin's lymphoma (Shibata et al., 1991). However, Dolcetti et al. (1995) only rarely observed monoclonal EBV episomes in PGL samples with a high content of EBV-infected cells.

(ii) *Cytokines*

Dysregulation of the normal 'steady-state' cytokine network is a key feature of HIV infection (Fauci et al., 1991). However, data regarding the role of cytokines in AIDS-related lymphomagenesis are restricted to IL-6 and IL-10.

IL-6

The role of IL-6 is schematically depicted in Figure 13. IL-6 may be particularly important to both pre-malignant polyclonal B-cell expansion and malignant transformation.

Monocytes appear to be responsible for the major portion of IL-6 produced by PBMCs isolated from HIV-infected individuals (Birx et al., 1990). The production of

IL-6 by HIV-infected monocytes promotes the proliferation of B-cells activated by, for example, EBV, thereby driving immunoglobulin synthesis and causing the non-specific hyperimmunoglobulinaemia commonly seen in early HIV infection (Birx *et al.*, 1986, 1990). Therefore, IL-6 excess in HIV infection seems to contribute to B-cell hyperstimulation and to hypergammaglobulinaemia (reviewed by Martínez-Maza, 1992) (Figure 13). Moreover, AIDS-related large-cell lymphomas containing a high proportion of immunoblasts express high levels of IL-6 (Emilie *et al.*, 1992). This finding is consistent with the role of IL-6 in the terminal differentiation of B cells. Further evidence linking IL-6 to AIDS-related lymphomagenesis is that HIV-infected patients with elevated serum levels of IL-6 are at high risk for later developing large-cell lymphomas (Pluda *et al.*, 1993). It has also been suggested that, once the lymphoma is well established, continuous tumour growth may be sustained by IL-6 through paracrine loops (Emilie *et al.*, 1992). Thus, IL-6 could contribute to lymphomagenesis either by acting as a chronic stimulus to B cells in HIV-infected people and/or, more directly, as an autocrine or paracrine growth factor for lymphoma cells (Martínez-Maza, 1992).

Figure 13. Potential role of IL-6 in AIDS-related lymphomagenesis

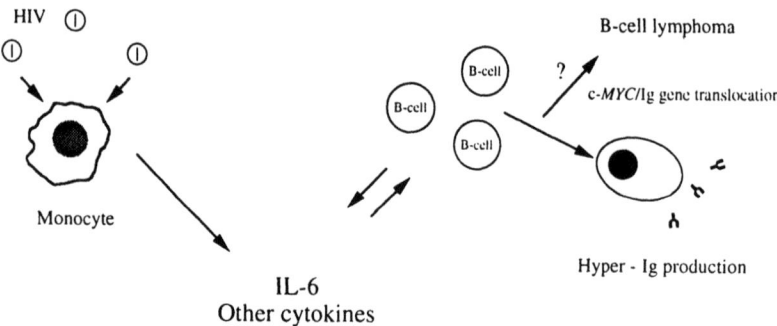

Contact between monocytes and HIV can cause IL-6 production. This increased IL-6 production could then induce B-cell hyperstimulation (hypergammaglobulinaemia) and, possibly, B-cell lymphoma.
Adapted from Martínez-Maza (1992)

An environment of dysregulated cytokines may also play a role in the pathogenesis of AIDS-related body cavity-based lymphomas that usually contain HHV-8 gene sequences. A recent study has demonstrated that IL-6 and IL-10 levels in lymphomatous effusions are much higher than those in normal plasma (Ng *et al.*, 1995). IL-6 protein has also been found in multicentric Castleman's disease (Yoshizaki *et al.*, 1989), another HHV-8-associated lymphoproliferative disorder (Soulier *et al.*, 1995). However, the functional relationship between IL-6 and HHV-8 needs to be clarified further (Levy, 1995).

In conclusion, it is clear that IL-6 is involved in B-cell lymphocyte expansion and could be involved at any stage during the development of B-cell lymphomas (Figure 13).

IL-10

IL-10, a potent B-cell stimulator, is a pleotropic cytokine sharing significant homology with the EBV protein BCRF1. Although the precise role of IL-10 in the development of AIDS-related lymphomagenesis is still unclear, a possible involvement is suggested by the finding that high levels of IL-10 are constitutively expressed by EBV-positive B-cell lines derived from patients with AIDS-related small non-cleaved-cell lymphoma (Benjamin *et al.*, 1992). Furthermore, an autocrine growth mechanism involving IL-10 can occur in AIDS-related lymphoma cells (Masood *et al.*, 1995).

(c) *Genetic abnormalities*

Various genetic abnormalities have been found in AIDS-related non-Hodgkin's lymphoma (Ballerini *et al.*, 1993; Gaidano *et al.*, 1993) (see Table 32 and Figures 11 and 12).

Table 32. Frequency of genetic lesions in AIDS-related non-Hodgkin's lymphomas

Histology	c-*myc*	p53	BCL-6	6q deletions	ras	EBV	HHV-8
Small non-cleaved-cell lymphomas (Ballerini *et al.*, 1993; Hamilton-Dutoit *et al.*, 1993a; Gaidano *et al.*, 1994b; Cesarman *et al.*, 1995; Carbone *et al.*, 1996b; Pastore *et al.*, 1996)[a]	100%	60%	Neg.	Neg.	15%	30%	Neg.
Diffuse large B-cell lymphomas (Ballerini *et al.*, 1993; Hamilton-Dutoit *et al.*, 1993a; Gaidano *et al.*, 1994b; Cesarman *et al.*, 1995; Pastore *et al.*, 1996)	20%	Neg.	20%	40%	15%	80%	Neg.
Anaplastic large-cell (CD30/Ki-1$^+$) lymphomas (Carbone *et al.*, 1993b; Chadburn *et al.*, 1993; Cesarman *et al.*, 1995; Carbone *et al.*, 1996b; Pastore *et al.*, 1996)	Neg.	Neg.	ND	Neg.	ND	90%	Neg.
Body cavity-based lymphomas (Cesarman *et al.*, 1995; Carbone *et al.*, 1996a)	Neg.	Neg.	ND	ND	Neg.	> 50%	> 70%

ND, not done
[a] Chromosome 1q abnormalities have been detected in AIDS-related small non-cleaved-cell lymphomas (Bernheim & Berger, 1988; Polito *et al.*, 1995)

(i) *c*-myc

Several reports have pointed to an association of AIDS-related non-Hodgkin's lymphoma with chromosomal translocations involving the c-*myc* oncogene. Activation of c-*myc* has been detected in 100% of AIDS-related small non-cleaved-cell lymphomas, including Burkitt's lymphoma (Figures 11 and 14). In diffuse large-cell lymphomas including large non-cleaved-cell lymphomas and large-cell immunoblastic plasmacytoid lymphomas, activation is restricted to a minority (approximately 20%) of tumours (Ballerini *et al.*, 1993; Delecluse *et al.*, 1993; Bhathia *et al.*, 1994). Tumours with an intermediate morphology between small non-cleaved-cell and large-cell immunoblastic lymphomas have been shown to harbour a c-*myc* rearrangement. This finding is consistent with the notion that such a tumour may represent a small non-cleaved-cell lymphoma that has adopted an immunoblastic morphotype in the context of AIDS (Delecluse *et al.*, 1993). In contrast, no AIDS-related anaplastic large-cell lymphoma or body cavity-based lymphoma has shown c-*myc* alterations (Chadburn *et al.*, 1993; Cesarman *et al.*, 1995).

As in sporadic Burkitt's lymphoma, c-*myc* activation in AIDS-related non-Hodgkin's lymphoma occurs through gene rearrangements following chromosomal translocations between 8q24, the site of the c-*myc* proto-oncogene, and an immunoglobulin chromosomal locus, most commonly the immunoglobulin heavy-chain genes at 14q32 (Chaganti *et al.*, 1983). B-lymphocyte clones harbouring similar translocations can persist and be detected in peripheral blood of lymphoma-free HIV-positive homosexual men but are rare in HIV-negative controls (Müller *et al.*, 1995).

(ii) BCL-6

Chromosomal translocations in AIDS-related non-Hodgkin's lymphoma also involve *BCL*-6, a proto-oncogene affecting B-cell maturation, that maps to 3q27 (Ye *et al.*, 1993). Gross rearrangements of *BCL*-6 are mostly associated with AIDS-related diffuse large-cell lymphomas (20%) (Figures 12 and 15), and are consistently absent in AIDS-related small non-cleaved-cell lymphomas. This is similar to the chromosomal aberrations seen in the same histological subtypes of non-HIV-related non-Hodgkin's lymphoma. In diffuse large-cell lymphoma, gross rearrangements of *BCL*-6 and of c-*myc* appear to be mutually exclusive genetic lesions (Gaidano *et al.*, 1994b).

(iii) ras

Other dominantly acting oncogenes commonly involved in the pathogenesis of lymphomas in immunocompetent hosts (e.g., *BCL*-1, *BCL*-2) do not seem to play a role in AIDS-related lymphomagenesis (reviewed by Gaidano & Dalla-Favera, 1992). On the other hand, mutations of K-*ras* or N-*ras* genes, which have not been detected in B-cell non-Hodgkin's lymphoma of immunocompetent hosts, were present in 4/27 (15%) of AIDS-related non-Hodgkin's lymphoma (Ballerini *et al.*, 1993).

(iv) p53

A role of tumour-suppressor gene inactivation in AIDS-related lymphomagenesis is supported by a number of observations. Mutations and/or losses of *p53* have been found in 60% of AIDS-related small non-cleaved-cell lymphomas (Ballerini *et al.*, 1993; Gaidano *et al.*, 1993), but not in the other types of AIDS-related non-Hodgkin's lymphoma (Gaidano *et al.*, 1991; Ballerini *et al.*, 1993; De Re *et al.*, 1994). In the small non-cleaved-cell lymphomas series examined (Ballerini *et al.*, 1993), *p53* mutations were

Figure 14

Small non-cleaved-cell lymphoma

Small non-cleaved-cell lymphoma with plasma cell differentiation

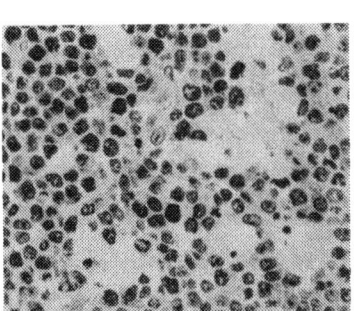

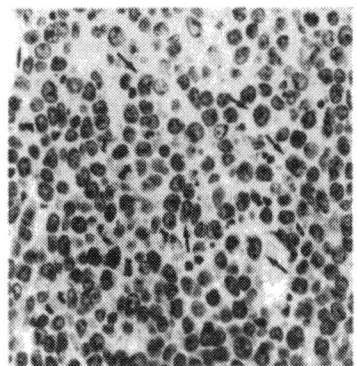

The tumour is composed of small to medium-sized monomorphic cohesive cells interspersed with large phagocytosine histiocytes (starry sky pattern). Haematoxylin–eosin, × 400

Tumour cells have round or irregular, frequently eccentric, nuclei containing randomly located nucleoli. Larger basophilic cells with large nucleoli are recognizable (arrows). Haematoxylin–eosin, × 400

Figure 15. Diffuse large-cell lymphoma of the immunoblastic type with plasmacytic features

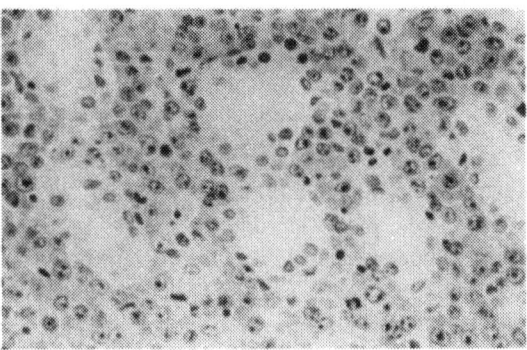

Gastric involvement by diffuse large-cell lymphoma of the immunoblastic type with plasmacytic features. Most tumour cells have large, solitary nucleoli. In this field mucosal glandular epithelium is surrounded, but not destroyed, by tumour growth. Haematoxylin–eosin, × 400.

seen only in tumours carrying a rearranged c-*myc* gene. p53 protein overexpression was observed in 3/3 lymphomas with a morphology intermediate between small non-cleaved-cell and large-cell immunoblastic lymphomas. It is unknown whether this overexpression was due to *p53* mutations (Carbone *et al.*, 1995b).

Little is known about the frequency of *p53* aberrations in anaplastic large-cell lymphomas. In contrast to small non-cleaved cell lymphoma, AIDS-related anaplastic large-cell lymphoma has been reported not to contain *p53* mutations, but accumulation of wild-type p53 protein has been observed by immunohistochemistry (Inghirami *et al.*, 1994; Carbone *et al.*, 1996b), as reported previously for this type of lymphoma in immunocompetent hosts (Cesarman *et al.*, 1993).

(v) *6q deletions*

Deletions of the long arm of chromosome 6 at band q27 occur in non-Hodgkin's lymphoma (both AIDS-related and -unrelated) and represent the putative site of a distinct tumour-suppressor gene. 6q deletions among AIDS-related non-Hodgkin's lymphoma were restricted to diffuse large-cell lymphomas (5/13 cases) (Pastore *et al.*, 1996), whereas, among non-Hodgkin's lymphoma in immunocompetent hosts, 6q deletions occur throughout the entire histological spectrum, including both diffuse large-cell and small non-cleaved-cell lymphomas (Gaidano *et al.*, 1992).

(vi) *Chromosome 1q abnormalities*

In AIDS-related small non-cleaved-cell lymphomas, structural changes of chromosome 1 have been found (Bernheim & Berger, 1988). Cell lines derived from such tumours have also been found to contain chromosome 1q abnormalities (Polito *et al.*, 1995). These chromosomal changes are very similar to those previously detected in AIDS-unrelated small non-cleaved-cell lymphomas or cell lines (Gurtsevitch *et al.*, 1988; Kornblau *et al.*, 1991). Owing to its very frequent involvement, chromosome 1q 21-25 is a site that should be examined in greater detail for genetic alterations that may play a pathogenetic role in small non-cleaved-cell lymphomas (Polito *et al.*, 1995).

4.3.2 *Lymphotropic viruses*

(a) *EBV*

EBV appears to play an important role in the development of some AIDS-related non-Hodgkin's lymphoma (Knowles, 1993; Herndier *et al.*, 1994b; Rabkin, 1994). The best evidence so far for its pathogenetic role is the ability of EBV-infected B cells to cause EBV-positive B-cell lymphomas in SCID mice (Mosier *et al.*, 1989; Rowe *et al.*, 1991). Other studies have demonstrated that the introduction of activated c-*myc* genes into EBV-transformed lymphoblasts confers tumorigenicity in nude mice (Lombardi *et al.*, 1987).

HIV-infected individuals possess abnormally high numbers of circulating EBV-infected B cells (Birx *et al.*, 1986). Moreover, EBV infection precedes the expansion of the tumour clone (Neri *et al.*, 1991), and a large fraction (see below) of AIDS-related non-Hodgkin's lymphoma cells contain EBV sequences and express at least some EBV latent proteins known to have transforming properties (Hamilton-Dutoit et al., 1989; Ballerini et al., 1993; Hamilton-Dutoit et al., 1993b).

It is likely that HIV-related immunosuppression permits the development of EBV-infected and immortalized B-cell clones. Such clones are susceptible to further genetic alterations resulting in the development of an EBV-containing monoclonal lymphoproliferation (Pelicci et al., 1986).

The frequency of EBV infection in AIDS-related non-Hodgkin's lymphoma has been a matter of controversy (reviewed by Gaidano et al., 1994a; Shibata, 1994). Discrepancies may depend on the different methods used for viral detection (Southern blot, PCR or in-situ hybridization) and on the different histological types or sites of disease investigated.

In contrast to systemic non-Hodgkin's lymphoma, AIDS-associated primary lymphomas of the central nervous system were positive for EBV in most studies (MacMahon et al., 1991; Hamilton-Dutoit et al., 1993a; Camilleri-Broët et al., 1995; Cinque et al., 1993) (see Table 20). However, Gunthel et al. (1994) reported a few primary lymphomas of the central nervous system that were negative for EBV by a sensitive PCR assay. Almost all lymphomas primarily involving body cavities contain clonal EBV genome (Knowles et al., 1989; Cesarman et al., 1995).

Most molecular studies have indicated that the presence of EBV within systemic AIDS-related non-Hodgkin's lymphoma varies according to the histopathological type (Table 21). EBV infection is found in the majority of diffuse large-cell lymphomas, particularly in the large-cell immunoblastic lymphoma subtype (80%), but in a much smaller fraction (30–50%) of small non-cleaved-cell lymphomas (Hamilton-Dutoit et al., 1991; Ballerini et al., 1993). A high frequency of EBV association has been shown in anaplastic large-cell lymphoma (80–90%) and Hodgkin's disease (90–100%) tissues from AIDS patients (Carbone et al., 1993a; Hamilton-Dutoit et al., 1993a; Tirelli et al., 1995b). The EBV genomes in such cases have been reported to be episomal and clonal (Boiocchi et al., 1993a), even when detected in multiple, independent lesions (Boiocchi et al., 1993b).

There are two EBV subtypes which differ in the genomic region encoding the EBV nuclear antigen-2 (EBNA-2) (Adldinger et al., 1985). Type 1 EBV is a more potent lymphocyte transformer than type 2 (Rickinson et al., 1987). While type 2 virus rarely occurs in immunocompetent hosts in developed countries, it is found in a much higher proportion of subjects with HIV-related immunosuppression. The elevated frequency of type 2 virus in AIDS-related lymphoproliferative diseases appears to mirror the excess seen in HIV-infected subjects without such disease (Boyle et al., 1991, 1993; De Re et al., 1993).

A role of EBV in the pathogenesis of AIDS-related non-Hodgkin's lymphoma is further supported by data showing that the EBV-transforming proteins, EBV-encoded latent membrane protein-1 (LMP-1) and/or EBNA-2 may be expressed in EBV-positive cases.

Expression of LMP-1 has been detected in AIDS-related lymphomas of various localizations and histological types. In primary AIDS-related immunoblastic lymphomas of the central nervous system, 10/11 (90%) of tumours expressed LMP-1 and 21/57 (54%) expressed EBNA-2, as assessed by immunohistochemistry. Expression of both *BCL*-2 and LMP-1 in EBV-positive AIDS-related primary brain lymphomas *in vivo* has been described (Camilleri-Broët *et al.*, 1995). This is in agreement with in-vitro findings showing that *BCL*-2 can be transactivated by LMP-1 in small non-cleaved-cell lymphoma cell lines. Also, *BCL*-2 expression induced by LMP-1 may protect tumour B cells from apoptosis and lead to a higher proliferative rate (Henderson *et al.*, 1991; Finke *et al.*, 1992). Body cavity-based lymphoma cells exhibiting pleomorphic and anaplastic morphology are also associated with LMP-1 expression (Carbone *et al.*, 1996a,c).

Regarding AIDS-related systemic lymphomas, some investigators have reported that LMP-1 expression is restricted to anaplastic large-cell lymphomas (Carbone *et al.*, 1993a, 1994) and Hodgkin's disease (Audouin *et al.*, 1992; Carbone *et al.*, 1993a; Siebert *et al.*, 1995), while AIDS-related large-cell immunoblastic lymphomas show heterogeneity in both EBV presence and latency patterns (Carbone *et al.*, 1993a; Hamilton-Dutoit *et al.*, 1993b). In Hodgkin's disease, EBV adopts a latency type 2 pattern (LMP-1$^+$, EBNA-2$^-$) (Boiocchi *et al.*, 1993a), while AIDS-associated anaplastic large-cell lymphomas appear to be heterogeneous and both the type 2 patterns and, less frequently, a type 3 pattern (LMP-1$^+$, EBNA-2$^+$ phenotype) have been described (Carbone *et al.*, 1996b).

In contrast, EBV-positive AIDS-related small non-cleaved-cell lymphomas usually show the restricted latency pattern of EBV gene expression (latency type 1 pattern; EBNA-1$^+$, EBNA-2$^-$, LMP-1$^-$) also found in endemic Burkitt's lymphoma (Carbone *et al.*, 1993a; Hamilton-Dutoit *et al.*, 1993a). However, in some EBV-positive cases of small non-cleaved-cell lymphoma, a limited number of tumour cells express LMP-1 but not EBNA-2 (Hamilton-Dutoit *et al.*, 1993b; Carbone *et al.*, 1996b). Furthermore, both EBV latency type 2 pattern and a new latency pattern (EBNA-2$^+$, LMP-1$^-$) have been found in endemic, sporadic and AIDS-related small non-cleaved-cell lymphomas (Niedobitek *et al.*, 1995; Carbone *et al.*, 1996c). Altogether, these data document heterogeneous expression of EBV latent proteins throughout the entire spectrum of small non-cleaved-cell lymphomas.

LMP-1 expression has not been found in cases of EBV-associated plasmacytomas (Voelkerding *et al.*, 1989; Carbone *et al.*, 1993a).

In summary, EBV is more frequently present in large-cell AIDS-related lymphomas, including body cavity-based lymphomas, large-cell immunoblastic lymphomas, either systemic or arising in the brain, and anaplastic large-cell lymphomas. The two subtypes of EBV (types 1 and 2) are almost equally represented, and three types of EBV latency pattern (latency 1 — EBNA-1$^+$, EBNA-2$^-$, LMP-1$^-$; latency 2 — EBNA-1$^+$, EBNA-2$^-$, LMP-1$^+$; latency 3 — EBNA-1$^+$, EBNA-2$^+$, LMP-1$^+$) have been detected. Therefore, a large fraction of AIDS-related diffuse large-cell lymphomas can be considered as EBV-driven lymphoproliferations arising in the absence of effective cell-mediated immunity against EBV. Since EBV-transforming antigens are expressed by EBV-positive AIDS-related diffuse large-cell lymphomas, it is plausible that EBV is indeed a driving force for tumour growth and expansion. Moreover, while Hodgkin's disease may not be more common in HIV-infected persons, it is more frequently associated with EBV infection in such individuals.

The grouping of the different pathological subtypes of AIDS-related lymphomas based on EBV association and EBV latent gene expression is shown in Table 33 (see also Figure 16).

Table 33. Grouping of pathological types of AIDS-related lymphomas based on EBV latent gene expression and genetic abnormalities

'Blastic'^{a} cell lymphomas not associated with expression of Epstein–Barr virus-encoded latent membrane protein-1
- Large non-cleaved cell
- Small non-cleaved cell (always associated with c-*myc* rearrangements and frequently with *p53* inactivation)
- Extramedullary (plasmacytoma)^b
- Blastic cells with 'intermediate' features

'Blastic'^{a} cell lymphomas that may be associated with expression of Epstein–Barr virus-encoded latent membrane protein-1 expression
- Immunoblastic (either systemic or arising in the brain as a primary site)
- Occasional cases of small non-cleaved cell

'Anaplastic'^{c} cell lymphomas associated with monoclonal Epstein–Barr virus infection and latent membrane protein-1 expression
- Anaplastic large-cell (CD30/Ki-1$^+$) lymphomas
- Body cavity-based lymphomas (associated with HHV-8 infection)^d
- Hodgkin's lymphoma (mixed cellularity and lymphocyte depletion)^b

Updated and adapted from Carbone *et al.* (1993b)
^{a} The term 'blastic' is used in analogy with the suffix 'blastic' used in the Kiel classification (Stansfeld *et al.*, 1988).
^{b} Whether extramedullary plasmacytomas and Hodgkin's lymphomas should be included among HIV-related lymphomas is still debated.
^{c} The term 'anaplastic' is used in analogy with the term used in the definition of CD30-positive anaplastic large-cell lymphomas; it indicates blastic large cells which display marked pleomorphism, with giant cells possessing bizarre and irregular nuclei and large nucleoli (Harris *et al.*, 1994).
^{d} The morphology of body cavity-based lymphoma cells includes both immunoblastic and anaplastic features (Ansari *et al.*, 1996)

The frequent association between EBV infection and some lymphomas in HIV-positive persons, including those arising primarily in the brain and body cavities, as well as anaplastic large-cell lymphoma and Hodgkin's disease types, suggests that EBV is an important cofactor in their pathogenesis. Thus, the presence of EBV in these lymphoma cells appears important for their neoplastic transformation as well as for the expression of certain morphological and immunophenotypic features in the context of HIV infection (Cesarman *et al.*, 1995; Gaidano & Carbone, 1995). This conclusion is consistent with the observation discussed in Section 3.2.2, indicating that B-cell lymphoma in SIV-infected macaques is frequently associated with an EBV-related virus.

Figure 16

EBV-encoded latent membrane protein-1 (LMP-1) expression in AIDS-related CD30⁺ anaplastic large cell lymphoma

EBV-encoded latent membrane protein-1 (LMP-1) expression in Hodgkin's disease

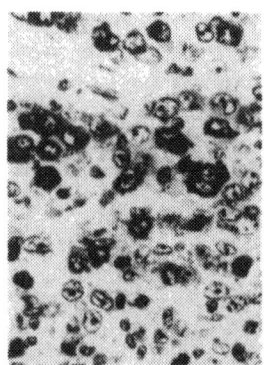

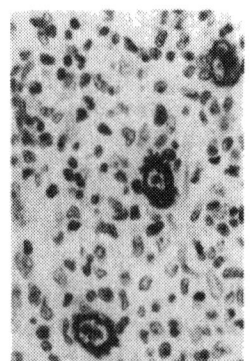

Several large tumour cells show a strong cytoplasmic staining. Bouin-fixed paraffin-embedded tissue section, APAAP method, haematoxylin counterstain, × 400

Reed–Sternberg cells of Hodgkin's disease, mixed cellularity subtype, show strong cytoplasmic staining for EBV-encoded LMP-1. Bouin-fixed paraffin-embedded tissue section, APAAP method, haematoxylin counterstain, × 400

(b) *HHV-6*

Human herpesvirus-6 (HHV-6) is a member of the herpesviridae family, and was originally isolated from peripheral blood mononuclear cells of patients with lymphoproliferative disorders or AIDS (Salahuddin *et al.*, 1986). HHV-6, like the human retroviruses HIV, HTLV-I and HTLV-II, predominantly infects T lymphocytes but can also infect other cell types including fibroblasts, epithelial cells, natural killer cells, megakaryocytes, neural cells and, occasionally, B lymphocytes.

Like other herpesviruses, HHV-6 is responsible for a latent, lifelong infection of the host and can reactivate during immunosuppression (Carrigan *et al.*, 1991; Knox & Carrigan, 1994).

The role of this virus in the pathogenesis of AIDS-related non-Hodgkin's lymphoma is still obscure. It has been hypothesized that HHV-6 may contribute to the development of lymphoproliferative disorders by stimulating polyclonal B-cell activation as a consequence of persistent active viral infection (Krueger *et al.*, 1989). A combined molecular and immunohistochemical study has shown that HHV-6 DNA sequences are significantly more prevalent in persistent generalized lymphadenopathy biopsies than in HIV-unrelated reactive lymphadenopathies. The presence of HHV-6 sequences closely correlates with follicular hyperplasia, while follicular involution is HHV-6-negative. Therefore, persistent generalized lymphadenopathy lymph nodes with B-cell hyperplasia constitute one of the sites where biologically relevant interactions between HHV-6 and HIV may occur (Dolcetti et al., 1996).

However, the prevalence of HHV-6 DNA in Hodgkin's disease and B-cell non-Hodgkin's lymphoma from HIV-infected patients is remarkably low (Carbone et al., 1996b) and similar to that observed in lymphoproliferative disorders from HIV-seronegative patients (Di Luca et al., 1994; Dolcetti et al., 1996). These results suggest that HHV-6 may have no direct role in the pathogenesis of AIDS-related non-Hodgkin's lymphoma and Hodgkin's disease.

(c) *HHV-8*

HHV-8 (see Section 4.2.4) has been associated with several lymphoproliferative disorders. It has been found in the majority of body cavity-based lymphomas arising in patients with or without HIV infection (Cesarman et al., 1995; Karcher & Alkan, 1995; Nador et al., 1995; Pastore et al., 1995) as well as in all (14/14) HIV-associated and a proportion (21/75) of HIV-unrelated multicentric Castleman's disease tissues (Soulier et al., 1995). Both in fresh body cavity-based lymphoma samples and in cell lines derived from such tumours, HHV-8 is present in multiple episomal copies. Body cavity-based lymphomas are frequently co-infected with EBV (Cesarman et al., 1995), but a few cases which contain only HHV-8 have been reported (Renne et al., 1996) and a few others do not contain HHV-8 (Carbone et al., 1996b; Hermine et al., 1996).

Cell lines latently infected with HHV-8 and several cases also with EBV have been established from body cavity-based lymphoma effusions (Cesarman et al., 1995; Gaidano et al., 1996). HHV-8 is also present in peripheral blood B cells in some HIV-infected individuals with neither lymphoma nor Kaposi's sarcoma (Whitby et al., 1995). In addition, HHV-8 has been detected in PMBCs and lymphoid tissue of less than 10% of HIV-uninfected individuals (Bigoni et al., 1996). The issue of how common HHV-8 is in the general population is discussed in Section 2.1.5.

Whether HHV-8 , like its close relative EBV, is oncogenic in its own right is not yet clear. Mechanisms of pathogenesis that might operate in HHV-8-positive lymphomas include cooperation with EBV, and participation of an HHV-8-encoded cyclin homologue or HHV-8-induced lymphokines (Levy, 1995; Hermine et al., 1996).

4.3.3 *Conclusion*

The putative role of cofactors differs substantially according to the pathological type and site of disease; moreover, several independent pathways in AIDS-related lymphomagenesis can be identified.

The first pathway of pathogenesis is associated with small non-cleaved-cell lymphomas (Figure 11). More than in other AIDS-related non-Hodgkin's lymphomas, antigen stimulation appears to play an important role in this form of non-Hodgkin's lymphoma (Riboldi et al., 1994). At the molecular level, genetic changes appear to be fairly homogeneous (Table 32). They are characterized by rearrangement of c-*myc* (100%), mutation of *p53* (60%) and the presence of EBV infection (30%) (Ballerini *et al.*, 1993; Gaidano *et al.*, 1993); however, expression of EBV transforming protein is usually absent (Carbone *et al.*, 1993a; Hamilton-Dutoit *et al.*, 1993b).

A second pathway of pathogenesis is associated with diffuse large-cell lymphomas (Figure 12 and Table 32). Because of the very high frequency of EBV infection (60–100%) (Hamilton-Dutoit *et al.*, 1991; MacMahon *et al.*, 1991; Ballerini *et al.*, 1993), AIDS-related diffuse large-cell lymphomas, including those arising primarily in the brain, can be considered as EBV-driven lymphoproliferations developing in the context of a disrupted immunosurveillance against EBV (Birx *et al.*, 1986). Viral transforming proteins EBNA-2 and LMP-1 may be expressed by EBV-positive diffuse large-cell lymphomas (Carbone *et al.*, 1993a; Hamilton-Dutoit *et al.*, 1993b). The vast majority (80–90%) of AIDS-related anaplastic large-cell lymphomas are also associated with EBV infection (Carbone *et al.*, 1993b) (Table 33) and EBV-infected tumour cells consistently express LMP-1 (Carbone *et al.*, 1994) (Figure 16).

A third pathway may apply in the pathogenesis of body cavity-based lymphomas. This pathway includes EBV infection and consistent presence of HHV-8, at least in most cases, but not other known genetic lesions (Cesarman *et al.*, 1995) (Table 32).

Finally, Hodgkin's disease in HIV-infected persons appears to be an EBV-related lymphoma expressing LMP-1 (Audouin *et al.*, 1992; Carbone *et al.*, 1994; Siebert *et al.*, 1995), whereas multicentric Castleman's disease seems to be an HHV-8-related disorder in the HIV setting (Soulier *et al.*, 1995).

In summary, understanding of the mechanisms of lymphomagenesis is hampered by the heterogeneity of non-Hodgkin's lymphoma and the substantial number of cofactors examined. These have been studied independently, generally on relatively small numbers of tumours. Seldom have different mechanisms of lymphomagenesis been examined in the same study.

4.4 Cofactors in anal and cervical carcinomas and other cancers

As discussed in Section 2.3, preneoplastic anogenital lesions and HPV-related changes (koilocytosis) are associated with HIV infection, whereas no such association has been convincingly demonstrated for invasive cancer. Dysregulation of the expression of early proteins E6 and E7 of high-risk HPV types is strongly suggested by in-vitro studies to be an important factor in malignant progression, as well as by data from human tumours (see IARC, 1995).

Little is known about the pathogenetic mechanisms involved in anogenital oncogenesis associated with other viral and chemical agents; indirect and/or direct modulation of HPV expression, however, seems to be the most relevant pathway. There are two possible, not mutually exclusive, ways in which HIV may contribute to HPV-related carcinogenesis: the major indirect mechanism is immunosuppression; possible direct mechanisms include transactivation of HPV oncogenic early-gene expression and abnormal expression of cellular genes.

4.4.1 *The role of HPV in the molecular pathogenesis of anogenital cancers in immunocompetent patients*

HPVs have been recognized as sexually transmitted etiological agents for human lower genital tract malignancies (zur Hausen, 1989; IARC, 1995). Over 70 types of HPV have been identified, of which only a small subset (HPV-16, -18, -31, -33, -35, -45 and, more recently, -51 and -52) have been associated with anogenital cancers. Many more subtypes are associated with benign, epithelial neoplasms. During the life cycle of HPV, most of the viral DNA is maintained episomally in the nucleus of the infected cells. Integration of viral DNA sequences is frequently associated with malignant progression (Schwarz *et al.*, 1985; Jeon *et al.*, 1995), being detected more frequently in carcinomas than in cervical intraepithelial neoplasia (CIN) (Cullen *et al.*, 1991). In CIN, the mainly episomal HPV actively replicates (productive infection), whereas in cervical epithelial cancers the HPV DNA is prevalently integrated (latent infection). This transition results in changes at the level of viral DNA as well as of RNA and protein.

(*a*) *Status and level of HPV DNA in the natural history of infection*

In CIN lesions, the level of predominantly episomal, infecting viral genome detected varies according to the techniques used. PCR, with a detection limit of 10 copies per sample, detects HPV genomes in 72–91% of 'low-grade lesions' and in 90–100% of 'high-grade lesions' (van den Brule *et al.*, 1991; Bergeron *et al.*, 1992; Lungu *et al.*, 1992); procedures with a lower sensitivity (3×10^5 viral genomes per sample or 0.1 viral copy per cell when testing 1.5×10^5 cells = 1 µg genomic DNA), such as Southern blot, dot blot and ViraPap™, detect HPV genomes in only 36–55% of 'low-grade lesions' and in 43–81% of 'high-grade lesions' (Fuchs *et al.*, 1988; Lim-Tan *et al.*, 1988; McNicol *et al.*, 1989).

In invasive cancer, HPV DNA is present at > 1 viral copy per cell, because of the predominantly integrated high-risk HPVs in genomic DNA and the homogeneity of the clonal neoplastic population. At this level, both high- and low-sensitivity analytical techniques detect HPV in > 90% of samples. Furthermore, the HPV-type specificity of PCR equals that of Southern blot hybridization, with HPV-16 identified in over 60% of cervical cancers (Riou *et al.*, 1990; van den Brule *et al.*, 1991; Higgins *et al.*, 1991b; Lörincz *et al.*, 1992). In penile cancers, 'high-risk' genital HPVs were detected in more than 48% of the biopsies by both techniques, with no major geographical differences in the detection frequency (McCance *et al.*, 1986; Tornesello *et al.*, 1992; Wiener *et al.*, 1992).

(*b*) *Expression of HPV proteins in the natural history of infection*

In benign lesions, late HPV proteins are expressed, with viral transcription patterns that vary by epithelial layer: weak expression of early genes occurs in the basal layers of low-grade cervical dysplasias induced by HPV-16 or HPV-33 and in some HPV-6- or HPV-11-induced condylomas; late genes are expressed in terminally differentiated keratinocytes of the superficial strata (Dürst *et al.*, 1992; Stoler *et al.*, 1992). Studies in HPV-16- and HPV-18-infected female renal transplant recipients demonstrate that, following immunosuppression, antibodies to the late proteins decrease, whereas antibodies against early proteins E2, E4 and E7 significantly increase. This pattern suggests reactivation of latent virus (Lewensohn-Fuchs *et al.*, 1993). The regulation of gene expression is complex and is controlled by various cellular and viral transcription factors, different promoter usage, differential splicing, differential transcription termination and stability of mRNA.

In malignant lesions, integration of HPV DNA, generally concomitant with the disruption of *E2/E1* gene sequences, determines the major transcriptional changes. *E6* and *E7* are always transcribed actively in tumour cells (Schwarz *et al.*, 1985). The *E2* and/or *E1* disruption could lead to derepression of the P97 promoter. This, in turn, would modulate the expression of transforming genes and increase the transforming potential of HPVs (Lambert & Howley, 1988; Schiller *et al.*, 1989; Romanczuk & Howley, 1992; Jeon *et al.*, 1995).

(c) *Molecular mechanisms of transforming activity of HPV*

The transforming activity of HPV seems to be associated mainly with E6 and E7 open reading frames, which are consistently expressed in cervical cancers and cell lines derived from them (Smotkin & Wettstein, 1986; Hsu *et al.*, 1993). HPV-16 and HPV-18 *E6* and *E7* early genes, when expressed by a LTR promoter and transduced into cells by retroviral infection, immortalize human primary keratinocytes *in vitro* (Pirisi *et al.*, 1987; Schlegel *et al.*, 1988; Halbert *et al.*, 1991).

(i) *Intrinsic properties of high-risk HPV E6 and E7*

The HPV strains associated with malignant tumours (mainly HPV-16, -18, -31, -33, -35) are designated 'high-risk' HPV (IARC, 1995).

The E6 zinc finger protein of HPV-16 and HPV-18, like SV40 T antigen and adenovirus 5E1B, interacts specifically with the p53 tumour-suppressor protein. The p53–E6 complexes are then targeted to destruction through the ubiquitin-mediated proteolysis pathway (Scheffner *et al.*, 1990; Crook *et al.*, 1991). Thus it has been shown that expression of E6 in transfected cells abrogates a p53-controlled G1/S cell-cycle checkpoint (Kessis *et al.*, 1993; Foster *et al.*, 1994; Gu *et al.*, 1994; Canman *et al.*, 1995).

The E7 protein of high-risk HPV shares sequence homology with conserved regions 1 and 2 of the adenovirus E1a 243- and 289-amino-acid proteins. Like E1a, it binds to the product of the retinoblastoma gene, pRB (Dyson *et al.*, 1989; Münger *et al.*, 1989; Gage *et al.*, 1990). The RB protein is a phosphoprotein which, in its underphosphorylated form, appears to negatively regulate entry into the S-phase of the cell cycle; the initiation of S-phase is accompanied by pRB phosphorylation, via cyclin-dependent kinases. Binding of HPV E7 to pRB indirectly enhances transcription of several genes involved in cycle control, such as c-*myc*, c-*myb*, *cdc2*, DNA polymerase alpha, ribonucleotide reductase and thymidylate synthetase (Mudryi *et al.*, 1990; Nevins, 1992).

(ii) *Regulation of E6 and E7 expression*

Early gene expression is controlled by the long control region (LCR), extending over 400–900 bp, which may be considered to consist of three functional units. The 5' region, adjacent to the L1 gene, contains the first E2 binding site as well as negative regulatory elements acting at the level of late mRNA stability (Kennedy et al., 1991). The 3' segment contains a single E1 binding site (which identifies the origin of replication), an Sp1 transcription binding site, two E2 binding sites and the E6/E7 transcription promoter (Phelps & Howley, 1987; Swift et al., 1987; Guis et al., 1988). Between these two regions lies the HPV enhancer, the activity of which depends on cellular nuclear factors (Nakshatri et al., 1990). In particular, the HPV-16 and HPV-18 enhancers contain recognition sites for cellular transcription factors such as *jun/fos* (Cripe et al., 1990; Thierry et al., 1992), nuclear factor I (NFI), transcription factor Sp1, activator protein AP1, glucocorticoid receptor and other papillomavirus enhancer-associated, but not yet characterized, factors (Chong et al., 1990; Hoppe-Seyler & Butz, 1992). The activities of individual *cis*-acting elements contribute to the full enhancer activity. Published data suggest that HPV enhancer function depends on the cooperative interaction of multiple factors. Short segments of the enhancer have only a weak transactivating function. Frequently, recognition sites bind multiple proteins, and individual factors can interact with different recognition sequences (Chong et al., 1990; Cripe et al., 1990; Hoppe-Seyler & Butz, 1992; Thierry et al., 1992).

Thus the expression of E6 and E7 could be enhanced by several mechanisms: mutational inactivation of *E2* or *E1* genes during HPV integration events; extracellular stimuli (growth factors, promoting agents, cytokines, etc.) via membrane receptors; or intracellular factors that bind the regulatory LCR, either directly or through activation of nuclear factors. For example, expression of HPV E6 and E7 can be modulated by the tumour promoter 12-*O*-tetradecanoylphorbol 13-acetate, which activates protein kinase C in the plasma membrane, eventually activating the nuclear transcription factor AP1 (Chan et al., 1990).

4.4.2 Interactions between HIV and HPV

HIV is transmitted sexually (see Section 1.3.1). Although infection of squamous and colorectal epithelial cell lines or primary cultures has been reported (Adachi et al., 1987; Tan et al., 1993; Phillips et al., 1994b), there is no convincing evidence of infection of epithelial cells by HIV *in vivo*.

Epithelial Langerhans' cells and related antigen-presenting cells in the layers beneath the mucosal epithelium are thought to be a major route of genital infection by HIV or SIV (Spira et al., 1996). It is thus unlikely that the same cells *in vivo* will be co-infected by HIV and HPV. Even where HIV has been detected in CIN II biopsies, immunohistochemical evidence indicates that the HIV is localized to cells resembling lymphocytes or macrophages in the subepithelial stromal layer (Vernon et al., 1994).

Infection and malfunction of Langerhans' cells could affect the local immune control of other HIV-infected cells. Furthermore, Spinillo et al. (1993) reported that counts of Langerhans' cells in CIN biopsies from HIV-infected women with CDC stage IV disease were significantly lower than those in CIN biopsies from HIV-negative matched controls.

(a) *Effects of HIV-related immunosuppression on HPV replication and HPV-associated anogenital lesions*

There are no experimental data addressing the effects of HIV-induced immunosuppression on HPV replication and transformation.

The epidemiological data reviewed in Section 2.3 suggest an increase in HPV genome copy numbers with immunosuppression. Higher HPV load may increase the probability of chromosomal integration of viral DNA and subsequent neoplastic events, as described above. Besides the increase in the number of HPV copies, HIV-infected immunosuppressed homosexual men as well as female transplant recipients often have multiple types of HPV (Palefsky *et al.*, 1992; Brown *et al.*, 1994b). However, the role of multiple HPV infection in the pathogenesis of anogenital neoplasia is unknown.

(b) *HIV Tat stimulation of cytokines and their role in genital lesions*

Cytokines have been shown to stimulate HPV-transformed epithelial cells. In particular, the pro-inflammatory cytokines IL-1α and TNFα, the expression of which is induced by Tat (Philippon *et al.*, 1994; Biswas *et al.*, 1995), inhibit proliferation of normal epithelial cells cultured from human cervix. However, they also significantly stimulate proliferation of cervical cell lines immortalized by transfection with HPV-16 or HPV-18 DNAs and of HPV-positive cell lines derived from cervical carcinoma. Growth stimulation by IL-1α or TNFα is accompanied by a 6–10-fold increase in RNA encoding amphiregulin, an epidermal growth factor receptor ligand (Woodworth *et al.*, 1995). However, whether this chain of events occurs *in vivo* is not known.

(c) *Possible effect of HIV-1 Tat on HPV E6/E7 expression*

Tornesello *et al.* (1991) reported that transfection of HIV-1 *tat* increased the expression of HPV-18 E7 in HeLa cells constitutively harbouring 10–20 copies of HPV-18. Expression of the HPV-16 LCR is also enhanced by HIV-1 Tat (Tornesello *et al.*, 1993; Vernon *et al.*, 1993). In addition, Tat increased the efficiency of E6/E7-mediated transformation of NIH 3T3 cells (Buonaguro *et al.*, 1994). Vogel *et al.* (1995) reported that transgenic mice carrying the HIV-1 *tat* gene express Tat protein in their keratinocytes. This is not sufficient to cause epidermal tumours, but is able to promote tumours after a single subthreshold dose of a carcinogenic initiator. Such tumour promotion has an effect additive to that of phorbol esters.

Although, as discussed above, HIV-1 and HPV are unlikely to co-infect the same cell, HIV-1 Tat has been shown to be released from infected cells (Frankel & Pabo, 1988). Extracellular Tat can be taken up by cervical epithelial cell lines (Frankel & Pabo, 1988; Frankel *et al.*, 1989; Ensoli *et al.*, 1993) and could thus allow the direct transactivation of HPV promoters.

In conclusion, both the immunosuppressive effect of HIV-1 infection and the secretion of HIV-1 Tat could promote the development of HIV-related precancerous anogenital lesions. Similar mechanisms might account for the increased incidence of other HPV-related and unrelated neoplasms in HIV infection.

5. Summary of Data Reported and Evaluation

5.1 Exposure data

The human immunodeficiency viruses (HIV-1 and HIV-2), the etiological agents of the acquired immune deficiency syndrome (AIDS), belong to the lentivirus subfamily of the *Retroviridae* family. Sequence analysis of viral DNA indicates a separate ancestral lineage for HIV-1 and HIV-2. Phylogenetic analysis of diverse geographical isolates has shown HIV-1 to cluster into two distinct major groups and HIV-2 into another. Multiple viral clades (subtypes) exist on the basis of sequence diversity within these groups, but these are not the same as virus serotypes which are based on antigenic diversity.

HIV-1 interaction with the cellular receptor (CD4) and its co-receptor helps to explain why the virus is tropic for $CD4^+$ lymphocytes and macrophages.

HIV-1 and HIV-2 have similar, but not identical, complex genomes consisting of three genes encoding structural proteins, two genes which are essential for virus replication and four accessory genes which contribute to the efficiency of replication. Once the virus has bound to its receptor on the cell membrane, it internalizes by fusion and releases its core in which the RNA undergoes reverse transcription. The resultant proviral DNA, once integrated into the host cell DNA, exploits the biochemical machinery of the cell to synthesize new viral proteins which assemble intracytoplasmically, mature and are released at the cell membrane.

Diagnosis of infection with HIV-1 and HIV-2 relies on the identification of specific antibodies to, or the direct detection of, the viruses. The direct detection of virus or viral protein provides the definitive diagnosis for HIV-1 and HIV-2.

The main routes of HIV-1 transmission are sexual intercourse, blood–blood contact and from mother to infant, including breast-feeding. The risk of transmission through all routes is associated with viral load in the infected person. Other factors which increase the rate of sexual transmission are the presence of other sexually transmitted diseases, especially genital ulcerative disease, and the type of sexual intercourse. Transmission from mother to child is associated with vaginal delivery and with breast-feeding.

Patterns of HIV-1 transmission vary substantially with time and geographical area. Most developed countries experienced early waves of HIV-1 infection among homosexual men, and in some of these countries intravenous drug use is an important mode of transmission. In Africa, heterosexual contact has remained the predominant mode of transmission, with transmission from mother to child also occurring extensively. There have been substantial increases in HIV-1 transmission in certain Asian countries in the past decade, initially through homosexual contact between men and through injecting drug use, but increasingly through heterosexual contact.

Infection with HIV-1 and HIV-2 has protean clinical manifestations. As early as one to six weeks after HIV-1 infection, many adult patients have a seroconversion syndrome. The timing of HIV-1-related symptoms and diseases reflects virological and immunological changes that occur. In the first few weeks after HIV-1 infection, the level of $CD4^+$

lymphocytes and the $CD4^+$ cell : $CD8^+$ cell ratio decrease and viral load increases. Generally the immunological parameters stabilize, although not to normal levels, after the initial phase of infection. This is followed by a long period of clinical latency, marked by gradually declining $CD4^+$ counts, and then the appearance of a range of symptoms (constitutional, oral, pulmonary or skin conditions). The development of AIDS is defined by the occurrence of one or more specific opportunistic infections, malignancies and related diseases occurring in patients with HIV-1 and HIV-2 infection. The median incubation period (from infection to AIDS) for HIV-1 in developed countries is 10 years, and may be longer for persons infected with HIV-2.

In the absence of an effective treatment or vaccine, control and prevention of HIV-1 and HIV-2 infection continue to rely mainly on behavioural interventions. In preventing sexual transmission, reducing the number and modifying the types of sexual contact, and the consistent and correct use of condoms are essential. Drug-dependence treatment programmes and improving the availability of sterile needles are putatively effective ways of stemming the HIV epidemic among intravenous drug users.

Screening the blood of donors for HIV-1 and HIV-2 antibody has virtually eliminated transmission of these viruses in blood products in many countries. A significant reduction in perinatal transmission of HIV-1 can be achieved by maternal use of zidovudine during pregnancy and delivery, and by treatment of newborns immediately after delivery. This has become clinical practice in many countries. Delivery by Caesarian section has been associated with a reduction in mother-to-child transmission in most studies.

New approaches to the treatment of HIV-1-infected people include combination therapy and use of new classes of drugs such as protease inhibitors. The development of a safe, effective and economical preventive vaccine for HIV-1 and HIV-2 faces many obstacles.

5.2 Human carcinogenicity data

Epidemiological evidence indicates that the incidence of Kaposi's sarcoma is greatly increased in persons infected with HIV-1. Some studies in developed countries point to a relative risk of more than 1000-fold. The incidence increases markedly as HIV-1-related immunosuppression progresses. Within developed countries, the risk varies between HIV-1-transmission categories, with homosexual and bisexual men having a 5–10-fold greater risk than other HIV-1-infected groups. In parts of Africa, Kaposi's sarcoma incidence is rapidly increasing, probably as a result of HIV-1 infection. These variations suggest the existence of cofactor(s), for which human herpesvirus type 8 (HHV-8) is the leading candidate.

Non-Hodgkin's lymphoma incidence is greatly increased in persons with HIV-1-infection. Case–control and cohort studies of HIV-1-infected individuals have consistently demonstrated large increases in risk for non-Hodgkin's lymphoma in developed countries. In AIDS patients, the rate may be at least 100-fold increased. This increased risk has been found to be similar in all HIV-1-transmission groups. It appears that the association is mediated by HIV-1-related immune dysregulation. Co-infections with specific viruses are associated with primary lymphoma of the brain (Epstein–Barr virus; EBV) and body-cavity lymphomas and multicentric Castleman's disease (HHV-8). Viruses may be involved in some other cases of HIV-1-associated lymphomagenesis.

In HIV-1-infected persons, total cancer incidence does not appear to be increased, after exclusion of Kaposi's sarcoma and non-Hodgkin's lymphoma. However, increases have been observed for several specific cancers. Studies of women with HIV show increases in cervical carcinoma *in situ* among HIV-1-infected women. The risk increases with increasing immunodeficiency. However, there may be confounding due to common exposure factors between HIV-1 and human papillomavirus (HPV). This confounding has made assessment of the relationship between HIV-1 and carcinoma *in situ* difficult. To date, there is no association between invasive cervical cancer and HIV-1 infection.

Anal cancer incidence has been increasing for several decades and the trend has not increased in the AIDS era. However, homosexual men have a high risk for anal HPV infection and anal cancer, which appears to be associated with their lifestyle.

There are several reports suggesting an association with HIV-1-infection with leiomyosarcoma in children, conjunctival squamous-cell tumours in Africa and, to a lesser extent, Hodgkin's disease. Studies reported to date have not documented a relationship between HIV-1 and any other form of cancer.

Kaposi's sarcoma has also been seen in some HIV-2-infected persons, but the strength of any association has not been determined.

There are a few case reports and one case–control study suggesting that HIV-2 infection may be associated with non-Hodgkin's lymphoma.

There are no reports of an association of HIV-2 with cancers other than Kaposi's sarcoma and non-Hodgkin's lymphoma.

5.3 Animal carcinogenicity data

In nonhuman primates infected with HIV-1 or HIV-2, a single case of fibromatosis has been observed in a baboon infected with HIV-2.

Lymphomas occur more frequently in simian immunodeficiency virus (SIV)-infected macaques than in uninfected macaques. Most malignant lymphomas are of B-cell origin and are associated with an EBV-like simian herpesvirus and with immunodeficiency.

Lymphosarcoma in the cat is associated with experimental and naturally acquired feline immunodeficiency virus (FIV) infection. Lymphosarcoma is a B-cell lymphoma which has similar morphological, immunophenotypic and molecular characteristics to HIV- and SIV-associated lymphomas. There is no evidence of FIV sequence integration into tumour cells, indicating that the role of the virus in tumour development is possibly indirect.

5.4 Other relevant data and mechanistic considerations on HIV-1-associated neoplasms

Patients with non-HIV-associated forms of acquired immunodeficiency — primarily as a result of organ transplantation — have a substantially increased risk for neoplastic lesions. These include consistent excesses of non-Hodgkin's lymphoma, Kaposi's sarcoma and skin cancers, particularly of squamous-cell origin. The increased relative risk for most of these malignancies is seen within the first few years after initiation of treatment and remains relatively constant over time. The exception to this is that the relative risk for skin cancer increases with time. Removal of the immunosuppressive therapy can lead to regression of both non-Hodgkin's lymphoma and Kaposi's sarcoma. Among patients with a variety of inborn immune dysfunctions, a substantial excess of haematopoietic malignancies is also documented. It may therefore be concluded that, in these patients, immunosuppression causes this excess of neoplastic lesions. Inherited immunodeficiencies of various kinds are also limited to increased cancer incidence.

It is likely that the immunosuppressive effect of HIV-1 is a major factor in the development of Kaposi's sarcoma. Kaposi's sarcoma lesions are composed of various cellular lineages, probably mainly endothelial cells and fibroblastoid cells, which proliferate in response to several growth factors. The HIV-1 Tat protein has been shown to have angiogenic properties in animal models and to stimulate the growth of Kaposi's sarcoma spindle cells *in vitro*, and may therefore be a factor for the development of Kaposi's sarcoma lesions. In addition to extracellular Tat, increased cytokine levels found in AIDS patients may be responsible for this effect. The production of these growth factors and the proliferation of spindle and endothelial cells may be associated with an additional infectious agent. HHV-8 seems the best candidate reported so far, but its role in the pathogenesis of Kaposi's sarcoma remains to be clarified.

Regarding non-Hodgkin's lymphoma, consistent failure to unequivocally detect HIV-1 sequences within the tumour clone suggests that HIV-1 does not directly cause transformation of B-cell lymphocytes. Its role in lymphomagenesis seems to be indirect and related to an effect of HIV-1 on immunoregulation. Several host factors (disrupted immunosurveillance, chronic antigen stimulation and cytokine dysregulation) play a role in lymphoma pathogenesis in HIV-1-infected persons. This results in oligoclonal expansion, which commonly occurs in the early phases of HIV-1 infection, corresponding to B-cell proliferation.

The potential role of cofactors in AIDS-related lymphomagenesis differs depending on the histopathological type and site of disease. Pathological and molecular data show that somatic genetic changes are frequently involved in the development of AIDS-related non-Hodgkin's lymphomas. These genetic changes cluster in distinct molecular pathways which correlate with different pathological types.

The frequent association of *c-myc* deregulation and *p53* inactivation in small non-cleaved-cell lymphoma may imply a synergistic involvement of these two events in the pathogenesis of this tumour. The striking association between EBV infection and specific types of lymphomas in HIV-1-infected persons (those arising primarily in the brain and body cavities as well as $CD30^+$ anaplastic large-cell lymphoma and Hodgkin's disease) suggests that EBV may be important in their pathogenesis. The putative transforming role of EBV is further strengthened by data showing that the transforming genes of EBV, encoding EBV nuclear antigen-2 and EBV latent membrane protein-1, are expressed in EBV-positive tumour cells.

Preliminary evidence suggests that HHV-8 has a role in inducing some AIDS-related lymphoproliferative disorders in HIV-1-infected persons such as body cavity-based lymphoma and multicentric Castleman's disease.

The immunosuppressive effect of HIV-1 infection may promote the development of HPV-related precancerous and anogenital lesions. HIV-1 *tat* may also enhance their development.

5.5 Evaluation[1]

There is *sufficient evidence* in humans for the carcinogenicity of infection with HIV-1.

There is *inadequate evidence* in humans for the carcinogenicity of infection with HIV-2.

Overall evaluation

Infection with HIV-1 is *carcinogenic to humans (Group 1)*.

Infection with HIV-2 is *possibly carcinogenic to humans (Group 2B)*.

In making this evaluation, the Working Group took into account data indicating that HIV-2 infection can show the same clinical manifestations, including severe immune deficiency, as HIV-1 infection.

6. References

Abrams, D.I. (1988) The pre-AIDS syndromes. Asymptomatic carriers, thrombocytopenic purpura, persistent generalized lymphadenopathy, and AIDS-related complex. *Infect. Dis. Clin. N. Am.*, **2**, 343–351

Abrams, D.I., Goldman, A.I., Launer, C., Korvick, J.A., Neaton, J.D., Crane, L.R., Grodesky, M., Wakefield, S., Muth, K., Kornegay, S., Cohn, D.L., Harris, A., Luskin-Hawk, R., Markowitz, N., Sampson, J.H., Thompson, M., Deyton, L. & The Terry Beirn Community Programs for Clinical Research on AIDS (1994) A comparative trial of didanosine or zalcitabine after treatment with zidovudine in patients with human immunodeficiency virus infection. *New Engl. J. Med.*, **330**, 657–662

Adachi, A., Koening, S., Gendelman, H.E., Daugherty, D., Gattoni-Celli, S., Fauci, A.S. & Martin, M.A. (1987) Productive, persistent infection of human colorectal cell lines with human immunodeficiency virus. *J. Virol.*, **61**, 209–213

---

[1] For definition of the italicized terms, see Preamble, pp. 22–25.

Adachi, A., Fleming, I., Burk, R.D., Ho, G.Y.F. & Klein, R.S. (1993) Women with human immunodeficiency virus infection and abnormal Papanicolaou smears: a prospective study of colposcopy and clinical outcome. *Obstet. Gynecol.*, **81**, 372–377

Adams, V., Kempf, W., Hassam, S., Briner, J., Schmid, M., Moos, R. & Pfaltz, M. (1995) Detection of several types of human papilloma viruses in AIDS-associated Kaposi's sarcoma. *J. med. Virol.*, **46**, 189–193

Adamson, R.H., McIntire, K.R., Sieber, S.M., Correa, P. & Dalgard, D.W. (1975) Nonhuman primate models for lymphoma, leukemia and other neoplasms. *Bibl. haematol.*, **40**, 723–730

Adldinger, H.K., Delius, H., Freese, U.K., Clarke, J. & Bornkamm, G.W. (1985) A putative transforming gene of Jijoye virus differs from that of Epstein-Barr virus prototypes. *Virology*, **141**, 221–234

Agut, H., Guetard, D., Collandre, H., Dauguet, C., Montagnier, L., Miclea, J.-M., Baurmann, H. & Gessain, A. (1988) Concomitant infection by human herpesvirus 6, HILV-I, and HIV-2 (Letter to the Editor). *Lancet*, **i**, 712

Aiken, C., Konner, J., Landau, N.R., Lenburg, M.E. & Trono, D. (1994) Nef induces CD4 endocytosis: requirement for a critical dileucine motif in the membrane-proximal CD4 cytoplasmic domain. *Cell*, **76**, 853–864

Akashi, K., Eizuru, Y., Sumiyoshi, Y., Minematsu, T., Hara, S., Harada, M., Kikuchi, M., Niho, Y. & Minamishima, Y. (1993) Brief report: severe infectious mononucleosis-like syndrome and primary human herpesvirus 6 infection in an adult. *New Engl. J. Med.*, **329**, 168–171

van den Akker, R., van den Hoek, J.A.R., van den Akker, W.M.R., Kooy, H., Vijge, E., Roosendaal, G., Coutinho, R.A. & van Loon, A.M. (1992) Detection of HIV antibodies in saliva as a tool for epidemiological studies. *AIDS*, **6**, 953–957

Al-Bahar, S., Pandita, R., Dhabhar, B. & Al-Bahar, E. (1994) Human immunodeficiency virus (HIV) infection associated with acute myeloblastic leukemia in a low HIV prevalence area. *Acta haematol.*, **91**, 52–53

Albini, A., Mitchell, C.D., Thompson, E.W., Seeman, R., Martin, G.R., Wittek, A.E. & Quinnan, G.V. (1988) Invasive activity and chemotactic response to growth factors by Kaposi's sarcoma cells. *J. cell. Biochem.*, **36**, 369–376

Albini, A., Fontanini, G., Masiello, L., Tacchetti, C., Bigini, D., Luzzi, P., Noonan, D.M. & Stetler-Stevenson, W.G. (1994) Angiogenic potential *in vivo* by Kaposi's sarcoma cell-free supernatants and HIV-1 *tat* product: inhibition of KS-like lesions by tissue inhibitor of metalloproteinase-2. *AIDS*, **8**, 1237–1244

Alcabes, P., Schoenbaum, E.E. & Klein, R.S. (1993a) $CD4^+$ Lymphocyte level and rate of decline as predictors of AIDS in intravenous drug users with HIV infection. *AIDS*, **7**, 513–517

Alcabes, P., Muñoz, A., Vlahov, D. & Friedland, G.H. (1993b) Incubation period of human immunodeficiency virus. *Epidemiol. Rev.*, **15**, 303–318

Ali, M., Taylor, G.P., Pitman, R.J., Parker, D., Rethwilm, A., Cheingson-Popov, R., Weber, J.N., Bieniasz, P.D., Bradley, R. & McClure, M.O. (1996) No evidence of antibody to human foamy virus in widespread human populations. *AIDS Res. hum. Retroviruses*, **12** (in press)

Alkhatib, G., Combadiere, C., Broder, C.C., Feng, Y., Kennedy, P.E., Murphy, P.M. & Berger, E.A. (1996) CC CKR 5: A RANTES, MIP-1α, MIP-1β receptor as a fusion cofactor for macrophage-tropic HIV-1. *Science*, **272**, 1955–1958

Allen, S., Van de Perre, P., Serufilira, A., Lepage, P., Carael, M., DeClercq, A., Tice, J., Black, D., Nsengumuremyi, F., Ziegler, J., Levy, J. & Hulley, S. (1991) Human immunodeficiency virus and malaria in a representative sample of childbearing women in Kigali, Rwanda. *J. infect. Dis.*, **164**, 67–71

Alonso, M.L., Richardson, M.E., Metroka, C.E., Mouradian, J.A., Koduru, P.R.K., Filippa, D.A. & Chaganti, R.S.K. (1987) Chromosome abnormalities in AIDS-associated lymphadenopathy. *Blood*, **69**, 855–858

Ambinder, R.F., Newman, C., Hayward, G., Biggar, R.J., Melbye, M., Kestens, L., Marck, E.V., Piot, P., Gigase, P., Wright, P.B. & Quinn, T.C. (1987) Lack of association of cytomegalovirus with endemic African Kaposi's sarcoma. *J. infect. Dis.*, **156**, 193–197

Ambroziak, J.A., Blackbourn, D.J., Herndier, B.G., Glogau, R.G., Gullett, J.H., McDonald, A.R., Lennette, E.T. & Levy, J.A. (1995) Herpes-like sequences in HIV-infected and uninfected Kaposi's sarcoma patients. *Science*, **268**, 582–583

van Ameijden, E.J.C., van den Hoek, A.(J)A.R. & Coutinho, R.A. (1994) Injecting risk behavior among drug users in Amsterdam, 1986 to 1992, and its relationship to AIDS prevention programs. *Am. J. public Health*, **84**, 275–281

Ancelle, R., Bletry, O., Baglin, A.C., Brun-Vézinet, F., Rey, M.-A. & Godeau, P. (1987) Long incubation period for HIV-2 infection (Letter to the Editor). *Lancet*, **i**, 688–689

Anderson, D.J., O'Brien, T.R., Politch, J.A., Martinez, A., Seage, G.R., III, Padian, N., Horsburgh, C.R., Jr & Mayer, K.H. (1992) Effects of disease stage and zidovudine therapy on the detection of human immunodeficiency virus type 1 in semen. *J. Am. med. Assoc.*, **267**, 2769–2774

Andrieu, J.M., Roithmann, S., Tourani, J.M., Levy, R., Desablens, B., Le Maignan, C., Gastaut, J.A., Brice, P., Raphael, M. & Taillan, B. (1993) Hodgkin's disease during HIV-1-infection: the French registry experience. *Ann. Oncol.*, **4**, 635–641

Anon. (1992a) *Pneumocystis carinii* pneumonia amongst persons with hemophilia A. *Morbid. Mortal. Wkly Rep.*, **31**, 365–367, 644–646, 665–667

Anon. (1992b) Opportunistic infections and Kaposi's sarcoma among Haitians in the United States. *Morbid. Mortal. Wkly Rep.*, **31**, 353–361

Anon. (1994) Human immunodeficiency virus transmission in household settings — United States. *Morbid. Mortal. Wkly Rep.*, **43**, 347–356

Anon. (1995) Case-control study of HIV seroconversion in health-care workers after percutaneous exposure to HIV-infected blood — France, United Kingdom, and United States, January 1988–August 1994. *Morbid. Mortal. Wkly Rep.*, **44**, 929–933

Ansari, M.Q., Dawson, D.B., Nador, R., Rutherford, C., Schneider, N.R., Latimer, M.J., Picker, L., Knowles, D.M. & Mckenna, R.W. (1996) Primary body cavity-based AIDS-related lymphomas. *Am. J. clin. Pathol.*, **105**, 221–229

Archibald, C.P., Schechter, M.T., Craib, K.J.P., Le, T.N., Douglas, B., Willoughby, B. & O'Shaughnessy, M. (1990) Risk factors for Kaposi's sarcoma in the Vancouver Lymphadenopathy-AIDS study. *J. acquir. Immun. Defic. Syndr.*, **3** (Suppl. 1), S18–S23

Archibald, C.P., Schechter, M.T., Le, T.N., Craib, K.J.P., Montaner, J.S.G. & O'Shaughnessy, M.V. (1992) Evidence for a sexually transmitted cofactor for AIDS-related Kaposi's sarcoma in a cohort of homosexual men. *Epidemiology*, **3**, 203–209

Armenian, H.K., Hoover, D.R., Rubb, S., Metz, S., Kaslow, R., Visscher, B., Chmiel, J., Kingsley, L. & Saah, A. (1993) Composite risk score for Kaposi's sarcoma based on a case–control and longitudinal study in the multicenter AIDS cohort study (MACS) population. *Am. J. Epidemiol.*, **138**, 256–265

Armstrong, J.A. & Horne, R. (1984) Follicular dendritic cells and virus-like particles in AIDS-related lymphadenopathy. *Lancet*, **ii**, 370–372

Arribas, J.R., Clifford, D.B., Fichtenbaum, C.J., Roberts, R.L., Powderly, W.G. & Storch, G.A. (1995) Detection of Epstein-Barr virus DNA in cerebrospinal fluid for diagnosis of AIDS-related central nervous system lymphoma. *J. clin. Microbiol.*, **33**, 1580–1583

Astrin, S.M., Schattner, E., Laurence, J., Lebman, R.I. & Rodriguez-Alfageme, C. (1992) Does HIV infection of B lymphocytes initiate AIDS lymphoma? Detection by PCR of viral sequences in lymphoma tissue. *Current Topics Microbiol. Immunol.*, **182**, 399–407

Ateenyi-Agaba, C. (1995) Conjunctival squamous-cell carcinoma associated with HIV infection in Kampala, Uganda. *Lancet*, **345**, 695-696

Athale, U.H., Patil, P.S., Chintu, C. & Elem, B. (1995) Influence of HIV epidemic on the incidence of Kaposi's sarcoma in Zambian children. *J. acquir. Immune Defic. Syndr. hum. Retrovirol.*, **8**, 96–100

Audouin, J., Diebold, J. & Pallesen, G. (1992) Frequent expression of Epstein-Barr virus latent membrane protein-1 in tumour cells of Hodgkin's disease in HIV-positive patients. *J. Pathol.*, **167**, 381–384

Baba, T.W., Jeong, Y.S., Penninck, D., Bronson, R., Greene, M.F. & Ruprecht, R.M. (1995) Pathogenicity of live, attenuated SIV after mucosal infection of neonatal macaques. *Science*, **267**, 1820–1825

Bacchetti, P. & Moss, A.R. (1989) Incubation period of AIDS in San Francisco. *Nature*, **338**, 251–253

Ballerini, P., Gaidano, G., Gong, J.Z., Tassi, V., Saglio, G., Knowles, D.M. & Dalla-Favera, R. (1993) Multiple genetic lesions in acquired immunodeficiency syndrome-related non-Hodgkin's lymphoma. *Blood*, **81**, 166–176

Balsam, D. & Segal, S. (1992) Two smooth muscle tumors in the airway of an HIV-infected child. *Pediatr. Radiol.*, **22**, 552–553

Baltimore, D. (1970) Viral RNA-dependent DNA polymerase. *Nature*, **226**, 1209–1211

Baltimore, D. (1995) Lessons from people with nonprogressive HIV infection. *New Engl. J. Med.*, **332**, 259–260

Barbé, F., Klein, M. & Badonnel, Y. (1994) Early detection of antibodies to human immunodeficiency virus 1 by third-generation enzyme immunoassay. A comparative study with the results of second-generation immunoassays and western blot. *Ann. Biol. clin.*, **52**, 341–345

Barchielli, A., Buiatti, E., Galanti, C. & Lazzeri, V. (1995) Linkage between AIDS surveillance system and population-based cancer registry data in Italy: a pilot study in Florence, 1985–90. *Tumori*, **81**, 169–172

Barillari, G., Buonaguro, L., Fiorelli, V., Hoffman, J., Michaels, F., Gallo, R.C. & Ensoli, B. (1992) Effects of cytokines from activated immune cells on vascular cell growth and HIV-1 gene expression. Implications for AIDS–Kaposi's sarcoma pathogenesis. *J. Immunol.*, **149**, 3727–3734

Barillari, G., Gendelman, R., Gallo, R.C. & Ensoli, B. (1993) The Tat protein of human immunodeficiency virus type 1, a growth factor for AIDS Kaposi sarcoma and cytokine-activated vascular cells, induces adhesion of the same cell types by using integrin receptors recognizing the RGD amino acid sequence. *Proc. natl Acad. Sci. USA*, **90**, 7941–7945

Barker, E., Barnett, S.W., Stamatatos, L. & Levy, J.A. (1995) The human immunodeficiency virus. In: Levy, J.A., ed., *The Retroviridae*, Vol. 4, New York, Plenum Press, pp. 1–61

Barnett, S.W., Barboza, A., Wilcox, C.M., Forsmark, C.E. & Levy, J.A. (1991) Characterization of human immunodeficiency virus type 1 strains recovered from the bowel of infected individuals. *Virology*, **182**, 802–809

Barnett, S.W., Murthy, K.K., Herndier, B.G. & Levy, J.A. (1994) An AIDS-like condition induced in baboons by HIV-2. *Science*, **266**, 642-646

Baroni, C.D., Pezzella, F., Stoppacciaro, A., Mirolo, M., Pescarmona, E., Vitolo, D., Cassano, A.M., Barsotti, P., Nicoletti, L., Ruco, L.P & Uccini, S. (1985) Systemic lymphadenopathy (LAS) in intravenous drug abusers. Histology, immunohistochemistry and electron microscopy: pathogenic correlations. *Histopathology*, **9**, 1275–1293

Baroni, C.D., Pezzella, F., Mirolo, M., Ruco, L.P. & Rossi, G.B. (1986) Immunohistochemical demonstration of p24 HTLV III major core protein in different cell types within lymph nodes from patients with lymphadenopathy syndrome (LAS). *Histopathology*, **10**, 5–13

Barr, B.B.B., Benton E.C., McLaren K., Bunney, M.H., Smith, I.W., Blessing, K. & Hunter, J.A.A. (1989) Human papillomavirus infection and skin cancer in renal allograft recipients. *Lancet*, **i**, 124–129

Barr, M.C., Butt, M.T., Anderson, K.L., Lin, D.-S., Kelleher, T.F. & Scott, F.W. (1993) Spinal lymphosarcoma and disseminated mastocytoma associated with feline immunodeficiency virus infection in a cat. *J. Am. vet. Med. Assoc.*, **202**, 1978–1980

Barré-Sinoussi, F., Chermann, J.C., Rey, F., Nugeyre, M.T., Chamaret, S., Gruest, J., Dauguet, C., Axler-Blin, C., Vézinet-Brun, F., Rouzioux, C., Rozenbaum, W. & Montagnier, L. (1983) Isolation of a T-lymphotropic retrovirus from a patient at risk for acquired immunodeficiency syndrome (AIDS). *Science*, **220**, 868–871

Barrett, W.L., First, M.R., Aron, B.S. & Penn, I. (1993) Clinical course of malignancies in renal transplant recipients. *Cancer*, **72**, 2186–2189

Barzan, L., Carbone, A., Saracchini, S., Vaccher, G., Tirelli, U. & Comoretto, R. (1989) Nasopharyngeal lymphatic tissue hypertrophy in HIV-infected patients (Letter to the Editor). *Lancet*, **i**, 42–43

Barzan, L., Carbone, A., Tirelli, U., Crosato, I.M., Vaccher, E., Volpe, R. & Comoretto, R. (1990) Nasopharyngeal lymphatic tissue in patients infected with human immunodeficiency virus. A prospective clinicopathologic study. *Arch. Otolaryngol. Head Neck Surg.*, **116**, 928–931

Baskerville, A., Ramsay, A., Cranage, M.P., Cook, N., Cook, R.W., Dennis, M.J., Greenaway, P.J., Kitchin, P.A. & Stott, E.J. (1990) Histopathological changes in simian immunodeficiency virus infection. *J. Pathol.*, **162**, 67–75

Baskin, G.B., Martin, L.N., Rangan, S.R.S., Gormus, B.J., Murphey-Corb, M., Wolf, R.H. & Soike, K.F. (1986) Transmissible lymphoma and simian acquired immunodeficiency syndrome in rhesus monkeys. *J. natl Cancer Inst.*, **77**, 127–139

Baskin, G.B., Murphey-Corb, M., Watson, E.A. & Martin, L.N. (1988) Necropsy findings in rhesus monkeys experimentally infected with cultured simian immunodeficiency virus (SIV)/delta. *Vet. Pathol.*, **25**, 456–467

Bassett, M.T., Chokunonga, E., Mauchaza, B., Levy, L., Ferlay, J. & Parkin, D.M. (1995) Cancer in the African population of Harare, Zimbabwe, 1990–1992. *Int. J. Cancer*, **63**, 29–36

Bauer, F.A., Wear, D.J., Angritt, P. & Lo, S.-C. (1991) *Mycoplasma fermentans* (incognitus strain) infection in the kidneys of patients with acquired immunodeficiency syndrome and associated nephropathy: a light microscopic, immunohistochemical and ultrastructural study. *Hum. Pathol.*, **22**, 63–69

Baum, L.G. & Vinters, HV. (1989) Lymphadenopathic Kaposi's sarcoma in a pediatric patient with acquired immune deficiency syndrome. *Pediatr. Pathol.*, **9**, 459–465

Bautch, V.L., Toda, S., Hassel, J.A. & Hanahan, D. (1987) Endothelial cell tumours develop in transgenic mice carrying polyomavirus middle T oncogene. *Cell*, **51**, 529–538

Bayley, A.C. (1984) Aggressive Kaposi's sarcoma in Zambia, 1983. *Lancet*, **i**, 1318–1320

Bayley, A.C., Downing, R.G., Cheinsong-Popov, R., Tedder, R.S., Dalgleish, A.G. & Weiss, R.A. (1985) HTLV-III serology distinguishes atypical and endemic Kaposi's sarcoma in Africa. *Lancet*, **i**, 359-361

Behets, F.M., Edidi, B., Quinn, T.C., Atikala, L., Bishagara, K., Nzila, N., Laga, M., Piot, P., Ryder, R.W. & Brown, C.C. (1991) Detection of salivary HIV-1-specific IgG antibodies in high-risk populations in Zaire. *J. acquir. Immun. Defic. Syndr.*, **4**, 183–187

Behling, C.A., Wolf, P.L. & Haghighi, P. (1993) AIDS and malignant mesothelioma — Is there a connection? *Chest*, **103**, 1268–1269

Bendsöe, N., Dictor, M., Blomberg, J., Ågren, S. & Merk, K. (1990) Increased incidence of Kaposi's sarcoma in Sweden before the AIDS epidemic. *Eur. J. Cancer*, **26**, 699–702

Benedetti, P., Greco, D., Figoli, F. & Tirelli, U. (1991) Epidemic Kaposi's sarcoma in female AIDS-patients — a report of 23 Italian cases. *AIDS*, **5**, 466–467

Benichou, S., Bomsel, M., Bodéus, M., Durand, H., Douté, M., Letourneur, F., Camonis, J. & Benarous, R. (1994) Physical interaction of the HIV-1Nef protein with β-COP, a component of non-clathrin-coated vesicles essential for membrane traffic. *J. biol.Chem.*, **269**, 30073-30076

Benjamin, D., Knobloch, T.J. & Dayton, M.A. (1992) Human B-cell interleukin-10: B-cell lines derived from patients with acquired immunodeficiency syndrome and Burkitt's lymphoma constitutively secrete large quantities of interleukin-10. *Blood*, **80**, 1289–1298

Bentwich, Z. & Bar-Yehuda, S. (1994) HIV specific immunity in seronegative Ethiopian immigrants: evidence for HIV exposure, silent infection or immune cross reactivity. *AIDS Res. hum. Retroviruses*, **10** (Suppl. 3), S143

Benveniste, R.E., Arthur, L.O., Tsai, C.-C., Sowder, R., Copeland, T.D., Henderson, L.E. & Oroszlan, S. (1986) Isolation of a lentivirus from a macaque with lymphoma: comparison to HTLV-III/LAV and other lentiviruses. *J. Virol.*, **60**, 483–490

Beral, V. (1991a) Epidemiology of Kaposi's sarcoma. *Cancer Surv.*, **10**, 5–23

Beral, B. (1991b) The epidemiology of cancer in AIDS patients. *AIDS*, **5** (Suppl. 2), S99–S103

Beral, V., Peterman, T.A., Berkelman, R.L. & Jaffe, H.W. (1990) Kaposi's sarcoma among persons with AIDS: a sexually transmitted infection? *Lancet*, **335**, 123–128

Beral, V., Bull, D., Jaffe, H., Evans, B., Gill, N., Tillett, H. & Swerdlow, A.J. (1991a) Is risk of Kaposi's sarcoma in AIDS patients in British Isles increased if sexual partners come from USA or Africa? *Br. med. J.*, **302**, 624–625

Beral, V., Peterman, T.A., Berkelman, R. & Jaffe, H. (1991b) AIDS-associated non-Hodgkin lymphoma. *Lancet*, **337**, 805–809

Beral, V., Bull, D., Darby, S., Weller, I., Carne, C., Beecham, M. & Jaffe, H. (1992) Risk of Kaposi's sarcoma and sexual practices associated with faecal contact in homosexual or bisexual men with AIDS. *Lancet*, **339**, 632–635

Berger, P. & Dirnhofer, S. (1995) Kaposi's sarcoma in pregnant women (Letter to the Editor). *Nature*, **377**, 21–22

Bergeron, C., Barrasso, R., Beaudenon, S., Flamant, P., Croissant, O. & Orth, G. (1992) Human papillomaviruses associated with cervical intraepithelial neoplasia. Great diversity and distinct distribution in low- and high-grade lesions. *Am. J. surg. Pathol.*, **16**, 641–649

Berkhout, R.J.M., Tieben, L.M., Smits, H.L., Bouwes Bavinck, J.N., Vermeer, B.J. & ter Schegget, J. (1995) Nested PCR approach for detection and typing of epidermodysplasia verruciformis-associated human papillomavirus types in cutaneous cancers from renal transplant recipients. *J. clin. Microbiol.*, **33**, 690–695

Berkley, S.F., Widy-Wirski, R., Okware, S.I., Downing, R., Linnan, M.J., White, K.E. & Sempala, S. (1989) Risk factors associated with HIV infection in Uganda. *J. infect. Dis.*, **160**, 22–30

Bernard, C., Mougin, C., Madoz, L., Drobacheff, C., van Landuyt, H., Laurent, R. & Lab, M. (1992) Viral co-infections in human papillomavirus-associated anogenital lesions according to the serostatus for the human immunodeficiency virus. *Int. J. Cancer*, **52**, 731–737

Bernardi, D., Salvioni, R., Vaccher, E., Repetto, L., Piersantelli, N., Marini, B., Talamini, R., & Tirelli, U. (1995) Testicular germ cell tumors and human immunodeficiency virus infection: a report of 26 cases. *J. clin. Oncol.*, **13**, 2705–2711

Bernheim, A. & Berger, R. (1988) Cytogenetic studies of Burkitt lymphoma-leukemia in patients with acquired immunodeficiency syndrome. *Cancer Genet. Cytogenet.*, **32**, 67–74

Bernstein, L., Levin, D., Menck, H. & Ross, R.K. (1989) AIDS-related secular trends in cancer in Los Angeles County men: a comparison by marital status. *Cancer Res.*, **49**, 466–470

Besnier, J.-M., Barin, F., Baillou, A., Liard, F., Choutet, P. & Goudeau, A. (1990) Symptomatic HIV-2 primary infection (Letter to the Editor). *Lancet*, **335**, 798

Bhatia, K., Spangler, G., Gaidano, G., Hamdy, N., Dalla-Favera, R. & Magrath, I. (1994) Mutations in the coding region of c-*myc* occur frequently in acquired immunodeficiency syndrome-associated lymphomas. *Blood*, **84**, 883–888

Biberfeld, P., Porwit-Ksiazek, A., Böttiger, B., Morfeldt-Månsson, L. & Biberfeld, G. (1985) Immunohistopathology of lymph nodes in HLTV-III infected homosexuals with persistent adenopathy or AIDS. *Cancer Res.* (Suppl.), **45**, 4665s–4670s

Biberfeld, P., Chayt, K.J., Marselle, L.M., Biberfeld, G., Gallo, R.C. & Harper, M.E. (1986) HTLV-III expression in infected lymph nodes and relevance to pathogenesis of lymphadenopathy. *Am. J. Pathol.*, **125**, 436–442

Biberfeld, P., Öst, Å., Porwit, A., Sandstedt, B., Pallesen, G., Böttiger, B., Morfelt-Månsson, L. & Biberfeld, G. (1987) Histopathology and immunohistology of HTLV-III/LAV related lymphadenopathy and AIDS. *Acta pathol. microbiol. immunol. scand.*, Sect. A, **95**, 47–65

Biggar, R.J. & Rabkin, C.S. (1992) The epidemiology of acquired immunodeficiency syndrome-related lymphomas. *Curr. Opin. Oncol.*, **4**, 883–893

Biggar, R.J. & the International Registry of Seroconverters (1990) AIDS incubation in 1891 HIV seroconverters from different exposure groups. *AIDS*, **4**, 1059–1066

Biggar, R.J., Horm, J., Fraumeni, J.F., Jr, Greene, M.H. & Goedert, J.J. (1984a) Incidence of Kaposi's sarcoma and mycosis fungoides in the United States including Puerto Rico, 1973–81. *J. natl Cancer Inst.*, **73**, 89–94

Biggar, R.J., Melbye, M., Kestems, L., Sarngadharan, M.G., de Feyter, M., Blattner, W.A., Gallo, R.C. & Gigase, P.L. (1984b) Kaposi's sarcoma in Zaire is not associated with HTLV-III infection (Letter to the Editor). *New Engl. J. Med.*, **311**, 1051–1052

Biggar, R.J., Horm, J., Lubin, J.H., Goedert, J.J., Greene, M.H. & Fraumeni, J.F., Jr (1985) Cancer trends in a population at risk of acquired immunodeficiency syndrome. *J. natl Cancer Inst.*, **74**, 793–797

Biggar, R.J., Horm, J., Goedert, J.J. & Melbye, M. (1987) Cancer in a group at risk of acquired immunodeficiency syndrome (AIDS) through 1984. *Am. J. Epidemiol.*, **126**, 578–586

Biggar, R.J., Burnett, W., Mikl, J. & Nasca, P. (1989) Cancer among New York men at risk of acquired immunodeficiency syndrome. *Int. J. Cancer*, **43**, 979–985

Biggar, R.J., Dunsmore, N., Kurman, R.J., Shah, K.V., Kordor, J., Cottoni, F., Hatzakis, A. & Gigase, P.L. (1992) Failure to detect human papillomavirus in Kaposi's sarcoma (Letter to the Editor). *Lancet*, **339**, 1604–1605

Biggar, R.J., Curtis, R.E., Coté, T.R., Rabkin, C.S. & Melbye, M. (1994) Risk of other cancers following Kaposi's sarcoma: relation to acquired immunodeficiency syndrome. *Am. J. Epidemiol.*, **139**, 362–368

Bignall, J. (1993) Rochalimaeas from cat-scratch to Kaposi. *Lancet*, **342**, 359

Bigoni, B., Dolcetti, R., de Lellis, L., Carbone, A., Boiocchi, M., Cassai, E. & Di Luca, D. (1996) Human herpesvirus 8 is present in the lymphoid system of healthy persons and can reactivate in the course of AIDS. *J. infect. Dis.*, **173**, 542–549

Birkeland, S.A., Storm, H.H., Lamm, L.U., Barlow, L., Blohmé, I., Forsberg, B., Eklund, B., Fjeldbord, O., Friedberg, M., Frödin, L., Glattre, E., Halvorsen, S., Holm, N.V., Jakobsen, A., Jørgensen, H.E., Ladefoged, J., Lindholm, T., Lundgren, G. & Pukkala, E. (1995) Cancer risk after renal transplantation in the Nordic countries, 1964–1986. *Int. J. Cancer*, **60**, 183–189

Birx, D.L., Redfield, R.R. & Tosato, G. (1986) Defective regulation of Epstein-Barr virus infection in patients with acquired immunodeficiency syndrome (AIDS) or AIDS-related disorders. *New Engl. J. Med.*, **314**, 874–879

Birx, D.L., Redfield, R.R., Tencer, K., Fowler, A., Burke, D.S. & Tosato, G. (1990) Induction of interleukin-6 during human immunodeficiency virus infection. *Blood*, **76**, 2303–2310

Biswas, P., Smith, C.A., Goletti, D., Hardy, E.C., Jackson, R.W. & Fauci, A.S. (1995) Cross-linking of CD30 induces HIV expression in chronically infected T cells. *Immunity*, **2**, 587–596

Blatt, S.P., Hendrix, C.W., Butzin, C.A., Freeman, T.M., Ward, W.W., Hensley, R.E., Melcher, W.P., Donovan, D.J. & Boswell, R.N. (1993) Delayed-type hypersensitivity skin testing predicts progression to AIDS in HIV-infected patients. *Ann. intern. Med.*, **119**, 177–184

Blum, S., Singh, T.P., Gibbons, J., Fordyce, E.J., Lassner, L., Chaisson, M.A., Weisfuse, I.B. & Thomas, P.A. (1994) Trends in survival among persons with acquired immunodeficiency syndrome in New York City. The experience of the first decade of the epidemic. *Am. J. Epidemiol.*, **139**, 351–361

Blumberg, P.M. (1988) Protein kinase C as the receptor for the phorbol ester tumor promoters: Sixth Rhoads Memorial Award Lecture. *Cancer Res.*, **48**, 1–8

Bobkov, A., Cheingsong-Popov, R., Garaev, M., Salminen, M., McCutchan, F., Louwagie, J., Arioshi, K., Whittle, H. &Weber, J.N. (1996) Complex mosaic structure of the partial envelope sequence from a Gambian HIV Type 1 isolate. *AIDS Res. hum. Retroviruses*, **12**, 169-171

Boiocchi, M., Carbone, A., De Re, V., Dolcetti, R., Volpe, R. & Tirelli, U. (1990) AIDS-related B-cell non-Hodgkin's lymphomas in direct blood-stream HIV-infected patients: pathogenesis and differentiation features. *Int. J. Cancer*, **45**, 883–888

Boiocchi, M., De Re, V., Gloghini, A., Vaccher, E., Dolcetti, R., Marzotto, A., Bertola, G. & Carbone, A. (1993a) High incidence of monoclonal EBV episomes in Hodgkin's disease and anaplastic large-cell Ki-1-positive lymphomas in HIV-1-positive patients. *Int. J. Cancer*, **54**, 53–59

Boiocchi, M., Dolcetti, R., De Re, V., Gloghini, A. & Carbone, A. (1993b) Demonstration of a unique Epstein-Barr virus-positive cellular clone in metachronous multiple localizations of Hodgkin's disease. *Am. J. Pathol.*, **142**, 33–38

Bollinger, R.C., Jr, Kline, R.L., Francis, H.L., Moss, M.W., Bartlett, J.G. & Quinn, T.C. (1992) Acid dissociation increases the sensitivity of p24 antigen detection for the evaluation of antiviral therapy and disease progression in asymptomatic human immunodeficiency virus-infected persons. *J. infect. Dis.*, **165**, 913–916

Booth, R.E. & Watters, J.K. (1994) How effective are risk-reduction interventions targeting injecting drug users? *AIDS*, **8**, 1515–1524

Borisch Chappuis, B., Müller, H., Stutte, J., Hey, M.M., Hübner, K. & Müller-Hermelink, H.K. (1990) Identification of EBV-DNA in lymph nodes from patients with lymphadenopathy and lymphomas associated with AIDS. *Virchows Arch. (B) Cell Pathol.*, **58**, 199–205

Borman, A.M., Quillent, C., Charneau, P., Dauguet, D. & Clavel, F. (1995) Human immuno-deficiency virus type 1 *vif* mutant particles from restrictive cells: role of *vif* in correct particle assembly and infectivity. *J. Virol.*, **69**, 2058–2067

Boshoff, C., Whitby, D., Hatziioannou, T., Fisher, C., van der Walt, J., Hatzakis, A.,Weiss, R. & Schulz, T. (1995a) Kaposi's-sarcoma-associated herpesvirus in HIV-negative Kaposi sarcoma (Letter to the Editor). *Lancet*, **345**, 1043–1044

Boshoff, C., Schulz, T.F., Kennedy, M.M., Graham, A.K., Fisher, C., Thomas, A., McGee, J., Weiss, R.A. & O'Leary, J.J. (1995b) Kaposi's sarcoma-associated herpes virus (KSHV) infects endothelial and spindle cells. *Nature Med.*, **1**, 1274–1278

Bouscarat, F., Samuel, D., Simon, F., Debat, P., Bismuth, H. & Saimot, A.G. (1994) An observational study of 11 French liver transplant recipients infected with human immuno-deficiency virus type 1. *Clin. infect. Dis.*, **19**, 854–859

Bouwes Bavinck, J.N., Vermeer, B.J., van der Woude, F.J., Vandenbroucke, J.P., Schreuder, G.M.T., Thorogood, J., Persijn, G.G. & Claas, F.H.J. (1991) Relation between skin cancer and HLA antigens in renal-transplant recipients. *New Engl. J. Med.*, **325**, 843–848

Bovenzi, P., Mirandola, P., Secchiero, P., Strumia, R., Cassai, E. & Di Luca, D. (1993) Human herpesvirus 6 (variant A) in Kaposi's sarcoma (Letter to the Editor). *Lancet*, **341**, 1288–1289

Boyle, M.J., Sewell, W.A., Sculley, T.B., Apolloni, A., Turner, J.J., Swanson, C.E., Penny, R. & Cooper, D.A. (1991) Subtypes of Epstein-Barr virus in human immunodeficiency virus-associated non-Hodgkin lymphoma. *Blood*, **78**, 3004–3011

Boyle, M.J., Vasak, E., Tschuchnigg, M., Turner, J.J., Sculley, T., Penny, R., Cooper, D.A., Tindall, B. & Sewell, W.A. (1993) Subtypes of Epstein-Barr virus (EBV) in Hodgkin's disease: association between B-type EBV and immunocompromise. *Blood*, **81**, 468–474

Bradbeer, C. (1987) Is infection with HIV a risk factor for cervical intraepithelial neoplasia? (Letter to the Editor). *Lancet*, **ii**, 1277–1278

Braun, L. (1994) Role of human immunodeficiency virus infection in the pathogenesis of human papillomavirus-associated cervical neoplasia. *Am. J. Pathol.*, **144**, 209–214

Breese, P.L., Judson, F.N., Penley, K.A. & Douglas, J.M., Jr (1995) Anal human papillomavirus infection among homosexual and bisexual men: prevalence of type-specific infection and association with human immunodeficiency virus. *Sex. transm. Dis.*, **22**, 7–14

Breimer, L. (1994) Original description of Kaposi's sarcoma (Letter to the Editor). *Br. med. J.*, **308**, 1303-1304

Brown, T., Sittitrai, W., Vanichseni, S. & Thisyakorn, U. (1994a) The recent epidemiology of HIV/AIDS in Thailand. *AIDS*, **8** (Suppl 2), S131–S141

Brown, D.R., Bryan, T.J., Cramer, H., Katz, B.P., Handy, V. & Fife, K.H. (1994b) Detection of multiple human papillomavirus types in condylomata acuminata from immunosuppressed patients. *J. infect. Dis.*, **170**, 759–765

Browning, P.J., Sechler, J.M.G., Kaplan, M., Washington, R.H., Gendelman, R., Yarchoan, R., Ensoli, B. & Gallo, R.C. (1994) Identification and culture of Kaposi's sarcoma-like spindle cells from the peripheral blood of human immunodeficiency virus-1-infected individuals and normal controls. *Blood*, **84**, 2711–2720

Brücker, G., Brun-Vézinet, F., Rosenheim, M., Rey, M.A., Katlama, C. & Gentilini, M. (1987) HIV-2 infection in two homosexual men in France (Letter to the Editor). *Lancet*, **i**, 223

van den Brule, A.J.C., Walboomers, J.M.M., Du Maine, M., Kenemans, P. & Meijer, C.J.L.M. (1991) Difference in prevalence of human papillomavirus genotypes in cytomorphologically normal cervical smears is associated with a history of cervical intraepithelial neoplasia. *Int. J. Cancer*, **48**, 404–408

Brun-Vézinet, F., Rey, M.A., Katlama, C., Girard, P.M., Roulot, D., Yeni, P., Lenoble, L., Clavel, F., Alizon, M., Gadelle, S., Madjar, J.J. & Harzic, M. (1987) Lymphadenopathy-associated virus type 2 in AIDS and AIDS-related complex. *Lancet*, **i**, 128–132

Brunson, M.E., Balakrishnan, K. & Penn, I. (1990) HLA and Kaposi's sarcoma in solid organ transplantation. *Hum. Immunol.*, **29**, 56–63

Brusamolino, E., Pagnucco, G. & Bernasconi, C. (1989) Secondary lymphomas: a review on lymphoproliferative diseases arising in immunocompromized hosts: prevalence, clinical features and pathogenetic mechanisms. *Haematologica*, **74**, 605–622

Buchbinder, S.P., Katz, M.H., Hessol, N.A., Liu, J.Y., O'Malley, P.M., Underwood, R. & Holmberg, S.D. (1992) Herpes zoster and human immunodeficiency virus infection. *J. infect. Dis.*, **166**, 1153–1156

Buchbinder, S.P., Katz, M.H., Hessol, N.A., O'Malley, P.M. & Holmberg, S.D. (1994) Long-term HIV-1 infection without immunologic progression. *AIDS*, **8**, 1123–1128

Buehler, J.W., Berkelman, R.L. & Curran, J.W. (1989) Reporting of AIDS: tracking HIV morbidity and mortality. *J. Am. med. Assoc.*, **262**, 2896–2897

Bukrinsky, M.I., Haggerty, S., Dempsey, M.P., Sharova, N., Adzhubei, A., Spitz, L., Lewis, P., Goldfarb, D., Emerman, M. & Stevenson, M. (1993) A nuclear localization signal within HIV-1 matrix protein that governs infection of non-dividing cells. *Nature*, **365**, 666–669

Buonaguro, F.M., Tornesello, M.L., Buonaguro, L., Del Gaudio, E., Beth-Giraldo, E. & Giraldo, G. (1994) Role of HIV as cofactor in HPV oncogenesis: in-vitro evidences of virus interactions. In: Giraldo, G., Salvatore, M., Chieco-Bianchi, L. & Beth-Giraldo, E., eds, *Advanced Technologies in Research, Diagnosis and Treatment of AIDS and in Oncology*, Basel, Karger, pp. 102–109

Buonaguro, F.M., Tornesello, M.L., Beth-Giraldo, E., Hatzakis, A., Mueller, N., Downing, R., Biryamwaho, B., Sempala, S.D.K. & Giraldo, G. (1996) Herpesvirus-like DNA sequences detected in endemic, classic, iatrogenic and epidemic Kaposi's sarcoma (KS) biopsies. *Int. J. Cancer*, **65**, 25-28

Burin Des Roziers, N., Bruet, A., Leger, J.-P., Collet, C., Aufeuvre, J.-P., Fendler, J.-P, Chamaret, S. & Montagnier, L. (1987) HIV-2 infection with long incubation period. *Presse méd.*, **16**, 1981 (in French)

Burke, A.P., Benson, W., Ribas, J.L., Anderson, D., Chu, W.-S., Smialek, J. & Virmani, R. (1993) Postmortem localization of HIV-1 RNA by in situ hybridization in lymphoid tissues of intravenous drug addicts who died unexpectedly. *Am. J. Pathol.*, **142**, 1701–1713

Busch, M.P., Young, M.J., Samson, S.M., Mosley, J.W., Ward, J.W. & Perkins, H.A. (1991) Risk of human immunodeficiency virus (HIV) transmission by blood transfusion before the implementation of HIV-1 antibody screening. *Transfusion*, **31**, 4–11

Buzelin, F., Karam, G., Moreau, A., Wetzel, O. & Gaillard, F. (1994) Testicular tumor and the acquired immunodeficiency syndrome. *Eur. Urol.*, **26**, 71–76

Byrne, M.A., Taylor-Robinson, D., Munday, P.E. & Harris, J.R.W. (1989) The common occurrence of human papillomavirus infection and intraepithelial neoplasia in women infected by HIV. *AIDS*, **3**, 379–382

Cáceres, C.F. & Hearst, N. (1996) HIV/AIDS in Latin America and the Caribbean: an update. *AIDS*, **10** (Suppl A), S43–S49

Caiaffa, W.T., Graham, N.M.H. & Vlahov, D. (1993) Bacterial pneumonia in adult populations with human immunodeficiency virus (HIV) infection. *Am. J. Epidemiol.*, **138**, 909–922

Callanan, J.J., McCandlish, I.A.P., O'Neil, B., Lawrence, C.E., Rigby, M., Pacitti, A.M. & Jarrett, O. (1992) Lymphosarcoma in experimentally induced feline immunodeficiency virus infection. *Vet. Rec.*, **130**, 293–295

Callanan, J.J., Rácz, P., Thompson, H. & Jarrett, O. (1993) Morphological characterisation of the lymph node changes in feline immunodeficiency virus infection as an animal model of AIDS. In: Rácz, P., Letvin, N.L. & Gluckmann, J.C., eds, *Animal Models of HIV and Other Retroviral Infections*, Basel, Karger, pp. 115–136

Callanan, J.J., Jones, B.A., Irvine, J., Willett, B.J., McCandlish, I.A.P. & Jarrett, O. (1996) Histological classification and immunophenotype of lymphosarcomas in cats with naturally and experimentally acquired feline immunodeficiency virus infections. *Vet. Pathol.*, **33**, 264-272

Cameron, D.W., Simonsen, J.N., D'Costa, L.J., Ronald, A.R., Maitha, G.M., Gakinya, M.N., Cheang, M., Ndinya-Achola, J.O., Piot, P., Brunham, R.C. & Plummer, F.A. (1989) Female-to-male transmission of human immunodeficiency virus type 1: risk factors for seroconversion in men. *Lancet*, **ii**, 403–407

Camilleri-Broët, S., Davi, F., Feuillard, J., Bourgeois, C., Seilhean, D., Hauw, J.-J. & Raphaël, M. (1995) High expression of latent membrane protein 1 of Epstein-Barr virus and BCL-2 oncoprotein in acquired immunodeficiency syndrome-related primary brain lymphomas. *Blood*, **86**, 432–435

Campioni, D., Corallini, A., Zauli, G., Possati, L., Altavilla, G. & Barbanti-Brodano, G. (1995) HIV type 1 extracellular Tat protein stimulates growth and protects cells of BK virus/*tat* transgenic mice from apoptosis. *AIDS Res. hum. Retroviruses*, **11**, 1039–1048

Canman, C.E., Gilmer, T.M., Coutts, S.B. & Kastan, M.B. (1995) Growth factor modulation of p53-mediated growth arrest versus apoptosis. *Genes Dev.*, **9**, 600–611

Cao, Y., Qin, L., Zhang, L., Safrit, J. & Ho, D.D. (1995) Virologic and immunologic characterization of long-term survivors of human immunodeficiency virus type 1 infection. *New Engl. J. Med.*, **332**, 201–208

Cappell, M.S., Yao, F. & Cho, K.C. (1988) Colonic adenocarcinoma associated with the acquired immunodeficiency syndrome. *Cancer*, **62**, 616–619

Carbone, A., Manconi, R., Poletti, A., Tirelli, U., De Paoli, P., Santini, G., Diodato, S., Manconi, P.E., Grigoletto, E., Santi, L. & Volpe, R. (1985) Lymph node immunohistology in intravenous drug abusers with persistent generalized lymphadenopathy. *Arch. Pathol. Lab. Med.*, **109**, 1007–1012

Carbone, A., Manconi, R., Poletti, A. & Volpe, R. (1986) A histopathologic study of persistent generalized lymphadenopathy in intravenous drug abusers. *Pathol. Res. Pract.*, **181**, 195–199

Carbone, A., De Re, V., Gloghini, A., Volpe, R., Tavian, M., Tirelli, U., Monfardini, S. & Boiocchi, M. (1989) Immunoglobulin and T cell receptor gene rearrangements and in situ immunophenotyping in lymphoproliferative disorders. *Virchows Arch. (A) Pathol. Anat.*, **414**, 233–230

Carbone, A., Tirelli, U., Vaccher, E., Volpe, R., Gloghini, A., Bertola, G., De Re, V., Rossi, C., Boiocchi, M. & Monfardini, S. (1991) A clinicopathologic study of lymphoid neoplasias associated with human immunodeficiency virus infection in Italy. *Cancer*, **68**, 842–852

Carbone, A., Gloghini, A., Zanette, I., Canal, B. & Volpe, R. (1993a) Demonstration of Epstein-Barr viral genomes by in situ hybridization in acquired immune deficiency syndrome-related high grade and anaplastic large cell CD30$^+$ lymphomas. *Am. J. clin. Pathol.*, **99**, 289–297

Carbone, A., Tirelli, U., Gloghini, A., Volpe, R. & Boiocchi, M. (1993b) Human immunodeficiency virus-associated systemic lymphomas may be subdivided into two main groups according to Epstein-Barr viral latent gene expression. *J. clin. Oncol.*, **11**, 1674–1681

Carbone, A., Gloghini, A., Volpe, R., Boiocchi, M., Tirelli, U. & the Italian Cooperative Group on AIDS & Tumors (1994) High frequency of Epstein-Barr virus latent membrane protein-1 expression in acquired immunodeficiency syndrome-related Ki-1 (CD30) — positive anaplastic large cell lymphomas. *Am. J. clin. Pathol.*, **101**, 768–772

Carbone, A., Gloghini, A., Gaidano, G., Cilia, A.M., Bassi, P., Polito, P., Vaccher, E., Saglio, G. & Tirelli, U. (1995a) AIDS-related Burkitt's lymphoma. Morphologic and immunophenotypic study of biopsy specimens. *Am. J. clin. Pathol.*, **103**, 561–567

Carbone, A., Gloghini, A., Vaccher, E., Barzan, L. & Tirelli, U. (1995b) Nasopharyngeal lymphoid tissue masses in patients with human immunodeficiency virus-1 (Letter to the Editor). *Cancer*, **76**, 527–528

Carbone, A., Dolcetti, R., Gloghini, A., Maestro, R., Vaccher, E., Di Luca, D., Tirelli, U. & Boiocchi, M. (1996a) Immunophenotypic and molecular analyses of acquired immune deficiency syndrome-related and Epstein-Barr virus-associated lymphomas: a comparative study. *Hum. Pathol.*, **27**, 133–146

Carbone, A., Tirelli, U., Gloghini, A., Pastore, C., Vaccher, E. & Gaidano, G. (1996b) Herpesvirus-like DNA sequences selectively cluster with body cavity-based lymphomas throughout the spectrum of AIDS-related lymphomatous effusions. *Eur. J. Cancer*, **32A**, 555–556

Carbone, A., Gloghini, A., Zagonel, V. & Tirelli, U. (1996c) Expression of Epstein-Barr virus-encoded latent membrane protein 1 in nonendemic Burkitt's lymphomas. *Blood*, **86**, 1202–1204

Carrigan, D.R., Drobyski, W.R., Russler, S.K., Tapper, M.A., Knox, K.K. & Ash, R.C. (1991) Interstitial pneumonitis associated with human herpesvirus-6 infection after marrow transplantation. *Lancet*, **338**, 147–149

Casabona, J., Salas, T., Lacasa, C., Melbye, M. & Segura, A. (1990) Kaposi's sarcoma in people with AIDS from an area in southern Europe [letter]. *J. acquir. Immun. Defic. Syndr.*, **3**, 929–930

Casabona, J., Melbye, M., Biggar, R.J. & the AIDS Registry Contributors (1991) Kaposi's sarcoma and non-Hodgkin's lymphoma in European AIDS cases. No excess risk of Kaposi's sarcoma in Mediterranean countries. *Int. J. Cancer*, **47**, 49–53

Casabona, J., Salas, T. & Salinas, R. (1993) Trends and survival in AIDS-associated malignancies. *Eur. J. Cancer*, **29A**, 877–881

Castro, B.A., Nepomuceno, M., Lerche, N.W., Eichberg, J.W. & Levy, J.A. (1991) Persistent infection of baboons and rhesus monkeys with different strains of HIV-2. *Virology*, **184**, 219–226

Catania, J.A., Coates, T.J., Stall, R., Turner, H., Peterson, J., Hearst, N., Dolcini, M.M., Hudes, E., Gagnon, J., Wiley, J. & Groves, R. (1992) Prevalence of AIDS-related risk factors and condom use in the United States. *Science*, **258**, 1101–1106

Caussy, D., Goedert, J.J., Palefsky, J., Gonzales, J., Rabkin, C.S., DiGioia, R.A., Sanchez, W.C, Grossman, R.J., Colclough, G., Wiktor, S.Z., Krämer, A., Biggar, R.J. & Blattner, W.A. (1990) Interaction of human immunodeficiency and papilloma viruses: association with anal epithelial abnormality in homosexual men. *Int. J. Cancer*, **46**, 214–219

Celum, C.L., Coombs, R.W., Lafferty, W., Inui, T.S., Louie, P.H., Gates, C.A., McCreedy, B.J., Egan, R., Grove, T., Alexander, S., Koepsell, T., Weiss, N., Fisher, L., Corey, L. & Holmes, K.K. (1991) Indeterminate human immunodeficiency virus type-1 western blots: seroconversion risk, specificity of supplemental tests, and an algorithm for evaluation. *J. infect. Dis.*, **164**, 656–664

Centers for Disease Control (CDC) (1982) Persistent, generalized lymphadenopathy among homosexual males. *Morbid. Mortal. Wkly Rep.*, **31**, 249–251

Centers for Disease Control (CDC) (1988) AIDS due to HIV-2 infection — New Jersey. *Morbid. Mortal. Wkly Rep.*, **37**, 33–35

Centers for Disease Control (CDC) (1989a) Interpretation and use of the western blot assay for serodiagnosis of human immunodeficiency virus type-1 infections. *Morbid. Mortal. Wkly Rep.*, **38** (No. S-7), 1–7

Centers for Disease Control (CDC) (1989b) Update: HIV-2 infection — United States. *Morbid. Mortal. Wkly Rep.*, **38**, 572–580

Centers for Disease Control and Prevention (1992a) 1993 revised classification system for HIV infection and expanded surveillance case definition for AIDS among adolescents and adults. *Morbid. Mortal. Wkly Rep.*, **41** (RR-17), 1–19

Centers for Disease Control and Prevention (1992b) Recommendations for prophylaxis against *Pneumocystis carinii* pneumonia for adults and adolescents infected with human immunodeficiency virus. *Morbid. Mortal. Wkly Rep.*, **41**, 1–11

Centers for Disease Control and Prevention (1992c) Changes in sexual behavior and condom use associated with a risk-reduction program — Denver, 1988–1991. *Morbid. Mortal. Wkly Rep.*, **41**, 412–415

Centers for Disease Control and Prevention (1994a) *HIV/AIDS Surveillance Report*, Vol. 6, Atlanta, GA, US Department of Health and Human Services

Centers for Disease Control and Prevention (1994b) Knowledge and practices among injecting-drug users of bleach use for equipment disinfection — New York City, 1993. *Morbid. Mortal. Wkly Rep.*, **43**, 439, 445–446

Centers for Disease Control and Prevention (1995a) US HIV and AIDS cases reported through June 1995. *HIV/AIDS Surv. Rep.*, **7**, 1–34

Centers for Disease Control and Prevention (1995b) USPHS/IDSA guidelines for the prevention of opportunistic infections in persons infected with human immunodeficiency virus: a summary. *Morbid. Mortal. Wkly Rep.*, **44**, 1–34

Centers for Disease Control and Prevention (1995c) Syringe exchange programs — United States, 1994–1995. *Morbid. Mortal. Wkly Rep.*, **44**, 684–685, 691

Centers for Disease Control and Prevention (1995d) U.S. Public Health Service recommendations for human immunodeficiency virus counseling and voluntary testing for pregnant women. *Morbid. Mortal. Wkly Rep.*, **44** (No. RR-7), 1–15

Centers for Disease Control and Prevention (1995e) Recommendations of the U.S. Public Health Service Task Force on the use of zidovudine to reduce perinatal transmission of human immunodeficiency virus. *Morbid. Mortal. Wkly Rep.*, **43** (No. RR-11)

Cesarman, E., Inghirami, G., Chadburn, A. & Knowles, D.M. (1993) High levels of p53 protein expression do not correlate with p53 gene mutations in anaplastic large cell lymphoma. *Am. J. Pathol.*, **143**, 845–856

Cesarman, E., Chang, Y., Moore, P.S., Said, J.W. & Knowles, D.M. (1995) Kaposi's sarcoma-associated herpesvirus-like DNA sequences in AIDS-related body-cavity-based lymphomas (Letter to the Editor). *New Engl. J. Med.*, **332**, 1186–1191

Cesarman, E., Nador, R. & Knowles, D.M. (1996) Body-cavity-based lymphoma in an HIV-seronegative patient without Kaposi's sarcoma-associated herpesvirus-like DNA sequences (Letter to the Editor). *New Engl. J. Med.*, **334**, 272–273

Chadburn, A., Cesarman, E., Jagirdar, J., Subar, M., Mir, R.N. & Knowles, D.M. (1993) CD30 (Ki-1) positive anaplastic large cell lymphomas in individuals infected with the human immunodeficiency virus. *Cancer*, **72**, 3078–3090

Chadha, M., Rosenblatt, E.A., Malamud, S., Pisch, J. & Berson, A. (1994) Squamous-cell carcinoma of the anus in HIV-positive patients. *Dis. Colon Rectum*, **37**, 861–865

Chadwick, E.G., Connor, E.J., Guerra Hanson, I.C., Joshi, V.V., Abu-Farsakh, H., Yogev, R., McSherry, G., McClain, K. & Murphy, S.B. (1990) Tumors of smooth-muscle origin in HIV-infected children. *J. Am. med. Assoc.*, **263**, 3182–3184

Chaganti, R.S.K., Jhanwar, S.C., Koziner, B., Arlin, Z., Mertelsmann, R. & Clarkson, B.D. (1983) Specific translocations characterize Burkitt's-like lymphoma of homosexual men with the acquired immunodeficiency syndrome. *Blood*, **61**, 1265–1268

Chalifoux, L.V., King, N.W., Daniel, M.D., Kannagi, M., Desrosiers, R.C., Sehgal, P.K., Waldron, L.M., Hunt, R.D. & Letvin, N.L. (1986) Lymphoproliferative syndrome in an immunodeficient rhesus monkey naturally infected with an HTLV-III-like virus (STLV-III). *Lab. Invest.*, **55**, 43–50

Chamberlain, M.C. (1994) Gliomas in patients with acquired immune deficiency syndrome. *Cancer*, **74**, 1912–1914

Chan, W.-K., Chong, T., Bernard, H.-U. & Klock, G. (1990) Transcription of the transforming genes of the oncogenic human papillomavirus-16 is stimulated by tumor promoters through AP1 binding sites. *Nucleic Acids Res.*, **18**, 763–769

Chan, T.K., Aranda, C.P. & Rom, W.N. (1993) Bronchogenic carcinoma in young patients at risk for acquired immunodeficiency syndrome. *Chest*, **103**, 862–864

Chang, Y., Cesarman, E., Pessin, M.S., Lee, F., Culpepper, J., Knowles, D.M. & Moore, P.S. (1994) Identification of herpesvirus-like DNA sequences in AIDS-associated Kaposi's sarcoma. *Science*, **266**, 1865–1869

Chang, Y., Ziegler, J., Wabinga, H., Katangole-Mbidde, E., Boshoff, C., Schulz, T., Whitby, D., Maddalena, D., Jaffe, H.W., Weiss, R.A., the Uganda Kaposi's Sarcoma Study Group & Moore, P.S. (1996) Kaposi's sarcoma-associated herpesvirus and Kaposi's sarcoma in Africa. *Arch. intern. Med.*, **156**, 202–204

Chant, K., Lowe, D., Rubin, G., Manning, W., O'Donoughue, R., Lyle, D., Levy, M., Morey, S., Kaldor, J., Garsia, R., Penny, R., Marriott, D., Cunningham, A. & Tracy, G.D. (1993) Patient-to-patient transmission of HIV in private surgical consulting rooms. *Lancet*, **342**, 1548–1549

Chen, Z., Telfer, P., Reed, P., Zhang, L., Gettie, A., Ho, D.D. & Marx, P.A. (1995) Isolation and characterization of the first simian immunodeficiency virus from a feral sooty mangabey (*Cerocebus atys*) in West Africa. *J. med. Primatol.* **24**, 108-115

Chen, Z., Telfer, P., Gettie, A., Reed, P., Zhang, L., Ho, D.D. & Marx, P.A. (1996) Genetic characterization of new west African simian immunodeficiency virus SIVsm: geographic clustering of household-derived SIV strains with human immunodeficiency virus type 2 subtypes and genetically diverse viruses from a single feral sooty mangabey troop. *J. Virol.*, **70**, 3617–3627

Chin, J. (1995) Scenarios for the AIDS epidemic in Asia. *Asia-Pacific Pop. Res. Rep.*, **2**, 1–15

Chintu, C., Malek, A., Nyumbu, M., Luo, C., Masona, J., DuPont, M.L. & Zumla, A. (1993) Case definitions for paediatric AIDS: the Zambian experience. *Int. J. STD AIDS*, **4**, 83–85

Chitwood, D.D. (1994) Annotation: HIV risk and injection drug users — evidence for behavioral change. *Am. J. public Health*, **84**, 350

Choi, K.-H. & Coates, T.J. (1994) Prevention of HIV infection. *AIDS*, **8**, 1371–1389

Chong, T., Chan, W.-K. & Bernard, H.-U. (1990) Transcriptional activation of human papillomavirus 16 by nuclear factor 1, AP1, steroid receptors and a possibly novel transcription factor, PVF: a model for the composition of genital papillomavirus enhancers. *Nucleic Acids Res.*, **18**, 465–470

Christeff, N., Winter, C., Gharakhanian, S., Thobie, N., Wirbel, E., Costagliola, D., Nunez, E.A. & Rozenbaum, W. (1995) Differences in androgens of HIV positive patients with and without Kaposi sarcoma. *J. Clin. Pathol.*, **48**, 513–518

Ciesiclski, C., Marianos, D., Ou, C.-Y., Dumbaugh, R., Witte, J., Berkelman, R., Gooch, B., Myers, G., Luo, C.-C., Schochetman, G., Howell, J., Lasch, A., Bell, K., Economou, N., Scott, B., Furman, L., Curran, J. & Jaffe, H. (1992) Transmission of human immunodeficiency virus in a dental practice. *Ann. intern. Med.*, **116**, 798–805

Cinque, P., Brytting, M., Vago, L., Castagna, A., Parravicini, C., Zanchetta, N., Monforte, A.D'A., Wahren, B., Lazzarin, A. & Linde, A. (1993) Epstein-Barr virus DNA in cerebrospinal fluid from patients with AIDS-related primary lymphoma of the central nervous system. *Lancet*, **342**, 398–401

Clapham, P.R., Blanc, D. & Weiss, R.A. (1991) Specific cell surface requirements for the infection of CD4-positive cells by human immunodeficiency virus types 1 and 2 and by Simian immunodeficiency virus. *Virology*, **181**, 703–715

Clark, S.J., Saag, M.S., Don Decker, W., Campbell-Hill, S., Roberson, J.L., Veldkamp, P.J., Kappes, J.C., Hahn, B.H. & Shaw, G.M. (1991) High titers of cytopathic virus in plasma of patients with symptomatic primary HIV-1 infection. *New Engl. J. Med.*, **324**, 954–960

Clavel, F., Guétard, D., Brun-Vézinet, F., Chamaret, S., Rey, M.-A., Santos-Ferreira, M.O., Laurent, A.G., Dauguet, C., Katlama, C., Rouzioux, C., Klatzmann, D., Champalimaud, J.L. & Montagnier, L. (1986) Isolation of a new human retrovirus from West African patients with AIDS. *Science*, **233**, 343–346

Clavel, F., Mansinho, K., Chamaret, S., Guetard, D., Favier, V., Nina, J., Santos-Ferreira, M.-O., Champalimaud, J.-L. & Montagnier, L. (1987) Human immunodeficiency virus type 2 infection associated with AIDS in West Africa. *New Engl. J. Med.*, **316**, 1180–1185

Clumeck, N., Sonnet, J., Taelman, H., Mascart-Lemone, F., De Bruyere, M., Vandeperre, P., Dasnoy, J., Marcelis, L., Lamy, M., Jonas, C., Eyckmans, L., Noel, H., Vanhaeverbeek, M. & Butzler, J.-P. (1984) Acquired immunodeficiency syndrome in African patients. *New Engl. J. Med.*, **310**, 492–497

Cockerell, C.J. (1991) Histopathological features of Kaposi's sarcoma in HIV infected individuals. *Cancer Surv.*, **10**, 73–89

Coffin, J.M. (1986) Genetic variation in AIDS viruses. *Cell*, **46**, 1–4

Coffin, J.M. (1992) Classification and nomenclature of viruses. *Arch. Virol.*, **Suppl. 2**, 290–298

Coffin, J.M. (1996) Retroviridae: the viruses and their replication. In: Fields, B.N., Knipe, P.M., Howley, P.M., Chanock, R.M., Melnick, J.L., Monath, T.P. & Roizman, B., eds, *Fields Virology*, 3rd Ed., Vol. 2, Philadelphia, Lippincott-Raven Publishers, pp. 1767–1847

Cohen, E.A., Terwilliger, E.F., Jalinoos, Y., Proulx, J., Sodroski, J.G. & Haseltine, W.A. (1990a) Identification of HIV-1 *vpr* product and function. *J. acquir. Immun. Defic. Syndr.*, **3**, 11–18

Cohen, E.A., Dehni, G., Sodroski, J.G. & Haseltine, W.A. (1990b) Human immunodeficiency virus *vpr* product is a virion-associated regulatory protein. *J. Virol.*, **64**, 3097–3099

Coleman, M.P., Estève, J., Damiecki, P., Arslan, A. & Renard, H., eds (1993) *Trends in Cancer Incidence and Mortality* (IARC Scientific Publications No. 121), Lyon, IARC, pp. 641–672

Collandre, H., Ferris, S., Grau, O., Montagnier, L. & Blanchard, A. (1995) Kaposi's sarcoma and new herpesvirus (Letter to the Editor). *Lancet*, **345**, 1043

Collier, A.C., Coombs, R.W., Schoenfeld, D.A., Bassett, R.L., Timpone, J., Baruch, A., Jones, M., Facey, K., Whitacre, C., McAuliffe, V.J., Friedman, H.M., Merigan, T.C., Reichman, R.C., Hooper, C. & Corey, L. for the AIDS Clinical Trials Group (1996) Treatment of human immunodeficiency virus infection with saquinavir, zidovudine and zalcitabine. *New Engl. J. Med.*, **334**, 1011–1017

Colombini-Hatch, S., Biberfeld, P., Reitz, M.S., Jr, Sadowska, M., Franchini, G., Ensoli, B. & Gallo, R.C. (1995) Detection of HHV-8-like DNA sequences in cynomolgus monkeys developing B-cell lymphomas. LTCB-Annual Lab-Meeting, NCI/NIH, Bethesda, USA, Sept. 1995 (Abstract 45). *AIDS Res. hum. Retroviruses*, **11** (Suppl. 1), S75

Concorde Coordinating Committee (1994) Concorde: MRC/ANRS randomised double-blind controlled trial of immediate and deferred zidovudine in symptom-free HIV infection. *Lancet*, **343**, 871–881

Connor, E.M., Sperling, R.S., Gelber, R., Kiselev, P., Scott, G., O'Sullivan, M.J., VanDyke, R., Bey, M., Shearer, W., Jacobson, R.L., Jimenez, E., O'Neill, E., Bazin, B., Delfraissy, J.-F., Culnane, M., Coombs, R., Elkins, M., Moye, J., Stratton, P. & Balsley, J. for the Pediatric AIDS Clinical Trials Group Protocol 076 Study Group (1994) Reduction of maternal-infant transmission of human immunodeficiency virus type 1 with zidovudine treatment. *New Engl. J. Med.*, **331**, 1173–1180

Connor, R.I., Chen, B.K,. Choe, S. & Landau, N.R. (1995) Vpr is required for efficient replication of human immunodeficiency virus type-1 in mononuclear phagocytes. *Virology*, **206**, 935–944

Conti, M., Agarossi, A., Parazzini, F., Muggiasca, M.L., Boschini, A., Negri, E. & Casolati, E. (1993) HPV, HIV infection, and risk of cervical intraepithelial neoplasia in former intravenous drug abusers. *Gynecol. Oncol.*, **49**, 344–348

Contu, L., Cerimele, D., Pintus, A., Cottoni, F. & La Nasa, G. (1984) HLA and Kaposi's sarcoma in Sardinia. *Tissu. Anti.*, **23**, 240–245

Cooper, D.A., Gold, J., Maclean, P., Donovan, B., Finlayson, R., Barnes, T.G., Michelmore, H.M., Brooke, P. & Penny, R. for the Sydney AIDS Study Group. (1985) Acute AIDS retrovirus infection: definition of a clinical illness associated with seroconversion. *Lancet*, **i**, 537–540

Corallini, A., Altavilla, G., Pozzi, L., Bignozzi, F., Negrini, M., Rimessi, P., Gualandi, F. & Barbanti-Brodano, G. (1993) Systemic expression of HIV-1 tat gene in transgenic mice induces endothelial proliferation and tumors of different histotypes. *Cancer Res.*, **53**, 5569–5575

Corbeil, J., Evans, L.A., Vasak, E., Cooper, D.A. & Penny, R. (1991) Culture and properties of cells derived from Kaposi's sarcoma. *J. Immunol.*, **146**, 2972–2976

Cornford, M.E., Said, J.W. & Vinters, H.V. (1991) Immunohistochemical localization of human immunodeficiency virus (HIV) in central nervous system lymphoproliferative disorders of patients with AIDS. *Mod. Pathol.*, **4**, 232–238

Coté, T.R. & Biggar, R.J. (1995) Does zidovudine cause non-Hodgkin's lymphoma? *AIDS*, **9**, 404–405

Coté, T.R., Howe, H.L., Anderson, S.P., Martin, R.J., Evans, B. & Francis, B.J. (1991) A systematic consideration of the neoplastic spectrum of AIDS: registry linkage in Illinois. *AIDS*, **5**, 49–53

Coté, T., Schiffmann, M., Biggar, R., Goedert, J., Blattner, W. & the NACMR Study Group (1993) Invasive cervical cancer among women with AIDS: results of registry linkage (Abstract no. A1546). *Proc. Am. Assoc. Cancer Res.*, **34**, 259

Coté, T.R., O'Brien, T.R., Ward, J.W., Wilson, S.E. & Blattner, W.A. (1995) AIDS and cancer registry linkage: measurement and enhancement of registry completeness. *Prev. Med.*, **24**, 375–377

Cripe, T.P., Alderborn, A., Anderson, R.D., Pakkinen, S., Bergman, P., Haugen, T.H., Petterson, U. & Turek, L. (1990) Transcriptional activation of the human papillomavirus-16 p97 promoter by an 88-nucleotide enhancer containing distinct cell-dependent and AP-1-responsive modules. *New Biol.*, **2**, 450–463

Critchlow, C.W., Holmes, K.K., Wood, R., Krueger, L., Dunphy, C., Vernon, D.A., Daling, J.R. & Kiviat, N.B. (1992) Association of human immunodeficiency virus and anal human papillomavirus infection among homosexual men. *Arch. intern. Med.*, **152**, 1673–1676

Critchlow, C.W., Surawicz, C.M., Holmes, K.K., Kuypers, J., Daling, J.R., Hawes, S.E., Goldbaum, G.M., Sayer, J., Hurt, C., Dunphy, C. & Kiviat, N.B. (1995) Prospective study of high-grade anal squamous intraepithelial neoplasia in a cohort of homosexual men: influence of HIV infection, immunosuppression and human papillomavirus infection. *AIDS*, **9**, 1255–1262

Crofts, N., Ballard, J., Chetwynd, J., Dickson, N., Lindberg, W. & Watson, C. (1994) Involving the communities: AIDS in Australia and New Zealand. *AIDS*, **8** (Suppl. 2), S45–S53

Crook, T., Tidy, J.A. & Vousden, K.H. (1991) Degradation of p53 can be targeted by HPV E6 sequences distinct from those required for p53 binding and trans-activation. *Cell*, **67**, 547–556

Csiszar, J.W. & Zimmern, P.E. (1993) Sertoli cell tumor in an HIV+ man. *J. Urol.*, **99**, 183–185

Cullen, B.R. (1991) Human immunodeficiency virus as a prototypic complex retrovirus. *J. Virol.*, **65**, 1053–1056

Cullen, B.R. (1993) *Human Retroviruses*, Oxford, IRL Press

Cullen, B.R. (1994) The role of Nef in the replication cycle of the human and simian immunodeficiency viruses. *Virology*, **205**, 1–6

Cullen, A.P., Reid, R., Campion, M. & Lörincz, A.T. (1991) Analysis of the physical state of different human papillomavirus DNAs in intraepithelial and invasive cervical neoplasms. *J. Virol.*, **65**, 606–612

Currie, B.P. & Casadevall, A. (1994) Estimation of the prevalence of cryptococcal infection among patients infected with the human immunodeficiency virus in New York City. *Clin. infect. Dis.*, **19**, 1029–1033

Daar, E.S., Moudgil, T., Meyer, R.D. & Ho, D.D. (1991) Transient high levels of viremia in patients with primary human immunodeficiency virus type 1 infection. *New Engl. J. Med.*, **324**, 961–964

Dabis, F., Mandelbrot, L., Msellati, P. & Van de Perre, P. (1995) Zidovudine to decrease mother-to-child transmission of HIV-1: is it good for developing countries? *AIDS*, **9**, 204–206

Dalgleish, A.G., Beverley, P.C.L., Clapham, P.R., Crawford, D.H., Greaves, M.F. & Weiss, R.A. (1984) The CD4 (T4) antigen is an essential component of the receptor for the AIDS retrovirus. *Nature*, **312**, 763–767

Dal Maso, L., Franceschi, S., Negri, E., Serraino, D., La Vecchia, C. & Ancelle-Park, R.A. (1995) Trends of AIDS incidence in Europe and the United States. *Soz. Präventivmed.*, **40**, 239–265

Daniel, M.D., Letvin, N.L., King, N.M., Kannagi, M., Sehgal, P.K., Hunt, R.D., Kanki, P.J., Essex, M. & Desrosiers, R.C. (1985) Isolation of T-cell tropic HTLV-III-like retrovirus from macaques. *Science*, **228**, 1201–1204

Danner, S.A., Carr, A., Leonard, J.M., Lehman, L.M., Gudiol, F., Gonzales, J., Raventos, A., Rubio, R., Bouza, E., Pintado, V., Aguado, A.G., Garcia de Lomas, J., Delgado, R., Borleffs, J.C.C., Hsu, A., Valdes, J.M., Boucher, C.A.B. & Cooper, D.A. for the European-Australian Collaborative Ritonavir Study Group (1995) A short-term study of the safety, pharmacokinetics, and efficacy of ritonavir, an inhibitor of HIV-1 protease. *New Engl. J. Med.*, **333**, 1528–1533

Darby, S.C., Ewart, D.W., Giangrande, P.L.F., Dolin, P.J., Spooner, R.J.D. & Rizza, C.R. (1995) Mortality before and after HIV infection in the complete UK population of haemophiliacs. *Nature*, **377**, 79–82

Darby, S.C., Ewart, D.W., Giangrande, P.L.F., Spooner, R.J.D. & Rizza, C.R. (1996) Importance of age at infection with HIV-1 for survival and development of AIDS in UK haemophilia population. *Lancet*, **347**, 1573–1579

Darrow, W.W., Peterman, T.A., Jaffe, H.W., Rogers, M.F., Curran, J.W. & Beral, V. (1992) Kaposi's sarcoma and exposure to faeces (Letter to the Editor). *Lancet*, **339**, 685–686

Deacon, N.J., Tsykin, A., Solomon, A., Smith, K., Ludford-Menting, M., Hooker, D.J., McPhee, D.A., Greenway, A.L., Ellett, A., Chatfield, C., Lawson, V.A., Crowe, S., Maerz, A., Sonza, S., Learmont, J., Sullivan, J.S., Cunningham, A., Dwyer, D., Dowton, D. & Mills, J. (1995) Genomic structure of an attenuated quasi species of HIV-1 from a blood transfusion donor and recipients. *Science*, **270**, 988–991

DeAngelis, L.M., Wong, E., Rosenblum, M. & Furneaux, H. (1992) Epstein-Barr virus in acquired immune deficiency syndrome (AIDS) and non-AIDS primary central nervous system lymphoma. *Cancer*, **70**, 1607–1611

De Cock, K.M. & Brun-Vézinet, F. (1989) Epidemiology of HIV-2 infection. *AIDS*, **3** (Suppl. 1), S89–S95

DeHovitz, J.A., Pape, J.W., Boncy, M. & Johnson, W.D., Jr (1986) Clinical manifestations and therapy of *Isospora belli* infection in patients with acquired immunodeficiency syndrome. *New Engl. J. Med.*, **315**, 87–90

Delecluse, H.J., Raphael, M., Magaud, J.P., Felman, P., the French Study Group of Pathology for Human Immunodeficiency Virus-Associated Tumors, Abd Alsamad, I., Bornkamm, G.W. & Lenoir, G.M. (1993) Variable morphology of human immunodeficiency virus-associated lymphomas with c-*myc* rearrangements. *Blood*, **82**, 552–563

Delli-Bovi, P., Donti, E., Knowles, D.M., II, Friedman-Kien, A., Luciw, P.A., Dina, D., Dalla-Favera, R. & Basilico, C. (1986) Presence of chromosomal abnormalities and lack of AIDS retrovirus DNA sequences in AIDS-associated Kaposi's sarcoma. *Cancer Res.*, **46**, 6333–6338

Deng, H.K., Liu, R., Ellmeier, W., Choe, S., Unutmaz, D., Burkhart, M., Di Marzio, P., Marmon, S., Sutton, R.E., Hill, C.M., David, C.B., Peiper, S.C., Schall, T.J., Littman, D.R. & Landau, N.R. (1996) Identification of a major co-receptor for primary isolates of HIV-1. *Nature*, **381**, 661–666

Denis, B.J., May, T., Bigard, M.-A. & Canton, P. (1992) Anal and perianal lesions in symptomatic HIV infections. *Gastroenterol. clin. biol.*, **16**, 148–154 (in French)

De Re, V., Boiocchi, M., De Vita, S., Dolcetti, R., Gloghini, A., Uccini, S., Baroni, C., Scarpa, A., Cattoretti, G. & Carbone, A. (1993) Subtypes of Epstein-Barr virus in HIV-1-associated and HIV-1-unrelated Hodgkin's disease cases. *Int. J. Cancer*, **54**, 895–898

De Re, V., Carbone, A., De Vita, S., Gloghini, A., Maestro, R., Gasparotto, D., Vukosavljevic, T. & Boiocchi, M. (1994) p53 Protein overexpression and p53 gene abnormalities in HIV-1-related non-Hodgkin's lymphomas. *Int. J. Cancer*, **56**, 662–667

Des Jarlais, D.C., Padian, N.S. & Winkelstein, W., Jr (1994) Targeted HIV-prevention programs. *New Engl. J. Med.*, **331**, 1451–1453

Desrosiers, R.C. & Letvin, N.L. (1987) Animal models for acquired immunodeficiency syndrome. *Rev. infect. Dis.*, **9**, 438–446

Devesa, S.S., Silverman, D.T., Young, J.L., Pollack, E.S., Brown, C.C., Horm, J.W., Percy, C.L., Myers, M.H., McKay, F.W. & Fraumeni, J.F., Jr (1987) Cancer incidence and mortality trends among whites in the United States, 1947–84. *J. natl Cancer Inst.*, **79**, 701–770

Diaz, T., Chu, S.Y., Conti, L., Sorvillo, F., Checko, P.J., Hermann, P., Fann, S.A., Frederick, M., Boyd, D., Mokotoff, E., Rietmeijer, C.A., Herr, M. & Samuel, M.C. (1994) Risk behaviors of persons with heterosexually acquired HIV infection in the United States: results of a multistate surveillance project. *J. acquir. Immun. Defic. Syndr.*, **7**, 958–963

DiCarlo, F.J., Jr, Joshi, V.V., Oleske, J.M. & Connor, E.M. (1990) Neoplastic diseases in children with acquired immunodeficiency syndrome. *Progr. AIDS Pathol.*, **2**, 163–185

Dictor, M. & Attewell, R. (1988) Epidemiology of Kaposi's sarcoma in Sweden prior to the acquired immunodeficiency syndrome. *Int. J. Cancer*, **42**, 346–351

Dik, J., Habbema, F. & de Vlas, S.J. (1995) Impact of improved treatment of sexually transmitted disease on HIV infection (Letter to the Editor). *Lancet*, **346**, 1157–1160

Di Luca, D., Dolcetti, R., Mirandola, P., De Re, V., Secchiero, P., Carbone, A., Boiocchi, M. & Cassai, E. (1994) Human herpesvirus 6: a survey of presence and variant distribution in normal peripheral lymphocytes and lymphoproliferative disorders. *J. infect. Dis.*, **170**, 211–215

Dimitrov, D.S., Willey, R.L., Sato, H., Chang, L.-J., Blumethal, R. & Martin, M.A. (1993) Quantitation of human immunodeficiency virus type 1 infection kinetics. *J. Virol.*, **67**, 2182–2190

Dock, N.L., Kleinman, S.H., Rayfield, M.A., Schable, C.A., Williams, A.E. & Dodd, R.Y. (1991) Human immunodeficiency virus infection and indeterminate western blot patterns. Prospective studies in a low prevalence population. *Arch. intern. Med.*, **151**, 525–530

Dolcetti, R., Di Luca, D., Mirandola, P., De Vita, S., De Re, V., Carbone, A., Tirelli, U., Cassai, E. & Boiocchi, M. (1994) Frequent detection of human herpesvirus 6 DNA in HIV-associated lymphadenopathy (Letter to the Editor). *Lancet*, **344**, 543

Dolcetti, R., Gloghini, A., De Vita, S., Vaccher, E., De Re, V., Tirelli, U., Carbone, A. & Boiocchi, M. (1995) Characteristics of EBV-infected cells in HIV-related lymphadenopathy: implications for the pathogenesis of EBV-associated and EBV-unrelated lymphomas of HIV-seropositive individuals. *Int. J. Cancer*, **63**, 652–659

Dolcetti, R., Di Luca, D., Carbone, A., Mirandola, P., De Vita, S., Vaccher, E., Sighinolfi, L., Gloghini, A., Tirelli, U., Cassai, E. & Boiocchi, M. (1996) Human herpesvirus 6 in human immunodeficiency virus-infected individuals: association with early histologic phases of lymphadenopathy syndrome but not with malignant lymphoproliferative disorders. *J. med. Virol.*, **48**, 344–353

Dolin, R. (1995) Human studies in the development of human immunodeficiency virus vaccines. *J. infect. Dis.*, **172**, 1175–1183

Donaldson, Y.K., Bell, J.E., Ironside, J.W., Brettle, R.P., Robertson, J.R., Busuttil, A. & Simmonds, P. (1994) Redistribution of HIV outside the lymphoid system with onset of AIDS. *Lancet*, **343**, 382–385

Dondero, T.J. & Gill, O.N. (1991) Large-scale HIV serologic surveys: what has been learned? *AIDS*, **5** (Suppl. 2), S63–S69

Dondero, T.J., Jr, Pappaioanou, M. & Curran, J.W. (1988) Monitoring the levels and trends of HIV infection: the Public Health Service's HIV Surveillance Program. *Public Health Rep.*, **103**, 213–220

Donegan, E., Stuart, M., Niland, J.C., Sacks, H.S., Azen, S.P., Dietrich, S.L., Faucett, C., Fletcher, M.A., Kleinman, S.H., Operskalski, E.A., Perkins, H.A., Pindyck, J., Schiff, E.R., Stites, D.P., Tomasulo, P.A., Mosley, J.W. & the Transfusion Safety Group (1990) Infection with human immunodeficiency virus type 1 (HIV-1) among recipients of antibody-positive blood donations. *Ann. intern. Med.*, **113**, 733–739

Donoghoe, M.C., Stimson, G.V., Dolan, K. & Alldritt, L. (1989) Changes in HIV risk behaviour in clients of syringe-exchange schemes in England and Scotland. *AIDS*, **3**, 267–272

Dore, G.J., Li, Y., Grulich, A., Hoy, J.F., Mallal, S.A., Mijch, A.-M., French, M.A., Cooper, D.A. & Kaldor, J.M. (1996) Declining incidence and later occurrence of Kaposi's sarcoma among people with AIDS in Australia: the Australian AIDS cohort. *AIDS* (in press)

Dörffel, J. (1932) Histogenesis of multiple idiopathic hemorrhagic sarcoma of Kaposi. *Arch. Dermatol. Syph.*, **26**, 608–634

Downs, A.M., Ancelle, R.A., Jager, H.J.C. & Brunet, J.-B. (1987) AIDS in Europe: current trends and short-term predictions estimated from surveillance data, January 1981–June 1986. *AIDS*, **1**, 53–57

Dragic, T., Litwin, V., Allaway, G.P., Martin, S.R., Huang, Y., Nagashima, K.A., Cayanan, C., Maddon, P.J., Koup, R.A., Moore, J.P. & Paxton, W.A. (1996) HIV-1 entry into CD4+ cells is mediated by the chemokine receptor CC-CKR-5. *Nature*, **381**, 667–673

Dresdale, A.R., Lutz, S., Drost, C., Levine, T.B., Fenn, N., Paone, G., del Busto, R. & Silverman, N.A. (1993) Prospective evaluation of malignant neoplasms in cardiac transplant recipients uniformly treated with prophylactic antilymphocyte globulin. *J. thorac. cardiovasc. Surg.*, **106**, 1202–1207

Drew, W.L., Conant, M.A., Miner, R.C., Huang, E.-S., Ziegler, J.L., Groundwater, J.R., Gullett, J.H., Volberding, P., Abrams, D. & Mintz, L. (1982) Cytomegalovirus and Kaposi's sarcoma in young homosexual men. *Lancet*, **ii**, 125–127

Du, Z., Lang, S.M., Sasseville, V.G., Lackner, A.A., Ilyinskii, P.O., Daniel, M.D., Jung, J.U. & Desrosiers, R.C. (1995) Identification of a *nef* allele that causes lymphocyte activation and acute disease in macaque monkeys. *Cell*, **82**, 665–674

Dumitrescu, O., Kalish, M.L., Kliks, S.C., Bandea, C.I. & Levy, J.A. (1994) Characterization of human immunodeficiency virus type 1 isolates from children in Romania: identification of a new envelope subtype. *J. infect. Dis.*, **169**, 281–288

Dupin, N., Grandadam, M., Calvez, V., Gorin, I., Aubin, J.T., Havard, S., Lamy, F., Leibowitch, M., Huraux, J.M., Escande, J.P. & Agut, H. (1995) Herpesvirus-like DNA sequences in patients with Mediterranean Kaposi's sarcoma. *Lancet*, **345**, 761–762

DuPont, H.L. & Marshall, G.D. (1995) HIV-associated diarrhoea and wasting. *Lancet*, **346**, 352–356

Dürst, M., Glitz, D., Schneider, A. & zur Hausen, H. (1992) Human papillomavirus type 16 (HPV 16) gene expression and DNA replication in cervical neoplasia: analysis by in situ hybridization. *Virology*, **189**, 132–140

Dyson, N., Howley, P.M., Münger, K. & Harlow, E. (1989) The human papillomavirus-16 E7 oncoprotein is able to bind to the retinoblastoma gene product. *Science*, **243**, 934–937

Eeles, R., Warren, W. & Stamps, A. (1992) The PCR revolution. *Eur. J. Cancer*, **28**, 289–293

Einhorn, L.H., Richie, J.P. & Shipley, W.U. (1993) Cancer of the testis. In: DeVita, V.T., Jr, Hellman, S. & Rosenberg, S.A., eds, *Cancer: Principles and Practice of Oncology*, 4th Ed., Philadelphia, Lippincott, pp. 1126–1151

Elford, J., Tindall, B. & Sharkey, T. (1992) Kaposi's sarcoma and insertive rimming (Letter to the Editor). *Lancet*, **339**, 938

Elford, J., McDonald, A., Kaldor, J. & the National HIV Surveillance Committee (1993) Kaposi's sarcoma as a sexually transmissible infection: an analysis of Australian AIDS surveillance data. *AIDS*, **7**, 1667–1671

Elias, C.J. & Meise, L. (1993) *The Development of Microbicides: A New Method of HIV Prevention for Women* (Working Paper No. 60), New York, Population Council

Ellerbrock, T.V., Harrington, P.E., Bush, T.J., Schoenfisch, S.A., Oxtoby, M.J. & Witte, J.J. (1995) Risk of human immunodeficiency virus infection among pregnant crack cocaine users in a rural community. *Obstet. Gynecol.*, **86**, 400–404

Emau, P., McClure, H.M., Isahakia, M., Else, J.G. & Fultz, P.N. (1991) Isolation from African Sykes' monkeys (*Cercopithecus mitis*) of a lentivirus related to humans and simian immunodeficiency viruses. *J. Virol.*, **65**, 2135–2140

Embretson, J., Zupancic, M., Ribas, J.L., Burke, A., Rácz, P., Tenner-Racz, K. & Haase, A.T. (1993) Massive covert infection of helper T lymphocytes and macrophages by HIV during the incubation period of AIDS. *Nature*, **362**, 359–362

Emilie, D., Coumbaras, J., Raphael, M., Devergne, O., Delecluse, H.J., Gisselbrecht, C., Michiels, J.F., Van Demme, J., Taga, T., Kishimoto, T., Crevon, M.C. & Galanaud, P. (1992) Interleukin-6 production in high-grade B lymphomas: correlation with the presence of malignant immunoblasts in acquired immunodeficiency syndrome and in human immunodeficiency virus-seronegative patients. *Blood*, **80**, 498–504

English, R.V., Nelson, P., Johnson, C.M., Nasisse, M., Tompkins, W.A. & Tompkins, M.B. (1994) Development of clinical disease in cats experimentally infected with feline immunodeficiency virus. *J. infect. Dis.*, **170**, 543–552

Ensoli, B., Nakamura, S., Salahuddin, S.Z., Biberfeld, P., Larsson, L., Beaver, B., Wong-Staal, F. & Gallo, R.C. (1989) AIDS-Kaposi's sarcoma-derived cells express cytokines with autocrine and paracrine growth effects. *Science*, **243**, 223–226

Ensoli, B., Barillari, G., Salahuddin, S.Z., Gallo, R.C. & Wong-Staal, F. (1990) Tat protein of HIV-1 stimulates growth of cells derived from Kaposi's sarcoma lesions of AIDS patients. *Nature*, **345**, 84–86

Ensoli, B., Buonaguro, L., Barillari, G., Fiorelli, V., Gendelman, R., Morgan, R.A., Wingfield, P. & Gallo, R.C. (1993) Release, uptake and effects of extracellular HIV-1 Tat protein on cell growth and viral transactivation. *J. Virol.*, **67**, 277–287

Ensoli, B., Markham, P., Kao, V., Barillari, G., Fiorelli, V., Gendelman, R., Raffeld, M., Zon, G. & Gallo, R.C. (1994a) Block of AIDS-Kaposi's sarcoma (KS) cell growth, angiogenesis, and lesion formation in nude mice by antisense oligonucleotide targeting basic fibroblast growth factor. A novel strategy for the therapy of KS. *J. clin. Invest.*, **94**, 1736–1746

Ensoli, B., Gendelman, R., Markham, P., Fiorelli, V., Colombini, S., Raffeld, M., Cafaro, A., Chang, H.-K., Brady, J.N. & Gallo, R.C. (1994b) Synergy between basic fibroblast growth factor and HIV-1 Tat protein in induction of Kaposi's sarcoma. *Nature*, **371**, 674–680

Epstein, L.G., Kuiken, C., Blumberg, B.M., Hartman, S., Sharer, L.R., Clement, M. & Doudsmit, J. (1991) HIV-1 V3 domain variation in brain and spleen of children with AIDS: tissue-specific evolution within host-determined quasispecies. *Virology*, **180**, 583–590

Ernberg, I. & Altiok, E. (1989) The role of Epstein-Barr virus in lymphomas of HIV-carriers. *APMIS Suppl.*, **8**, 58–61

Errante, D., Zagonel, V., Vaccher E., Serraino, D., Bernardi, D., Sorio, R., Trovò, M., Carbone, A., Monfardini, S. & Tirelli, U. (1994) Hodgkin's disease in patients with HIV infection and in the general population: comparison of clinicopathological features and survival. *Ann. Oncol.*, **5** (Suppl. 2), S37–S40

European Centre for the Epidemiological Monitoring of AIDS (1994) *AIDS Surveillance in Europe*, Quart. Rep. No. 44, *HIV Seroprevalence in Pregnant Women: Unlinked Anonymous, Voluntary, and Mandatory HIV Testing*, 94 Saint-Maurice, France, Hôpital National de Saint-Maurice, pp. 41–51

European Centre for the Epidemiological Monitoring of AIDS (1995a) *HIV/AIDS Surveillance in Europe*, Quart. Rep. No. 46, *AIDS Cases Reported by 30 June 1995*, 94 Saint-Maurice, France, Hôpital National de Saint-Maurice, pp. 20–21

European Centre for the Epidemiological Monitoring of AIDS (1995b) *HIV/AIDS Surveillance in Europe*, Quart. Rep. No. 47, *AIDS Cases Reported by 30 September 1995*, 94 Saint-Maurice, France, Hôpital National de Saint-Maurice, pp. 1–30

European Collaborative Study (1992) Risk factors for mother-to-child transmission of HIV-1. *Lancet*, **339**, 1007–1012

European Collaborative Study (1994) Caesarean section and risk of vertical transmission of HIV-1 infection. *Lancet*, **343**, 1464–1467

European Study Group on Heterosexual Transmission of HIV (1992) Comparison of female to male and male to female transmission of HIV in 563 stable couples. *Br. med. J.*, **304**, 809–813

Evans, L.A., McHugh, T.M., Stites, D.P. & Levy, J.A. (1987) Differential ability of human immunodeficiency virus isolates to productively infect human cells. *J. Immunol.*, **138**, 3415–3418

Eyster, M.E., Gail, M.H., Ballard, J.O., Al-Mondhiry, H. & Goedert, J.J. (1987) Natural history of human immunodeficiency virus infections in hemophiliacs: effects of T-cell subsets, platelet counts, and age. *Ann. intern. Med.*, **107**, 1–6

Fahey, J.L., Taylor, J.M.G., Detels, R., Hofmann, B., Melmed, R., Nishanian, P. & Giorgi, J.V. (1990) The prognostic value of cellular and serologic markers of infection with human immunodeficiency virus type 1. *New Engl. J. Med.*, **322**, 166–172

Fanjul, A., Dawson, M.I., Hobbs, P.D., Jong, L., Cameron, J.F., Harlev, E., Graupner, G., Lu, X.-P. & Pfahl, M. (1994) A new class of retinoids with selective inhibition of AP-1 inhibits proliferation. *Nature*, **372**, 107–111

Farizo, K.M., Buehler, J.W., Chamberland, M.E., Whyte, B.M., Froelicher, E.S., Hopkins, S.G., Reed, C.M., Mokotoff, E.D., Cohn, D.L., Troxler, S., Phelps, A.F. & Berkelman, R.L. (1992) Spectrum of disease in persons with human immunodeficiency virus infection in the United States. *J. Am. med. Assoc.*, **267**, 1798–1805

Farr, G., Gabelnick, H., Sturgen, K. & Dorflinger, L. (1994) Contraceptive efficacy and acceptability of the female condom. *Am. J. public Health*, **84**, 1960–1964

Fauci, A.S. (1992) Combination therapy for HIV infection: getting closer. *Ann. intern. Med.*, **116**, 85–86

Fauci, A.S., Schnittman, S.M., Poli, G., Koenig, S. & Pantaleo, G. (1991) Immunopathogenic mechanisms in human immunodeficiency virus (HIV) infection. *Ann. intern. Med.*, **114**, 678–693

Feachem, R., Musgrove, P. & Elmendorf, A.E. (1995) Comment from the World Bank (Letter to the Editor). *AIDS*, **9**, 982–984

Feder, B.M. & Hurvitz, A.I. (1990) Feline immunodeficiency virus infection in 100 cats and association with lymphoma. Proceedings 8th ACVIM Forum (Abstract no. 17), p. 1112

Feichtinger, H., Putkonen, P., Parravicini, C., Li, S.-L., Kaaya, E.E., Böttiger, D., Biberfeld, G. & Biberfeld, P. (1990) Malignant lymphomas in cynomolgus monkeys infected with SIV. *Am. J. Pathol.*, **137**, 1311–1315

Feichtinger, H., Kaaya, E.E., Putkonen, P., Li, S.-L., Ekman, M., Gendelman, R., Biberfeld, G. & Biberfeld, P. (1992a) Malignant lymphoma associated with human AIDS and with SIV-induced immunodeficiency in macaques. *AIDS Res. hum. Retroviruses*, **8**, 339–348

Feichtinger, H., Li, S-L., Kaaya, E.E., Putkonen, P., Grünewald, K., Weyrer, K., Böttiger, D., Ernberg, I., Line, A., Biberfeld, G. & Biberfeld, P. (1992b) A monkey model for Epstein-Barr virus-associated lymphomagenesis in human acquired immunodeficiency syndrome. *J. exp. Med.*, **176**, 281–286

Feingold, A.R., Vermund, S.H., Burk, R.D., Kelley, K.F., Schrager, L.K., Schreiber, K., Munk, G., Friedland, G.H. & Klein, R.S. (1990) Cervical cytologic abnormalities and papillomavirus in women infected with human immunodeficiency virus. *J. acquir. Immun. Defic. Syndr.*, **3**, 896–903

Feng, Y., Broder, C.C., Kennedy, P.E. & Berger, E.A. (1996) HIV-1 entry cofactor: functional cDNA cloning of a seven-transmembrane G protein-coupled receptor. *Science*, **272**, 872–876

Feorino, P., Forrester, C., Schable, C., Warfield, D. & Schochetman, G. (1987) Comparison of antigen assay and reverse transcriptase assay for detecting human immunodeficiency virus in culture. *J. clin. Microbiol.*, **25**, 2344–2346

Ficarra, G. & Eversole, L.E. (1994) HIV-related tumors of the oral cavity. *Crit. Rev. oral Biol. Med.*, **5**, 159–185

Filice, G., Cereda, P.M. & Varnier, O.E. (1988) Infection of rabbits with human deficiency virus. *Nature*, **335**, 366–369

Filipovich, A.H., Mathuir, A., Kamat, D., Kersey, J.H. & Shapiro, R.S. (1994) Lymphoproliferative disorders and other tumours complicating immunodeficiencies. *Immunodeficiency*, **5**, 91–112

Fillet, A.-M., Raphael, M., Visse, B., Audouin, J., Poirel, L., Agut, H. & the French Study Group for HIV-associated Tumours (1995) Controlled study of human herpesvirus 6 detection in acquired immunodeficiency syndrome-associated non-Hodgkin's lymphoma. *J. med. Virol.*, **45**, 106–112

Finke, J., Fritzen, R., Ternes, P., Trivedi, P., Bross, K.J., Lange, W., Mertelsmann, R. & Dölken, G. (1992) Expression of *BCL*-2 in Burkitt's lymphoma cell lines: Induction by latent Epstein-Barr virus genes. *Blood*, **80**, 459–469

Finn, D.G. (1995) Lymphoma of the head and neck and acquired immunodeficiency syndrome: clinical investigation and immunohistological study. *Laryngoscope*, **105**, 1–18

Fischl, M.A., Richman, D.D., Griego, M.H., Gottlieb, M.S., Volberding, P.A., Laskin, O.L., Leedom, J.M., Groopman, J.E., Mildvan, D., Schooley, R.T., Jackson, G.G., Durack, D.T., King, D. & the AZT Collaborative Working Group (1987) The efficacy of azidothymidine (AZT) in the treatment of patients with AIDS and AIDS-related complex. A double-blind, placebo-controlled trial. *New Engl. J. Med.*, **317**, 185–191

Fitzgibbon, J.E., Gaur, S., Frenkel, L.D., Laraque, F., Edlin, B.R. & Dubin, D.T. (1993) Transmission from one child to another of human immunodeficiency virus type 1 with a zidovudine-resistance mutation. *New Engl. J. Med.*, **329**, 1835–1841

Flanigan, T.P., Imam, N., Lange, N., Fiore, T., Hoy, J., Stein, M. & Carpenter, C.C.J. (1992) Decline of CD4 lymphocyte counts from the time of seroconversion in HIV-positive women. *AIDS Res. hum. Retroviruses*, **1**, 231–234

Flores, R.M., Sridhar, K.S., Thurer, R.J., Saldana, M., Raub, W.A., Jr & Klimas, N.G. (1995) Lung cancer in patients with human immunodeficiency virus infection. *Am. J. clin. Oncol.*, **18**, 59–66

Flynn, J.N., Cannon, C.A., Lawrence, C.E. & Jarrett, O. (1994) Polyclonal B-cell activation in cats infected with feline immunodeficiency virus. *Immunology*, **81**, 626–630

Fong, I.W., Toma, E. & the Canadian PML Study Group (1995) The natural history of progressive multifocal leukoencephalopathy (PML) in patients with AIDS. *Clin. infect. Dis.*, **20**, 1305–1310

Forjaz Lacerda, M.J., Santos-Ferreira, M.O., Lourenço, M.H. & Forjaz Lacerda, J.M. (1990) Incidence of HIV infection in patients treated for lymphoma (Abstract No. 2042). *Int. Conf. AIDS*, **6**, 364

Foster, S.A., Demers, G.W., Etscheid, B.G. & Galloway, D.A. (1994) The ability of human papillomavirus E6 proteins to target p53 for degradation *in vivo* correlates with their ability to abrogate actinomycin D-induced growth arrest. *J. Virol.*, **68**, 5698–5705

Foulkes, M.A., Rida, W.N. & Hoff, R. (1995) Impact of improved treatment of sexually transmitted disease on HIV infection (Letter to the Editor). *Lancet*, 1157–1160

Fox, R., Eldred, L.J., Fuchs, E.J., Kaslow, R.A., Visscher, B.R., Ho, M., Phair, J.P. & Polk, B.F. (1987) Clinical manifestations of acute infection with human immunodeficiency virus in a cohort of gay men. *AIDS*, **1**, 35–38

Fox, C.H., Tenner-Rácz, K., Rácz, P., Firpo, A., Pizzo, P.A. & Fauci, A.S. (1991) Lymphoid germinal centers are reservoirs of human immunodeficiency virus type 1 RNA. *J. infect. Dis.*, **164**, 1051–1057

Franceschi, S. & Geddes, M. (1995) Epidemiology of classic Kaposi's sarcoma, with special reference to Mediterranean population. *Tumori*, **81**, 308–314

Franceschi, S. & Serraino, D. (1995) Kaposi's sarcoma and KSHV (Letter to the Editor). *Lancet*, **346**, 1360–1361

Franceschi, S., Levi, F., Rolland-Portal, I. & La Vecchia, C. (1992) Linkage of death certification of AIDS and cancer registration in Vaud, Switzerland. *Eur. J. Cancer*, **28A**, 1487–1490

Franceschi, S., Dal Maso, L., La Vecchia, C., Negri, E. & Serraino, D. (1994) AIDS incidence rates in Europe and the United States. *AIDS*, **8**, 1173–1177

Franceschi, S., Del Maso, L. & La Vecchia, C. (1995a) Trends in incidence of AIDS associated with transfusion of blood and blood products in Europe and the United States, 1985–93. *Br. med. J.*, **311**, 1534–1536

Franceschi, S., Rezza, G., Serraino, D., Cozzi Lepri, A., Geddes, M. & Coté, T. (1995b) Risk for Kaposi's sarcoma among Italian women with AIDS (Letter to the Editor). *J. acquir. Immune Defic. Syndr. hum. Retrovirol.*, **9**, 313–314

Frankel, A.D. & Pabo, C.O. (1988) Cellular uptake of the Tat protein from human immunodeficiency virus. *Cell*, **55**, 1189–1193

Frankel, A.D., Biancalana, S. & Hudson, D. (1989) Activity of synthetic peptides from the Tat protein of human immunodeficiency virus type 1. *Proc. natl. Acad. Sci. USA*, **86**, 7397–7401

Frazer, I.H., Medley, G., Crapper, R.M., Brown, T.C. & Mackay, I.R. (1986) Association between anorectal dysplasia, human papillomavirus, and human immunodeficiency virus infection in homosexual men. *Lancet*, **ii**, 657–660

Freed, E.O., Myers, D.J. & Risser, R. (1991) Identification of the principal neutralizing determinant of human immunodeficiency virus type 1 as a fusion domain. *J. Virol.*, **65**, 190–194

Frieden, T.R., Sterling, T., Pablos-Mendez, A., Kilburn, J.O., Cauthen, G.M. & Dooley, S.M. (1993) The emergence of drug-resistant tuberculosis in New York City. *New Engl. J. Med.*, **328**, 521–526

Friedland, G., Kahl, P., Saltzman, B., Rogers, M., Feiner, C., Mayers, M., Schable, C. & Klein, R.S. (1990) Additional evidence for lack of transmission of HIV infection by close interpersonal (casual) contact. *AIDS*, **4**, 639–644

Friedman, S.R. & Des Jarlais, D.C. (1991) HIV among drug injectors: the epidemic and the response. *AIDS Care*, **3**, 239–250

Frisch, M., Melbye, M. & Møller, H. (1993) Trends in incidence of anal cancer in Denmark. *Br. med. J.*, **306**, 419–422

Frizzera, G. (1994) Immunosuppression, autoimmunity, and lymphoproliferative disorders. *Hum. Pathol.*, **25**, 627–629

Fruchter, R.G., Maiman, M., Sillman, F.H., Camilien, L., Webber, C.A. & Kim, D.S. (1994) Characteristics of cervical intraepithelial neoplasia in women infected with the human immunodeficiency virus. *Am. J. Obstet. Gynecol.*, **171**, 531–537

Frumkin, L.R., Agy, M.B., Coombs, R.W., Panther, L., Morton, W.R., Koehler, J., Florey, M.J., Dragavon, J., Schmidt, A., Katze, M.G. & Corey, L. (1993) Acute infection of *Macaca nemestrina* by human immunodeficiency virus type-1. *Virology*, **195**, 422–431

Fuchs, P.G., Girardi, F. & Pfister, H. (1988) Human papillomavirus DNA in normal, metaplastic, preneoplastic and neoplastic epithelia of the cervix uteri. *Int. J. Cancer*, **41**, 41–45

Gage, J.R., Meyers, C. & Wettstein, F.O. (1990) The E7 proteins of the nononcogenic human papillomavirus type 6b (HPV-6b) and of the oncogenic HPV-16 differ in retinoblastoma protein binding and other properties. *J. Virol.*, **64**, 723–730

Gaidano, G. & Carbone, A. (1995) AIDS-related lymphomas: from pathogenesis to pathology. *Br. J. Haematol.*, **90**, 235–243

Gaidano, G. & Dalla-Favera, R. (1992) Biologic aspects of human immunodeficiency virus-related lymphoma. *Curr. Opin. Oncol.*, **4**, 900–906

Gaidano, G., Ballerini, P., Gong, J.Z., Inghirami, G., Neri, A., Newcomb, E.W., Magrath, I.T., Knowles, D.M. & Dalla-Favera, R. (1991) p53 Mutations in human lymphoid malignancies: association with Burkitt lymphoma and chronic lymphocytic leukemia. *Proc. natl Acad. Sci. USA*, **88**, 5413–5417

Gaidano, G., Hauptschein, R.S., Parsa, N.Z., Offit, K., Rao, P.H., Lenoir, G., Knowles, D.M., Chaganti, R.S.K., & Dalla-Favera, R. (1992) Deletions involving two distinct regions of 6q in B-cell non-Hodgkin lymphoma. *Blood*, **80**, 1781–1787

Gaidano, G., Parsa, N.Z., Tassi, V., Della-Latta, P., Chaganti, R.S.K., Knowles, D.M. & Dalla-Favera, R. (1993) In vitro establishment of AIDS-related lymphoma cell lines: phenotypic characterization, oncogene and tumor suppressor gene lesions, and heterogeneity in Epstein-Barr virus infection. *Leukemia*, **7**, 1621–1629

Gaidano, G., Pastore, C., Lanza, C., Mazza, U. & Saglio, G. (1994a) Molecular pathology of AIDS-related lymphomas. Biologic aspects and clinicopathologic heterogeneity. *Ann. Hematol.*, **69**, 281–290

Gaidano, G., Lo Coco, F., Ye, B.H., Shibata, D., Levine, A., Knowles, D.M. & Dalla-Favera, R. (1994b) Rearrangements of the *BCL-6* gene in acquired immunodeficiency syndrome-associated non-Hodgkin's lymphoma: association with diffuse large-cell subtype. *Blood*, **84**, 397–402

Gaidano, G., Cechova, K., Chang, Y., Moore, P.S., Knowles, D.M. & Dalla-Favera, R. (1996) Establishment of AIDS-related lymphoma cell lines from lymphomatous effusions. *Leukemia* (in press)

Gaines, H., von Sydow, M., Sönnerborg, A., Albert, J., Czajkowski, J., Pehrson, P.O., Chiodi, F., Moberg, L., Fenyö, E.M., Åsjö, B. & Forsgren, M. (1987) Antibody response in primary human immunodeficiency virus infection. *Lancet*, **i**, 1249–1253

Galai, N., Muñoz, A., Chen, K., Carey, V.J., Chmiel, J. & Zhou, S.Y.J. (1993) Tracking the markers and onset of disease among HIV-1 seroconverters. *Statistics Med.*, **12**, 2133–2145

Galgiani, J.N & Ampel, N.M. (1990) Coccidiomycosis in human immunodeficiency virus-infected patients. *J. infect. Dis.*, **162**, 1165–1169

Gallo, R.C., Salahuddin, S.Z., Popovic, M., Shearer, G.M., Kaplan, M., Haynes, B.F., Palker, T.J., Redfield, R., Oleske, J., Safai, B., White, G., Foster, P. & Markham, P.D. (1984) Frequent detection and isolation of cytopathic retroviruses (HTLV-III) from patients with AIDS and at risk for AIDS. *Science*, **224**, 500–503

Gao, F., Yue, L., White, A.T., Pappas, P.G., Barchue, J,. Hanson, A.P., Greene, B.M., Sharp, P.M., Shaw, G.M. & Hahn, B.H. (1992) Human infection by genetically diverse SIVSM-related HIV-2 in West Africa. *Nature*, **358**, 495–499

Gao, F., Yue, L., Robertson, D.L., Hill, S.C., Hui, H., Biggar, R.J., Neequaye, A.E., Whelan, T.M., Ho, D.D., Shaw, G.M., Sharp, P.M. & Hahn, B.H. (1994) Genetic diversity of human immunodeficiency virus type 2: evidence for distinct sequence subtypes with differences in virus biology. *J. Virol.*, **68**, 7433–7447

Gao, S.-J., Kingsley, L., Hoover, D.R., Spira, T.J., Rinaldo, C.R., Saah, A., Phair, J., Detels, R., Preston, P., Chang, Y. & Moore, P.S. (1996a) Seroconversion to antibodies against Kaposi's sarcoma-associated herpesvirus-related latent nuclear antigens before the development of Kaposi's sarcoma. *New Engl. J. Med.*, **335**, 233–241

Gao, S.-J., Kingsley, L., Li, M., Zheng, W., Parravicini, C., Ziegler, J., Newton, R., Rinaldi, C.R., Saah, A., Phair, J., Detels, R., Chang, Y. & Moore, P.S. (1996b) KSHV antibodies among Americans, Italians and Ugandans with and without Kaposi's sarcoma. *Nature Med.*, **2**, 925–928

Garcia, J.V. & Miller, A.D. (1991) Serine phosphorylation-independent downregulation of cell-surface CD4 by *nef. Nature*, **350**, 508–511

Gardner, M.B., Endres, M. & Barry, P.A. (1994) The simian retroviruses: SIV and SRV. In: Levy, J.A., ed., *The Retroviridae*, Vol. 3, New York, Plenum Press, pp. 133–276

Gartner, S., Liu, Y., Lewis, M.G., Polonis, V., Elkins, W.R., Zack, P.M., Miao, J., Hunter, E.A., Greenhouse, J. & Eddy, G.A. (1994) HIV-1 infection in pigtailed macaques. *AIDS Res. hum. Retroviruses*, **10** (Suppl. 2), S129–S133

Garza, B.W., Drotman, D.P., Martin, L.S., McDougal, J.S., Bond, W.W. & Jones, T.S. (1994) Brief communication: HIV-1 and bleach. *J. acquir. Immun. Defic. Syndr.*, **7**, 169–170

Gaya, S.B.M., Rees, A.J., Lechler, R.I., Williams, G. & Mason, P.D. (1995) Malignant disease in patients with long-term renal transplants. *Transplantation*, **59**, 1705–1709

Geddes, M., Franceschi, S., Barchielli, A., Falcini, F., Carli, S., Cocconi, G., Conti, E., Crosignani, P., Gafà, L., Giarelli, L., Vercelli, M. & Zanetti, R. (1994) Kaposi's sarcoma in Italy before and after the AIDS epidemic. *Br. J. Cancer*, **69**, 333–336

Geddes, M., Franceschi, S., Balzi, D., Arniani, S., Gafà, L. & Zanetti, R. (1995) Birthplace and classic Kaposi's sarcoma in Italy. *J. natl Cancer Inst.*, **87**, 1015–1017

Gelderblom, H.R. (1991) Assembly and morphology of HIV: potential effect of structure on viral function. *AIDS*, **5**, 617–637

Gentile, G., Formelli, G., Costigliola, P., Busacchi, P. & Pelusi, G. (1993) Cervical intra-epithelial neoplasia in HIV seropositive patients. *Eur. J. Gynaec. Oncol.*, **14**, 246–248

Gershon, R.R.M., Vlahov, D. & Nelson, K.E. (1990) The risk of transmission of HIV-1 through non-percutaneous, non-sexual modes — a review. *AIDS*, **4**, 645–650

Gessain, A., Sudaka, A., Brière, J., Fouchard, N., Nicola, A.-M., Rio, B., Arborio, M., Troussard, X., Audouin, J., Diebold, J. & de Thé, G. (1996) Kaposi sarcoma-associated herpes-like virus (human herpesvirus type 8) DNA sequences in multicentric Castleman's disease: is there any relevant association in non-human immunodeficiency virus-infected patients? (Letter to the Editor), *Blood*, **86**, 414–416

Giddens, W.E., Jr, Tsai, C.-C., Morton, W.R., Ochs, H.D., Knitter, G.H. & Blakley, G.A. (1985) Retroperitoneal fibromatosis and acquired immunodeficiency syndrome in macaques. Pathogenic observations and transmission studies. *Am. J. Pathol.*, **119**, 253–263

Giesecke, J., Scalia-Tomba, G., Håkansson, C., Karlsson, A. & Lidman, K. (1990) Incubation time of AIDS: progression of disease in a cohort of HIV-infected homo- and bisexual men with known dates of infection. *Scand. J. infect. Dis.*, **22**, 407–411

Gill, O.N., Adler, M.W. & Day, N.E. (1989) Monitoring the prevalence of HIV. Foundations for a programme of unlinked anonymous testing in England and Wales. *Br. med. J.*, **299**, 1295–1298

Gillitzer, R. & Berger, R. (1991) High mRNA levels of macrophage chemotactic protein 1 and IL-6 in lesions of Kaposi's sarcoma *in situ* (Abstract no. CF-411). *J. cell. Biochem.*, **Suppl. 15F**, 249

Giraldo, G., Beth, E. & Hagenau, F. (1972) Herpes-type virus particles in tissue culture of Kaposi's sarcoma from different geographic regions. *J. natl Cancer Inst.*, **49**, 1509–1526

Giraldo, G., Beth, E., Kourilsky, F.M., Henle, W., Henle, G., Miké, V., Huraux, J.M., Andersen, H.K., Gharbi, M.R., Kyalwazi, S.K. & Puissant, A. (1975) Antibody patterns to herpesviruses in Kaposi's sarcoma: serological association of European Kaposi's sarcoma with cytomegalovirus. *Int. J. Cancer*, **15**, 839–848

Giraldo, G., Beth, E., Henle, W., Henle, G., Miké, V., Safai, B., Huraux, J.M., McHardy, J. & de Thé, G. (1978) Antibody patterns to herpesviruses in Kaposi's sarcoma. II. Serological association of American Kaposi's sarcoma with cytomegalovirus. *Int. J. Cancer*, **22**, 126–131

Giraldo, G., Beth, E. & Huang, E.-S. (1980) Kaposi's sarcoma and its relationship to cytomegalovirus (CMV). III. CMV DNA and CMV early antigens in Kaposi's sarcoma. *Int. J. Cancer*, **26**, 23–29

Girard, M. (1995) Present status of vaccination against HIV-1 infection. *Int. J. Immunopharmacol.*, **17**, 75–78

Glaser, S.L. & Swartz, W.S. (1990) Time trends in Hodgkin's disease incidence. The role of diagnostic accuracy. *Cancer*, **66**, 2196–2204

Gleghorn, A.A., Doherty, M.C., Vlahov, D., Celentano, D.D. & Jones, T.S. (1994) Inadequate bleach contact times during syringe cleaning among injection drug users. *J. acquir. Immun. Defic. Syndr.*, **7**, 767–772

Goedert, J.J. & Coté, T.R. (1995) Conjunctival malignant disease with AIDS in USA (Letter to the Editor). *Lancet*, **346**, 257–258

Goedert, J.J., Neuland, C.Y., Wallen, W.C., Greene, M.H., Mann, D.L., Murray, C., Strong, D.M., Fraumeni, J.F., Jr & Blattner, W.A. (1982) Amyl nitrite may alter T-lymphocytes in homosexual men. *Lancet*, **i**, 412–416

Goedert, J.J., Biggar, R.J., Melbye, M., Mann, D.L., Wilson, S., Gail, M.H., Grossman, R.J., DiGioia, R.A., Sanchez, W.C., Weiss, S.H. & Blattner, W.A. (1987) Effect of T4 count and cofactors on the incidence of AIDS in homosexual men infected with human immunodeficiency virus. *J. Am. med. Assoc.*, **257**, 331–334

Goedert, J.J., Duliège, A.-M., Amos, C.I., Felton, S., Biggar, R.J. & the International Registry of HIV-exposed Twins (1991) High risk of infection with HIV-1 for first-born twins. *Lancet*, **338**, 1471–1475

Goldman, S., Glimelius, B., Nilsson, B. & Páhlman, L. (1989) Incidence of anal epidermoid carcinoma in Sweden, 1970–1984. *Acta chir. Scand.*, **155**, 191–197

Gordin, F.M., Hartigan, P.M., Klimas, N.G., Zolla-Pazner, S.B., Simberkoff, M.S. & Hamilton, J.D., for the Department of Veterans Affairs Cooperative Study Group (1994) Delayed-type hypersensitivity skin tests are an independent predictor of human immunodeficiency virus disease progression. *J. infect. Dis.*, **169**, 893–897

Gottlieb, M.S., Schroff, R., Schanker, H.M., Weisman, J.D., Fan, P.T., Wolf, R.A. & Saxon, A. (1981) *Pneumocystis carinii* pneumonia and mucosal candidiasis in previously healthy homosexual men: evidence of a new acquired cellular immunodeficiency. *New Engl. J. Med.*, **305**, 1425–1431

Graham, B.S. & Wright, P.F. (1995) Candidate AIDS vaccines. *New Engl. J. Med.*, **333**, 1331–1339

Greenberg, A.E., Thomas, P.A., Landesman, S.H., Mildvan, D., Seidlin, M., Friedland, G.H., Holzman, R., Starrett, B., Braun, J., Bryan, E.L., Evans, R.F. & The Expanded Outpatient Surveillance Project (1992) The spectrum of HIV-1-related disease among outpatients in New York City. *AIDS*, **6**, 849–859

Grez, M., Dietrich, U., Balfe, P., von Briesen, H., Maniar, J.K., Mahambre, G., Delwart, E.L., Mullins, J.I. & Rübsamen-Waigmann, H. (1994) Genetic analysis of human immunodeficiency virus type 1 and 2 (HIV-1 and HIV-2) mixed infections in India reveals a recent spread of HIV-1 and HIV-2 from a single ancestor for each of these viruses. *J. Virol.*, **68**, 2161–2168

van Griensven, G.J.P., Hessol, N.A., Koblin, B.A., Byers, R.H., O'Malley, P.M., Albercht-van Lent, N., Buchbinder, S.P., Taylor, P.E., Stevens, C.E. & Coutinho, R.A. (1993) Epidemiology of human immunodeficiency virus type 1 infection among homosexual men participating in hepatitis B vaccine trials in Amsterdam, New York City, and San Francisco, 1978–1990. *Am. J. Epidemiol.*, **137**, 909–915

Grindem, C.B., Corbett, W.T., Ammerman, B.E. & Tompkins, M.T. (1989) Seroepidemiologic survey of feline immunodeficiency virus infection in cats of Wake County, North Carolina. *J. Am. vet. Med. Assoc.*, **194**, 226–228

Grosskurth, H., Mosha, F., Todd, J., Mwijarubi, E., Klokke, A., Senkoro, K., Mayaud, P., Changalucha, J., Nicoll, A., ka-Gina, G., Newell, J., Mugeye, K., Mabey, D. & Hayes, R. (1995) Impact of improved treatment of sexually transmitted diseases on HIV infection in rural Tanzania: randomised controlled trial. *Lancet*, **346**, 530–536

Gruffydd-Jones, T.J., Hopper, C.D., Harbour, D.A. & Lutz, H. (1988) Serological evidence of feline immunodeficiency virus infection in UK cats from 1975–76. *Vet. Rec.*, **123**, 569–570

Grulich, A.E., Beral, V. & Swerdlow, A.J. (1992) Kaposi's sarcoma in England and Wales before the AIDS epidemic. *Br. J. Cancer*, **66**, 1135–1137

Grunfeld, C. (1995) What causes wasting in AIDS? *New Engl. J. Med.*, **333**, 123–124

Gruters, R.A., Terpstra, F.G., De Goede, R.E.Y., Mulder, J.W., De Wolf, F., Schellekens, P.T.A., Van Lier, R.A.W., Tersmette, M. & Miedema, F. (1991) Immunologic and virologic markers in individuals progressing from seroconversion to AIDS. *AIDS*, **5**, 837–844

Gu, Z., Pim, D., Labrecque, S., Banks, L. & Matlashewski, G. (1994) DNA damage induced p53 mediated transcription is inhibited by human papillomavirus type 18 E6. *Oncogene*, **9**, 629–633

Guettier, C., Hamilton-Dutoit, S., Guillemain, R., Farge, D., Amrein, C., Vulser, C., Hofman, P., Carpentier, A. & Diebold, J. (1992) Primary gastrointestinal malignant lymphomas associated with Epstein-Barr virus after heart transplantation. *Histopathology*, **20**, 21–28

Guis, D., Grossman, S., Bedell, M.A. & Laimins, L.A. (1988) Inducible and constitutive enhancer domains in the noncoding region of human papillomavirus type 18. *J. Virol.*, **62**, 665–672

Gunthel, C.J. & Northfelt, D.W. (1994) Cancers not associated with immunodeficiency in HIV infected persons. *Oncology*, **8**, 59–64

Gunthel, C.J., Ng, V., McGrath, M., Herndier, B. & Shiramizu, B. (1994) Association of Epstein–Barr virus types 1 and 2 with acquired immunodeficiency syndrome-related primary central nervous system lymphomas. *Blood*, **83**, 618–619

Gürtler, L.G., Hauser, P.H., Eberle, J., von Brunn, A., Knapp, S., Zekeng, L., Tsague, J.M. & Kaptue, L. (1994) A new subtype of human immunodeficiency virus type 1 (MVP-5180) from Cameroon. *J. Virol.*, **68**, 1581–1585

Gurtsevitch, V.E., O'Conor, G.T. & Lenoir, G.M. (1988) Burkitt's lymphoma cell lines reveal different degrees of tumorigenicity in nude mice. *Int. J. Cancer*, **41**, 87–95

Gyorkey, F., Sinkovics, J.G., Melnick, L. & Gyorkey, P. (1984) Retroviruses in Kaposi's sarcoma cells in AIDS. *New Engl. J. Med.*, **311**, 1183–1184

Ha, C., Haller, J.O. & Rollins, N.K. (1993) Smooth muscle tumors in immunocompromised (HIV negative) children. *Pediatr. Radiol.*, **23**, 413–414

van den Haesevelde, M., Decourt, J.L., De Leys, R.J., Vanderborght, B., van der Groen, G., van Heuverswijn, H. & Saman, E. (1994) Genomic cloning and complete sequence analysis of a highly divergent African human immunodeficiency virus isolate. *J. Virol.*, **68**, 1586–1596

Hagan, H., Des Jarlais, D.C., Friedman, S.R., Purchase, D. & Alter, M.J. (1995) Reduced risk of hepatitis B and hepatitis C among injection drug users in the Tacoma Syringe Exchange Program. *Am. J. public Health*, **85**, 1531–1537

Hahn, B.H. (1994) Viral genes and their products. In: Broder, S., Merigan, T. & Bolognesi, D., eds, *Textbook of AIDS Medicine*, New York, Williams & Wilkins, pp. 21–43

Hahn, B.H., Shaw, G.M., Taylor, M.E., Redfield, R.R., Markham, P.D., Salahuddin, S.Z., Wong-Staal, F., Gallo, R.C., Parks, E.S. & Parks, W.P. (1986) Genetic variation in HTLV-III/LAV over time in patients with AIDS or at risk for AIDS. *Science*, **232**, 1548–1553

Halbert, C.L., Demers, G.W. & Galloway, D.A. (1991) The E7 gene of human papillomavirus type 16 is sufficient for immortalization of human epithelial cells. *J. Virol.*, **65**, 473–478

Hamilton-Dutoit, S.J., Pallesen, G., Karkov, J., Skinhøj, P., Franzmann, M.B. & Pedersen, C. (1989) Identification of EBV-DNA in tumour cells of AIDS-related lymphomas by in situ hybridization (Letter to the Editor). *Lancet*, **i**, 554–555

Hamilton-Dutoit, S.J., Pallesen, G., Franzmann, M.B., Karkov, J., Black, F., Skinhøj, P. & Pedersen, C. (1991) AIDS-related lymphoma. Histopathology, immunophenotype, and association with Epstein-Barr virus as demonstrated by in situ nucleic acid hybridization. *Am. J. Pathol.*, **138**, 149–163

Hamilton-Dutoit, S.J., Raphael, M., Audouin, J., Diebold, J., Lisse, I., Pedersen, C., Oksenhendler, E., Marelle, L. & Pallesen, G. (1993a) In situ demonstration of Epstein-Barr virus small RNAs (EBER 1) in acquired immunodeficiency syndrome-related lymphomas: correlation with tumor morphology and primary site. *Blood*, **82**, 619–624

Hamilton-Dutoit, S.J., Rea, D., Raphael, M., Sandvej, K., Delecluse, H.J., Gisselbrecht, C., Marelle, L., van Krieken, J.H.J.M. & Pallesen, G. (1993b) Epstein-Barr virus-latent gene expression and tumor cell phenotype in acquired immunodeficiency syndrome-related non-Hodgkin's lymphoma. Correlation of lymphoma phenotype with three distinct patterns of viral latency. *Am. J. Pathol.*, **143**, 1072–1085

Hardy, W.D., Jr (1981) Hematopoietic tumors of cats. *J. Am. An. Hosp. Assoc.*, **17**, 921–940

Harnly, M.E., Swan, S.H., Holly, E.A., Kelter, A. & Padian, N. (1988) Temporal trends in the incidence of non-Hodgkin's lymphoma and selected malignancies in a population with a high incidence of acquired immunodeficiency syndrome (AIDS). *Am. J. Epidemiol.*, **128**, 261–267

Harris, P.J. (1995) Treatment of Kaposi's sarcoma and other manifestations of AIDS with human chorionic gonadotropin (Letter to the Editor). *Lancet*, **346**, 118–119

Harris, N.L., Jaffe, E.S., Stein, H., Banks, P.M., Chan, J.K.C., Cleary, M.L., Delsol, G., De Wolf-Peeters, C., Falini, B., Gatter, K.C., Grogan, T.M., Isaacson, P.G., Knowles, D.M., Mason, D.Y., Muller-Hermelink, H.-K., Pileri, S., Piris, M.A., Ralfkiaer, E. & Warnke, R.A. (1994) A revised European-American classification of lymphoid neoplasms: a proposal from the International Lymphoma Study Group. *Blood*, **84**, 1361–1392

Hart, G.J., Carvell, A.L.M., Woodward, N., Johnson, A.M., Williams, P. & Parry, J.V. (1989) Evaluation of needle exchange in central London: behaviour change and anti-HIV status over one year. *AIDS*, **3**, 261–265

Hartge, P. & Devesa, S.S. (1992) Quantification of the impact of known risk factors on time trends in non-Hodgkin's lymphoma incidence. *Cancer Res.*, **52**, 5566s–5569s

Hartgers, C., Buning, E.C., van Santen, G.W., Verster, A.D. & Coutinho, R.A. (1989) The impact of the needle and syringe-exchange programme in Amsterdam on injecting risk behavior. *AIDS*, **3**, 571–576

Haseltine, W.A. (1992) Molecular biology of the AIDS virus: ten years of discovery — Hope for the future. In: Rossi, G.B., Beth-Giraldo, E., Chieco-Bianchi, L., Dianzani, F., Giraldo, G. & Verani, P., eds, *Science Challenging AIDS*, Basel, Karger, pp. 71–106

Hattori, N., Michaels, F., Fargnoli, K., Marcon, L., Gallo, R.C. & Franchini, G. (1990) The human immunodeficiency virus type 2 *vpr* gene is essential for productive infection of human macrophages. *Proc. natl Acad. Sci. USA*, **87**, 8080–8084

Haverkos, H.W., Pinsky, P.F., Drotman, D.P. & Bregman, D.J. (1985) Disease manifestation among homosexual men with acquired immunodeficiency syndrome: a possible role of nitrites in Kaposi's sarcoma. *Sex. transm. Dis.*, **12**, 203–208

Hayes, R., Grosskurth, H. & ka-Gina, G. (1995) Impact of improved treatment of sexually transmitted disease on HIV infection (Letter to the Editor). *Lancet*, **346**, 1157–1160

Heimer, R., Kaplan, E.H., O'Keefe, E., Khoshnood, K. & Altice, F. (1994) Three years of needle exchange in New Haven: what have we learned? *AIDS public Policy J.*, **9**, 59–74

Heinzinger, N.K., Bukrinsky, M.I., Haggerty, S.A., Ragland, A.M., Kewalramani, V., Lee, M.-A., Gendelman, H.E., Ratner, L., Stevenson, M. & Emerman, M. (1994) The Vpr protein of human immunodeficiency virus type 1 influences nuclear localization of viral nucleic acids in non-dividing host cells. *Proc. natl Acad. Sci. USA*, **91**, 7311–7315

Henderson, L.E., Benveniste, R.E., Sowder, R., Copeland, T.D., Schultz, A.M. & Oroszlan, S. (1988) Molecular characterization of Gag proteins from simian immunodeficiency virus (SIV_{Mne}). *J. Virol.*, **62**, 2587–2595

Henderson, D.K., Fahey, B.J., Willy, M., Schmitt, J.M., Carey, K., Koziol, D.E., Lane, H.C., Fedio, J. & Saah, A.J. (1990) Risk for occupational transmission of human immunodeficiency virus type 1 (HIV-1) associated with clinical exposures. A prospective evaluation. *Ann. intern. Med.*, **113**, 740–746

Henderson, S., Rowe, M., Gregory, C., Croom-Carter, D., Wang, F., Longnecker, R., Kieff, E. & Rickinson, A. (1991) Induction of *bcl*-2 expression by Epstein-Barr virus latent membrane protein 1 protects infected B cells from programmed cell death. *Cell*, **65**, 1107–1115

Henrard, D.R., Daar, E., Farzadegan, H., Clark, S.J., Phillips, J., Shaw, G.M. & Busch, M.P. (1995) Virologic and immunologic characterization of symptomatic and asymptomatic primary HIV-1 infection. *J. acquir. Immun. Defic. Syndr.*, **9**, 305–310

Henry, M.J., Stanley, M.W., Cruikshank, S. & Carson, L. (1989) Association of human immunodeficiency virus-induced immunosuppression with human papillomavirus infection and cervical intaepithelial neoplasia. *Am. J. Obstet. Gynecol.*, **160**, 352–353

Hermine, O., Michel, M., Buzyn-Veil, A. & Gessain, A. (1996) Body-cavity-based lymphoma in an HIV-seronegative patient without Kaposi's sarcoma-associated herpesvirus-like DNA sequences (Letter to the Editor). *New Engl. J. Med.*, **334**, 272

Herndier, B.G. & Friedman, S.L. (1992) Neoplasms of the gastrointestinal tract and hepatobiliary system in acquired immunodeficiency syndrome. *Sem. Liver Dis.*, **12**, 128–141

Herndier, B.G., Shiramizu, B.T. & McGrath, M.S. (1992) AIDS associated non-Hodgkin's lymphomas represent a broad spectrum of monoclonal and polyclonal lymphoproliferative processes. *Curr. Topics Microbiol. Immunol.*, **182**, 385–394

Herndier, B.G., Werner, A., Arnstein, P., Abbey, N.W., Demartis, F., Cohen, R.L., Shuman, M.A. & Levy, J.A. (1994a) Characterization of a human Kaposi's sarcoma cell line that induces angiogenic tumours in animals. *AIDS*, **8**, 575–581

Herndier, B.G., Kaplan, L.D. & McGrath, M.S. (1994b) Pathogenesis of AIDS lymphomas. *AIDS*, **8**, 1025–1049

Hersh, B.S., Popovici, F., Apetrei, R.C., Zolotusca, L., Beldescu, N., Calomfirescu, A., Jezek, Z., Oxtoby, M.J., Gromyko, A. & Heymann, D.L. (1991) Acquired immunodeficiency syndrome in Romania. *Lancet*, **338**, 645–649

Hessol, N.A., Lifson, A.R., O'Malley, P.M., Doll, L.S., Jaffe, H.W. & Rutherford, G.W. (1989) Prevalence, incidence, and progression of human immunodeficiency virus infection in homosexual and bisexual men in hepatitis B vaccine trials, 1978–1988. *Am. J. Epidemiol.*, **130**, 1167–1175

Hessol, N.A., Katz, M.H., Liu, J.Y., Buchbinder, S. P., Rubino, C.J. & Holmberg, S.D. (1992) Increased incidence of Hodgkin disease in homosexual men with HIV infection. *Ann. intern. Med.*, **117**, 309–311

Higgins, D.L., Galavotti, C., O'Reilly, K.R., Schnell, D.J., Moore, M., Rugg, D.L. & Johnson, R. (1991a) Evidence for the effects of HIV antibody counseling and testing on risk behaviors. *J. Am. med. Assoc.*, **266**, 2419–2429

Higgins, G.D., Davy, M., Roder, D., Uzelin, D.M., Phillips, G.E. & Burrell, C.J. (1991b) Increased age and mortality associated with cervical carcinomas negative for human papillomavirus RNA. *Lancet*, **338**, 910–913

Hilleman, M.R. (1995) Whether and when an AIDS vaccine? *Nat. Med.*, **1**, 1126–1129

Hintner, H. & Fritsch, P. (1989) Skin neoplasia in the immunodeficient host. The clinical spectrum: Kaposi's sarcoma, lymphoma, skin cancer and melanoma. In: Fritsch, P., Schuler, G. & Hintner, H., eds, *Current Problems in Dermatology*, Vol. 18, *Immunodeficiency and Skin*, Basel, Karger, pp. 210–217

Hirsch, M.S. & D'Aquila, R.T. (1993) Therapy for human immunodeficiency virus infection. *New Engl. J. Med.*, **328**, 1686–1695

Hirsch, V.M., Olmsted, R.A., Murphey-Corb, M., Purcell, R.H. & Johnson, P.R. (1989) An African primate lentivirus (SIV_{SM}) closely related to HIV-2. *Nature*, **339**, 389–392

Hjalgrim, H., Melbye, M., Pukkala, E., Langmark, F., Frisch, M., Dictor, M. & Ekbom, A. (1996) Epidemiology of Kaposi's sarcoma in the Nordic countries prior to the AIDS epidemic. *Br. J. Cancer* (in press)

Ho, D.D., Sarngadharan, M.G., Resnick, L., Dimarzo-Veronese, F., Rota, T.R. & Hirsch, M.S. (1985a) Primary human T-lymphotropic virus type III infection. *Ann. intern. Med.*, **103**, 880–883

Ho, M., Miller, G., Atchison, R.W., Breinig, M.K., Dummer, J.S., Andiman, W., Starzl, T.E., Eastman, R., Griffith, B.P., Hardesty, R.L., Bahnson, H.T., Hakala, T.R. & Rosenthal, J.T. (1985b) Epstein-Barr virus infections and DNA hybridization studies in posttransplantation lymphoma and lymphoproliferative lesions: the role of primary infection. *J. infect. Dis.*, **152**, 876–886

Ho, G.Y.F., Burk, R.D., Fleming, I. & Klein, R.S. (1994) Risk of genital human papillomavirus infection in women with human immunodeficiency virus-induced immunosuppression. *Int. J. Cancer*, **56**, 788–792

Ho, D.D., Neumann, A.U., Perelson, A.S., Chen, W., Leonard, J.M. & Markowitz, M. (1995) Rapid turnover of plasma virions and CD4+ lymphocytes in HIV-1 infection. *Nature*, **373**, 123–125

Hogervorst, E., Jurriaans, S., de Wolf, F., van Wijk, A., Wiersma, A., Valk, M., Roos, M., van Gemen, B., Coutinho, R., Miedema, F. & Goudsmit, J. (1995) Predictors for non- and slow progression in human immunodeficiency virus (HIV) type 1 infection: low viral RNA copy numbers in serum and maintenance of high HIV-1 p24-specific but not V3-specific antibody levels. *J. infect. Dis.*, **171**, 811–821

Holmberg, S.D. & Byers, R.H. (1993) Does zidovudine delay development of AIDS? Analysis of data from observational cohorts (Letter to the Editor). *Lancet*, **342**, 558–559

Holmberg, S.D., Conley, L.J., Luby, S.P., Cohn, S., Wong, L.C. & Vlahov, D. (1995a) Recent infection with human immunodeficiency virus and possible rapid loss of CD4 T lymphocytes. *J. acquir. Immun. Defic. Syndr.*, **9**, 291–296

Holmberg, S.D., Buchbinder, S.P., Conley, L.J., Wong, L.C., Katz, M.H., Penley, K.A. Hershow, R.C. & Judson, F.N. (1995b) The spectrum of medical conditions and symptoms before acquired immunodeficiency syndrome in homosexual and bisexual men infected with the human immunodeficiency virus. *Am. J. Epidemiol.*, **141**, 395–404

Holodniy, M., Katzenstein, D.A., Sengupta, S., Wang, A.M., Casipit, C., Schwartz, D.H., Konrad, M., Groves, E. & Merigan, T.C. (1991) Detection and quantification of human immunodeficiency virus RNA in patient serum by use of the polymerase chain reaction. *J. infect. Dis.*, **163**, 862–866

Holtgrave, D.R., Qualls, N.L., Curran, J.W., Valdiserri, R.O., Guinan, M.E. & Parra, W.C. (1995) An overview of the effectiveness and efficiency of HIV prevention programs. *Public Health Rep.*, **110**, 134–146

Hoover, D.R., Saah, A.J., Bacellar, H., Murphy, R., Visscher, B., Anderson, R. & Kaslow, R.A. for the Multicenter AIDS Cohort Study (1993) Signs and symptoms of 'asymptomatic' HIV-1 infection in homosexual men. *J. acquir. Immune Defic. Syndr.*, **6**, 66–71

Hoppe-Seyler, F. & Butz, K. (1992) Activation of human papillomavirus type 18 E6-E7 oncogene expression by transcription factor Sp1. *Nucleic Acids Res.*, **20**, 6701–6706

Hopper, C.D., Sparkes, A.H., Gruffydd-Jones, T.J., Crispin, S.M., Muir, P., Harbour, D.A. & Stokes, C.R. (1989) Clinical and laboratory findings in cats infected with feline immunodeficiency virus. *Vet. Rec.*, **125**, 341–346

Horowitz, M.E. & Pizzo, P.A. (1990) Pediatric AIDS: a perspective for the oncologist. *Oncol.-Huntingt.*, **4**, 21–27

Horsburgh, C.R., Jr (1991) *Mycobacterium avium* complex infection in the acquired immunodeficiency syndrome. *New Engl. J. Med.*, **324**, 1332–1338

Hosie, M.J., Robertson, C. & Jarrett, O. (1989) Prevalence of feline leukaemia virus and antibodies to feline immunodeficiency virus in cats in the United Kingdom. *Vet. Rec.*, **128**, 293–297

Howard, M., Brink, N., Miller, R. & Tedder, R. (1995) Association of human herpes virus with pulmonary Kaposi's sarcoma (Letter to the Editor). *Lancet*, **346**, 712

Hsu, E.M., McNicol, P.J., Guijon, F.B. & Paraskevas, M. (1993) Quantification of HPV-16 E6-E7 transcription in cervical intraepithelial neoplasia by reverse transcriptase polymerase chain reaction. *Int. J. Cancer*, **55**, 397–401

Htoon, M.T., Lwin, H.H., San, K.O., Zan, E. & Thwe, M. (1994) HIV/AIDS in Myanmar. *AIDS*, **8** (Suppl. 2), S105–S109

Huang, Y.Q., Li, J.J., Rush, M.G., Poiesz, B.J., Nicolaides, A., Jacobson, M., Zhang, W.G., Coutavas, E., Abbott, M.A. & Friedman-Kien, A.E. (1992) HPV-16-related DNA sequences in Kaposi's sarcoma. *Lancet*, **339**, 515–518

Huang, Y.Q., Li, J.J., Kaplan, M.H., Poiesz, B., Katabira, E., Zhang, W.C., Feiner, D. & Friedman-Kien, A.E. (1995) Human herpesvirus-like nucleic acid in various forms of Kaposi's sarcoma. *Lancet*, **345**, 759–761

Huet, T., Cheynier, R., Meyerhans, A., Roelants, G. & Wain-Hobson, S. (1990) Genetic organization of a chimpanzee lentivirus related to HIV-1. *Nature*, **345**, 356-359

Hughes, P.A. (1995) Opportunistic infections in HIV-infected children. *Immunol. Allergy Clin. N. Am.*, **15**, 261–284

Hughes, R.G., Norval, M. & Howie, S.E.M. (1988) Expression of major histocompatibility class II antigens by Langerhans' cells in cervical intraepithelial neoplasia. *J. clin. Pathol.*, **41**, 253–259

Hugon, J., Giordano, C., Dumas, M., Denis, F., Barin, F., Vallat, J.M. & Sonan, T. (1988) HIV-2 antibodies in African with spastic paraplegia (Letter to the Editor). *Lancet*, **i**, 189

Hunt, R.D., Blake, B.J., Chalifoux, L.V., Sehgal, P.K., King, N.W. & Letvin, N.L. (1983) Transmission of naturally occurring lymphoma in macaque monkeys. *Proc. natl Acad. Sci. USA*, **80**, 5085–5090

Hunter, D.J., Maggwa, B.N., Mati, J.K.G., Tukei, P.M. & Mbugua, S. (1994) Sexual behavior, sexually transmitted diseases, male circumcision and risk of HIV infection among women in Nairobi, Kenya. *AIDS*, **8**, 93–99

Hurtrel, M., Ganière, J.-P., Guelfi, J.-F., Chakrabarti, L., Maire, M.-A., Gray, F., Montagnier, L. & Hurtrel, B. (1992) Comparsion of early and late feline immunodeficiency virus encephalopathies. *AIDS*, **6**, 399–406

Hutson, C.A., Rideout, B.A. & Pedersen, N.C. (1991) Neoplasia associated with feline immunodeficiency virus infection in cats of Southern California. *J. Am. vet. Med. Assoc.*, **199**, 1357–1362

Hutt, M.S.R. (1984) Classical and endemic form of Kaposi's sarcoma. A review. *Antibiot. Chemother.*, **32**, 12–17

Hutt, M.S.R. & Burkitt, D. (1965) Geographical distribution of cancer in East Africa: a new clinicopathological approach. *Br. med. J.*, **ii**, 719–722

Hymes, K.B., Cheung, T., Greene, J.B., Prose, N.S., Marcus, A., Ballard, H., William, D.C. & Laubenstein, L.J. (1981) Kaposi's sarcoma in homosexual men — A report of eight cases. *Lancet*, **ii**, 598–600

IARC (1990) *IARC Monographs on the Evaluation of Carcinogenic Risks to Humans*, Vol. 50, *Pharmaceutical Drugs*, Lyon

IARC (1994) *IARC Monographs on the Evaluation of Carcinogenic Risks to Humans*, Vol. 59, *Hepatitis Viruses*, Lyon

IARC (1995) *IARC Monographs on the Evaluation of Carcinogenic Risks to Humans*, Vol. 64, *Human Papillomaviruses*, Lyon

Inghirami, G., Macri, L., Cesarman, E., Chadburn, A., Zhong, J. & Knowles, D.M. (1994) Molecular characterization of $CD30^+$ anaplastic large-cell lymphoma: high frequency of c-*myc* proto-oncogene activation. *Blood*, **83**, 3581–3590

Ioachim, H.L., Lerner, C.W. & Tapper, M.L. (1983) The lymphoid lesions associated with the acquired immunodeficiency syndrome. *Am. J. Surg. Pathol.*, **7**, 543–553

Ioachim, H.L., Cronin, W., Roy, M. & Maya, M. (1990) Persistent lymphadenopathies in people at high risk for HIV infection. Clinicopathologic correlations and long-term follow-up in 79 cases. *Am. J. clin. Pathol.*, **93**, 208–218

Ioannidis, J.P.A., Skolnik, P.R., Chalmers, T.C. & Lau, J. (1995) Human leukocyte antigen associations of epidemic Kaposi's sarcoma. *AIDS*, **9**, 649–651

Ishida, T., Washizu, T., Toriyabe, K., Motoyoshi, S., Tomoda, I. & Pedersen, N.C. (1989) Feline immunodeficiency virus infection in cats of Japan. *J. Am. vet. Med. Assoc.*, **194**, 221–225

Israel, A.M., Koziner, B. & Strauss, D.J. (1983) Plasmacytoma and the acquired immunodeficiency syndrome. *Ann. intern. Med.*, **99**, 635–636

Italian Cooperative Group for AIDS-Related Tumours (GICAT) (1988) Malignant lymphomas in patients with or at risk for AIDS in Italy. *J. natl Cancer Inst.*, **80**, 855–860

Jacobson, L.P., Muñoz, A., Fox, R., Phair, J.P., Dudley, J,. Obrams, G.I., Kingsley, L.A., Polk, B.F. & the Multicenter AIDS Cohort Study Group (1990) Incidence of Kaposi's sarcoma in a cohort of homosexual men infected with the human immunodeficiency virus type 1. *J. acquir. Immun. Defic. Syndr.*, **3** (Suppl. 1), S24–S31

Jacobson, L.P., Kirby, A.J., Polk, S., Phair, J.P., Besley, D.R., Saah, A.J., Kingsley, L.A. & Schrager, L.K. (1993) Changes in survival after acquired immunodeficiency syndrome (AIDS): 1984–1991. *Am. J. Epidemiol.*, **138**, 952–964

Jaffe, E.S. (1996) Primary body-cavity-based AIDS-related lymphomas. Evolution of a new disease entity. *Am. J. clin. Pathol.*, **105**, 141–143

Jaffe, H.W., Choi, K., Thomas, P.A., Haverkos, H.W., Auerbach, D.M., Guinan, M.E., Rogers, M.F., Spira, T.J., Darrow, W.W., Kramer, M.A., Friedman, S.M., Monroe, J.M., Friedman-Kien, A.E., Laubenstein, L.J., Marmor, M., Safal, B., Dritz, S.K., Crispi, S.J., Fannin, S.L., Orkwis, J.P., Kelter, A., Rushing, W.R., Thacker, S.B. & Curran, J.W. (1983) National case–control study of Kaposi's sarcoma and *Pneumocystis carinii* pneumonia in homosexual men: Part 1, epidemiological results. *Ann. intern. Med.*, **99**, 145–151

Jain, M.K., John, T.J. & Keusch, G.T. (1994) Epidemiology of HIV and AIDS in India. *AIDS*, **8**, (Suppl. 2), S61–S75

Janossy, G., Pinching, A.J., Bofill, M., Weber, J., McLaughlin, J.E., Ornstein, M., Ivory, K., Harris, J.R.W., Favrot, M. & MacDonald-Burns, D.C. (1985) An immunohistological approach to persistent lymphadenopathy and its relevance to AIDS. *Clin. exp. Med.*, **59**, 257–266

Janssen, R.S., Saykin, A.J., Cannon, L., Campbell, J., Pinsky, P., Hessol, N.A., O'Malley, P.M., Lifson, A.R., Doll, L.S., Rutherford, G.W. & Kaplan, J.E. (1989) Neurological and neuropsychological manifestations of HIV-1 infection: association with AIDS-related complex but not asymptomatic HIV-1 infection. *Ann. Neurol.*, **26**, 592–600

Jebakumar, S.P.R., Mandal, B.K. & Hamour, A. (1994) Anal carcinoma in an HIV-positive female acquired through blood transfusion: presentation of a rare case report and review of the literature. *Int. J. STD AIDS*, **5**, 223–224

Jeon, S., Allen-Hoffmann, L. & Lambert, P.F. (1995) Integration of human papillomavirus type 16 into the human genome correlates with a selective growth advantage of cells. *J. Virol.*, **69**, 2989–2997

Jochmus-Kudielka, I., Bouwes Bavinck, J.N., Claas, F.H.J., Schneider, A., Van der Woude, F.J. & Gissmann, L. (1992) Seroreactivity against HPV 16 E4 and E7 proteins in renal transplant recipients and pregnant women (Letter to the Editor). *J. invest. Dermatol.*, **98**, 389–390

Johnson, A.M. (1994) Condoms and HIV transmission. *New Engl. J. Med.*, **331**, 391–392

Johnson, J.C., Burnett, A.F., Willet, G.D., Young, M.A. & Doniger, J. (1992) High frequency of latent and clinical human papillomavirus cervical infections in immunocompromised human immunodeficiency virus-infected women. *Obstet. Gynecol.*, **79**, 321–327

Johnston, G.S., Jockusch, J., McMurtry, L.C. & Shandera, W.X. (1990) Cytomegalovirus (CMV) titers among acquired immunodeficiency syndrome (AIDS) patients with and without a history of Kaposi's sarcoma (KS). *Cancer Detect. Prev.*, **14**, 337–341

Johnston, M., Fast, P., Schultz, A. & Hoth, D. (1993) Progress toward development of a vaccine to prevent AIDS. *AIDS Res. hum. Retroviruses*, **9** (Suppl 1), S117–S122

Johnstone, F.D., McGoogan, E., Smart, G.E., Brettle, R.P. & Prescott, R.J. (1994) A population-based, controlled study of the relation between HIV infection and cervical neoplasia. *Br. J. Obstet. Gynaecol.*, **101**, 986–991

Jonas, M.M. Roldan, E.O., Lyons, H.J., Fojaco, R.M. & Reddy, R.K. (1989) Histopathologic features of the liver in pediatric acquired immune deficiency syndrome. *J. Pediatr. Gastroenterol. Nutr.*, **9**, 73–81

Jørgensen, K.A. & Lawesson, S.-O. (1982) Amyl nitrite and Kaposi's sarcoma in homosexual men (Letter to the Editor). *New Engl. J. Med.*, **307**, 893–894

Kaaya, E.E., Voevodin, A., Szalecki, P., Biberfeld, P., von Krogh, G., Dillner, J. & Parravicini, C. (1993a) No evidence of HPV in epidemic and endemic Kaposi's sarcoma (Letter to the Editor). *J. acquir. Immune Defic. Syndr.*, **6**, 964–965

Kaaya, E.E., Li, S.-L., Feichtinger, H., Stahmer, I., Putkonen, P., Mandache, E., Mgaya, E., Biberfeld, G. & Biberfeld, P. (1993b) Accessory cells and macrophages in the histopathology of SIVsm-infected cynomolgus monkeys. *Res. Virol.*, **144**, 81–92

Kaaya, E.E., Parravicini, C., Ordonez, C., Gendelman, R., Berti, E., Gallo, R.C. & Biberfeld, P. (1995) Heterogeneity of spindle cells in Kaposi's sarcoma: comparison of cells in lesions and in culture. *J. acquir. Immune Defic. Syndr. hum. Retrovirol.*, **10**, 295–305

Kahn, J.O., Lagakos, S.W., Richman, D.D., Cross, A., Pettinelli, C., Liou, S.-H., Brown, M., Volberding, P.A., Crumpacker, C.S., Beall, G., Sacks, H.S., Merigan, T.C., Beltangady, M., Smaldone, L., Dolin, R. & the NIAID AIDS Clinical Trials Group (1992) A controlled trial comparing continued zidovudine with didanosine in human immunodeficiency virus infection. *New Engl. J. Med.*, **327**, 581–587

Kahn, J.O., Steimer, K.S., Baenziger, J., Duliege, A.-M., Feinberg, M., Elbeik, T., Chesney, M., Murcar, N., Chernoff, D. & Sinangil, F. (1995) Clinical, immunologic, and virologic observations related to human immunodeficiency virus (HIV) type 1 infection in a volunteer in an HIV-1 vaccine clinical trial. *J. infect. Dis.*, **171**, 1343–1347

Kaldor, J.M., Tindall, B., Williamson, P., Elford, J. & Cooper, D.A. (1993) Factors associated with Kaposi's sarcoma in a cohort of homosexual and bisexual men. *J. acquir. Immun. Defic. Syndr.*, **6**, 1145–1149

Kaldor, J.M., Effler, P., Sarda, R., Petersen, G., Gertig, D.M. & Narain, J.P. (1994) HIV and AIDS in Asia and the Pacific: an epidemiological review. *AIDS*, **8** (Suppl. 1), S165–S172

Kaleebu, P., Bobkov, A., Cheingsong-Popov, R., Bieniasz, P., Garaev, M. & Weber, J. (1995) Identification of HIV-1 subtype G from Uganda. *AIDS Res. hum. Retroviruses*, **11**, 657–659

Kanki, P.J., Travers, K.U., MBoup, S., Hsieh, C.-C., Marlink, R.G., Gueye-NDiaye, A., Siby, T., Thior, I., Hernandez-Avila, M., Sankalé, J.L., NDoye, I. & Essex, M.E. (1994) Slower heterosexual spread of HIV-2 than HIV-1. *Lancet*, **343**, 943–946

Kaplan, L. (1995) Human immunodeficiency virus-associated neoplasia: changing spectrum? *J. clin. Oncol.*, **13**, 2684–2687

Kaplan, M.H., Susin, M., Pahwa, S.G., Fetten, J., Allen, S.L., Lichtman, S., Sarngadharan, M.G. & Gallo, R.C. (1987) Neoplastic complications of HTLV-III infection: lymphomas and solid tumors. *Am. J. Med.*, **82**, 389–396

Kaplan, J.E., Spira, T.J., Fishbein, D.B., Bozeman, L.H., Pinsky, P.F. & Schonberger, L.B. (1988) A six-year follow-up of HIV-infected homosexual men with lymphadenopathy. Evidence for an increased risk for developing AIDS after the third year of lymphadenopathy. *J. Am. med. Assoc.*, **260**, 2694–2697

Kaposi, M. (1872) Idiopathic, multiple, pigmented sarcoma of the skin. *Arch. Dermatol. Syph.*, **2**, 265–273 (in German)

Karcher, D.S. & Alkan, S. (1995) Herpes-like DNA sequences, AIDS-related tumors, and Castleman's disease. *New Engl. J. Med.*, **333**, 797–798

Karn, J. (1991) Control of human immunodeficiency virus replication by the *tat*, *rev*, *nef* and protease genes. *Curr. Opin. Immunol.*, **3**, 526–536

Karp, J.E. & Broder, S. (1992) The pathogenesis of AIDS lymphomas: a foundation for addressing the challenges of therapy and prevention. *Leuk. Lymphoma*, **8**, 167–188

Kashala, O., Marlink, R., Ilunga, M., Diese, M., Gormus, B., Xu, K., Mukeba, P., Kasongo, K. & Essex, M. (1994) Infection with human immunodeficiency virus type 1 (HIV-1) and human T cell lymphotropic viruses among leprosy patients and contacts: correlation between HIV-1 cross-reactivity and antibodies to liparabinomannan. *J. infect. Dis.*, **169**, 296–304

Katseni, V.L., Gilroy, C.B., Ryait, B.K., Ariyoshi, K., Bieniasz, P.D., Weber, J.N. & Taylor-Robinson, D. (1993) *Mycoplasma fermentans* in individuals seropositive and seronegative for HIV-1. *Lancet*, **341**, 271–273

Katz, R.A. & Skalka, A.M. (1994) The retroviral enzymes. *Annu. Rev. Biochem.*, **63**, 133–173

Katz, M.H., Hessol, N.A., Buchbinder, S.P., Hirozawa, A., O'Malley, P. & Holmberg, S.D. (1994) Temporal trends of opportunistic infections and malignancies in homosexual men with AIDS. *J. infect. Dis.*, **170**, 198–202

Kelly, J.A., Murphy, D.A., Washington, C.D., Wilson, T.S., Koob, J.J., Davis, D.R., Ledezma, G. & Davantes, B. (1994) The effects of HIV/AIDS intervention groups for high-risk women in urban clinics. *Am. J. public Health*, **84**, 1918–1922

Kempf, W., Adams, V., Pfaltz, M., Briner, J., Schmid, M., Moos, R. & Hassam, S. (1995) Human herpesvirus type 6 and cytomegalovirus in AIDS-associated Kaposi's sarcoma: no evidence for an etiological association. *Hum. Pathol.*, **26**, 914–919

Kennedy, I.M., Haddow, J.K. & Clements, J.B. (1991) A negative regulatory element in the human papillomavirus type 16 genome acts at the level of late mRNA stability. *J. Virol.*, **65**, 2093–2097

Kessis, T.D., Slebos, R.J., Nelson, W.G., Kastan, M.B., Plunkett, B.S., Han, S.M., Lörincz, A.T., Hedrick, L. & Cho, K.R. (1993) Human papillomavirus 16 E6 expression disrupts the p53-mediated cellular response to DNA damage. *Proc. natl. Acad. Sci. USA*, **90**, 3988–3992

Kessler, H.A., Blaauw, B., Spear, J., Paul, D.A., Falk, L.A. & Landay, A. (1987) Diagnosis of human immunodeficiency virus infection in seronegative homosexuals presenting with an acute viral syndrome. *J. Am. med. Assoc.*, **258**, 1196–1199

Kestelyn, P., Stevens, A.-M., Ndayambaje, A., Hanssens, M. & van de Perre, P. (1990) HIV and conjunctival malignancies (Letter to the Editor). *Lancet*, **336**, 51–52

Kestler, H.W., III, Ringler, D.J., Mori, K., Panicali, D.L., Sehgal, P.K., Daniel, M.D. & Desrosiers, R.C. (1991) Importance of the *nef* gene for maintenance of high virus loads and for development of AIDS. *Cell*, **65**, 651–662

Kim, R.Y., Seiff, S.R., Howes, E.L. & O'Donnel, J.J. (1990) Necrotizing scleritis secondary to conjunctival squamous cell carcinoma in acquired immunodeficiency syndrome. *Am. J. Ophthalmol.*, **109**, 231–233

King, N.W., Hunt, R.D. & Letvin, N.L. (1983) Histopathologic changes in macaques with an acquired immunodeficiency syndrome (AIDS). *Am. J. Pathol.*, **113**, 382–388

Kingsley, L.A., Zhou, S.Y.J., Bacellar, H., Rinaldo, C.R., Jr, Chmiel, J., Detels, R., Saah, A., VanRaden, M., Ho, M., Muñoz, A. & the Multicenter AIDS Cohort Study Group (1991) Temporal trends in human immunodeficiency virus type 1 seroconversion 1984–1989. A report from the Multicenter AIDS Cohort Study (MACS). *Am. J. Epidemiol.*, **134**, 331–339

Kinlen, L.J., (1992) Immunosuppression and cancer. In: Vainio, H., Magee, P.N., McGregor, D.B. & McMichael, A.J., eds, *Mechanisms of Carcinogenesis in Risk Identification* (IARC Scientific Publications No. 116), Lyon, IARC, pp. 237–253

Kinlen, L.J., Sheil, A.G.R., Peto, J. & Doll, R. (1979) Collaborative United Kingdom–Australasian study of cancer in patients treated with immunosuppressive drugs. *Br. Med. J.*, **2**, 1461–1466

Kinloch-de Loës, S., de Saussure, P., Saurat, J.-H., Stadler, H., Hirschel, B. & Perrin, L.H. (1993) Symptomatic primary infection due to human immunodeficiency virus type 1: review of 31 cases. *Clin. infect. Dis.*, **17**, 59–65

Kitchen, V.S., Skinner, C., Ariyoshi, K., Lane, E.A., Duncan, I.B., Burckhardt, J., Burger, H.U., Bragman, K., Pinching, A.J. & Weber, J.N. (1995) Safety and efficacy of saquinavir in HIV infection. *Lancet*, **345**, 952–955

Kiviat, N.B., Rompalo, A., Bowden, R., Galloway, D., Holmes, K.K., Corey, L., Roberts, P.L. & Stamm, W.E. (1990) Anal human papillomavirus infection among human immunodeficiency virus-seropositive and -seronegative men. *J. infect. Dis.*, **162**, 358–361

Kiviat, N.B., Critchlow, C.W., Holmes, K.K., Kuypers, J., Sayer, J., Dunphy, C., Surawicz, C., Kirby, P., Wood, R. & Daling, J.R. (1993) Association of anal dysplasia and human papillomavirus with immunosuppression and HIV infection among homosexual men. *AIDS*, **7**, 43–49

Klasse, P.J., Moore, J.P. & Jameson, B.A. (1993) The interplay of HIV-1 envelope complex gp120 and gp41 with CD4. In: Morrow, W.J.W. & Haigwood, N.L., eds, *HIV: Molecular Organization, Pathogenicity and Treatment*, Amsterdam, Elsevier, pp. 241–266

Klatzmann, D., Champagne, E., Chamaraet, S., Gruest, J., Guetard, D., Hercend, T., Gluckman, J.-C. & Montagnier, L. (1984) T-lymphocyte T4 molecule behaves as the receptor for human retrovirus LAV. *Nature*, **312**, 767–768

Klauke, S., Schoefer, H., Althoff, P.H., Michels, B. & Helm, E.B. (1995) Sex hormones as a cofactor in the pathogenesis of epidemic Kaposi's sarcoma. *AIDS*, **9**, 1295–1296

Klein, R.S., Ho, G.Y.F., Vermund, S.H., Fleming, I. & Burk, R.D. (1994) Risk factors for squamous intraepithelial lesions on pap smear in women at risk for human immunodeficiency virus infection. *J. infect. Dis.*, **170**, 1404–1409

Klimkait, T., Strebel, K., Hoggan, M.D., Martin, M.A. & Orenstein, J.M. (1990) The human immunodeficiency virus type 1-specific protein Vpu is required for efficient virus maturation and release. *J. Virol.*, **64**, 621–629

Knopf, K.B. & Locker, G.Y. (1995) Hodgkin's disease and HIV infection (Letter to the Editor). *New Engl. J. Med.*, **333**, 65–66

Knowles, D.M. (1993) Biologic aspects of AIDS-associated non-Hodgkin's lymphoma. *Curr. Opin. Oncol.*, **5**, 845–851

Knowles, D.M., Inghirami, G., Ubriaco, A. & Dalla-Favera, R. (1989) Molecular genetic analysis of three AIDS-associated neoplasms of uncertain lineage demonstrates their B-cell derivation and the possible pathogenetic role of the Epstein-Barr virus. *Blood*, **73**, 792–799

Knox, K.K. & Carrigan, D.R. (1994) Disseminated active HHV-6 infections in patients with AIDS. *Lancet*, **343**, 577–578

Kolb, H.J., Guenther, W., Duell, T., Socie, G., Schaeffer, E., Holler, E., Schumm, M., Horowitz, M.M., Gale, R.P. & Fliedner, T.M. (1992) Cancer after bone marrow transplantation. *Bone Marrow Transplant.*, **10** (Supp. 1), 135–138

Korn, A.P., Autry, M., DeRemer, P.A. & Tan, W. (1994) Sensitivity of the Papanicolaou smear in human immunodeficiency virus-infected women. *Obstet. Gynecol.*, **83**, 401–404

Kornblau, S.M., Goodacre, A. & Cabanillas, F. (1991) Chromosomal abnormalities in adult non-endemic Burkitt's lymphoma and leukemia: 22 new reports and a review of 148 cases from the literature. *Hematol. Oncol.*, **9**, 63–78

Koup, R.A., Safrit, J.T., Cao, Y., Andrews, C.A., McLeod, G., Borkowsky, W., Farthing, C. & Ho, D.D. (1994) Temporal association of cellular immune responses with the initial control of viremia in primary human immunodeficiency virus type 1 syndrome. *J. Virol.*, **68**, 4650-4655

Krämer, A., Biggar, R.J., Hampl, H., Friedman, R.M., Fuchs, D., Wachter, H. & Goedert, J.J. (1992) Immunologic markers of progression to acquired immunodeficiency syndrome are time-dependent and illness-specific. *Am. J. Epidemiol.*, **136**, 71–80

Kraus, G., Werner, A., Baier, M., Binniger, D., Ferdinand, F.J., Norley, S. & Kurth, R. (1989) Isolation of human immunodeficiency virus-related simian immunodeficiency viruses from African green monkeys. *Proc. natl Acad. Sci. USA*, **86**, 2892–2896

Kreiss, J.K., Kiviat, N.B., Plummer, F.A., Roberts, P.L., Waiyaki, P., Ngugi, E. & Holmes, K.K. (1992) Human immunodeficiency virus, human papillomavirus, and cervical intraepithelial neoplasia in Nairobi prostitutes. *Sex. transm. Dis.*, **19**, 54–59

Kristal, A.R., Nasca, P.C., Burnett, W.S. & Mikl, J. (1988) Changes in the epidemiology of non-Hodgkin's lymphoma associated with epidemic human immunodeficiency virus (HIV) infection. *Am. J. Epidemiol.*, **128**, 711–718

Kroegel, C., Hess, G. & Meyer zum Büschenfelde, K.-H. (1987) Routes of HIV-2 transmission in western Europe (Letter to the Editor). *Lancet*, **i**, 1150

Krogh-Jensen, M., d'Amore, F., Jensen, M.K., Christensen, B.E., Thorling, K., Pedersen, M., Johansen, P., Boesen, A.M. & Andersen, E. (1994) Incidence, clinicopathological features and outcome of primary central nervous system lymphomas. Population-based data from a Danish lymphoma registry. *Ann. Oncol.*, **5**, 349–354

Krueger, G.R.F., Koch, B., Ramon, A., Ablashi, D.V., Salahuddin, S.Z., Josephs, S.F., Streicher, H.Z., Gallo, R.C. & Habermann, U. (1988) Antibody prevalence to HBLV (human herpesvirus-6, HHV-6) and suggestive pathogenicity in the general population and in patients with immune deficiency syndromes. *J. virol. Meth.*, **21**, 125–131

Krueger, G.R.F., Manak, M., Bourgeois, N., Ablashi, D.V., Salahuddin, S.Z., Josephs, S.S., Buchbinder, A., Gallo, R.C., Berthold, F. & Tesch, H. (1989) Persistent active herpes virus infection associated with atypical polyclonal lymphoproliferation (APL) and malignant lymphoma. *Anticancer Res.*, **9**, 1457–1476

Kulaga, H., Folks, T., Rutledge, R., Truckenmiller, M.E., Gugel, E. & Kindt, T.J. (1989) Infection of rabbits with human immunodeficiency virus 1. A small animal model for acquired immunodeficiency syndrome. *J. exp. Med.*, **169**, 321–326

Kumar, S., Kumar, D., Schnadig, V.J., Selvanayagam, P. & Slaughter, D.P. (1994) Plasma cell myeloma in patients who are HIV-positive. *Am. J. clin. Pathol.*, **102**, 633–639

Kuo, J.-M., Taylor, J.M.G. & Detels, R. (1991) Estimating the AIDS incubation period from a prevalent cohort. *Am. J. Epidemiol.*, **133**, 1050–1057

Lack, E.E. (1986) Leiomyosarcomas in childhood: a clinical and pathological study of 10 cases. *Pediatr. Pathol.*, **6**, 181–197

Lackritz, E.M., Satten, G.A., Aberle-Grasse, J., Dodd, R.Y., Raimondi, V.P., Janssen, R.S., Lewis, W.F., Notari, E.P., IV & Petersen, L.R. (1995) Estimated risk of transmission of the human immunodeficiency virus by screened blood in the United States. *New Engl. J. Med.*, **333**, 1721–1725

Lafferty, W.E., Glidden, D. & Hopkins, S.G. (1991) Survival trends of people with AIDS in Washington State. *Am. J. public Health*, **81**, 217–219

Laga, M., Icenogle, J.P., Marsella, R., Manoka, A.T., Nzila, N., Ryder, R.W., Vermund, S.H., Heyward, W.L., Nelson, A. & Reeves, W.C. (1992) Genital papillomavirus infection and cervical dysplasia — opportunistic complications of HIV infection. *Int. J. Cancer*, **50**, 45–48

Laga, M., Manoka, A., Kivuvu, M., Malele, B., Tuliza, M., Nzila, N., Goeman, J., Behets, F., Batter, V., Alary, M., Heyward, W., Ryder, R.W. & Piot, P. (1993) Non-ulcerative sexually transmitted diseases as risk factors for HIV-1 transmission in women: results from a cohort study. *AIDS*, **7**, 95–102

Lambert, P.F. & Howley, P.M. (1988) Bovine papillomavirus type 1 E1 replication-defective mutants are altered in their transcriptional regulation. *J. Virol.*, **62**, 4009–4015

Landay, A.L., Mackewicz, C.E. & Levy, J.A. (1993) An activated CD8$^+$ T cell phenotype correlates with anti-HIV activity and asymptomatic clinical status. *Clin. Immunol. Immunopathol.*, **69**, 106–116

Landman, P., Karsenty, E., Katz, L. & Saimot, A.G. (1984) Kaposi's sarcoma in Israel: epidemiological data 1960–1980. *Bull. Soc. Pathol. exp.*, **77**, 572–576 (in French)

Langley, C.L., Benga-De, E., Critchlow, C.W., Ndoye, I., Mbengue-Ly, M.D., Kuypers, J., Woto-Gaye, G., Mboup, S., Bergeron, C., Holmes, K.K. & Kiviat, N.B. (1996) HIV-1, HIV-2, human papillomavirus infection and cervical neoplasia in high-risk African women. *AIDS*, **10**, 413–417

LaRosa, G.J., Davide, J.P., Weinhold, K., Waterbury, J.A., Profy, A.T., Lewis, J.A., Langlois, A.J., Dreesman, G.R., Boswell, R.N., Shadduck, P., Holley, L.H., Karplus, M., Bolognesi, D.P., Matthews, T.J., Emini, E.A. & Putney, S.D. (1990) Conserved sequence and structural elements in the HIV-1 principal neutralizing determinant. *Science*, **249**, 932–935

Laurence, J. & Astrin, S.M. (1991) Human immunodeficiency virus induction of malignant transformation in human B-lymphocytes. *Proc. natl Acad. Sci. USA*, **88**, 7635–7639

Law, C.L.H., Quassim, M., Thompson, C.H., Rose, B.R., Grace, J., Morris, B.J. & Cossart, Y.E. (1991) Factors associated with clinical and sub-clinical anal human papillomavirus infection in homosexual men. *Genitourin. Med.*, **67**, 92–98

Lawrence, C.E., Callanan, J.J. & Jarrett, O. (1992) Decreased mitogen responsiveness and elevated tumour necrosis factor production in cats shortly after feline immunodeficiency virus infection. *Vet. Immunol. Immunopathol.*, **35**, 51–59

Lebbé, C., de Crémoux, P., Rybojad, M., Costa da Cunha, C., Morel, P. & Calvo, F. (1995) Kaposi's sarcoma and new herpesvirus (Letter to the Editor). *Lancet*, **345**, 1180

Lee, W. A. & Hutchins, G.M. (1992) Cluster analysis of the metastatic patterns of human immunodeficiency virus-associated Kaposi's sarcoma. *Hum. Pathol.*, **23**, 306–311

Lee, E.S., Locker, J., Nalesnik, M., Reyes, J., Jaffe, R., Alashari, M., Nour, B., Tzakis, A. & Dickman, P.S. (1995) The association of Epstein-Barr virus with smooth-muscle tumors occurring after organ transplantation. *New Engl. J. Med.*, **332**, 19–25

Leger-Ravet, M.B., Peuchmaur, M., Devergne, O., Audouin, J., Raphael, M., Van Damme, J., Galanaud, P., Diebold, J. & Emilie, D. (1991) Interleukin-6 gene expression in Castleman's disease. *Blood*, **78**, 2923–2930

Le Guenno, B., Jouan, A., Arborio, M., N'Diaye, B., Guiraud, M., Griffet, P., Seignot, P. & Digoutte, J.-P. (1987) HIV-2 is responsible for AIDS cases in Senegal. *Ann. Inst. Pasteur/Virol.*, **138**, 397–399

Lennert, K. & Feller, A.C. (1990) *Histopathology of Non-Hodgkin's Lymphomas (based on the Updated Kiel Classification)*, 2nd Ed., Berlin, Springer-Verlag, pp. 1–312

Leonard, J.M., Abramczuk, J.W., Pezen, D.S., Rutledge, R., Belcher, J.H., Hakim, F., Shearer, G., Lamperth, L., Travis, W., Fredrickson, T., Notkins, A.L. & Martin, M.A. (1988) Development of disease and virus recovery in transgenic mice containing HIV proviral DNA. *Science*, **242**, 1665–1670

Letvin, N.L. (1993) Vaccines against human immunodeficiency virus — progress and prospects. *New Engl. J. Med.*, **329**, 1400–1405

Letvin, N.L. & King, N.W. (1990) Immunologic and pathologic manifestations of the infection of rhesus monkeys with simian immunodeficiency virus of macaques. *J. acquir. Immun. Defic. Syndr.*, **3**, 1023–1040

Letvin, N.L., Eaton, K.A., Aldrich, W.R., Sehgal, P.K., Blake, B.J., Schlossman, S.F., King, N.W. & Hunt, R.D. (1983) Acquired immunodeficiency syndrome in a colony of macaque monkeys. *Proc. natl Acad. Sci.*, **80**, 2718-2722

Levin, T.L, Adam, H.M., van Hoeven, K.H. & Goldman, H.S. (1994) Hepatic spindle cell tumors in HIV positive children. *Pediatr. Radiol.*, **24**, 78–79

Levine, A.M. (1993) AIDS-related malignancies: the emerging epidemic. *J. natl Cancer Inst.*, **85**, 1382–1397

Levine, A.M., Bernstein, L., Sullivan-Halley, J., Shibata, D., Mahterian, S.B. & Nathwani, B.N. (1995) Role of zidovudine antiretroviral therapy in the pathogenesis of acquired immunodeficiency syndrome-related lymphoma. *Blood*, **86**, 4612–4616

Levy, J.A. (1993) Pathogenesis of human immunodeficiency virus infection. *Microbiol. Rev.*, **57**, 183–289

Levy, J.A. (1995) A new human herpesvirus: KSHV or HHV8? *Lancet*, **346**, 786

Levy, D.N., Fernandes, L.S., Williams, W.V. & Weiner, D.B. (1993a) Induction of cell differentiation by human immunodeficiency virus 1 *vpr*. *Cell*, **72**, 541–550

Levy, M., Backman, L., Husberg, B., Goldstein, R., McMillan, R., Gibbs, J., Gonwa, T.A., Holman, M. & Klintmalm, G. (1993b) De novo malignancy following liver transplantation: a single-center study. *Transplant. Proc.*, **25**, 1397–1399

Lévy, R., Colonna, P., Tourani, J.-M., Gastaut, J.A., Brice, P., Raphaël, M., Taillan, B. & Andrieu, J.-M. (1995) Human immunodeficiency virus associated Hodgkin's disease: Report of 45 cases from the French registry of HIV-associated tumours. *Leuk. Lymph.*, **16**, 451–456

Lewensohn-Fuchs, I., Wester, D., Bistoletti, P., Elfgren, K., Ohlman, S., Dillner, J. & Dalianis, T. (1993) Serological responses to human papillomavirus type 16 antigens in women before and after renal transplantation. *J. med. Virol.*, **40**, 188–192

Li, S.L., Feichtinger, H., Kaaya, E.E., Migliorini, P., Putkonen, P., Biberfeld, G., Middeldorp, J.M., Biberfeld, P. & Ernberg, I. (1993a) Expression of Epstein-Barr virus related nuclear antigens and B-cell markers in lymphomas of SIV immunosuppressed monkeys. *Int. J. Cancer*, **55**, 609–615

Li, J.J., Huang, Y.Q., Moscatelli, D., Nicolaides, A., Zhang, W.C., Friedman-Kien, A.E. (1993b) Expression of fibroblast growth factors and their receptors in acquired immunodeficiency syndrome-associated Kaposi sarcoma tissue and derived cells. *Cancer*, **72**, 2253–2259

Li, S.L., Biberfeld, P. & Ernberg, I. (1994) DNA of lymphoma-associated herpes virus (HVMF-1) in SIV-infected monkeys (*Macaca fascicularis*) shows homologies to EBNA-1, -2 and -5 genes. *Int. J. Cancer*, **59**, 287–295

Li, J.J., Huang, Y.Q. & Friedman-Kien, A.E. (1995) Detection of DNA sequences of KSHV in blood semen, KS tumor, and uninvolved skin of AIDS-KS patients (Abstract no. 136). *AIDS Res. hum. Retroviruses*, **11** (Suppl.1), S98

Lifson, A.R., Darrow, W.W., Hessol, N.A., O'Malley, P.M., Barnhart, J.L., Jaffe, H.W. & Rutherford, G.W. (1990a) Kaposi's sarcoma in a cohort of homosexual and bisexual men. Epidemiology and analysis for cofactors. *Am. J. Epidemiol.*, **131**, 221–31

Lifson, A.R., Darrow, W.W., Hessol, N.A., O'Malley, P.M., Barnhart, L., Jaffe, H.W. & Rutherford, G.W. (1990b) Kaposi's sarcoma among homosexual and bisexual men enrolled in the San Francisco City Clinic Cohort Study. *J. acquir. Immun. Defic. Syndr.*, **3** (Suppl. 1), S32–S37

Lifson, A.R., Buchbinder, S.P., Sheppard, H.W., Mawle, A.C., Wilber, J.C., Stanley, M., Hart, C.E., Hessol, N.A. & Holmberg, S.D. (1991) Long-term human immunodeficiency virus infection in asymptomatic homosexual and bisexual men with normal CD4$^+$ lymphocyte counts: immunologic and virologic characteristics. *J. infect. Dis.*, **163**, 959–965

Lifson, A.R., Hessol, N.A., Buchbinder, S.P., O'Malley, P.M., Barnhart, L., Segal, M., Katz, M.H. & Holmberg, S.D. (1992) Serum β_2-microglobulin and prediction of progression to AIDS in HIV infection. *Lancet*, **339**, 1436–1440

Lim-Tan, S.K., Yoshikawa, H., Sng, I.T.Y., de Villiers, E.M., zur Hausen, H., Ho, T.H. & Yoong, T. (1988) Human papillomavirus in dysplasia and carcinoma of the cervix in Singapore. *Pathology*, **20**, 317–319

Lin, J.-C., Lin, S.-C., Mar, E.-C., Pellett, P.E., Stamey, F.R., Stewart, J.A. & Spira, T.J. (1995) Is Kaposi's sarcoma-associated herpesvirus detectable in semen of HIV-infected homosexual men? *Lancet*, **346**, 1601–1602

Little, D., Said,W., Siegel, R.J., Fealy, M. & Fishbein, M.C. (1986) Endothelial cell markers in vascular neoplasms: an immunohistochemical study comparing factor VIII-related antigen, blood group specific antigens, 6-keto-PGF1-α, and Ulex europaeus 1 lectin. *Am. J. Pathol.*, **149**, 89–95

Livartowski, J., Dormont, D., Boussin, F., Chamaret, S., Guetard, D., Vazeux, R., Lebon, P., Metivier, H. & Montagnier, L. (1992) Clinical and virological aspects of HIV2 infection in rhesus monkeys. *Cancer Detect. Prev.*, **16**, 341–345

Livingston, R.A., Hutton, N., Halsey, N.A., Kline, R.L., Joyner, M. & Quinn, T.C. (1995) Human immunodeficiency virus-specific IgA in infants born to human immunodeficiency virus-seropositive women. *Arch. pediatr. adolesc. Med.*, **149**, 503–507

Lo, S.-C., Shih, J.W.-K., Yang, N.-Y., Ou, C.-Y. & Wang, R.Y.-H. (1989) A novel virus-like infectious agent in patients with AIDS. *Am. J. trop. Med. Hyg.*, **40**, 213–216

Lo, S.-C., Hayes, M.M., Wang, R.Y.-H., Pierce, P.F., Kotani, H. & Shih, J.W.-K. (1991) Newly discovered mycoplasma isolated from patients infected with HIV. *Lancet*, **338**, 1415–1418

Lobo, D.V., Chu, P., Grekin, R.C. & Berger, T.G. (1992) Nonmelanoma skin cancers and infection with the human immunodeficiency virus. *Arch. Dermatol.*, **128**, 623–627

Loeb, D.D., Hutchison, C.A., III, Edgell, M.H., Farmerie, W.G. & Swanstrom, R. (1989) Mutational analysis of human immunodeficiency virus type 1 protease suggests functional homology with aspartic proteinases. *J. Virol.*, **63**, 111–121

Lombardi, L., Newcomb, E.W. & Dalla-Favera, R. (1987) Pathogenesis of Burkitt's lymphoma: expression of an activated c-*myc* oncogene causes the tumorigenic conversion of EBV-infected human B lymphoblasts. *Cell*, **49**, 161–170

Lopez, A.P. & Gorbach, S.L. (1988) Diarrhea in AIDS. *Infect. Dis. Clin. N. Am.*, **2**, 705–718

Lorenz, H.P., Wilson, W., Leigh, B., Crombleholme, T. & Schecter, W. (1991) Squamous cell carcinoma of the anus and HIV infection. *Dis. Colon Rectum*, **34**, 336–338

Lörincz, A.T., Reid, R., Jenson, A.B., Greenberg, M.D., Lancaster, W. & Kurman, R.J. (1992) Human papillomavirus infection of the cervix: relative risk associations of 15 common anogenital types. *Obstet. Gynecol.*, **79**, 328–337

Lowenstine, L.J., Pedersen, N.C., Higgins, J., Pallis, K.C., Uyeda, A., Marx, P., Lerche, N.W., Munn, R.J. & Gardner, M.B. (1986) Seroepidemiologic survey of captive Old-World primates for antibodies to human and simian retroviruses and isolation of a lentivirus from sooty mangabeys (*Cercocebus atys*). *Int. J. Cancer*, **38**, 563–574

Lowenstine, L.J., Lerche, N.W., Yee, J.L., Uyeda, A., Jennings, M.B., Munn, R.J., McClure, H.M., Anderson, D.C., Fultz, P.N. & Gardner, M.B. (1992) Evidence for a lentiviral etiology in an epizootic of immune deficiency and lymphoma in stump-tails macaques (*Macaca arctoides*). *J. med. Primatol.*, **21**, 1–14

Lowsky, R., Lipton, J., Fyles, G., Minden, M., Meharchand, J., Tejpar, I., Atkins, H., Sutcliffe, S. & Messner, H. (1994) Secondary malignancies after bone marrow transplantation in adults. *J. clin. Oncol.*, **12**, 2187–2192

Lucas, S.B., Diomande, M., Hounnou, A., Beaumel, A., Giordano, C., Kadio, A., Peacock, C.S., Honde, M. & De Cock, K.M. (1994) HIV-associated lymphoma in Africa: an autopsy study in Côte d'Ivoire. *Int. J. Cancer*, **59**, 20–24

Luciw, P.A. (1996) Human immunodeficiency viruses and their replication. In: Fields, B.N., Knipe, D.M., Howley, P.M., Chanock, R.M., Melnick, J.L., Monath, T.P., Roizman, B. & Straus, S.E., eds, *Fields Virology*, Vol. 2, 3rd Ed., Philadelphia, Lippincott-Raven, pp. 1881–1952

Lui, K.-J., Darrow, W.W. & Rutherford, G.W., III (1988) A model-based estimate of the mean incubation period for AIDS in homosexual men. *Science*, **240**, 1333–1335

Lunardi-Iskandar, Y., Bryant, J.L., Zeman, R.A., Lam, V.H., Samaniego, F., Besnier, J.M., Hermans, P., Thierry, A.R., Gill, P. & Gallo, R.C. (1995a) Tumorigenesis and metastasis of neoplastic Kaposi's sarcoma cell line in immunodeficient mice blocked by a human pregnancy hormone. *Nature*, **375**, 64–68

Lunardi-Iskandar, Y., Gill, P., Lam, V.H., Zeman, R.A., Michaels, F., Mann, D.L., Reitz, M.S., Jr, Kaplan, M., Berneman, Z.N., Carter, D., Bryant, J.L. & Gallo, R.C. (1995b) Isolation and characterization of an immortal neoplastic cell line (KS Y-1) from AIDS-associated Kaposi's sarcoma. *J. natl Cancer Inst.*, **87**, 974–981

Lundgren, J.D., Pedersen, C., Clumeck, N., Gatell, J.M., Johnson, A.M., Ledergerber, B., Vella, S., Phillips, A., Nielsen, J.O. & the AIDS in Europe Study Group (1994) Survival differences in European patients with AIDS, 1979-1989. *Br. med. J.*, **308**, 1068–1073

Lundgren, J.D., Melbye, M., Pedersen, C., Rosenberg, P.S. & Gerstoft, J. for the Danish Study Group for HIV Infection (DASHI) (1995) Changing patterns of Kaposi's sarcoma in Danish acquired immunodeficiency syndrome patients with complete follow-up. *Am. J. Epidemiol.*, **141**, 652–658

Lungu, O., Sun, X.W., Felix, J., Richart, R.M., Silverstein, S. & Wright, T., Jr (1992) Relationship of human papillomavirus type to grade of cervical intraepithelial neoplasia. *J. Am. med. Assoc.*, **267**, 2493–2496

Luo, K., Law, M., Kaldor, J.M., McDonald, A.M. & Cooper, D.A. (1995) The role of initial AIDS-defining illness in survival following AIDS. *AIDS*, **9**, 57–63

Lusso, P. & Gallo, R.C. (1995) Human herpesvirus 6 in AIDS. *Immunol. Today*, **16**, 67–71

Lusso, P., Markham, P.D., Ranki, A., Earl, P., Moss, B., Dorner, F., Gallo, R.C. & Krohn, K.J.E. (1988) Cell-mediated immune response toward viral envelope and core antigens in gibbon apes (*Hylobates lar*) chronically infected with human immunodeficiency virus-1. *J. Immunol.*, **141**, 2467–2473

Lyter, D.W., Bryant, J., Thackeray, R., Rinaldo, C.R. & Kingsley, L.A. (1995) Incidence of human immunodeficiency virus-related and nonrelated malignancies in a large cohort of homosexual men. *J. clin. Oncol.*, **13**, 2540–2546

Macallan, D.C., Noble, C., Baldwin, C., Jebb, S.A., Prentice, A.M., Coward, W.A., Sawyer, M.B., McManus, T.J. & Griffin, G.E. (1995) Energy expenditure and wasting human immunodeficiency virus infection. *New Engl. J. Med.*, **333**, 83–88

Mackewicz, C.E., Ortega, H.W. & Levy, J.A. (1991) $CD8^+$ cell anti-HIV activity correlates with the clinical state of the infected individual. *J. clin. Invest.*, **87**, 1462–1466

MacMahon, E.M.E., Glass, J.D., Hayward, S.D., Mann, R.B., Becker, P.S., Charache, H., McArthur, J.C. & Ambinder, R.F. (1991) Epstein–Barr virus in AIDS-related primary central nervous system lymphoma. *Lancet*, **338**, 969–973

Maggwa, B.N., Hunter, D.J., Mbugua, S., Tukei, P. & Mati, J.K. (1993) The relationship between HIV infection and cervical intraepithelial neoplasia among women attending two family planning clinics in Nairobi, Kenya. *AIDS*, **7**, 733–738

Maiman, M., Fruchter, R.G., Serur, E., Remy, J.C., Feuer, G. & Boyce, J. (1990) Human immunodeficiency virus infection and cervical neoplasia. *Gynecol. Oncol.*, **38**, 377–382

Maiman M., Tarricone, N., Vieira, J., Suarez, E & Boyce, J. (1991) Colposcopic evaluation of human immunodeficiency virus-positive women. *Obstet. Gynecol.*, **78**, 84–88

Maiman, M., Fruchther, R.G., Serur, E., Levine, P.A., Arrastia, C.D. & Sedlis, A. (1993a) Recurrent cervical intraepithelial neoplasia in human immunodeficiency virus-seropositive women. *Obstet. Gynecol.*, **82**, 170–174

Maiman, M., Fruchter, R.G., Guy, L., Cuthill, S., Levine, P. & Serur, E. (1993b) Human immunodeficiency virus infection and invasive cervical carcinoma. *Cancer*, **71**, 402–406

Malamba, S.S., Wagner, H.-U., Maude, G., Okongo, M., Nunn, A.J., Kengeya-Kayondo, J.F. & Mulder, D.W. (1994) Risk factors for HIV-1 infection in adults in a rural Ugandan community: a case-control study. *AIDS*, **8**, 253–257

Malau, C., O'Leary, M., Jenkins, C. & Faraclas, N. (1994) HIV/AIDS prevention and control in Papua New Guinea. *AIDS*, **8** (Suppl. 2), S117–S124

Mandelblatt, J.S., Fahs, M., Garibalbi, K., Senie, R.T. & Peterson, H.B. (1992) Association between HIV infection and cervical neoplasia: implications for clinical care of women at risk for both conditions. *AIDS*, **6**, 173–178

Mann, D.L., Murray, C., O'Donnell, M., Blattner, W.A. & Goedert, J.J. (1990) HLA antigen frequencies in HIV-1 related Kaposi's sarcoma. *J. acquir. Immun. Defic. Syndr.*, **3**, S51–S55

Margolick, J.B., Muñoz, A., Vlahov, D., Solomon, L., Astemborski, J., Cohn, S. & Nelson, K.E. (1992) Changes in T-lymphocyte subsets in intravenous drug users with HIV-1 infection. *J. Am. med. Assoc.*, **267**, 1631–1636

Margolick, J.B., Donnenberg, A.D., Muñoz, A., Park, L.P., Bauer, K.D., Giorgi, J.V., Saah, A.J. & the Multicenter AIDS Cohort Study (1993) Changes in T and non-T lymphocyte subsets following seroconversion to HIV-1: stable $CD3^+$ and declining CD3- populations suggest regulatory responses linked to loss of CD4 lymphocytes. *J. acquir. Immun. Defic. Syndr.*, **6**, 153–161

Margolick, J.B., Donnenberg, A.D. & Muñoz, A. (1994) T lymphocyte homeostasis after HIV seroconversion. *J. acquir. Immun. Defic. Syndr.*, **7**, 415–420

Mariotto, A.B., Mariotti, S., Pezzotti, P., Rezza, G. & Verdecchia, A. (1992) Estimation of the acquired immunodeficiency syndrome incubation period in intravenous drug users: a comparison with male homosexuals. *Am. J. Epidemiol.*, **135**, 428–437

Markowitz, D.M. (1993) Infection with the human immunodeficiency virus type 2. *Ann. intern. Med.*, **118**, 211–218

Marlink, R.G., Ricard, D., M'Boup, S., Kanki, P.J., Romet-Lemonne, J.-L., N'Doye, I., Diop, K., Simpson, M.A., Greco, F., Chou, M.-J., Degruttola, V., Hsieh, C.-C., Boye, C., Barin, F., Denis, F., McLane, M.F. & Essex, M. (1988) Clinical, hematologic, and immunologic cross-sectional evaluation of individuals exposed to human immunodeficiency virus type-2 (HIV-2). *AIDS Res. hum. Retroviruses*, **4**, 137–148

Marmor, M., Friedman-Kien, A.E., Laubenstein, L., Byrum, R.D., William, D.C., D'Onofrio, S. & Dubin, N. (1982) Risk factors for Kaposi's sarcoma in homosexual men. *Lancet*, **i**, 1083–1087

Martinez, S., Young, R., Moll, B., Balbi, H., Ciminera, P., Coren, C., Kosuri, S., Sabatino, D., Frieri, M. & Meadow, E. (1990) Simultaneous leiomyosarcoma and leiomyoma in pediatric HIV infection (Abstract no. 82). *Ann. Allergy*, **64**, 89

Martínez-Maza, O. (1992) IL6 and AIDS. *Res. Immunol.*, **143**, 764–769

Marx, P.A., Bryant, M.L., Osborn, K.G., Maul, D.H., Lerche, N.W., Lowenstine, L.J., Kluge, J.D., Zaiss, C.P., Henrickson, R.V., Shiigi, S.M., Wilson, B.J., Malley, A., Olson, L.C., McNulty, W.P., Arthur, L.O., Gilden, R.V., Barker, C.S., Hunter, E., Munn, R.J., Heidecker, G. & Gardner, M.B. (1985) Isolation of a new serotype of simian acquired immune deficiency syndrome type D retrovirus from Celebes black macaques (*Macaca nigra*) with immune deficiency and retroperitoneal fibromatosis. *J. Virol.*, **56**, 571–578

Mason, D.Y., Cordell, J.L., Tse, A.G.D., van Dongen, J.J.M., van Noesel, C.J.M., Micklem, K., Pulford, K.A.F., Valensi, F., Comans-Bitter, W.M., Borst, J. & Gatter, K.C. (1991) The IgM-associated protein mb-1 as a marker of normal and neoplastic B cells. *J. Immunol.*, **147**, 2474–2482

Masood, R., Zhang, Y., Bond, M.W., Scadden, D.T., Moudgil, T., Law, R.E., Kaplan, M.H., Jung, B., Espina, B.M., Lunardi-Iskandar, Y., Levine, A.M. & Gill, P.S. (1995) Interleukin-10 is an autocrine growth factor for acquired immunodeficiency syndrome-related B-cell lymphoma. *Blood*, **85**, 3423–3430

Mastro, T.D. & de Vincenzi, I. (1996) Probabilities of sexual HIV-1 transmission. *AIDS*, **10** (Suppl. A), S75–S82

Matheron, S., Courpotin, C., Simon, F., Di Maria, H., Balloul, H., Bartzack, S., Dormont, D., Brun-Vézinet, F., Saimont, A.G. & Coulaud, J.P. (1990) Vertical transmission of HIV-2 (Letter to the Editor). *Lancet*, **335**, 1103–1104

Mayer, K.H. & DeGruttola, V. (1987) Human immunodeficiency virus and oral intercourse (Letter to the Editor). *Ann. intern. Med.*, **107**, 428–429

McCance, D.J., Kalache, A., Ashdown, K., Andrade, L., Menzes, F., Smith, P. & Doll, R. (1986) Human papillomavirus type 16 and 18 in carcinomas of the penis from Brazil. *Int. J. Cancer*, **37**, 55–59

McClain, K.L., Leach, C.T., Jenson, H.B., Joshi, V.V., Pollock, B.H., Parmley, R.T., DiCarlo, F.J., Chadwick, E.G. & Murphy, S.B. (1995) Association of Epstein-Barr virus with leiomyosarcomas in young people with AIDS. *New Engl. J. Med.*, **332**, 12–18

McClure, M.O., Sommerfelt, M.A., Marsh, M. & Weiss, R.A. (1990) The pH independence of mammalian retrovirus infection. *J. gen. Virol.*, **71**, 767–773

McClure, M.O., Goulder, P.J., Ogg, G., McMichael, A.J. & Weber, J.N. (1996) HIV clearance in infants (Letter to the Editor). *Lancet*, **347**, 1122

McCutchan, F.E., Sanders-Buell, E., Oster, C.W., Redfield, R.R., Hira, S.K., Perine, P.L., Ungar, B.L.P. & Burke, D.S. (1991) Genetic comparison of human immunodeficiency virus (HIV-1) isolates by polymerase chain reaction. *J. Acquir. Immun. Defic. Syndr.*, **4**, 1241–1250

McCutchan, F.E., Ungar, B.L.P., Hegerich, P., Roberts, C.R., Fowler, A.K., Hira, S.K., Perine, P.L. & Burke, D.S. (1992) Genetic analysis of HIV-1 isolates from Zambia and an expanded phylogenetic tree for HIV-1. *J. Acquir. Immun. Defic. Syndr*, **5**, 441-449

McDonald, A.M., Crofts, N., Blumer, C.E., Gertig, D.M., Patten, J.J., Roberts, M., Davey, T., Mullins, S.E., Chuah, J.C., Bailey, K.A. & Kaldor, J.M. (1994) The pattern of diagnosed HIV infection in Australia, 1984–1992. *AIDS*, **8**, 513–519

McGrath, M.S., Shiramizu, B., Meeker, T.C., Kaplan, L.D. & Herndier, B. (1991) AIDS-associated polyclonal lymphoma: identification of a new HIV-associated disease process. *J. acquir. Immun. Defic. Syndr.*, **4**, 408–415

McLoughlin, L.C., Nord, K.S., Joshi, V.V., DiCarlo, F.J. & Kane, M.J. (1991) Disseminated leiomyosarcoma in a child with acquired immune deficiency syndrome. *Cancer*, **67**, 2618–2621

McMichael, A., Koup, R. & Ammann, A.J. (1996) Transient HIV infection in infants (Letter to the Editor). *Lancet*, **334**, 801–802

McNicol, P.J., Guijon, F.B., Paraskevas, M. & Brunham, R.C. (1989) Comparison of filter in situ deoxyribonucleic acid hybridization with cytologic, colposcopic, and histopathologic examination for detection of human papillomavirus infection in woman with cervical intra-epithelial neoplasia. *Am. J. Obstet. Gynecol.*, **160**, 265–270

Medeiros, L.J. & Greiner, T.C. (1995) Hodgkin's disease. *Cancer*, **75**, 357–369

Melbye, M., Biggar, R.J., Ebbesen, P., Andersen, H.K. & Vestergaard, B.F. (1983) Lifestyle and antiviral antibody studies among homosexual men in Denmark. *Acta pathol. microbiol. immunol. scand.*, **B91**, 357–364

Melbye, M., Njelesani, E.K., Bayley, A., Mukelabai, K., Manuwele, J.K., Bowa, F.J., Clayden, S.A., Levin, A., Blattner, W.A., Weiss, R.A., Tedder, R. & Biggar, R.J. (1986) Evidence for heterosexual transmission and clinical manifestations of human immunodeficiency virus infection and related conditions in Lusaka, Zambia. *Lancet*, **ii**, 1113–1115

Melbye, M., Kestens, L., Biggar, R.J., Schreuder, G.M.T. & Gigase, P.L. (1987) HLA studies of endemic African Kaposi's sarcoma patients and matched controls: no association with HLA-DR5. *Int. J. Cancer*, **39**, 182–184

Melbye, M., Palefsky, J., Gonzales, J., Ryder, L.P., Nielsen, H., Bergmann, O., Pindborg, J. & Biggar, R.J. (1990) Immune status as a determinant of human papillomavirus detection and its association with anal epithelial abnormalities. *Int. J. Cancer*, **46**, 203–206

Melbye, M., Rabkin, C., Frisch, M. & Biggar, R.J. (1994a) Changing patterns of anal cancer incidence in the United States, 1940-1989. *Am. J. Epidemiol.*, **139**, 772–780

Melbye, M., Coté, T.R., Kessler, L., Gail, M., Biggar, R.J. & the AIDS/Cancer Working Group (1994b) High incidence of anal cancer among AIDS patients. *Lancet*, **343**, 636–639

Melbye, M., Coté, T.R., West, D., Kessler, L., Biggar, R.J. & the AIDS/Cancer Working Group (1996) Nasopharyngeal carcinoma: an EBV-associated tumour not significantly influenced by HIV-induced immunosuppression. *Br. J. Cancer*, 73, 995–997

Melmed, R.N., Taylor, J.M.G., Detels, R., Bozorgmehri, M. & Fahey, J.L. (1989) Serum neopterin changes in HIV-infected subjects: indicator of significant pathology, CD4 T cell changes, and the development of AIDS. *J. acquir. Immun. Defic. Syndr.*, 2, 70–76

Mellors J.W., Rinaldo, C.R., Gupta, P., White, R.M., Todd, J.A. & Kingsley, L.A. (1996) Prognosis in HIV-1 infection predicted by the quantity of virus in plasma. *Science*, 272, 1167–1170

ter Meulen, J., Eberhardt, H.C., Luande, J., Mgaya, H.N., Chang-Claude, J., Mtiro, H., Mhina, M., Kashaija, P., Ockert, S., Yu, X., Meinhardt, G., Gissmann, L. & Pawlita, M. (1992) Human papillomavirus (HPV) infection, HIV infection and cervical cancer in Tanzania, East Africa. *Int. J. Cancer*, 51, 515–521

Michaels, F.H., Hattori, N., Gallo, R.C. & Franchini, G. (1993) The human immunodeficiency virus type 1 (HIV-1) Vif protein is located in the cytoplasm of infected cells and its effect on viral replication is equivalent in HIV-2. *AIDS Res. hum. Retroviruses*, 9, 1025–1030

Miles, S.A., Martinez-Maza, O., Rezai, A., Magpantay, L., Kishimoto, T., Nakamura, S., Radka, S.F. & Linsley, P.S. (1992) Oncostatin M as a potent mitogen for AIDS-Kaposi's sarcoma-derived cells. *Science*, 255, 32–430

Miller, G., Rigsby, M.O., Heston, L., Grogan, E., Sun, R., Metroka, C., Levy, J.A., Gao, S.-J., Chang, Y. & Moore, P. (1996) Antibodies to butyrate-inducible antigens of Kaposi's sarcoma-associated herpesvirus in patients with HIV-1 infection. *New Engl. J. Med.*, 334, 1292–1297

Ministério da Saúde (Brazilian Ministry of Health) (1993) *National Programme of Control of Sexually Transmitted Diseases/AIDS. AIDS Boletim Epidemiologico*, Vol. 6, Semane Epidemiológica (in Portuguese)

Ministry of Public Health (1994) *Trend of HIV Spreading from Sentinel Surveillance, June 1993, Thailand. Weekly Epidemiological Surveillance Report*, Bangkok, Division of Epidemiology

Mintz, L., Drew, W.L., Miner, R.C. & Braff, E.H. (1983) Cytomegalovirus infections in homosexual men. An epidemiological study. *Ann. intern. Med.*, 99, 326–329

Mittal, K., Neri, A., Feiner, H., Schinella, R. & Alfonso, F. (1990) Lymphomatoid granulomatosis in the acquired immunodeficiency syndrome. *Cancer*, 65, 1345–1349

Modlin, R.L., Hofman, F.M., Kempf, R.A., Taylor, C.R., Conant, M.A. & Rea, T.H. (1983a) Kaposi's sarcoma in homosexual men: an immunohistochemical study. *J. Am. Acad. Dermatol.*, 8, 620–627

Modlin, R.L., Meyer, P.R., Hofman, F.M., Mehlmauer, M., Levy, N.B., Lukes, R.J., Parker, J.W., Ammann, A.J., Conant, M.A., Rea, T.H. & Taylor, C.R. (1983b) T-lymphocyte subsets in lymph nodes from homosexual men. *J. Am. med. Assoc.*, 250, 1302–1305

Mølbak, K., Lauritzen, E., Fernandes, D., Böttiger, B. & Biberfeld, G. (1986) Antibodies to HTLV-IV associated with chronic, fatal illness resembling 'slim' disease (Letter to the Editor). *Lancet*, ii, 1214–1215

Monfardini, S., Vaccher, E., Pizzocaro, G., Stellini, R., Sinicco, A., Sabbatani, S., Marangolo, M., Zagni, R., Clerici, M., Foà, R. et al. (1989) Unusual malignant tumours in 49 patients with HIV infection. *AIDS*, 3, 449–452

Monfardini, S., Tirelli, U., Vaccher, E., Foà, R. & Gavosto, F. (1991) Hodgkin's disease in 63 intravenous drug users infected with human immunodeficiency virus. *Ann. Oncol.*, **2** (Suppl. 2), 201–205

Monini, P., de Lellis, L., Fabris, M., Rigolin, F. & Cassai, E. (1996) Kaposi's sarcoma-associated herpesvirus DNA sequences in prostate tissue and human semen. *New Engl. J. Med.*, **334**, 1168–1172

Montella, M., Franceschi, S., Geddes, M., Cocchiarella, G., Di Gennaro, F., Arniani, S., Balzi, D., Delfino, M. & Satriano, R.A. (1996) Classic Kaposi's sarcoma and volcanic soil in the south of Italy: a case–control study (Letter to the Editor). *Lancet*, **347**, 905

Montesano, R., Pepper, M.S., Mohle-Steinlein, U., Risau, W., Wagner, E.F. & Orci, L. (1990) Increased proteolytic activity is responsible for the aberrant morphogenetic behaviour of endothelial cells expressing the middle T oncogene. *Cell*, **62**, 435–455

Moore, J.P. & Nara, P.L. (1991) The role of the V3 loop of gp120 in HIV infection. *AIDS*, **5**, S21–S33

Moore, P.S. & Chang, Y. (1995) Detection of herpesvirus-like DNA sequences in Kaposi's sarcoma in patients with and without HIV infection. *New Engl. J. Med.*, **332**, 1181–1185

Moore, R.D., Kessler, H., Richman, D.D., Flexner, C. & Chaisson, R.E. (1991) Non-Hodgkin's lymphoma in patients with advanced HIV infection treated with zidovudine. *J. Am. med. Assoc.*, **265**, 2208–2211

Moore, J.P., Jameson, B.A., Weiss, R.A. & Sattentau, Q.J. (1993) The HIV-cell fusion reaction. In: Bentz, J., ed., *Viral Fusion Mechanisms*, Boca Raton, FL, CRC Press, pp. 233–289

Moore, J.S., Harrison, J.S. & Doll, L.S. (1994) Interventions for sexually active, heterosexual women in the United States. In: DiClemente, R.J. & Peterson, J.L., eds, *Preventing AIDS. Theories and Methods of Behavioral Interventions*, New York, Plenum Press, pp. 243–265

Moore, P.S., Gao, S.-J., Dominguez, G., Cesarman, E., Lungu, O., Knowles, D.M., Garber, R., Pellett, P.E., McGeoch D.J. & Chang Y. (1996) Primary characterization of a herpesvirus agent associated with Kaposi's sarcoma. *J. Virol.*, **70**, 549–558

Moran, C.A., Tuur, S., Angritt, P., Reid, A.H. & O'Leary T.J. (1992) Epstein-Barr virus in Hodgkin's disease from patients with human immunodeficiency virus infection. *Mod. Pathol.*, **5**, 85–88

Morgan, A.R., Miles, A.J. & Wastell, C. (1994) Anal warts and squamous carcinoma-*in-situ* of the anal canal. *J. R. Soc. Med.*, **87**, 15

Morgello, S. (1992) Epstein-Barr and human immunodeficiency viruses in acquired immunodeficiency syndrome-related primary central nervous system lymphoma. *Am. J. Pathol.*, **141**, 441–450

Morrow, W.J.W., Wharton, M., Lau, D. & Levy, J.A. (1987) Small animals are not susceptible to human immunodeficiency virus infection. *J. gen. Virol.*, **68**, 2253–2257

Morrow, W.J.W., Homsy, J., Eichberg, J.W., Krowka, J., Pan, L.-Z., Gaston, I., Legg, H., Lerche, N., Thomas, J. & Levy, J.A. (1989) Long-term observation of baboons, rhesus monkeys and chimpanzees inoculated with HIV and given periodic immunosuppressive treatment. *AIDS Res. hum. Retroviruses*, **5**, 233–245

Mosier, D.E., Gulizia, R.J., Baird, S.M., Spector, S., Spector, D., Kipps, T.J., Fox, R.I., Carson, D.A., Cooper, N., Richman, D.D. & Wilson, D.B. (1989) Studies of HIV infection and the development of Epstein–Barr virus-related B cell lymphomas following transfer of human lymphocytes to mice with severe combined immunodeficiency. *Curr. Topics Microbiol. Immunol.*, **152**, 195–199

Moss, G.B., Clemetson, D., D'Costa, L., Plummer, F.A., Ndinya-Achola, J.O., Reilly, M., Holmes, K.K., Piot, P., Maitha, G.M., Hillier, S.L., Kiviat, N.C., Cameron, C.W., Wamoler, I.A. & Kreiss, J.K. (1991) Association of cervical ectopy with heterosexual transmission of human immunodeficiency virus: results of a study of couples in Nairobi, Kenya. *J. infect. Dis.*, **164**, 588–591

Moulignier, A., Mikol, J., Pialoux, G., Eliaszewicz, M., Thurel C. & Thiebaut, J.-B. (1994) Cerebral glial tumors and human immunodeficiency virus-1 infection. *Cancer*, **74**, 686–692

Moyle, G., Hawkins, D.A. & Gazzard, B.G. (1991) Seminoma and HPV infections. *Int. J. STD AIDS*, **2**, 293–294

Mudryi, M., Hiebert, S.W. & Nevins, J.R. (1990) A role for the adenovirus inducible E2F transcription factor in a proliferation dependent signal transduction pathway. *EMBO J.*, **9**, 2179–2184

Mueller, N. (1996) Hodgkin's disease. In: Schottenfeld, D. & Fraumeni, J.S., Jr, *Cancer Epidemiology and Prevention*, 2nd Ed., New York, Oxford University Press (in press)

Mueller, B.U. & Pizzo, P.A. (1995) Cancer in children with primary or secondary immunodeficiencies. *J. Pediatr.*, **126**, 1–10

Mueller, B.U., Butler, K.M., Higham, M.C., Husson, R.N., Montrella, K.A., Pizzo, P.A., Feuerstein, I.M. & Manjunath, K. (1992) Smooth muscle tumors in children with human immunodeficiency virus infection. *Pediatrics*, **90**, 460–463

Müller, J.R., Janz, S., Goedert, J.J., Potter, M. & Rabkin, C.S. (1995) Persistence of immunoglobulin heavy chain/c-*myc* recombination-positive lymphocyte clones in the blood of human immunodeficiency virus-infected homosexual men. *Proc. natl Acad. Sci. USA*, **92**, 6577–6581

Münger, K., Werness, B.A., Dyson, N., Phelps, W.C., Harlow, E. & Howley, P.M. (1989) Complex formation of human papillomavirus E7 proteins with the retinoblastoma tumor suppressor gene product. *EMBO J.*, **8**, 4099–4105

Muñoz, A., Vlahov, D., Solomon, L., Margolick, J.B., Bareta, J.C., Cohn, S., Astemborski, J. & Nelson, K.E. (1992) Prognostic indicators for development of AIDS among intravenous drug users. *J. acquir. Immun. Defic. Syndr.*, **5**, 694–700

Muñoz, A., Schrager, L.K., Bacellar, H., Speizer, I., Vermund, S.H., Detels, R., Saah, A.J., Kingsley, L.A., Seminara, D. & Phair, J.P. (1993) Trends in the incidence of outcomes defining acquired immunodeficiency syndrome (AIDS) in the Multicenter AIDS Cohort Study: 1985–1991. *Am. J. Epidemiol.*, **137**, 423–438

Myers, G. (1993) Assimilating HIV sequences. *AIDS Res. Human Retroviruses*, **9**, 697–702

Myers, G., Korber, B., Berzofsky, J.A., Smith, R.F., Pavalkis, G.N. & Wain-Hobson, S. (1991) *Human Retroviruses and AIDS 1991*, Los Alamos, New Mexico, Los Alamos National Laboratory

Myers, G., Korber, B., Wain-Hobson, S., Smith, R.F. & Pavlakis, G.N. (1993) *Human retroviruses and AIDS*, Los Alamos, NMex, Los Alamos National Laboratory

Myers, G., Korber, B., Wain-Hobson, S., Jeang, K.T., Henderson, L.E. & Pavlakis, G.N. (1994) *Human Retroviruses and AIDS. A Compilation and Analysis of Nucleic Acid and Amino Acid Sequences*, Los Alamos, NMex, Los Alamos National Laboratory

Nadji, M., Morales, A.R., Ziegler-Weissman, J. & Penneys, N.S. (1981) Kaposi's sarcoma: immunohistological evidence for an endothelial origin. *Arch. Pathol. Lab. Med.*, **105**, 274–275

Nador, R.G., Cesarman, E., Knowles, D.M. & Said, J.W. (1995) Herpes-like DNA sequences in a body-cavity-based lymphoma in an HIV-negative patient (Letter to the Editor). *New Engl. J. Med.*, **333**, 943

Naidu, Y.M., Rosen, E.M., Zitnick, R., Goldberg, I., Park, M., Naujokas, M., Polverini, P.J. & Nickoloff, B.J. (1994) Role of scatter factor in the pathogenesis of AIDS-related Kaposi sarcoma. *Proc. natl. Acad. Sci. USA*, **91**, 5281–5285

Nair, B.C., DeVico, A.L., Nakamura, S., Copeland, T.D., Chen, Y., Patel, A., O'Neil, T., Oroszlan, S., Gallo, R.C. & Sarngadharan, M.G. (1992) Identification of a major growth factor for AIDS-Kaposi's sarcoma cells as oncostatin M. *Science*, **255**, 1430–1432

Nakahara, H., Moriya, Y., Shinkai, T. & Hirota, T. (1993) Small cell carcinoma of the anus in a human HIV carrier: report of a case. *Jpn. J. Surg.*, **23**, 85–88

Nakamura, S., Salahuddin, S.Z., Biberfeld, P., Ensoli, B., Markham, P.D., Wong-Staal, F. & Gallo, R.C. (1988) Kaposi's sarcoma cells: long-term culture with growth factor from retrovirus-infected $CD4^+$ T cells. *Science*, **242**, 426–430

Nakhlen, R.E., Manivel, J.C., Copenhaver, C.M., Sung, J.H. & Strickler, J.G. (1991) In situ hybridization for the detection of Epstein-Barr virus in central nervous system lymphomas. *Cancer*, **67**, 444–448

Nakshatri, H., Pater, M.M. & Pater, A. (1990) Ubiquitous and cell-type-specific protein interactions with human papillomavirus type 16 and type 18 enhancers. *Virology*, **178**, 92–103

Nasti, G., Santarossa, S., Vaccher, E., Serraino, D., Carbone, A. & Tirelli, U. (1994) Anal cancer in patients with HIV infection: a report of two cases without evidence of immunological dysfunction. *AIDS*, **8**, 1507–1508

Nauclér, A., Andreasson, P.-Å., Costa, C.M., Thorstensson, R. & Biberfeld, G. (1989) HIV-2-associated AIDS and HIV-2 seroprevalence in Bissau, Guinea-Bissau. *J. acquir. Immun. Defic. Syndr.*, **2**, 88–93

Nelson, J.A., Wiley, C.A., Reynolds-Kohler, C., Reese, C.E., Margaretten, W. & Levy, J.A. (1988) Human imunodeficiency virus detected in bowel epithelium from patients with gastrointestinal symptoms. *Lancet*, **i**, 259–262

Neri, A., Barriga, F., Inghirami, G., Knowles, D.M., Neequaye, J., Magrath, I.T. & Dalla-Favera, R. (1991) Epstein-Barr virus infection precedes clonal expansion in Burkitt's and acquired immunodeficiency syndrome-associated lymphoma. *Blood*, **77**, 1092–1095

Nevins, J.R. (1992) E2F: a link between the Rb tumor suppressor protein and viral oncoproteins. *Science*, **258**, 424–429

Newell, G.R., Adams, S.C., Mansell, P.W.A. & Hersh, E.M. (1984) Toxicity, immunosuppressive effects and carcinogenic potential of volatile nitrites: possible relationship to Kaposi's sarcoma. *Pharmacotherapy*, **4**, 284–291

Newton, R., Grulich, A., Beral, V., Sindikubwabo, B., Ngilimana, P.J., Nganyira, A. & Parkin, D.M. (1995) Cancer and HIV infection in Rwanda (Letter to the Editor). *Lancet*, **345**, 1378–1379

Newton, R., Ngilimana, P.-J., Grulich, A., Beral, V., Sindikubwabo, B., Nganyira, A. & Parkin, D.M. (1996) Cancer in Rwanda. *Int. J. Cancer*, **66**, 75–81

Ng, V.L., Hurt, M.H., Fein, C.L., Khayam-Bashi, F., Marsh, J., Nunes, W.M., McPhaul, L.W., Feigal, E., Nelson, P., Herndier, B.G., Shiramizu, B., Reyes, G.R., Fry, K.E. & McGrath, M.S. (1994) IgMs produced by two acquired immune deficiency syndrome lymphoma cell lines: Ig binding specificity and V_h — gene putative somatic mutation analysis. *Blood*, **83**, 1067–1078

Ng, V.L., Komanduri, K.V., Luce, J.A., Herndier, B.G. & McGrath, M.S. (1995) Clinical and laboratory features of HIV-associated body cavity based lymphomas (Abstract no. 1506), *Blood*, **86**, 379a

Ngendahayo, P., Mets, T., Bugingo, G. & Parkin, D.M. (1989) Kaposi's sarcoma in Rwanda: clinicopathological and epidemiological features. *Bull. Cancer*, **76**, 383–394 (in French)

Nickoloff, B.J. & Griffiths, C.E.M. (1989) Factor XIIIa-expressing dermal dendrocytes in AIDS-associated cutaneous Kaposi's sarcoma. *Science*, **243**, 1736–1737

Nickoloff, B.J., Huang, Y.Q., Li, J.J. & Friedman-Kien, A.E. (1992) Immunohistochemical detection of papillomavirus antigens in Kaposi's sarcoma (Letter to the Editor). *Lancet*, **339**, 548–549

Nicolosi, A., Leite, M.L.C., Musicco, M., Arici, C., Gavazzeni, G., Lazzarin, A. for the Italian Study Group on HIV Heterosexual Transmission (1994a) The efficiency of male-to-female and female-to-male sexual transmission of the human immunodeficiency virus: a study of 730 stable couples. *Epidemiology*, **5**, 570–575

Nicolosi, A., Musicco, M., Saracco, A. & Lazzarin, A. for the Italian Study Group on HIV Heterosexual Transmission (1994b) Risk factors for woman-to-man sexual transmission of the human immunodeficiency virus. *J. acquir. Immun. Defic. Syndr.*, **7**, 296–300

Niedobitek, G., Agathanggelou, A., Rowe, M., Jones, E.L., Jones, D.B., Turyaguma, P., Oryema, J., Wright, D.H. & Young, L.S. (1995) Heterogeneous expression of Epstein-Barr virus latent proteins in endemic Burkitt's lymphoma. *Blood*, **86**, 659–665

Nkowane, B.M. (1991) Prevalence and incidence of HIV infection in Africa: a review of data published in 1990. *AIDS*, **5** (Suppl. 1), S7–S15

Northfelt, D.W. & Palefsky, J.M. (1992) Human papillomavirus-associated anogenital neoplasia in persons with HIV infection. *AIDS clin. Rev.*, **??**, 241–259

N'tita, I., Mulanga, K., Dulat, C., Lusamba, D., Rehle, T., Korte, R. & Jäger, H. (1991) Risk of transfusion-associated HIV transmission in Kinshasa, Zaire. *AIDS*, **5**, 437–439

O'Brien, W.A., Hartigan, P.M., Martin, D., Esinhart, J., Hill, A., Benoit, S., Rubin, M., Simberkoff, M.S., Hamilton, J.D. & the Veterans Affairs Cooperative Study Group on AIDS (1996) Changes in plasma HIV-1 RNA and $CD4^+$ lymphocyte counts and the risk of progression to AIDS. *New Engl. J. Med.*, **334**, 426–431

O'Connor, T.P., Tonelli, Q.J. & Scarlett, J.M. (1991) Report of the National FeLV/FIV Awareness Project. *J. Am. vet. Med. Assoc.* **199**, 1348–1353

Odehouri, K., De Cock, K.M., Krebs, J.W., Moreau, J., Rayfield, M., McCormick, J.B., Schochetman, G., Bretton, R., Bretton, G., Ouattara, D., Heroin, P., Kanga, J.-M., Beda, B., Niamkey, E., Kadio, A., Gariepe, E. & Heyward, W.L. (1989) HIV-1 and HIV-2 infection associated with AIDS in Abidjan, Côte d'Ivoire. *AIDS*, **3**, 509–512

Oettlé, A.G. (1962) Geographical and racial differences in the frequency of Kaposi's sarcoma as evidence of environmental or genetic causes. *Acta unio. int. contra cancrum*, **18**, 330–363

Office of Technology Assessment (1995) *The Effectiveness of AIDS Prevention Efforts* (OTA Background Paper OTA-BP-H-172), Washington, DC, Congress of the United States

Oksenhendler E., Duarte M., Soulier J., Cacoub P., Welker Y., Cadranel J., Cazals-Hatem D., Autran B., Clauvel J.-P. & Raphael, M. (1996) Multicentric Castleman's disease in HIV infection: a clinical and pathological study of 20 patients. *AIDS*, **10**, 61–67

O'Reilly, K., Gerbase, A., Mertens, T. & Islam, M. (1995) Impact of improved treatment of sexually transmitted disease on HIV infection (Letter to the Editor). *Lancet*, **346**, 1157–1160

Orlow, S.J., Kamino, H. & Lawrence, R.L. (1992) Multiple subcutaneous leiomyosarcomas in an adolescent with AIDS. *Am. J. pediatr. Hematol. Oncol.*, **14**, 265–268

Orlow, S.J., Cooper, D., Petrea, S., Kamino, H., Popescu, V., Lawrence, R. & Leibovitz, E. (1993) AIDS-associated Kaposi's sarcoma in Romanian children. *J. Am. Acad. Dermatol.*, **28**, 449–453

Ottolenghi, F., Andreassi, L., Sbano, E. & Baiocchi, R. (1974) In-vitro culture of Kaposi's disease cells. *Arch. Dermatol. Forsch.*, **250**, 389–393

Otu, A.A. (1986) Kaposi's sarcoma and HTLV-III: a study in Nigerian adult males. *J. R. Soc. Med.*, **79**, 510–514

Ou, C.-Y., Takebe, Y., Luo, C.-C., Kalish, M., Auwanit, W., Bandea, C., de la Torre, N., Moore, J.L., Schochetman, G., Yamazaki, S., Gayle, H.D., Young, N.L. & Weniger, B.G. (1992) Wide distribution of two subtypes of HIV-1 in Thailand. *AIDS Res. hum. Retroviruses*, **8**, 1471–1472

Ou, C.-Y., Takebe, Y., Weniger, B.G., Luo, C.-C., Kalish, M.L., Auwanit, W., Yamazaki, S., Gayle, H.D., Young, N.L. & Schochetman, G. (1993) Independent introduction of two major HIV-1 genotypes into distinct high-risk populations in Thailand. *Lancet*, **341**, 1171–1174; **342**, 250

Padian, N.S. (1988) Prostitute women and AIDS: epidemiology. *AIDS*, **2**, 413–419

Page-Bodkin, K., Tappero, J., Samuel, M. & Winkelstein, W. (1992) Kaposi's sarcoma and faecal-oral exposure (Letter to the Editor). *Lancet*, **339**, 1490

Palasanthiran, P., Ziegler, J.B., Dwyer, D.E., Robertson, P., Leigh, D. & Cunningham, A.L. (1994) Early detection of human immunodeficiency virus type 1 infection in Australian infants at risk of perinatal infection and factors affecting transmission. *Pediatr. infect. Dis. J.*, **13**, 1083–1090

Palefsky, J.M. (1991) Human papillomavirus-associated anogenital neoplasia and other solid tumors in human immunodeficiency virus-infected individuals. *Curr. Opin. Oncol.*, **3**, 881–885

Palefsky, J.M. (1994) Anal human papillomavirus infection and anal cancer in HIV-positive individuals: an emerging problem. *AIDS*, **8**, 283–295

Palefsky, J.M., Gonzales, J., Greenblatt, R.M., Ahn, D.K. & Hollander, H. (1990) Anal intraepithelial neoplasia and anal papillomavirus infection among homosexual males with group IV HIV disease. *J. Am. med. Assoc.*, **263**, 2911–2916

Palefsky, J.M., Holly, E.A., Gonzales, J., Lamborn, K. & Hollander, H. (1992) Natural history of anal cytologic abnormalities and papillomavirus infection among homosexual men with group IV HIV disease. *J. acquir. Immun. Defic. Syndr.*, **5**, 1258–1265

Palefsky, J.M., Shiboski, S. & Moss, A. (1994) Risk factors for anal human papillomavirus infection and anal cytologic abnormalities in HIV-positive and HIV-negative homosexual men. *J. acquir. Immun. Defic. Syndr.*, **7**, 599–606

Pantaleo, G. & Fauci, A.S. (1995) New concepts in the immunopathogenesis of HIV infection. *Annu. Rev. Immunol.*, **13**, 487–512

Pantaleo, G., Graziosi, C., Demarest, J.F., Butini, L., Montroni, M., Fox, C.H., Orenstein, J.M., Kotler, D.P. & Fauci, A.S. (1993a) HIV infection is active and progressive in lymphoid tissue during the clinically latent stage of disease. *Nature*, **362**, 355–358

Pantaleo, G., Graziosi, C. & Fauci, A.S. (1993b) The role of lymphoid organs in the pathogenesis of HIV infection. *Sem. Immunol.*, **5**, 157–163

Pantaleo, G., Menzo, S., Vaccarezza, M., Graziosi, C., Cohen, O.J., Demarest, J.F., Montefiori, D., Orenstein, J.M., Fox, C., Schrager, L.K., Margolick, J.B., Buchbinder, S., Giorgi, J.V. & Fauci, A.S. (1995) Studies in subjects with long-term nonprogressive human immunodeficiency virus infection. *New Engl. J. Med.*, **332**, 209–216

Papadopoulos, E.B., Ladanyi, M., Emanuel, D., Mackinnon, S., Boulad, F., Carabasi, M.H., Castro-Malaspina, H., Childs, B.H., Gillio, A.P., Small, T.N., Young, J.W., Kernan, N.A. & O'Reilly, R.J. (1994) Infusions of donor leukocytes to treat Epstein–Barr virus-associated lymphoproliferative disorders after allogeneic bone marrow transplantation. *New Engl. J. Med.*, **330**, 1185–1191

Papasteriades, C., Kaloterakis, A., Filiotou, A., Economidou, J., Nicolis, G., Trichopoulos, D. & Stratigos, J. (1984) Histocompatibility antigens HLA-A, -B, -DR in Greek patients with Kaposi's sarcoma. *Tissu. Anti.*, **24**, 313–315

Parkin, D.M., Muir, C.S., Whelan, S.L., Gao, Y.T., Ferlay, J. & Powell, J., eds (1992) *Cancer Incidence in Five Continents*, Vol. VI (IARC Scientific Publications No. 120), Lyon, IARC

Pastore, C., Gloghini, A., Volpe, G., Nomdedeu, J., Leonardo, E., Mazza, U., Saglio, G., Carbone, A. & Gaidano, G. (1995) Distribution of Kaposi's sarcoma herpesvirus sequences among lymphoid malignancies in Italy and Spain. *Br. J. Haematol.*, **91**, 918–920

Pastore, C., Carbone, A., Gloghini, A., Volpe, G., Saglio, G. & Gaidano, G. (1996) Association of 6q deletions with AIDS-related diffuse large cell lymphoma. *Leukemia* (in press)

Patil, P., Elem, B. & Zumla, A. (1995) Pattern of adult malignancies in Zambia (1980–1989) in light of the human immunodeficiency virus type 1 epidemic. *J. trop. Med. Hyg.*, **98**, 281–284

Patrascu, I.V. & Dumitrescu, O. (1993) The epidemic of human immunodeficiency virus infection in Romanian children. *AIDS Res. hum. Retroviruses*, **9**, 99–104

Peckham, C. & Gibb, D. (1995) Mother-to-child transmission of the human immunodeficiency virus. *New Engl. J. Med.*, **333**, 298–302

Pedersen, N.C. & Barlough, J.E. (1991) Clinical overview of feline immunodeficiency virus. *J. Am. vet. Med. Assoc.*, **199**, 1298–1305

Pedersen, N.C., Ho, E.W., Brown, M.L. & Yamamoto, J.K. (1987) Isolation of a T-lymphotropic virus from domestic cats with an immunodeficiency-like syndrome. *Science*, **235**, 790–793

Pedersen, C., Barton, S.E., Chiesi, A., Skinhøj, P., Katlama, C., Johnson, A., van Lunzen, J., Hirschel, B., Maayan, S., Lundgren, J.D. & the AIDS in Europe Study Group (1995) HIV-related non-Hodgkin's lymphoma among European AIDS patients. *Eur. J. Haematol.*, **55**, 245–250

Peeters, M., Honore, C., Huet, T., Bedjaba, L., Ossari, S., Bussi, P., Cooper, R.W. & Delaporte, E. (1989) Isolation and partial characterization of an HIV-related virus occurring naturally in chimpanzees, in Gabon. *AIDS*, **3**, 625–630

Pelicci, P.-G., Knowles, D.M., II, Arlin, Z.A., Wieczorek, R., Luciw, P., Dina, D., Basilico, C. & Dalla-Favera, R. (1986) Multiple monoclonal B-cell expansions and *c-myc* oncogene rearrangements in acquired immune deficiency syndrome-related lymphoproliferative disorders. Implications for lymphomagenesis. *J. exp. Med.*, **164**, 2049–2060

Penn, I. (1983) Kaposi's sarcoma in immunosuppressed patients. *J. clin. Lab. Immunol.*, **12**, 1–10

Penn, I. (1988a) Secondary neoplasms as a consequence of transplantation and cancer therapy. *Cancer Detect. Prev.*, **12**, 39–57

Penn, I. (1988b) Tumors of the immunocompromised patient. *Ann. Rev. Med.*, **39**, 63–73

Penn, I. (1993) Neoplastic complications of transplantation. *Sem. resp. Infect.*, **8**, 233–239

Penn, I. (1994) De novo malignancy in pediatric organ transplant recipients. *J. pediatr. Surg.*, **29**, 221–228

Penn, I. & Porat, G. (1995) Central nervous system lymphomas in organ allograft recipients. *Transplantation*, **59**, 240–244

Pepin, J., Morgan, G., Dunn, D., Gevao, S., Mendy, M., Gaye, I., Scollen, N., Tedder, R. & Whittle, H. (1991) HIV-2-induced immunosuppression among asymptomatic West African prostitutes: evidence that HIV-2 is pathogenic, but less so than HIV-1. *AIDS*, **5**, 1165–1172

Peterlin, B.M. (1995) Molecular biology of HIV. In: Levy, J.A., ed., *The Retroviridae*, Vol. 4, New York, Plenum Press, pp. 185–238

Peterman, T.A., Jaffe, H.W. & Beral, V. (1993) Epidemiologic clues to the etiology of Kaposi's sarcoma. *AIDS*, **7**, 605–611

Peters, B.S., Beck, E.J., Coleman, D.G., Wadsworth, M.J.H., McGuinness, O., Harris, J.R.W. & Pinching, A.J. (1991) Changing disease patterns in patients with AIDS in a referral centre in the United Kingdom: the changing face of AIDS. *Br. med. J.*, **302**, 203–207

Petersen, L.R., Satten, G.A., Dodd, R., Busch, M., Kleinman, S., Grindon, A., Lenes, B. & the HIV Seroconversion Study Group (1994) Duration of time from onset of human immunodeficiency virus type 1 infectiousness to development of detectable antibody. *Transfusion*, **34**, 283–289

Phelps, W.C. & Howley, P.M. (1987) Transcriptional *trans*-activation by the human papillomavirus type 16 E2 gene product. *J. Virol.*, **61**, 1630–1638

Phelps, W.C., Yee, C.L., Münger, K. & Howley, P.M. (1988) The human papillomavirus type 16 E7 gene encodes transactivation and transformation functions similar to those of adenovirus E1A. *Cell*, **53**, 539–547

Philippon, V., Vellutini, C., Gambarelli, D., Harkiss, G., Arbuthnott, G., Metzger, D., Roubin, R. & Filippi, P. (1994) The basic domain of the lentivirus Tat protein is responsible for damages in mouse brain: involvement of cytokines. *Virology*, **205**, 519–529

Phillips, A., Lee, C.A., Elford, J., Janossy, G., Bofill, M., Timms, A. & Kernoff, P.B.A. (1989) Prediction of progression to AIDS by analysis of CD4 lymphocyte counts in a haemophilic cohort. *AIDS*, **3**, 737–741

Phillips, A.N., Lee, C.A., Elford, J., Janossy, G., Timms, A., Bofill, M. & Kernoff, P.B.A. (1991) Serial CD4 lymphocyte counts and development of AIDS. *Lancet*, **337**, 389–392

Phillips, A.N., Pezzotti, P., Cozzi Lepri, A., Rezza, G. & the Italian Seroconversion Study (1994a) CD4 lymphocyte count as a determinant of the time from HIV seroconversion to AIDS and death from AIDS: evidence from the Italian Seroconversion Study. *AIDS*, **8**, 1299–1305

Phillips, D.M., Zacharopoulos, V.R., Tan, X. & Pearce-Pratt, R. (1994b) Mechanisms of sexual transmission of HIV: does HIV infect intact epithelia? *Trends Microbiol.*, **2**, 454–458

PHLS (Public Health Laboratory Service) Communicable Diseases Surveillance Centre (1993) Unlinked anonymous monitoring of HIV prevalence in England and Wales: 1990–92. *CDR Rev.*, **3**, R1–R11

Piatak, M., Jr, Saag, M.S., Yang, L.C., Clark, S.J., Kappes, J.C., Luk, K.-C., Hahn, B.H., Shaw, G.M. & Lifson, J.D. (1993) High levels of HIV-1 in plasma during all stages of infection determined by competitive PCR. *Science*, **259**, 1749–1754

Piot, P., Quinn, T.C., Taelman, H., Feinsod, F.M., Minlangu, K.B., Wobin, O., Mbendi, N., Mazebo, P., Ndangi, K., Stevens, W., Kalambayi, K., Mitchell, S., Bridts, C. & McCormick, J.B. (1984) Acquired immunodeficiency syndrome in a heterosexual population in Zaire. *Lancet*, **ii**, 65–69

Pirisi, L., Yasumoto, S., Feller, M., Doniger, J. & DiPaolo, J.A. (1987) Transformation of human fibroblasts and keratinocytes with human papillomavirus type 16 DNA. *J. Virol.*, **61**, 1061–1066

Pitchenik, A.E. (1990) Tuberculosis control and the AIDS epidemic in developing countries. *Ann. intern. Med.*, **113**, 89–91

Pluda, J.M., Yarchoan, R., Jaffe, E.S., Feuerstein, I.M., Solomon, D., Steinberg, S.M., Wyvill, K.M., Raubitschek, A., Katz, D. & Broder, S. (1990) Development of non-Hodgkin lymphoma in a cohort of patients with severe human immunodeficiency virus (HIV) infection on long-term antiretroviral therapy. *Ann. intern. Med.*, **113**, 276–282

Pluda, J.M., Venzon, D.J., Tosato, G., Lietzau, J., Wyvill, K., Nelson, D.L., Jaffe, E.S., Karp, J.E., Broder, S. & Yarchoan, R. (1993) Parameters affecting the development of non-Hodgkin's lymphoma in patients with severe human immunodeficiency virus infection receiving antiretroviral therapy. *J. clin. Oncol.*, **11**, 1099–1107

Plummer, F.A., Simonsen, J.N., Cameron, D.W., Ndinya-Achola, J.O., Kreiss, J.K., Gakinya, M.N., Waiyaki, P., Cheang, M., Piot, P., Ronald, A.R. & Ngugi, E.N. (1991) Cofactors in male-female sex transmission of human immunodeficiency virus type 1. *J. infect. Dis.*, **163**, 233–239

Poli, A., Abramo, F., Baldinotti, F., Pistello, M., Da Prato, L. & Bendinelli, M. (1994) Malignant lymphoma associated with experimentally induced feline immunodeficiency virus infection. *J. comp. Pathol.*, **110**, 319–328

Polito, P., Cilia, A.M., Gloghini, A., Cozzi, M., Perin, T., De Paoli, P., Gaidano, G. & Carbone, A. (1995) High frequency of EBV association with non-random abnormalities of the chromosome region 1q21-25 in AIDS-related Burkitt's lymphoma-derived cell lines. *Int. J. Cancer*, **61**, 370–374

Pollack, M.S., Safai, B., Myskowski, P.L., Gold, J.W.M., Pandey, J. & Dupont, B. (1983a) Frequencies of HLA and Gm immunogenetic markers in Kaposi's sarcoma. *Tissue Antigens*, **21**, 1–8

Pollack, M.S., Safai, B. & Dupont, B. (1983b) HLA-DR5 and DR2 are susceptibility factors for acquired immunodeficiency syndrome with Kaposi's sarcoma in different ethnic subpopulations. *Dis. Markers*, **1**, 135–139

Pope, M., Betjes, M.G.H., Romani, N., Hirmand, H., Cameron, P.U., Hoffman, L., Gezelter, S., Schuler, G. & Steinman, R.M. (1994) Conjugates of dendritic cells and memory of T lymphocytes from skin facilitate productive infection with HIV-1. *Cell*, **78**, 389–398

Potterat, J.J., Spencer, N.E., Woodhouse, D.E. & Muth, J.B. (1989) Partner notification in the control of human immunodeficiency virus infection. *Am. J. public Health*, **79**, 874–876

Potts, K.E., Kalish, M.L., Lott, T., Orloff, G., Luo, C.C., Bernard, M.A., Alves, C.B., Badaro, R., Suleiman, J., Ferreira, O. et al. (1993) Genetic heterogeneity of the V3 region of the HIV-1 envelope glycoprotein in Brazil. *AIDS*, **7**, 1191–1197

Poulsen, A.-G., Kvinesdal, B., Aaby, P., Mølbak, K., Frederiksen, K., Dias, F. & Lauritzen, E. (1989) Prevalence of and mortality from human immunodeficiency virus type 2 in Bissau, West Africa. *Lancet*, **i**, 827–831

Prévot, S., Néris, J. & de Saint Maur, P.P. (1994) Detection of Epstein Barr virus in an hepatic leiomyomatous neoplasm in an adult human immunodeficiency virus 1-infected patient. *Virchows Arch.*, **425**, 321–325

Prince, H.E., Schroff, R.W., Ayoub, G., Han, S., Gottlieb, M.S. & Fahey, J.L. (1984) HLA studies in acquired immune deficiency syndrome patients with Kaposi's sarcoma. *J. clin. Immunol.*, **4**, 242–245

Putkonen, P., Böttiger, B., Warstedt, K., Thorstensson, R., Albert, J. & Biberfeld, G. (1989) Experimental infection of cynomolgus monkeys (*Macaca fascicularis*) with HIV-2. *J. acquir. Immun. Defic. Syndr.*, **2**, 366–373

Quinn, T.C., Mann, J.M., Curran, J.W. & Piot, P. (1986) AIDS in Africa: an epidemiologic paradigm. *Science*, **234**, 955–963

Qunibi, W., Akhtar, M., Sheth, K., Ginn, H.E., Al Furayh, O., DeVol, E.B. & Taher, S. (1988) Kaposi's sarcoma: the most common tumor after renal transplantation in Saudi Arabia. *Am. J. Med.*, **84**, 225–232

Qunibi, W.Y., Barri, Y., Alfurayh, O., Almeshari, K., Khan, B., Taher, S. & Sheth, K. (1993) Kaposi's sarcoma in renal transplant recipients: a report on 26 cases from a single institution. *Transplant. Proc.*, **25**, 1402–1405

Rabaud, C., Dorvaux, V., May, T., Paitel, J.F., Witz, B., Lederlin, P. & Canton, P. (1995) Acute myelogenous leukaemia followed by non-Hodgkin's lymphoma in a patient with AIDS. *J. Infect.*, **31**, 69–70

Rabkin, C.S. (1994) Epidemiology of AIDS-related malignancies. *Curr. Opin. Oncol.*, **6**, 492–496

Rabkin, C.S. & Blattner, W.A. (1991) HIV infection and cancers other than non-Hodgkin lymphoma and Kaposi's sarcoma. *Cancer Surv.*, **10**, 151–160

Rabkin, C.S. & Yellin, F. (1994) Cancer incidence in a population with a high prevalence of infection with human immunodeficiency virus type 1. *J. natl Cancer Inst.*, **86**, 1711–1716

Rabkin, C.S., Biggar, R.J. & Horm, J.W. (1991) Increasing incidence of cancers associated with the human immunodeficiency virus epidemic. *Int. J. Cancer*, **47**, 692–696

Rabkin, C.S., Hilgartner, M.W., Hedberg, K.W., Aledort, L.M., Hatzakis, A., Eichinger, S., Eyster, M.E., White, G.C., II, Kessler, C.M., Lederman, M.M., de Moerloose, P., Bray, G.L., Cohen, A.R., Andes, W.A., Manco-Johnson, M., Schramm, W., Kroner, B.L., Blattner, W.A. & Goedert, J.J. (1992) Incidence of lymphomas and other cancers in HIV-infected and HIV-uninfected patients with hemophilia. *J. Am. med. Assoc.*, **267**, 1090–1094

Rabkin, C.S., Biggar, R.J., Baptiste, M.S., Abe, T., Kohler, B.A. & Nasca, P.C. (1993a) Cancer incidence trends in women at high risk of human immunodeficiency virus (HIV) infection. *Int. J. Cancer*, **55**, 208–212

Rabkin, C.S., Devesa, S.S., Zahm, S.H. & Gail, M.H. (1993b) Increasing incidence of non-Hodgkin's lymphoma. *Semin. Hematol.*, **30**, 286–296

Rabkin, C.S., Wilson, S.E. & Goedert, J.J. (1993c) Changes in risks of opportunistic infections and cancer with CD4 lymphopenia in the therapy era (Abstract No. PO-C04-2663). *Int. Conf. AIDS*, **9**, 661

Rabkin, C.S., Chibwe, G., Muyunda, K. & Musaba, E. (1995a) Kaposi's sarcoma in pregnant women (Letter to the Editor). *Nature*, **377**, 21–22

Rabkin, C.S., Bedi, G., Musaba, E., Sunkutu, R., Mwansa, N., Sidransky, D. & Biggar, R.J. (1995b) AIDS-related Kaposi's sarcoma is a clonal neoplasm. *Clin. Cancer Res.*, **1**, 257–260

Radin, D.R. & Kiyabu, M. (1992) Multiple smooth-muscle tumors of the colon and adrenal gland in an adult with AIDS. *Am. J. Roentgenol.*, **159**, 545–546

Rady, P.L., Yen, A., Rollefson, J.L., Orengo, I., Bruce, S., Hughes, T.K. & Tyring, S.K. (1995) Herpesvirus-like DNA sequences in non-Kaposi's sarcoma skin lesions of transplant patients. *Lancet*, **345**, 1339–1340

Ragni, M.V., Belle, S.H., Jaffe R.A., Duerstein, S.L., Bass, D.C, McMillan, C.W., Lovrien, E.W., Aledort, L.M., Kisker, C.T., Stabler, S.P., Hoots, W.K., Hilgarther, M.W., Cox-Gill, J., Buchanan, G.R., Sanders, N.L., Brettler, D.B., Barron, L.E., Goldsmith, J.C., Ewenstein, B., Smith, K.J., Green, D., Addiego, J.E. & Kingsley, L.A. (1993) Acquired immuno-deficiency syndrome-associated non-Hodgkin's lymphomas and other malignancies in patients with hemophilia. *Blood*, **81**, 1889–1897

Rakowicz-Szulczynska, E.M., McIntosh, D.G., Morris, P. & Smith, M.L. (1994) Novel family of gynaecological cancer antigens detected by anti-HIV antibody. *Infect. Dis. Obstet. Gynecol.*, **2**, 171–178

Rakowicz-Szulczynska, E.M., McIntosh, D.G., Perry, M.J. & Smith, M.L. (1995) Mechanisms of cancer growth promotion by HIV-1 neutralizing antibodies. *Cancer J.*, **8**, 143–149

Ramsay, A.D., Giddings, J., Baskerville, A. & Cranage, M.P. (1991) Phenotypic analysis of malignant lymphoma in simian immunodeficiency virus infection using anti-human anti-bodies. *J. Pathol.*, **164**, 321–328

Ranki, A., Valle, S.-L., Krohn, M., Antonen, J., Allain, J.-P., Leuther, M., Franchini, G. & Krohn, K. (1987) Long latency precedes overt seroconversion in sexually transmitted human immunodeficiency-virus infection. *Lancet*, **ii**, 589–593

Raphael, M., Gentilhomme, O., Tulliez, M., Byron, P.-A. & Diebold, J., for the French Study Group of Pathology for Human Immunodeficiency Virus-Associated Tumors (1991) Histopathologic features of high-grade non-Hodgkin's lymphomas in acquired immuno-deficiency syndrome. *Arch. Pathol. Lab. Med.*, **115**, 15–20

Raphael, M.M., Audouin, J., Lamine, M., Delecluse, H.J., Vuillaume, M., Lenoir, G.M., Gisselbrecht, C., Lennert, K. & Diebold, J. (1994) Immunophenotypic and genotypic analysis of acquired immunodeficiency syndrome-related non-Hodgkin's lymphomas. Correlation with histologic features in 36 cases. French Study Group of Pathology for HIV-Associated Tumors. *Am. J. clin. Pathol.*, **101**, 773–782

Rappersberger, K., Tschachler, E., Zonzits, E., Gillitzer, R., Hatzakis, A., Kaloterakis, A., Mann, D.L., Popow-Kraupp, T., Biggar, R.J., Berger, R. et al. (1991) Endemic Kaposi's sarcoma in human immunodeficicency virus type I-seronegative persons: demonstration of retrovirus-like particles in cutaneous lesions. *J. invest. Dermatol.*, **95**, 371–381

Read, E.J., Orenstein, J.M., Chorba, T.L., Schwartz, A.M., Simon, G.L., Lewis, J.H. & Schulof, R.S. (1985) Listeria monocytogenes sepsis and small cell carcinoma of the rectum: an unusual presentation of the acquired immunodeficiency syndrome. *Am. J. clin. Pathol.*, **83**, 385–389

Ree, H.J., Strauchen, J.A., Khan, A.A., Gold, J.E., Crowley, J.P., Kahn, H. & Zalusky, R. (1991) Human immunodeficiency virus-associated Hodgkin's disease. Clinicopathologic studies of 24 cases and preponderance of mixed cellularity type characterized by the occurrence of fibrohistiocytoid stromal cells. *Cancer*, **67**, 1614–1621

Regezi, J.A., McPhail, L.A., Daniels, T.E., Greenspan, J.S., Greenspan, D., Dodd, C.L., Lozada-Nur, F., Heinic, G.S., Chinn, H., Silverman, S., Jr & Hansen, L.S. (1993) Oral Kaposi's sarcoma: a 10-year retrospective histopathologic study. *J. oral Pathol. Med.*, **22**, 292–297

Reitz, B.A., Burton, N.A., Jamieson, S.W., Bieber, C.P., Pennock, J.L., Stinson, E.B. & Shumway, N.E. (1980) Heart and lung transplantation: autotransplantation and allotransplantation in primates with extended survival. *J. thor. cardiovasc. Surg.*, **80**, 360–372

Remick, S.C., Diamond, C., Migliozzi, J.A., Solis, O., Wagner, H., Haase, R.F. & Ruckdeschel, J.C. (1990) Primary central nervous system lymphoma in patients with and without the acquired immune deficiency syndrome. A retrospective analysis and review of the literature. *Medicine*, **69**, 345–360

Remick, S.C., Boguniewicz, A. & Wolf, B. (1993) Solid tumors in HIV-infected patients other than AIDS-defining neoplasms. In: Friedman, H., Klein, T.W. & Specter, S., eds, *Drugs of Abuse, Immunity and AIDS*, New York, Plenum Press, pp. 219–224

Remis, R.S. & Sutherland, W.D. (1993) The epidemiology of HIV and AIDS in Canada: current perspectives and future needs. *Can. J. public Health*, **84** (Suppl. 1), S34–S38

Renzullo, P.O., McNeil, J.G., Gardner, L.I. & Brundage, J.F. (1991) Inpatient morbidity among HIV-infected male soldiers prior to their diagnosis of HIV infection. *Am. J. public Health*, **81**, 1280–1284

Reynolds, P., Layefsky, M.E., Saunders, L.D., Lemp, G.F. & Payne, S.F. (1990) Kaposi's sarcoma reporting in San Francisco: a comparison of AIDS and cancer surveillance systems. *J. acquir. Immun. Defic. Syndr.*, **3** (Suppl. 1), S8–S13

Reynolds, P., Saunders, L.D., Layefsky, M.E. & Lemp, G.F. (1993) The spectrum of acquired immunodeficiency syndrome (AIDS)-associated malignancies in San Francisco, 1980–1987. *Am. J. Epidemiol.*, **137**, 19–30

Rezikyan, S., Kaaya, E.E., Ekman, M., Voevodin, A.F., Feichtinger, H., Putkonen, P., Castaños-Velez, E., Biberfeld, G. & Biberfeld, P. (1995) B-cell lymphomagenesis in SIV-immunosuppressed cynomolgus monkeys. *Int. J. Cancer*, **61**, 574–579

Riboldi, P., Gaidano, G., Schettino, E.W., Steger, T.G., Knowles, D.M., Dalla-Favera, R. & Casali, P. (1994) Two acquired immunodeficiency syndrome-associated Burkitt's lymphomas produce specific anti-i IgM cold agglutinins using somatically mutated V_h 4-21 segments. *Blood*, **83**, 2952–2961

Ricard, D., Wilkins, A., N'Gum, P.T., Hayes, R., Morgan, G., Da Silva, A.P. & Whittle, H. (1994) The effects of HIV-2 infection in a rural area of Guinea-Bissau. *AIDS*, **8**, 977–982

Ricchetti, M. & Buc, H. (1990) Reverse transcriptases and genomic variability: the accuracy of DNA replication is enzyme specific and sequence dependent. *EMBO J.*, **9**, 1583–1593

Rickinson, A.B., Young, L.S. & Rowe, M. (1987) Influence of Epstein–Barr nuclear antigen 2 on the growth phenotype of virus-transformed B-cells. *J. Virol.*, **61**, 1310–1317

Rickinson, A.B., Murray, R.J., Brooks, J., Griffin, H., Moss, D.J. & Masucci, M.G. (1992) T cell recognition of Epstein–Barr virus associated lymphomas. *Cancer Surv.*, **13**, 53–80

Rideout, B.A., Lowenstine, L.J., Hutson, C.A., Moore, P.F. & Pedersen, N.C. (1992) Characterization of morphologic changes and lymphocyte subset distribution in lymph nodes from cats with naturally acquired feline immunodeficiency virus infection. *Vet. Pathol.*, **29**, 391–399

Rieckmann, P., Poli, G., Fox, C.H., Kehrl, J.H. & Fauci, A.S. (1991) Recombinant gp120 specifically enhances TNFα production and Ig secretion in B lymphocytes from HIV-infected individuals but not from seronegative donors. *J. Immunol.*, **147**, 2922–2927

Rinaldi, M.G. (1996) Epidemiology of mycoses in the HIV-infected patient — clinical aspects. *Int. J. antimicrob. Agents*, **6**, 131–134

Riou, G., Favre, M., Jeannel, D., Bourhis, J., Le Doussal, V. & Orth, G. (1990) Association between poor prognosis in early-stage invasive cervical carcinomas and non-detection of HPV DNA. *Lancet*, **335**, 1171–1174

Robertson, D.L., Hahn, B.H. & Sharp, P.M. (1995) Recombination in AIDS viruses. *J. mol. Evol.*, **40**, 249–259

Rogel, M.E., Wu, L.I. & Emerman, M. (1995) The human immunodeficiency virus type 1 *vpr* gene prevents cell proliferation during chronic infection. *J. Virol.*, **69**, 882–888

Rogers, M.F., Morens, D.M., Stewart, J.A., Kaminski, R.M., Spira, T.J., Feorino, P.M., Larsen, S.A., Francis, D.P., Wilson, M., Kaufman, L. & the Task Force on Acquired Immune Deficiency Syndrome (1983) National case–control study of Kaposi's sarcoma and *Pneumocystis carinii* pneumonia in homosexual men: Part 2, Laboratory results. *Ann. intern. Med.*, **99**, 151–158

Roithmann, S., Toledano, M., Tourani, J.M., Raphael, M., Gentilini, M., Gastaut, J.A., Armengaud, M., Morlat, P., Tilly, H., Dupont, B., Taillan, B., Theodore, C., Donadio, D. & Andrieu, J.-M. (1991) HIV-associated non-Hodgkin's lymphomas: clinical characteristics and outcome. The experience of the French Registry of HIV-associated tumors. *Ann. Oncol.*, **2**, 289–295

Roithmann, S., Tourani, J.M., Gastaut, J.A., Brice, P., Raphaël, M., Dujardin, P., Desablens, B. & Andrieu, J.M. (1992) HIV-associated Hodgkin's disease: characteristics and evolution. *Bull. Cancer*, **79**, 873–882 (in French)

Romanczuk, H. & Howley, P.M. (1992) Disruption of either the *E1* or the *E2* regulatory gene of human papillomavirus type 16 increases viral immortalization capacity. *Proc. natl Acad. Sci. USA*, **89**, 3159–3163

Roos, M.T.L., Lange, J.M.A., de Goede, R.E.Y., Coutinho, R.A., Schellekens, P.T.A., Miedma, F. & Tersmette, M. (1992) Viral phenotype and immune response in primary human immunodeficiency virus type 1 infection. *J. infect. Dis.*, **165**, 427–432

Roques, P., Marce, D., Courpotin, C., Mathieu, F.P., Herve, F., Boussin, F.-D., Narwa, R., Meyohas, M.-C., Dollfus, C. & Dormont, D. (1993) Correlation between HIV provirus burden and *in utero* transmission. *AIDS*, **7** (Suppl. 2), S39–S43

Rosenberg, P.S. (1995) Scope of the AIDS epidemic in the United States. *Science*, **270**, 1372–1375

Rosenberg, P.S., Gail, M.H. & Carroll, R.J. (1992) Estimating HIV prevalence and projecting AIDS incidence in the United States: a model that accounts for therapy and changes in the surveillance definition of AIDS. *Stat. Med.*, **11**, 1633–1655

Ross, R., Dworsky, R., Paganini-Hill, A., Levine, A. & Mack, T. (1985) Non-Hodgkin's lymphomas in never married men in Los Angeles. *Br. J. Cancer*, **52**, 785–787

Ross, J.S., Del Rosario, A., Bui, H.X., Sonbati, H. & Solis, O. (1992) Primary hepatic leiomyosarcoma in a child with the acquired immunodeficiency syndrome. *Hum. Pathol.*, **23**, 69–72

Roth, W.K. (1993) TGFβ and FGF-like growth factors involved in the pathogenesis of AIDS-associated Kaposi's sarcoma. *Res.Virol.*, **144**, 105–109

Roth, W.K., Werner, S., Risau, W., Remberger, K. & Hofschneider, P.H. (1988) Cultured, AIDS-related Kaposi's sarcoma cells express endothelial cell markers and are weakly malignant *in vitro*. *Int. J. Cancer*, **42**, 767–773

Roth, W.K., Werner, S., Schirren, C.G. & Hofschneider, P.H. (1989) Depletion of PDGF from serum inhibits growth of AIDS-related and sporadic Kaposi's sarcoma cells in culture. *Oncogene*, **4**, 483–487

Roth, W.K., Brandstetter, H. & Stürzl, M. (1992) Cellular and molecular features of HIV-associated Kaposi's sarcoma. *AIDS*, **6**, 895–913

Rowe, M., Young, L.S., Crocker, J., Stokes, H., Henderson, S. & Rickinson, A.B. (1991) Epstein-Barr virus (EBV)-associated lymphoproliferative disease in the *SCID* mouse model: implications for the pathogenesis of EBV-positive lymphomas in man. *J. exp. Med.*, **173**, 147–158

Rowland-Jones, S., Sutton, J., Ariyoshi, K., Dong, T., Gotch, F., McAdam, S., Whitby, D., Sabally, S., Gallimore, A., Corrah, T., Takiguchi, M., Schultz, T., McMichael, A. & Whittle, H. (1995) HIV-specific cytotoxic T-cells in HIV-exposed but uninfected Gambian women. *Nature Med.*, **1**, 59–64

Rozenbaum, W., Gharakhanian, S., Cardon, B., Duval, E. & Couland, J.P. (1988) HIV transmission by oral sex (Letter to the Editor). *Lancet*, **i**, 1395

Rubio, R. (1994) Hodgkin's disease associated with human immunodeficiency virus infection. A clinical study of 46 cases. *Cancer*, **73**, 2400–2407

Rüdlinger R. & Buchmann, P. (1989) HPV 16-positive Bowenoid papulosis and squamous-cell carcinoma of the anus in an HIV-positive man. *Dis. Colon Rectum*, **32**, 1042–1045

Rüger, R., Colimon, R. & Fleckenstein, B. (1984) Search for DNA sequences of human cytomegalovirus in Kaposi's sarcoma tissues with cloned probes. *Antibiot. Chemother.*, **32**, 43–47

Rutherford, G.W., Lifson, A.R., Hessol, N.A., Darrow, W.W., O'Malley, P.M., Buchbinder, S.P., Barnhart, J.L., Bodecker, T.W., Cannon, L., Doll, L.S., Holmberg, S.D., Harrison, J.S., Rogers, M.F., Werdegar, D. & Jaffe, H.W. (1990) Course of HIV-I infection in a cohort of homosexual and bisexual men: an 11 year follow up study. *Br. med. J.*, **301**, 1183–1188

Rwandan HIV Seroprevalence Study Group (1989) Nationwide community-based serological survey of HIV-1 and other human retrovirus infections in a Central African country. *Lancet*, **i**, 941–943

Rygnestad, T., Småbrekke, L. & Nesje, L. (1995) Impact of improved treatment of sexually transmitted disease on HIV infections (Letter to the Editor). *Lancet*, **346**, 1157–1160

Saag, M.S., Emini, E.A., Laskin, O.L., Douglas, J., Lapidus, W.J., Schleif, W.A., Whitley, R.J., Hildebrand, C., Byrnes, V.W., Kappes, J.C., Anderson, K.W., Massari, F.E., Shaw, G.M. & the L-697,661 Working Group (1993) A short-term clinical evaluation of L-697,661, a nonnucleoside inhibitor of HIV-1 reverse transcriptase. *New Engl. J. Med.*, **329**, 1065–1072

Safai, B., Mike, V., Giraldo, G., Beth, E. & Good, R.A. (1980) Association of Kaposi's sarcoma with second primary malignancies: possible etiopathogenic implications. *Cancer*, **45**, 1472–1479

Said, J.W., Shintaku, I.P., Teitelbaum, A., Chien, K. & Sassoon, A.F. (1984) Distribution of T-cell phenotypic subsets and surface immunoglobulin-bearing lymphocytes in lymph nodes from male homosexuals with persistent generalized adenopathy: an immunohistochemical and ultrastructural study. *Hum. Pathol.*, **15**, 785–790

Saikevych, I.A., Mayer, M., White, R.L. & Ho, R.C.S. (1988) Cytogenetic study of Kaposi's sarcoma associated with acquired immunodeficiency syndrome. *Arch Pathol. Lab. Med.*, **112**, 825–828

Saimot, A.G., Coulaud, J.P., Mechali, D., Matheron, S., Dazza, M.C., Rey, M.A., Brun-Vézinet, F. & Leibowitch, J. (1987) HIV-2/LAV-2 in Portuguese man with AIDS (Paris, 1978) who had served in Angola 1968–74 (Letter to the Editor). *Lancet*, **i**, 688

Salahuddin, S.Z., Ablashi, D.V., Markham, P.D., Josephs, S.F., Sturzenegger, S., Kaplan, M., Halligan, G., Biberfeld, P., Wong-Staal, F., Kramarsky, B. & Gallo, R.C. (1986) Isolation of a new virus, HBLV, in patients with lymphoproliferative disorders. *Science*, **234**, 596–601

Salahuddin, S.Z., Nakamura, S., Biberfeld, P., Kaplan, M.H., Markham, P.D., Larsson, L. & Gallo, R.C. (1988) Angiogenic properties of Kaposi's sarcoma-derived cells after long-term culture in vitro. *Science*, **242**, 430–433

Salas-Buzon, M.C. & Saez-Elegido, B. (1992) Squamous cell carcinoma of the tongue and HIV infection. *Rev. Clin. Esp.*, **190**, 359–360

Sande, M.A., Carpenter, C.C.J., Cobbs, C.G., Holmes, K.K. & Sanford, J.P. for the National Institute of Allergy and Infectious Diseases State-of-the-Art Panel on Anti-Retroviral Therapy for Adult HIV-Infected Patients (1993) Antiretroviral therapy for adult HIV-infected patients. Recommendations from a state-of-the-art conference. *J. Am. med. Assoc.*, **270**, 2583–2589

Sarkar, S., Das, N., Panda, S., Naik, T.N., Sarkar, K., Singh, B.C., Ralte, J.M., Ater, S.M. & Tripathy, S.P. (1993) Rapid spread of HIV among injecting drug users in north-eastern states of India. *Bull. Narcotics*, **45**, 91–105

Scappaticci, S., Cerimele, D., Cottoni, F., Pasquali, F. & Fraccaro, M. (1986) Chromosomal aberrations in lymphocyte and fibroblast cultures of patients with the sporatic type of Kaposi sarcoma. *Hum. Genet.*, **72**, 311–317

Schäfer, A., Friedmann, W., Mielke, M., Scwartländer, B. & Koch, M.A. (1991) The increased frequency of cervical dysplasia-neoplasia in women infected with the human immunodeficiency virus is related to the degree of immunosuppression. *Am. J. Obstet. Gynecol.*, **164**, 593–599

Schalling, M., Eukman, M., Kaaya, E.E., Linde, A. & Biberfeld, P. (1995) A role for a new herpesvirus (KSHV) in different forms of Kaposi's sarcoma. *Nature Med.*, **1**, 707–708

Schechter, M.T., Craib, K.J.P., Le, T.N., Willoughby, B., Douglas, B., Sestak, P., Montaner, J.S.G., Weaver, M.S., Elmslie, K.D. & O'Shaughnessy, M.V. (1989) Progression to AIDS and predictors of AIDS in seroprevalent and seroincident cohorts of homosexual men. *AIDS*, **3**, 347–353

Scheffner, M., Werness, B.A., Huibregtse, J.M., Levine, A.J. & Howley, P.M. (1990) The E6 oncoprotein encoded by human papillomavirus type 16 and 18 promotes the degradation of p53. *Cell*, **63**, 1129–1136

Schenk, P. (1986) Retroviruses in Kaposi's sarcoma in acquired immunodeficiency syndrome (AIDS). *Acta otolaryngol.*, **101**, 295–298

Schiller, J.T., Kleiner, E., Androphy, E.J., Lowy, D.R. & Pfister, H. (1989) Identification of bovine papillomavirus E1 mutants with increased transforming and transcriptional activity. *J. Virol.*, **63**, 1775–1782

Schlegel, R., Phelps, W.C., Zhang, Y.-L. & Barbosa, M. (1988) Quantitative keratinocyte assay detects two biological activities of human papillomavirus DNA and identifies viral types associated with cervical carcinoma. *EMBO J.*, **7**, 3181–3187

Schmidt, R., Stippel, D., Krings, F. & Pollok, M. (1995) Malignancies of the genito-urinary system following renal transplantation. *Br. J. Urol.*, **75**, 572–577

Schnittman, S.M., Vogel, S., Baseler, M., Lane, H.C. & Davey, R.T., Jr (1994) A phase I study of interferon-alpha 2b in combination with interleukin-2 in patients with human immunodeficiency virus infection. *J. infect. Dis.*, **169**, 981–989

Schoenbaum, E.E., Hartel, D., Selwyn, P.A., Klein, R.S., Davenny, K., Rogers, M., Feiner, C. & Friedland, G. (1989) Risk factors for human immunodeficiency virus infection in intravenous drug users. *New Engl. J. Med.*, **321**, 874–879

Schrager, L.K., Friedland, G.H., Maude, D., Schreiber, K., Adachi, A., Pizzuti, D.J,. Koss, L.G. & Klein, R.S. (1989) Cervical and vaginal squamous abnormalities in women infected with human immunodeficiency virus. *J. acquir. Immun. Defic. Syndr.*, **2**, 570–575

Schrier, R.D., McCutchan, J.A., Venable, J.C., Nelson, J.A. & Wiley, C.A. (1990) T-cell-induced expression of human immunodeficiency virus in macrophages. *J. Virol.*, **64**, 3280–3288

Schwarz, E., Freese, U.K., Gissmann, L., Mayer, W., Roggenbuck, B., Stremlau, A. & zur Hausen, H. (1985) Structure and transcription of human papillomavirus sequences in cervical carcinoma cells. *Nature*, **314**, 111–114

Schweizer, M., Turek, R., Reinhard, M. & Neumann-Haefelin, D. (1994) Absence of foamy virus DNA in Graves' disease. *AIDS Res. hum. Retroviruses*, **10**, 601–605

Scully, R.E., Mark, E.J., McNeely, W.F., McNeely, B.U., Kieff, E.D., Johnson, R.P. & Mark, E.J. (1989) Case records of the Massachusetts general hospital. Case 33-1989. Presentation of case. *New Engl. J. Med.*, **321**, 454–463

Selik, R.M., Chu, S.Y. & Ward, J.W. (1995) Trends in infectious diseases and cancers among persons dying of HIV infection in the United States from 1987 to 1992. *Ann. intern. Med.*, **123**, 933–936

Serraino, D. & Franceschi, S. (1996a) Kaposi's sarcoma and non-Hodgkin's lymphomas in children and adolescents with AIDS. *AIDS*, **10**, 643–647

Serraino, D. & Franceschi, S. (1996b) Kaposi's sarcoma in children with AIDS in Europe and the United States (Letter to the Editor). *Europ. J. Cancer*, **32A**, 650–651

Serraino, D., Zaccarelli, M., Franceschi, S. & Greco, D. (1992a) The epidemiology of AIDS-associated Kaposi's sarcoma in Italy. *AIDS*, **6**, 1015–1019

Serraino, D., Franceschi, S., Tirelli, U. & Monfardini, S. (1992b) The epidemiology of acquired immunodeficiency syndrome and associated tumours in Europe. *Ann. Oncol.*, **3**, 595–603

Serraino, D., Salamina, G., Franceschi, S., Dubois, D., La Vecchia, C., Brunet, J.B. & Ancelle-Park, R.A. (1992c) The epidemiology of AIDS-associated non-Hodgkin's lymphoma in the World Health Organization European Region. *Br. J. Cancer*, **66**, 912–916

Serraino, D., Carbone, A., Franceschi, S. & Tirelli, U. (1993) Increased frequency of lymphocyte depletion and mixed cellularity subtypes of Hodgkin's disease in HIV-infected patients. *Eur. J. Cancer.*, **29A**, 1948–1950

Serraino, D., Franceschi, S., Dal Maso L., Cozzi Lepri, A., Tirelli, U. & Rezza, G. (1995a) The classification of AIDS cases: concordance between two AIDS surveillance systems in Italy. *Am. J. public Health*, **85**, 1112–1114

Serraino, D., Franceschi, S., Dal Maso, L. & La Vecchia, C. (1995b) HIV transmission and Kaposi's sarcoma among European women. *AIDS*, **9**, 971–973

Serrano, M., Bellas, C., Campo, E., Ribera, J., Martín, C., Rubio, R., Ruiz, C., Ocaña, I., Buzón, L., Yebra, M., Font, M. & Martinez, M.A. (1990) Hodgkin's disease in patients with antibodies to human immunodeficiency virus. A study of 22 patients. *Cancer*, **65**, 2248–2254

Serwadda, D., Sewankambo, N.K., Carswell, J.W., Bayley, A.C., Tedder, R.S., Weiss, R.A., Mugerwa, R.D., Lwegaba, A., Kirya, G.B., Downing, R.G., Clayden, S.A. & Dalgleish, A.G. (1985) Slim disease: a new disease in Uganda and its association with HTLV-III infection. *Lancet*, **ii**, 849–852

Sha, B.E., Benson, C.A., Pottage, J.C., Jr, Urbanski, P.A., Daugherty, S.R. & Kessler, H.A. (1995) HIV infection in women: an observational study of clinical characteristics, disease progression, and survival for a cohort of women in Chicago. *J. acquir. Immune Defic. Syndr. hum. Retrovirol.*, **8**, 486–495

Shahab, I., Osborne, B.M. & Butler, J.J. (1994) Nasopharyngeal lymphoid tissue masses in patients with human immunodeficiency virus-1. Histologic findings and clinical correlation. *Cancer*, **74**, 3083–3088

Shapiro, R.S., McClain, K., Frizzera, G., Gajl-Peczalska, K.J., Kersey, J.H., Blazar, B.R., Arthur, D.C., Patton, D.F., Greenberg, J.S., Burke, B., Ramsay, N.K.C., McGlave, P. & Filipovich, A.H (1988) Epstein-Barr virus associated B-cell lymphoproliferative disorders following bone marrow transplantation. *Blood*, **71**, 1234–1243

Sharp, P.M., Robertson, D.L., Gao, F. & Hahn, B.H. (1994) Origins and diversity of human immunodeficiency viruses. *AIDS*, **8** (Suppl. 1), S27–S42

Sharp, P.M., Robertson, D.L. & Hahn, B.H. (1995) Cross-species transmission and recombination of 'AIDS' viruses. *Phil. Trans. R. Soc. London. B.*, **349**, 41–47

Shaunak, S. & Weber, J. (1992) The retroviruses: classification and molecular biology. *Baill. clin. Neurol.*, **1**, 1–21

Shaw, G.M., Harper, M.E., Hahn, B.H., Epstein, L.G., Gajdusek, D.C., Price, R.W., Navia, B.A., Petito, C.K., O'Hara, C.J., Groopman, J.E., Cho, E.-S., Oleske, J.M., Wong-Staal, F. & Gallo, R.C. (1985) HTLV-III infection in brains of children and adults with AIDS encephalopathy. *Science*, **227**, 177–182

Shelton, G.H., Waltier, R.M., Connor, S.C. & Grant, C.K. (1989) Prevalence of feline immunodeficiency virus and feline leukemia virus infections in pet cats. *J. Am. An. Hosp. Assoc.* **25**, 7–12

Shelton, G.H., Grant, C.K., Cotter, S.M., Gardner, M.B., Hardy, W.D., Jr & DiGiacomo, R.F. (1990) Feline immunodeficiency virus and feline leukemia virus infections and their relationships to lymphoid malignancies in cats: a retrospective study (1968–1988). *J. acquir. Immun. Defic. Syndr.*, **3**, 623–630

Shibata, D. (1994) Biologic aspects of AIDS-related lymphoma. *Curr. Opin. Oncol.*, **6**, 503–507

Shibata, D., Weiss, L.M., Nathwani, B.N., Brynes, R.K. & Levine, A.M. (1991) Epstein-Barr virus in benign lymph node biopsies from individuals infected with the human immunodeficiency virus is associated with concurrent or subsequent development of non-Hodgkin's lymphoma. *Blood*, **77**, 1527–1533

Shibata, D., Weiss, L.M., Hernandez, A.M., Nathwani, B.N., Bernstein, L. & Levine, A.M. (1993) Epstein–Barr virus-associated non-Hodgkin's lymphoma in patients infected with the human immunodeficiency virus. *Blood*, **81**, 2102–2109

Shiramizu, B. & McGrath, M.S. (1991) Molecular pathogenesis of AIDS-associated non-Hodgkin's lymphoma. *Hematol. oncol. Clin. North Am.*, **5**, 323–330

Shiramizu, B., Herndier, B.G. & McGrath, M.S. (1994) Identification of a common clonal human immunodeficiency virus integration site in human immunodeficiency virus-associated lymphomas. *Cancer Res.*, **54**, 2069–2072

Siebert, J.D., Ambinder, R.F., Napoli, V.M., Quintanilla-Martinez, L., Banks, P.M. & Gulley, M.L. (1995) Human immunodeficiency virus-associated Hodgkin's disease contains latent, not replicative, Epstein-Barr virus. *Hum. Pathol.*, **26**, 1191–1195

Siegal, B., Levinton-Kriss, S., Schiffer, A., Sayar, J., Engelberg, I., Vonsover, A., Ramon, Y. & Rubenstein, E. (1990) Kaposi's sarcoma in immunosuppression possibly the result of a dual infection. *Cancer*, **65**, 492–498

Sillman, F.H. & Sedlis, A. (1991) Anogenital papillomavirus infection and neoplasia in immunodeficient women: an update. *Dermatol.-Clin.*, **9**, 353–369

Simon, F., Pépin, J.M., Brun-Vézinet, F., Bouchaud, O., Casalino, H. & Gérard, L. (1992) Reliability of western blotting for the confirmation of HIV-1 seroconversion. *Lancet*, **340**, 1541–1542

Simpson, D.M. & Tagliati, M. (1994) Neurologic manifestations of HIV infection. *Ann. intern. Med.*, **121**, 769–785

Singh, J., Che'Rus, S., Chong, S., Chong, Y.K. & Crofts, N. (1994) AIDS in Malaysia. *AIDS*, **8** (Suppl. 2), S99–S103

Sinicco, A., Palestro, G., Caramello, P., Giacobbi, D., Giuliani, G., Paggi, G., Sciandra, M. & Gioannini, P. (1990) Acute HIV-1 infection: clinical and biological study of 12 patients. *J. acquir. Immun. Defic. Syndr.*, **3**, 260–265

Sinicco, A., Fora, R., Sciandra, M., Lucchini, A., Caramello, P. & Gioannini, P. (1993) Risk of developing AIDS after primary acute HIV infection. *J. acquir. Immun. Defic. Syndr.*, **6**, 575–581

Sirisanthana, V. & Sirisanthana, T. (1995) Disseminated *Penicillium marneffei* infection in human immunodeficiency virus-infected children. *Pediatr. Infect. Dis. J.*, **14**, 935–940

Sisk, J.E., Hatziandreu, E.J. & Hughes, R. (1990) *The Effectiveness of Drug Abuse Treatment: Implications for Controlling AIDS/HIV Infection* (Publ. OTA-BP-H-73, 1-11), Washington, DC, United States Congress, Office of Technology Assessment

Sitas, F., Levin, C.V., Spencer, D., Odes, R.A., Bezwoda, W., Windsor, I., Sher, R. & Wadee, A. A. (1993) HIV and cancer in South Africa. *S. Afr. med. J.*, **83**, 880–881

Sitas, F., Fleming, A.F. & Morris, J. (1994) Residual risk of transmission of HIV through blood transfusion in South Africa. *S. Afr. med. J.*, **84**, 142–144

Sitas, F., Terblanche, M. & Madhoo, J. (1996) *National Cancer Registry of South Africa. Incidence and Geographical Distribution of Histologically Diagnosed Cancer in South Africa, 1990 & 1991*, Johannesberg, South African Institute for Medical Research

Sloand, E.M., Pitt, E., Chiarello, R.J. & Nemo, G.J. (1991) HIV testing: state of the art. *J. Am. med. Assoc.*, **266**, 2861–2866

Sloand, E.M., Klein, H.G., Banks, S.M., Vareldzis, B., Merritt, S. & Pierce, P. (1992) Epidemiology of thrombocytopenia in HIV infection. *Eur. J. Haematol.*, **48**, 168–172

Small, C.B., Klein, R.S., Friedland, G.H., Moll, B., Emeson, E.E. & Spigland, I. (1983) Community-acquired opportunistic infections and defective cellular immunity in heterosexual drug abusers and homosexual men. *Am. J. Med.*, **74**, 433–441

Smith, P.D. (1994) Role of the mucosa in human immunodeficiency virus disease. *Mucosal Immun. Update*, **2**, 3–5

Smith, N. & Spittle, M. (1987) Tumours. Kaposi's sarcoma. *Br. med. J.*, **294**, 1274–1277

Smith, A.J., Srinivasakumar, N., Hammarskjold, M.L. & Rekosh, D. (1993a) Requirements for incorporation of Pr160gag-pol from human immunodeficiency virus type 1 into virus-like particles. *J. Virol.*, **67**, 2266–2275

Smith, J.R., Kitchen, V.S., Botcherby, M., Hepburn, M., Wells, C., Gor, D., Forster, S.M., Harris, J.R.W., Steer, P. & Mason, P. (1993b) Is HIV infection associated with an increase in the prevalence of cervical neoplasia? *Br. J. Obstet. Gynaecol.*, **100**, 149–153

Smith, K.J., Skelton, H.G., Yeager, J., Angritt, P. & Wagner, K.F. (1993c) Cutaneous neoplasms in a military population of HIV-1-positive patients. *J. Am. Acad. Dermatol.*, **29**, 400–406

Smith, C.A., Ng, C.Y., Heslop, H.E., Holladay, M.S., Richardson, S., Turner, E.V., Loftkin, S.K., Li, C., Brenner, M.K. & Rooney, C.M. (1995) Production of genetically modified Epstein–Barr virus-specific cytotoxic T cells for adoptive transfer to patients at high risk of EBV-associated lymphoproliferative disease. *J. Hematother.*, **4**, 73–79

Smitherman, M.H., Morris, L.E., Jr, Chang, B.K., Khankhanian, N.K. & Dunlap, D.B. (1990) Rectal small cell cancer in an HIV-positive man. *Am. J. Med.*, **89**, 239–240

Smotkin, D. & Wettstein, F.O. (1986) Transcription of human papillomavirus type 16 early genes in a cervical cancer and a cervical cancer-derived cell line and identification of the E7 protein. *Proc. natl Acad. Sci. USA*, **83**, 4680–4684

Socié, G., Henry-Amar, M., Cosset, J.M., Devergie, A., Girinsky, T. & Gluckman, E. (1991) Increased incidence of solid malignant tumors after bone marrow transplantation for severe aplastic anemia. *Blood*, **78**, 277–279

Socié, G., Henry-Amar, M., Bacigalupo, A., Hows, J., Tichelli, A., Ljungman, P., McCann, S.R., Frickhofen, N., Van't Veer-Korthof, E. & Gluckman, E. (1993) Malignant tumors occurring after treatment of aplastic anemia. *New Engl. J. Med.*, **329**, 1152–1157

Soulier, J., Grollet, L., Oksenhendler, E., Cacoub, P., Cazals-Hatem, D., Babinet, P., d'Agay, M.-F., Clauvel, J.-P., Raphael, M., Degos, L. & Sigaux, F. (1995) Kaposi's sarcoma-associated herpesvirus-like DNA sequences in multicentric Castleman's disease. *Blood*, **86**, 1276–1280

Sova, P. & Volsky, D.J. (1993) Efficiency of viral DNA synthesis during infection of permissive and nonpermissive cells with *vif*-negative -negative human immunodeficiency virus type 1. *J. Virol.*, **67**, 6322–6326

Spinillo, A., Tenti, P., Zappatore, R., De Seta, F., Silini, E. & Guaschino, S. (1993) Langerhans' cell counts and cervical intraepithelial neoplasia in women with human immunodeficiency virus infection. *Gynecol. Oncol.*, **48**, 210–213

Spira, A.I., Marx, P.A., Patterson, B.K., Mahoney, J., Koup, R.A., Wolinsky, S.M. & Ho, D.D. (1996) Cellular targets of infection and route of viral dissemination after an intravaginal inoculation of simian immunodeficiency virus into rhesus macaques. *J. exp. Med.*, **183**, 215–225

Stafford, M.K., Byrne, G., Sayers, J., Rosenstein, I., McClure, M., Flanagan, A.M., Smith, J.R., Weber, J. & Kitchen, V.S. (1995) *Dextrine Sulphate Gel — A Novel Potential Intravaginal Virucide: Safety, Tolerance and Residence Time*, The Medical Society for the Study of Venereal Diseases, Spring Meeting 1995, Vienna 18th–21st May

Stahl-Hennig, C., Herchenröder, O., Nick, S., Evers, M., Stille-Siegener, M., Jentsch, K.-D., Kirchhoff, F., Tolle, T., Gatesman, T.J., Lüke, W. & Hunsmann, G. (1990) Experimental infection of macaques with HIV-2_{ben}, a novel HIV-2 isolate. *AIDS*, **4**, 611–617

Stahmer, I., Ordonez, C., Popovic, M., Mesquita, R., Ekman, M., Albert, J., Putkonen, P., Böttiger, D., Biberfeld, G. & Biberfeld, P. (1996) SIV infection of monkey spleen cells including follicular dendritic cells in different stages of disease. *J. acquir. Immune Defic. Syndr. hum. Retrovirol.*, **11**, 1–9

Stansfeld, A.G., Diebold, J., Kapanci, Y., Kelényi, G., Lennert, K., Mioduszewska, O., Noel, H., Rilke, F., Sundstom, C., van Unnik, J.A.M. & Wright, D.H. (1988) Updated Kiel classification for lymphomas (Letter to the Editor). *Lancet*, **i**, 292–293

Steel, T.R., Pell, M.F., Turner, J.J. & Lim, G.H.K. (1993) Spinal epidural leiomyoma occuring in an HIV-infected man. *J. Neurosurg.*, **79**, 442–445

Stevens, D.A. (1995) Coccidiomycosis. *New Engl. J. Med.*, **332**, 1077–1082

Stewart, G.J., Tyler, J.P.P., Cunningham, A.L., Barr, J.A., Driscoll, G.L., Gold, J. & Lamont, B.J. (1985) Transmission of human T-lymphotropic virus type III (HTLV-III) by artificial insemination by donor. *Lancet*, **ii**, 581–584

Stimson, G.V. (1989) Syringe-exchange programmes for injecting drug users. *AIDS*, **3**, 253–260

Stoica, G., Hoffman, J. & Yuen, P.H. (1990). Moloney murine sarcoma virus 349 induces Kaposi's sarcoma-like lesions in Balb/c mice. *Am. J. Pathol.*, **136**, 933–947

Stoler, M.H., Rhodes, C.R., Whitbeck, A., Wolinsky, S.M., Chow, L.T. & Broker, T.R. (1992) Human papillomavirus type 16 and 18 gene expression in cervical neoplasias. *Hum. Pathol.*, **23**, 117–128

Stowell, R.E., Smith, E.K., España, C. & Nelson, V.G. (1971) Outbreak of malignant lymphoma in rhesus monkeys. *Lab. Invest.*, **25**, 476–479

Stratton, P. & Ciacco, K.H. (1994) Cervical neoplasia in the patient with HIV infection. *Current Opin. Obstet.*, **6**, 86–91

Strichman-Almashanu, L., Weltfriend, S., Gideoni, O., Friedman-Birnbaum, R. & Pollack, S. (1995) No significant association between HLA antigens and classic Kaposi's sarcoma: molecular analysis of 49 Jewish patients. *J. clin. Immunol.*, **15**, 205–209

Stryker, J., Coates, T.J., DeCarlo, P., Haynes-Sanstad, K., Shriver, M. & Makadon, H.J. (1995) Prevention of HIV infection. Looking back, looking ahead. *J. Am. med. Assoc.*, **273**, 1143–1148

Stürzl, M., Brandstetter, H. & Roth, W.K. (1992a) Kaposi's sarcoma: a review of gene expression and ultrastructure of KS spindle cells *in vivo*. *AIDS Res. hum. Retroviruses*, **8**, 1753–1763

Stürzl, M., Roth, W.K., Brockmeyer, N.H., Zietz, C., Speiser, B. & Hofschneider, P.H. (1992b) Expression of platelet-derived growth factor and its receptors in AIDS-related Kaposi sarcoma *in vitro* suggests paracrine and autocrine mechanisms of tumor maintenance. *Proc. natl Acad. Sci. USA*, **89**, 7046–7050

Su, I.-J., Hsu, Y.-S., Chang, Y.-C. & Wang, I.-W. (1995) Herpesvirus-like DNA sequence in Kaposi's sarcoma from AIDS and non-AIDS patients in Taiwan (Letter to the Editor). *Lancet*, **345**, 722–723

Subbramanian, R.A. & Cohen, E.A. (1994) Molecular biology of the human immunodeficiency virus accessory proteins. *J. Virol.*, **68**, 6831–6835

Sun, X.-W., Ellerbrock, T.V., Lungu, O., Chiasson, M.A., Bush, T.J. & Wright, T.C., Jr (1995) Human papillomavirus infection in human immunodeficiency virus-seropositive women. *Obstet. Gynecol.*, **85**, 680–686

Surawicz, C.M., Kirby, P., Critchlow, C., Sayer, J., Dunphy, C. & Kiviat, N. (1993) Anal dysplasia in homosexual men: role of anoscopy and biopsy. *Gastroenterology*, **105**, 658–666

Swift, F.V., Bhat, K., Younghusband, H.B. & Hamada, H. (1987) Characterization of a cell type-specific enhancer found in the human papillomavirus type 18 genome. *EMBO J.*, **6**, 1339–1344

Tan, X., Pearce-Pratt, R. & Phillips, D.M. (1993) Productive infection of a cervical epithelial cell line with human immunodeficiency virus: implications for sexual transmission. *J. Virol.*, **67**, 6447–6452

Tappero, J.W., Conant, M.A., Wolfe, S.F. & Berger, T.G. (1993) Kaposi's sarcoma. Epidemiology, pathogenesis, histology, clinical spectrum, staging criteria and therapy. *J. Am. Acad. Dermatol.*, **28**, 371–395

Taylor, J.F. (1971) *The Skeletal Lesions of Kaposi's Sarcoma*, Thesis, Liverpool

Taylor, A.G., Birtles, R. & Harrison, T.G. (1993) Cat-scratch, Kaposi's sarcoma, and bacillary angiomatosis (Letter to the Editor). *Lancet*, **342**, 688

Telzak, E.E., Chiasson, M.A., Bevier, P.J., Stoneburner, R.L., Castro, K.G. & Jaffe, H.W. (1993) HIV-1 seroconversion in patients with and without genital ulcer disease. A prospective study. *Ann. intern. Med.*, **119**, 1181–1186

Temin, H.M. (1976) The DNA provirus hypothesis. *Science*, **192**, 1075–1080

Templeton, A.C. (1972) Studies in Kaposi's sarcoma. Postmortem findings and disease patterns in women. *Cancer*, **30**, 854–867

Templeton, A.C. (1973) Tumours of a tropical country: a survey of Uganda 1964–1968. *Rec. Results Cancer Res.*, **41**, 203–214

Templeton, A.C. (1981) Kaposi's sarcoma. In: Sommers, S.C. & Rosen P.P., eds, *Pathology Annual,* New York, Appleton: Century-Crofts, pp. 315–336

Tenner-Rácz, K., Rácz, P., Dietrich, M. & Kern, P. (1985) Altered follicular dendritic cells and virus-like particles in AIDS and AIDS-related lymphadenopathy (Letter to the Editor). *Lancet*, **i**, 105–106

Tenner-Rácz, K., Rácz, P., Bofill, M., Schulz-Meyer, A., Dietrich, M., Kern, P., Weber, J., Pinching, A.J., Veronese-Dimarzo, F., Popovic, M., Klatzmann, D., Gluckman, J.C. & Janossy, G. (1986) HTLV-III/LAV viral antigens in lymph nodes of homosexual men with persistent generalized lymphadenopathy and AIDS. *Am. J. Pathol.*, **123**, 9–15

Terry, A., Callanan, J.J., Fulton, R., Jarrett, O. & Neil, J.C. (1995) Molecular analysis of tumours from feline immunodeficiency virus (FIV)-infected cats: an indirect role for FIV? *Int. J. Cancer*, **61**, 227–232

Thierry, F., Spyrou, G., Yaniv, M. & Howley, P.M. (1992) Two AP1 sites binding JunB are essential for human papillomavirus type 18 transcription in keratinocytes. *J. Virol.*, **66**, 3740–3748

Timmerman, J.M., Northfelt, D.W. & Small, E.J. (1995) Malignant germ cell tumors in men infected with the human immunodeficiency virus: natural history and results of therapy. *J. clin. Oncol.*, **13**, 1391–1397

Tindall, B., Barker, S., Donovan, B., Barnes, T., Roberts, J., Kronenberg, C., Gold, J., Penny, R., Cooper, D. & the Sydney AIDS Study Group (1988a) Characterization of the acute clinical illness associated with human immunodeficiency virus infection. *Arch. intern. Med.*, **148**, 945–949

Tindall, B., Cooper, D.A., Donovan, B. & Penny, R. (1988b) Primary human immunodeficiency virus infection. Clinical and serologic aspects. *Infect. Dis. Clin. N. Am.*, **2**, 329–341

Tirelli, U., Pizzoccaro, G., Vaccher, E., Parrinello, A.E., Zagonel, V., Carbone, A., Rezza, G., Monfardini, S. & Palmierim, G. (1988) Malignant tumors other than lymphoma and Kaposi's sarcoma in association with HIV infection. *Cancer Detect. Prevent.*, **12**, 267–272

Tirelli, U., Errante, D., Vaccher, E., Repetto, L., Rizzardini, G., Spina, M., Gastaldi, R., Bertola, G., Serraino, D., Carbone, A. & Monfardini, S. (1992) Hodgkin's disease in 92 patients with HIV infection: the Italian experience. *Ann. Oncol.*, **3** (Suppl. 4), S69–S72

Tirelli, U., Vaccher, E., Zagonel, V., Talamini, R., Bernardi, D., Tavio, M., Gloghini, A., Merola, M.C., Monfardini, S. & Carbone, A. (1995a) CD30 (Ki-1)-positive anaplastic large-cell lymphomas in 13 patients with and 27 patients without human immunodeficiency virus infection: the first comparative clinicopathologic study from a single institution that also includes 80 patients with other human immunodeficiency virus-related systemic lymphomas. *J. clin. Oncol.*, **13**, 373–380

Tirelli, U., Errante, D., Dolcetti, R., Gloghini, A., Serraino, D., Vaccher, E., Franceschi, S., Boiocchi, M. & Carbone, A. (1995b) Hodgkin's disease and human immmunodeficiency virus infection: clinicopathologic and virologic features of 114 patients from the Italian Cooperative Group on AIDS and Tumors. *J. clin. Oncol.*, **13**, 1758–1767

Titus, S., Marmor, M., Des Jarlais, D., Kim, M., Wolfe, H. & Beatrice, S. (1994) Bleach use and HIV seroconversion in New York City injection drug users. *J. acquir. Immun. Defic. Syndr.*, **7**, 700–704

Tornesello, M.L., Beth-Giraldo, E., Galloway, D.A., McDougall, J.K., Buonaguro, F.M. & Giraldo, G. (1991) Interaction between HIV and HPV in the development of penile cancers (Abstract). *7th Int. Conf. on AIDS, Florence,* 29

Tornesello, M.L., Buonaguro, F.M., Beth-Giraldo, E., Kyalwazi, S.K. & Giraldo, G. (1992) Human papillomavirus (HPV) DNA in penile carcinomas and in two cell lines from high-incidence areas for genital cancers in Africa. *Int. J. Cancer,* **51**, 587–592

Tornesello, M.L., Buonaguro, F.M., Beth-Giraldo, E. & Giraldo, G. (1993) Human immunodeficiency virus type 1 *tat* gene enhances human papillomavirus early gene expression. *Intervirology,* **36**, 57–64

Torpey, D., III, Huang, X.-L., Armstrong, J., Ho, M., Whiteside, T., McMahon, D., Pazin, G., Herberman, R., Gupta, P., Tripoli, C., Moody, D., Okarma, T., Elder, E. & Rinaldo, C., Jr (1993) Effects of adoptive immunotherapy with autologous $CD8^+$ T lymphocytes on immunologic parameters: lymphocyte subsets and cytotoxic activity. *Clin. Immunol. Immunopathol.,* **68**, 263–272

Tristem, M., Marshall, C., Karpas, A. & Hill, F. (1992) Evolution of the primate lentiviruses: evidence from *vpx* and *vpr*. *EMBO J.,* **11**, 3405–3412

Trono, D. (1995) HIV accessory proteins: leading roles for the supporting cast. *Cell,* **82**, 189–192

Trovato, R., Luppi, M., Vago, L., Torelli, G., Moroni, M. & Ceccherini-Nelli, L. (1995) Frequency of human herpesvirus type 6 (HHV-6) genome detection in AIDS-related lymphoproliferative disorders. *J. acquir. Immune Defic. Syndr. hum. Retrovirol.,* **9**, 311–312

Tsai, C.-C., Wu, H. & Meng, F. (1995) Immunocytochemistry of Kaposi's sarcoma-like tumor cells from pigtailed macaques with simian AIDS. *J. med. Primatol.,* **24**, 43–48

Tsujimoto, H., Cooper, R.W., Kodama, T., Fukasawa, M., Miura, T, Ohta, Y., Ishikawa, K.-I., Nakai, M., Frost, E., Roelants, G.E., Roffi, J. & Hayami, M. (1988) Isolation and characterization of simian immunodeficiency virus from mandrills in Africa and its relationship to other human and simian immunodeficiency viruses. *J. Virol.,* **62**, 4044–4050

Turnock, B.J. & Kelly, C.J. (1989) Mandatory premarital testing for human immunodeficiency virus. The Illinois experience. *J. Am. med Assoc.,* **261**, 3415–3418

Urmacher, C., Myskowski, P., Ochoa, M., Jr, Kris, M. & Safai, B. (1982) Outbreak of Kaposi's sarcoma with cytomegalovirus infection in young homosexual men. *Am. J. Med.,* **72**, 569–575

Van de Perre, P., Rouvroy, D., Lepage, P., Bogaerts, J., Kestelyn, P., Kayihigi, J., Hekker, A.C., Butzler, J.-P. & Clumeck, N. (1984) Acquired immunodeficiency syndrome in Rwanda. *Lancet,* **ii**, 62–65

Van de Perre, P., Simonon, A., Msellati, P., Hitimana, D.-G., Vaira, D., Bazubagira, A., Van Goethem, C., Stevens, A.-M., Karita, E., Sondag-Thull, D., Dabis, F. & Lepage, P. (1991) Postnatal transmission of human immunodeficiency virus type 1 from mother-to-infant. A prospective cohort study in Kigali, Rwanda. *New Engl. J. Med.,* **325**, 593–598

Vandermolen, L.A., Fehir, K.M. & Rice, L. (1985) Multiple myeloma in a homosexaul man with chronic lymphadenopathy. *Arch. intern. Med.,* **145**, 745–746

Van Doornum, G.J.J., Van den Hoek, J.A.R., Van Ameijden, H.J.C., Van Haastrecht, H.J.C., Roos, M.T.L., Henquet, C.J.M., Quint, W.G.V. & Coutinho, R.A. (1993) Cervical HPV infection among HIV-infected prostitutes addicted to hard drugs. *J. med. Virol.,* **41**, 185–190

Vermund, S.H., Kelley, K.F., Klein, R.S., Feingold, A.R., Schreiber, K., Munk, G. & Burk, R.D. (1991) High risk of human papillomavirus infection and cervical squamous intraepithelial lesions among women with symptomatic human immunodeficiency virus infection. *Am. J. Obstet. Gynecol.*, **165**, 392–400

Vernon, S.D., Hart, C.E., Reeves, W.C. & Icenogle, J.P. (1993) The HIV-1 Tat protein enhances E2-dependent human papillomavirus 16 transcription. *Virus Res.*, **27**, 133–145

Vernon, S.D., Zaki, S.R. & Reeves, W.C. (1994) Localisation of HIV-1 to human papillomavirus associated cervical lesions. *Lancet*, **344**, 954–955

Veronesi, R., Mazza, C.C., Santos-Ferreira, M.O. & Lourenço, M.H. (1987) HIV-2 in Brazil (Letter to the Editor). *Lancet*, **ii**, 402

Veugelers, P.J., Schechter, M.T., Tindall, B., Moss, A.R., Page, K.A., Craib, K.J.P., Cooper, D.A., Coutinho, R.A., Charlebois, E., Winkelstein, W., Jr & van Griensven, G.J.P. (1993) Differences in time from HIV seroconversion to $CD4^+$ lymphocyte end-points and AIDS in cohorts of homosexual men. *AIDS*, **7**, 1325–1329

Veugelers, P.J., Strathdee, S.A., Tindall, B., Page, K.A., Moss, A.R., Schechter, M.T., Montaner, J.S.G. & van Griensven, G.J.P. (1994) Increasing age is associated with faster progression to neoplasms but not opportunistic infections in HIV-infected homosexual men. *AIDS*, **8**, 1471–1475

Veugelers, P.J., Strathdee, S.A., Moss, A.R., Page, K.A., Tindall, B., Schechter, M.T., Coutinho, R.A. & van Griensven, G.J.P. (1995) Is the human immunodeficiency virus-related Kaposi's sarcoma epidemic coming to an end? Insights from the Tricontinental Seroconverter Study. *Epidemiology*, **6**, 382–386

Viac, J., Guérin-Reverchon, I., Chardonnet, Y. & Brémond, A. (1990) Langerhans cells and epithelial cell modifications in cervical intraepithelial neoplasia: correlation with human papillomavirus infection. *Immunobiology*, **180**, 328–338

Victor, M. & Jarplid, B. (1988) The cause of Kaposi's sarcoma: an avian retroviral analog. *J. Am. Acad. Dermatol.*, **18**, 398–402

de Vincenzi, I. for the European Study Group on Heterosexual Transmission of HIV (1994) A longitudinal study of human immunodeficiency virus transmission by heterosexual partners. *New Engl. J. Med.*, **331**, 341–346

Vittecoq, D., Ferchal, F., Chamaret, S., Benbunan, M., Gerber, M., Hirsch, A. & Montagnier, L. (1987) Routes of HIV-2 transmission in western Europe (Letter to the Editor). *Lancet*, **i**, 1150–1151

Vlahov, D. (1995) Deregulation of the sale and possession of syringes for HIV prevention among injection drug users. *J. acquir. Immune Defic. Syndr. Hum. Retrovirol.*, **10**, 71–72

Voelkerding, K.V., Sandhaus, L.M., Kim, H.C., Wilson, J., Chittenden, T., Levine, A.J. & Raska, K., Jr (1989) Plasma cell malignancy in the acquired immune deficiency syndrome. Association with Epstein-Barr virus. *Am. J. clin. Pathol.*, **92**, 222–228

Vogel, J., Hinrichs, S.H., Reynolds, R.K., Luciw, P.A. & Jay, G. (1988) The HIV *tat* gene induces dermal lesions resembling Kaposi's sarcoma in transgenic mice. *Nature*, **335**, 606–611

Vogel, J., Cepeda, M., Enk, A.H., Ngo, L. & Jay, G. (1995) The HIV *tat* gene is a promoter of epidermal skin tumors. *Int. J. Oncol.*, **7**, 727–733

Volberding, P.A., Lagakos, S.W., Grimes, J.M., Stein, D.S., Balfour, H.H., Jr, Reichman, R.C., Bartlett, J.A., Hirsch, M.S., Phair, J.P., Mitsuyasu, R.T., Fischl, M.A. & Soeiro, R. for the AIDS Clinical Trials Group of the National Institute of Allergy and Infectious Diseases (1994) The duration of zidovudine benefit in persons with asymptomatic HIV infection. Prolonged evaluation of protocol 019 of the AIDS Clinical Trials Group. *J. Am. med. Assoc.*, **272**, 437–442

Volberding, P.A., Lagakos, S.W., Grimes, J.M., Stein, D.S., Rooney, J., Meng, T.-C., Fischl, M.A., Collier, A.C., Phair, J.P., Hirsch, M.S., Hardy, W.D., Balfour, H.H., Jr & Reichman, R.C. for the AIDS Clinical Trials Group (1995) A comparison of immediate with deferred zidovudine therapy for asymptomatic HIV-infected adults with CD4 cell counts of 500 or more per cubic millimeter. *New Engl. J. Med.*, **333**, 401–407

Vos, J., Gumodoka, B., van Asten, H.A., Berege, Z.A., Dolmans, W.M. & Borgdorff, M.W. (1994) Changes in blood transfusion practices after the introduction of consensus guidelines in Mwanza region, Tanzania. *AIDS*, **8**, 1135–1140

Wabinga, H.R., Parkin, D.M., Wabwire-Mangen, F. & Mugerwa, J.W. (1993) Cancer in Kampala, Uganda, in 1989-91: changes in incidence in the era of AIDS. *Int. J. Cancer*, **54**, 26–36

Wahman, A., Melnick, S.L., Rhame, F.S. & Potter, J.D. (1991) The epidemiology of classic, African and immunosuppressed Kaposi's sarcoma. *Epidemiol. Rev.*, **13**, 178–199

Wain-Hobson, S. (1993) The fastest genome evolution ever described: HIV variation *in situ*. *Curr. Opin. genet. Dev.*, **3**, 878–883

Walter, P.R., Philippe, E., Nguemby-Mbina, C. & Chamlian, A. (1984) Kaposi's sarcoma: presence of herpes-type virus particles in a tumor specimen. *Hum. Pathol.*, **15**, 1145–1146

Wang, R.Y.-H., Shih, J.W.-K., Grandinetti, T., Pierce, P.F., Hayes, M.M., Wear, D.J., Alter, H.J. & Lo, S.-C. (1992) High frequency of antibodies to *Mycoplasma penetrans* in HIV-infected patients. *Lancet*, **340**, 1312–1316

Wang, R.Y.-H., Shih, J.W.-K., Weiss, S.H., Grandinetti, T., Pierce, P.F., Lange, M., Alter, H.J., Wear, D.J., Davies, C.L., Mayur, R.-K. & Lo, S.-C. (1993) *Mycoplasma penetrans* infection in male homosexuals with AIDS: high seroprevalence and association with Kaposi's sarcoma. *Clin. infect. Dis.*, **17**, 724–729

Wang, J.J., Lu, Y.-L. & Ratner, L. (1994) Particle assembly and Vpr expression in human immunodeficiency virus type 1-infected cells demonstrated by immunoelectron microscopy. *J. gen. Virol.*, **75**, 2607–2614

Wang, F., So, Y., Vittinghoff, E., Malani, H., Reingold, A., Lewis, E., Giordano, J. & Janssen, R. (1995) Incidence proportion of and risk factors for AIDS patients diagnosed with HIV dementia, central nervous system toxoplasmosis, and cryptococcal meningitis. *J. acquir. Immune Defic. Syndr. hum. Retrovirol.*, **8**, 75–82

Ward, J.W., Holmberg, S.D., Allen, J.R., Cohn, D.L., Critchley, S.E., Kleinman, S.H., Lenes, B.A., Ravenholt, O., Davis, J.R., Quinn, M.G. & Jaffe, H.W. (1988) Transmission of human immunodeficiency virus (HIV) by blood transfusions screened as negative for HIV antibody. *New Engl. J. Med.*, **318**, 473–478

Ward, J.W., Bush, T.J., Perkins, H.A., Lieb, L.E., Allen, J.R., Goldfinger, D., Samson, S.M., Pepkowitz, S.H., Fernando, L.P., Holland, P.V., Kleinman, S.H., Grindon, A.J., Garner, J.L., Rutherford, G.W. & Holmberg, S.D. (1989) The natural history of transfusion-associated infection with human immunodeficiency virus. Factors influencing the progression of disease. *New Engl. J. Med.*, **321**, 947–952

Watters, J.K. (1994) Trends in risk behavior and HIV seroprevalence in heterosexual injection drug users in San Francisco, 1986–1992. *J. acquir. Immun. Defic. Syndr.*, **7**, 1276–1281

Watters, J.K., Estilo, M.J., Clark, G.L. & Lorvick, J. (1994) Syringe and needle exchange as HIV/AIDS prevention for injection drug users. *J. Am. med. Assoc.*, **271**, 115–120

Wei, X., Ghosh, S.K., Taylor, M.E., Johnson, V.A., Emini, E.A., Deutsch, P., Lifson, J.D., Bonhoeffer, S., Nowak, M.A., Hahn, B.H., Saag, M.S. & Shaw, G.M. (1995) Viral dynamics in human immunodeficiency virus type 1 infection. *Nature*, **373**, 117–122

Weich, H.A., Salahuddin, S.Z., Gill, P., Nakamura, S., Gallo, R.C. & Folkmann, J. (1991) AIDS-associated Kaposi's sarcoma-derived cells in long-term culture express and synthesize smooth muscle alpha-actin. *Am. J. Pathol.*, **139**, 1251–1258

Weiss, R.A. (1993a) Cellular receptors and viral glycoproteins involved in retrovirus entry. In: Levy, J., ed., *The Retroviridae*, Vol. 2, New York, Plenum Press, pp. 1–108

Weiss, R.A. (1993b) Cancers related to immunodeficiency. In: Iverson, O.H., ed., *New Frontiers in Cancer Causation*, Washington, Taylor & Francis, pp. 301–310

Weiss, S.H. & Biggar, R.J. (1986) The epidemiology of human retrovirus-associated illness. *Mt Sinai J. Med.*, **53**, 579–591

Weiss, R.A., Teich, N.M., Varmus, H.E. & Coffin, J.M. (1985) *RNA Tumor Viruses*, Cold Spring Harbor, NY, Cold Spring Harbor Laboratory

Weiss, R.A., Clapham, P.R., Weber, J.N., Dalgleish, A.G., Lasky, L.A. & Berman, P.W. (1986) Variable and conserved neutralization antigens of human immunodeficiency virus. *Nature*, **324**, 572–575

Weiss, P.J., Brodine, S.K., Goforth, R.R., Kennedy, C.A., Wallace, M.R., Olson, P.E., Garland, F.C., Hall, F.W., Ito, S.I. & Oldfield, E.C., III (1992) Initial low CD4 lymphocyte counts in recent human immunodeficiency virus infection and lack of association with identified coinfections. *J. infect. Dis.*, **166**, 1149–1153

Weniger, B.G., Limpakarnjanarat, K., Ungchusak, K., Thanprasertsuk, S., Choopanya, K., Vanichseni, S., Uneklabh, T., Thongcharoen, P. & Wasi, C. (1991) The epidemiology of HIV infection and AIDS in Thailand. *AIDS*, **5** (Suppl. 2), S71–S85

Werner, S., Hofschneider, P.H., Sturzl, M., Dick, I. & Roth, W.K. (1989) Cytochemical and molecular properties of simian virus 40 transformed Kaposi's sarcoma-derived cells: evidence for the secretion of a member of the fibroblast growth factor family. *J. cell. Physiol.*, **141**, 490–502

Werner, S., Hofschneider, P.H., Heldin, C.-H., Östman, A. & Roth, W.K. (1990) Cultured Kaposi's sarcoma-derived cells express functional PDGF A-type and B-type receptors. *Exp. Cell Res.*, **187**, 98–103

Werness, B.A., Levine, A.J. & Howley, P.M. (1990) Association of human papillomavirus type 16 and 18 E6 proteins with p53. *Science*, **248**, 76–79

Westmoreland, D. & Watkins, J.F. (1974) The IgG receptor induced by herpes simplex virus: studies using radioiodinated IgG. *J. gen. Virol.*, **24**, 167–178

Whimbey, E., Gold, J.W.M., Polsky, B., Dryjanski, J., Hawkins, C., Blevins, A., Brannon, P., Kiehn, T.E., Brown, A.E. & Armstrong, D. (1986) Bacteremia and fungemia in patients with the acquired immunodeficiency syndrome. *Ann. intern. Med.*, **104**, 511–514

Whitaker, L. & Renton, A. (1995) Impact of improved treatment of sexually transmitted disease on HIV infection (Letter to the Editor). *Lancet*, **346**, 1157–1160

Whitby, D., Howard, M.R., Tenant-Flowers, M., Brink, N.S., Copas, A., Boshoff, C., Hatzioannou, T., Suggett, F.E.A., Aldam, D.M., Denton, A.S., Miller, R.F., Weller, I.V.D., Weiss, R.A., Tedder, R.S. & Schulz, T.F. (1995) Detection of Kaposi's sarcoma-associated herpesvirus in peripheral blood of HIV-infected individuals and progression to Kaposi's sarcoma. *Lancet*, **346**, 799–802

Whitmore-Overton, S.E., Tillett, H.E., Evans, B.G. & Allardice, G.M. (1993) Improved survival from diagnosis of AIDS in adult cases in the United Kingdom and bias due to reporting delays. *AIDS*, **7**, 415–420

Whittle, H., Morris, J., Todd, J., Corrah, T., Sabally, S., Bangali, J., Ngom, P.T., Rolfe, M. & Wilkins, A. (1994) HIV-2-infected patients survive longer than HIV-1-infected patients. *AIDS*, **8**, 1617–1620

WHO (1986) Acquired immunodeficiency syndrome (AIDS) — WHO/CDC case definition for AIDS. *Wkly Epidemiol. Rec.*, **61**, 69–76

WHO (1988) Acquired immunodeficiency syndrome (AIDS). 1987 revision of the CDC/WHO case definition for AIDS. *Wkly epidemiol. Rec.*, **63**, 1–8

WHO (1993) *Global Programme on AIDS: Operational Characteristics of Commercially Available Assays to Detect Antibodies to HIV-1 and/or HIV-2 in Human Sera* (GPA/RES/DIA/93.4), Geneva

WHO (1995) *Global Programme on AIDS. The Current Global Situation of the HIV/AIDS Pandemic*, Geneva

Wieland, U., Hartman, J., Suhr, H., Salzberger, B., Eggers, H.J. & Kühn, J. (1994) *In vivo* genetic variability of the HIV-1 vif gene. *Virology*, **203**, 43–51

Wiener, J.S., Effert, P.J., Humphrey, P.A., Yu, L., Liu, E.T. & Walther, P.J. (1992) Prevalence of human papillomavirus types 16 and 18 in squamous-cell carcinoma of the penis: a retrospective analysis of primary and metastatic lesions by differential polymerase chain reaction. *Int. J. Cancer*, **50**, 694–701

Wilkenson, D.A., Mager, D. & Leong, J.-A. (1994) Endogenous human retroviruses. In: Levy, J.A., ed., *The Retroviridae*, New York, Plenum Press, pp. 465–536

Williams, G.R. & Talbot, I.C. (1994) Anal carcinoma — a histological review. *Histopathology*, **25**, 507–516

Williams, A.B., Darragh, T.M., Vranizan, K., Ochia, C., Moss, A.R. & Palefsky, J.M. (1994) Anal and cervical human papillomavirus infection and risk of anal and cervical epithelial abnormalities in human immunodeficiency virus-infected women. *Obstet. Gynecol.*, **83**, 205–211

Williams, A.O., Ward, J.M., Li, J.F., Jackson, M.A. & Flanders, K.C. (1995) Immunochemical localization of transforming growth factor-$\beta 1$ in Kaposi's sarcoma. *Hum. Pathol.*, **26**, 469–473

Winkelstein, W., Jr, Samuel, M., Padian, N.S., Wiley, J.A., Lang, W., Anderson, R.E. & Levy, A. (1987) The San Francisco Men's Health Study. III. Reduction in human immunodeficiency virus transmission among homosexual/bisexual men, 1982–1986. *Am. J. public Health*, **76**, 685–689

Winward, K.E. & Curtin, V.T. (1989) Conjunctival squamous cell carcinoma in a patient with human immunodeficiency virus infection. *Am. J. Ophthalmol.*, **107**, 554

Wittek, A.E., Mitchell, C.D., Armstrong, G.R., Albini, A., Martin, G.R., Seemann, R., Levenbook, I.S., Wierenga, D.E., Ridge, J., Dunlap, R.C., Lundquist, M.L., Steis, R.G., Congo, D.L., Muller, J. & Quinnan, G.V., Jr (1991) Propagation and properties of Kaposi's sarcoma-derived cell lines obtained from patients with AIDS: similarity of cultured cells to smooth muscle cells. *AIDS*, **5**, 1485–1493

Wood, G.S., Garcia, C.F., Dorfman, R.F. & Warnke, R.A. (1985) The immunohistology of follicle lysis in lymph node biopsies from homosexual men. *Blood*, **66**, 1092–1097

Wood, G.S., Burns, B.F., Dorfman, R.F. & Warnke, R.A. (1986) In situ quantitation of lymph node helper, suppressor, and cytotoxic T cell subsets in AIDS. *Blood*, **67**, 596–603

Woodworth, C.D., McMullin, E., Iglesias, M. & Plowman, G.D. (1995) Interleukin 1α and tumor necrosis factor α stimulate autocrine amphiregulin expression and proliferation of human papillomavirus-immortalized and carcinoma-derived cervical epithelial cells. *Proc. natl Acad. Sci. USA*, **92**, 2840–2844

Wright, T.C., Jr, Koulos, J., Schnoll, F., Swanbeck, J., Ellerbrock, T.V., Chiasson, M.A. & Richart, R.M. (1994) Cervical intraepithelial neoplasia in women infected with the human immunodeficiency virus: outcome after loop electrosurgical excision. *Gynecol. Oncol.*, **55**, 253–258

Wu, X., Tu, X., He, F., Shi, H., Chen, Z., Wei, Q., Jiang, H. & Shi, J. (1991) Studies on the monitoring of viruses in Chinese rhesus monkeys (*Macaca mulatta*). *Chin. J. Lab. Anim. Sci*, **1**, 179–183

Xerri, L., Hassoun, J., Planche, J., Guigou, V., Grob, J.-J., Parc, P., Birnbaum, D. & de Lapeyriere, O. (1991) Fibroblast growth factor gene expression in AIDS-Kaposi's sarcoma detected by in situ hybridization. *Am. J. Pathol.*, **138**, 9–15

Xinhua, S., Junhua, N. & Qili, G. (1994) AIDS and HIV infection in China. *AIDS*, **8** (Suppl. 2), S55–S60

Yamamoto, J.K., Sparger, E., Ho, E.W., Andersen, P.R., O'Connor, T.P., Mandell, C.P., Lowenstine, L., Munn, R. & Pedersen, N.C. (1988) Pathogenesis of experimentally induced feline immunodeficiency virus infection. *Am. J. vet. Res.*, **49**, 1246–1258

Yamamoto, J.K., Hansen, H., Ho, E.W., Morishita, T.Y., Okuda, T., Sawa, T.R., Nakamura, R.M. & Pedersen, N.C. (1989) Epidemiologic and clinical aspects of feline immunodeficiency virus infection in cats from the continental United States and Canada and possible mode of transmission. *J. Am. vet. Med. Assoc.*, **194**, 213–220

Yamanishi, K., Okuno, T., Shiraki, K., Takahashi, M., Kondo, T., Asano, Y. & Kurata, T. (1988) Identification of human herpesvirus-6 as a causal agent for exanthem subitum. *Lancet*, **i**, 1065–1067

Yarchoan, R., Lietzau, J.A., Nguyen, B.-Y., Brawley, O.W., Pluda, J.M., Saville, M.W., Wyvill, K.M., Steinberg, S.M., Agbaria, R., Mitsuya, H. & Broder, S. (1994) A randomized pilot study of alternating or simultaneous zidovudine and didanosine therapy in patients with symptomatic human immunodeficiency virus infection. *J. infect. Dis.*, **169**, 9–17

Ye, B.H., Rao, P.H., Chaganti, R.S.K. & Dalla-Favera, R. (1993) Cloning of *bcl*-6, the locus involved in chromosome translocations affecting band 3q27 in B-cell lymphoma. *Cancer Res.*, **53**, 2732–2735

Yoshizaki, K., Matsuda, T., Nishimoto, N., Kuritani, T., Taeho, L., Aozasa, K., Nakahata, T., Kawai, H., Tagoh, H., Komori, T., Kishimoto, S., Hirano, T. & Kishimoto, T. (1989) Pathogenetic significance of interleukin-6 (IL-6/BSF-2) in Castleman's disease. *Blood*, **74**, 1360–1367

Young, L.S., Finerty, S., Brooks, L., Scullion, F., Rickinson, A.B. & Morgan, A.J. (1989) Epstein–Barr virus gene expression in malignant lymphomas induced by experimental virus infection of cottontop tamarins. *J. Virol.*, **63**, 1967–1974

Yu, G. & Felsted, R.L. (1992) Effect of myristoylation on p27*nef* subcellular distribution and suppression of HIV-LTR transcription. *Virology*, **187**, 46–55

Zahger, D., Lotan, C., Admon, D., Klapholz, L., Kaufman, B., Shimon, D., Woolfson, N. & Gotsman, M.S. (1993) Very early appearance of Kaposi's sarcoma after cardiac transplantation in Sephardic Jews. *Am. Heart J.*, **126**, 999–1000

Zanetta, G., Maneo, A., Colombo, A., Ragusa, A., Gabriele, A., Placa, F. & Mangioni, C. (1995) HIV infection and invasive cervical carcinoma in an Italian population: the need for closer screening programmes in seropositive patients. *AIDS*, **9**, 909–912

Zangerle, R., Fuchs, D., Reibnegger, G., Fritsch, P. & Wachter, H. (1991) Markers for disease progression in intravenous drug users infected with HIV-1. *AIDS*, **5**, 985–991

Zaunders, J., Carr, A., McNally, L., Penny, R. & Cooper, D.A. (1995) Effects of primary HIV-1 infection on subsets of $CD4^+$ and $CD8^+$ T lymphocytes. *AIDS*, **9**, 561–566

Zhang, J. & Temin, H.M. (1994) Retrovirus recombination depends on the length of sequence identity and is not error prone. *J. Virol.*, **68**, 2409–2414

Zhang, Y.-M., Bachmann, S., Hemmer, C., van Lunzen, J., von Stemm, A., Kem, P., Dietrich, M., Ziegler, R., Waldherr, R. & Nawroth, P.P. (1994) Vascular origin of Kaposi's sarcoma: expression of leukocyte adhesion molecule-1, thrombomodulin, and tissue factor. *Am. J. Pathol.*, **144**, 51–59

Zhao, L.-J., Wang, L., Mukherjee, S. & Narayan, O. (1994) Biochemical mechanism of HIV-1 Vpr function: oligomerization mediated by the N-terminal domain. *J. biol. Chem.*, **269**, 32131–32137

Ziegler, J.L. (1993) Endemic Kaposi's sarcoma in Africa and local volcanic soils. *Lancet*, **342**, 1348–1351

Ziegler, J.L. & Katongole-Mbidde, E. (1996) Kaposi's sarcoma in childhood: an analysis of 100 cases from Uganda and relationship to HIV infection. *Int. J. Cancer*, **65**, 200–203

Ziegler, J.B., Cooper, D.A., Johnson, R.O. & Gold, J. for the Sydney AIDS Study Group (1985) Postnatal transmission of AIDS-associated retrovirus from mother to infant. *Lancet*, **i**, 896–898

zur Hausen, H. (1989) Papillomaviruses in anogenital cancer as a model to understand the role of viruses in human cancers. *Cancer Res.*, **49**, 4677–4881

HUMAN T-CELL LYMPHOTROPIC VIRUSES

1. Exposure Data

1.1 Structure, taxonomy and biology

1.1.1 *Structure*

The structure of retroviruses is reviewed in the monograph on human immunodeficiency viruses (HIV) in this volume. The human T-cell lymphotropic (T-cell leukaemia/lymphoma) viruses (HTLV) are enveloped viruses with a diameter of approximately 80–100 nm (Figure 1). The HTLV virions contain two covalently bound genomic RNA strands, which are complexed with the viral enzymes reverse transcriptase (RT; with associated RNase H activity), integrase and protease and the capsid proteins. The outer part of the virions consists of a membrane-associated matrix protein and a lipid layer intersected by the envelope proteins (Gelderblom, 1991).

Figure 1. An electron micrograph of HTLV-I virus

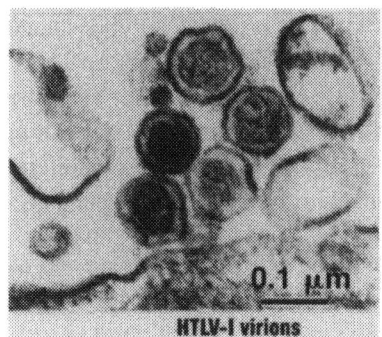

Courtesy of Dr Bernard Kramarsky, Advanced Biotechnologies, Inc., Columbia, MD, USA

1.1.2 *Taxonomy and phylogeny*

Traditionally, retroviruses (family *Retroviridae*) have been classified according to a combination of criteria including disease association, morphology and cytopathic effects *in vitro*. On this basis three subfamilies were defined. The oncoviruses (Greek, *onkos* = mass, swelling) consist of four morphological subtypes which are associated with tumours in naturally or experimentally infected animals, and non-oncogenic related viruses. The second group, the lentiviruses (Latin, *lentus* = slow), cause a variety of diseases including immunodeficiency and wasting syndromes, usually after a long period of clinical latency. The third subfamily, the spumaviruses (Latin, *spuma* = foam), so called because of the characteristic 'foamy' appearance induced in infected cells *in vitro*, have not been conclusively linked to any disease. More recently, the International Committee on the Taxonomy of Viruses has divided the *Retroviridae* family into seven genera on the basis of genetic structure. The lentiviruses and spumaviruses each constitute a genus; the oncoviruses have been subdivided into five genera (Coffin, 1996). The HTLVs form one of these genera, along with the related bovine and simian viruses (see Section 1.1.4), and in turn can be divided into type I (HTLV-I) and type II (HTLV-II) according to their genetic composition and serotype. The genotypes of HTLV types I and II are related to each other; within these types, genetic variability is greater in the type I group. By the use of the polymerase chain reaction (PCR) and sequencing, strain variation within types has been characterized in viruses from humans residing in different geographical areas.

The term HTLV-III was assigned to a virus which was later defined as HIV-1 (see the monograph in this volume).

Three subtypes of HTLV-I (known as clades (Myers *et al.*, 1993), which are defined as groups of viral strains with common nucleotides at any given position in the DNA sequence analysed) can be recognized using several analytical methods and by studying different viral genes (Figure 2) (Koralnik *et al.*, 1994).

The cosmopolitan clade (HTLV-I_{Cosm}), found in many populations across the world (also known as HTLV-IA), represents a very homogeneous group of viruses. In the New World, HTLV-I_{Cosm} was probably introduced by the slave trade (Gallo *et al.*, 1983; Gessain *et al.*, 1992a; Koralnik *et al.*, 1994) (see Figure 2).

The second clade (HTLV-I_{Zaire}), also known as HTLV-IB, was identified in central African populations in the Zairian basin (Figure 2) (Gessain *et al.*, 1992a).

The third clade (HTLV-I_{Mel}) was identified in inhabitants of Papua-New Guinea and the Solomon Islands and later in Australian Aboriginals (Bastian *et al.*, 1993; Gessain *et al.*, 1993). Phylogenetic analysis has shown that this clade (also known as HTLV-IC) and HTLV-I_{Cosm} probably evolved independently from a common ancestor (Figure 2). Analysis of sequence variations among these viral strains suggests that the HTLV-I_{Mel} clade diverged earliest, before the split between the HTLV-I_{Zaire} and HTLV-I_{Cosm} groups.

Two other subgroups have been proposed within the HTLV-I_{Cosm} clade, but rigorous phylogenetic analysis does not appear to support this notion.

Phylogenetically, HTLV-II separates into three clades: IIa, IIb and IIc. HTLV-IIa and b can be further divided into several subgroups (Dube *et al.*,1993; Neel *et al.*, 1994; Eiraku *et al.*, 1995; Gessain *et al.*, 1995a; Switzer *et al.*, 1995; Biggar *et al.*, 1996; Eiraku *et al.*, 1996). Approximately 70% of HTLV-II from intravenous drug users has been found to be HTLV-IIa. Amerindian tribes from Central and North America have the distinct type IIb, whereas remote Amazonian tribes harbour mainly subtype IIa (Biggar *et al.*, 1996; Eiraku *et al.*, 1996). These findings suggest that ancestral Amerindians who migrated to the New World brought at least two and possibly three genetic subtypes of HTLV-II (Neel *et al.*, 1994; Biggar *et al.*, 1996; Eiraku *et al.*, 1996).

Figure 2. Relationships between HTLV and STLV clades

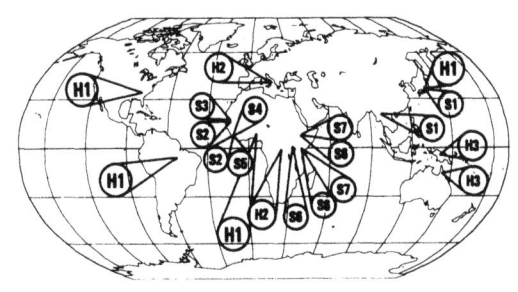

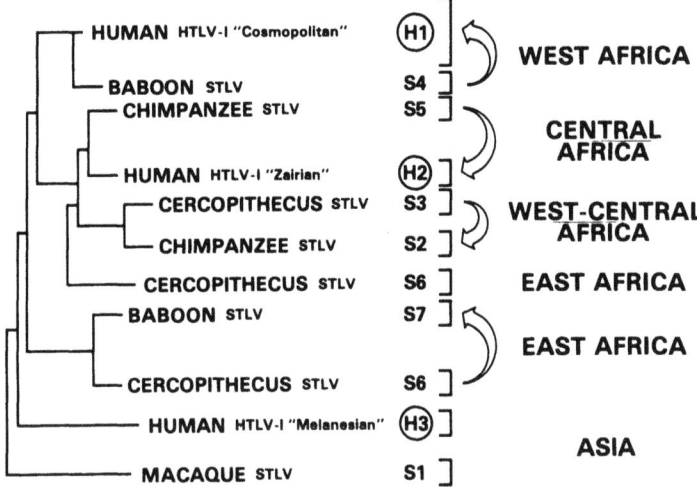

Top: Geographical origin of the samples studied. H1 corresponds to the HTLV-I$_{Cosm}$ clade, H2 to the HTLV-I$_{Zaire}$ and H3 to HTLV-I$_{Mel}$. The simian clades (S) are numbered according to the species of origin and their geographical origin.
Based on the data presented by Koralnik et al. (1994)

1.1.3 Host range

HTLV-I and HTLV-II have been isolated from humans (Poiesz et al., 1980; Kalyanaraman et al., 1982). Under experimental conditions, both HTLV-I and HTLV-II infect rabbits (Miyoshi et al., 1985; Cockerell et al., 1991) and HTLV-I can also infect rats (Yoshiki et al., 1987; Ibrahim et al., 1994). Among non-human primates, HTLV-I isolates have been shown to infect rhesus macaques (*Macaca mulatta*) (Lerche et al., 1987), cynomolgus monkeys (*M. fascicularis*) and squirrel monkeys (*Saimiri sciureus*) (Yamamoto et al., 1984; Nakamura et al., 1986). (See also Section 3).

1.1.4 *Related non-human primate viruses*

Viruses related to HTLV have been isolated from non-human primates. These are known as simian T-cell lymphotropic viruses (STLVs). DNA analysis of STLV-I strains of African and Asian origin has led to several conclusions. STLV-I from a single species can be sorted into genetically distinct clades. The distribution of STLV-I phylogenetic clades from *Cercopithecus aethiops* (African green monkey), *Pan troglodytes* (the common chimpanzee) and *Papio* (baboon) (respectively S3 and S6; S2 and S5; S4 and S7 in Figure 2) indicates that these retroviruses did not evolve within each species and suggests interspecies transfer within the primate genera, including man.

The human HTLV-I$_{Zaire}$ and the common chimpanzee clade S5 are closely related (Figure 2), suggesting that the human clade may have resulted from cross-species transmission of chimpanzee STLV-I to humans. Two additional examples of interspecies transmission which are suggested by the phylogenetic analysis of STLV-I from African primates with different geographical origins (Koralnik *et al.*, 1994) are shown in Figure 2. In the equatorial region of Africa, the STLV-I clades S2, S3 and S5 and HTLV-I$_{Zaire}$ are grouped by geographical region rather than species. Similarly, STLV-I clades S6 and S7 cluster in the eastern part of the continent. In addition, viral strains obtained from a West African baboon also cluster with the HTLV-I$_{Cosm}$ clade.

The S1 clade, from Asia, contains heterogeneous members and is closely related to HTLV-I$_{Mel}$. These results indicate the evolution of three clades in the human species and suggest that at least three independent introductions of HTLV-I into humans occurred during the evolution of these retroviruses. A simple interpretation of the global dissemination of these retroviruses might be the following. Ancestors of HTLV-I and STLV-I entered primates in Asia and were transmitted to several species. Primates infected with STLVs migrated to Africa, where the viruses were transmitted to local primate genera (*Cercopithecus, Papio, Pan* and humans). Meanwhile, HTLV-I$_{Mel}$ emerged by a separate primate-to-human transfer in Melanesia. More recent human migratory patterns, including the slave trade, led to the dissemination of the cosmopolitan HTLV-I clade worldwide. This hypothesis implies the existence of STLV for over 30 000 000 years, at least since the end of the Oligocene epoch and the beginning of the Miocene era, when the continents were linked, favouring contacts between primate species (Martin, 1990).

The recent description of STLVs in two species of African primates, the pygmy chimpanzees (*Pan paniscus*) and baboons from Ethiopia, adds further complexity to our picture of the evolution of the STLVs and HTLVs. Two closely related viruses (Giri *et al.*, 1994; Liu *et al.*, 1994) isolated from pygmy chimpanzees that live exclusively in central Africa (Kano, 1984; de Waal, 1995) are nearer to HTLV-II than to HTLV-I (Giri *et al.*, 1994; Liu *et al.*, 1994). This finding, in addition to the discovery of sporadic cases of HTLV-II infection in human pygmies (Goubau *et al.*, 1992; Gessain *et al.*, 1995a), raises questions concerning the origin and evolution of HTLV-II, previously thought to be a New World virus. Another STLV, designated primate T-lymphotropic virus-L (PTLV-L) (Goubau *et al.*, 1994), appears to be phylogenetically equidistant between HTLV-I and HTLV-II.

The observations of interspecies transmission of these phylogenetically distinct viruses among non-human primates (Saksena *et al.*, 1994) (see Section 3.2) and of indeterminate serological profiles of HTLVs (see Section 1.2) found in some human populations raise the question of the existence of other HTLV-related viruses in addition to HTLV-I and HTLV-II in humans (see also Figure 3).

Figure 3. Phylogenetic analysis of HTLV-I/STLV-I and HTLV-II/STLV-II

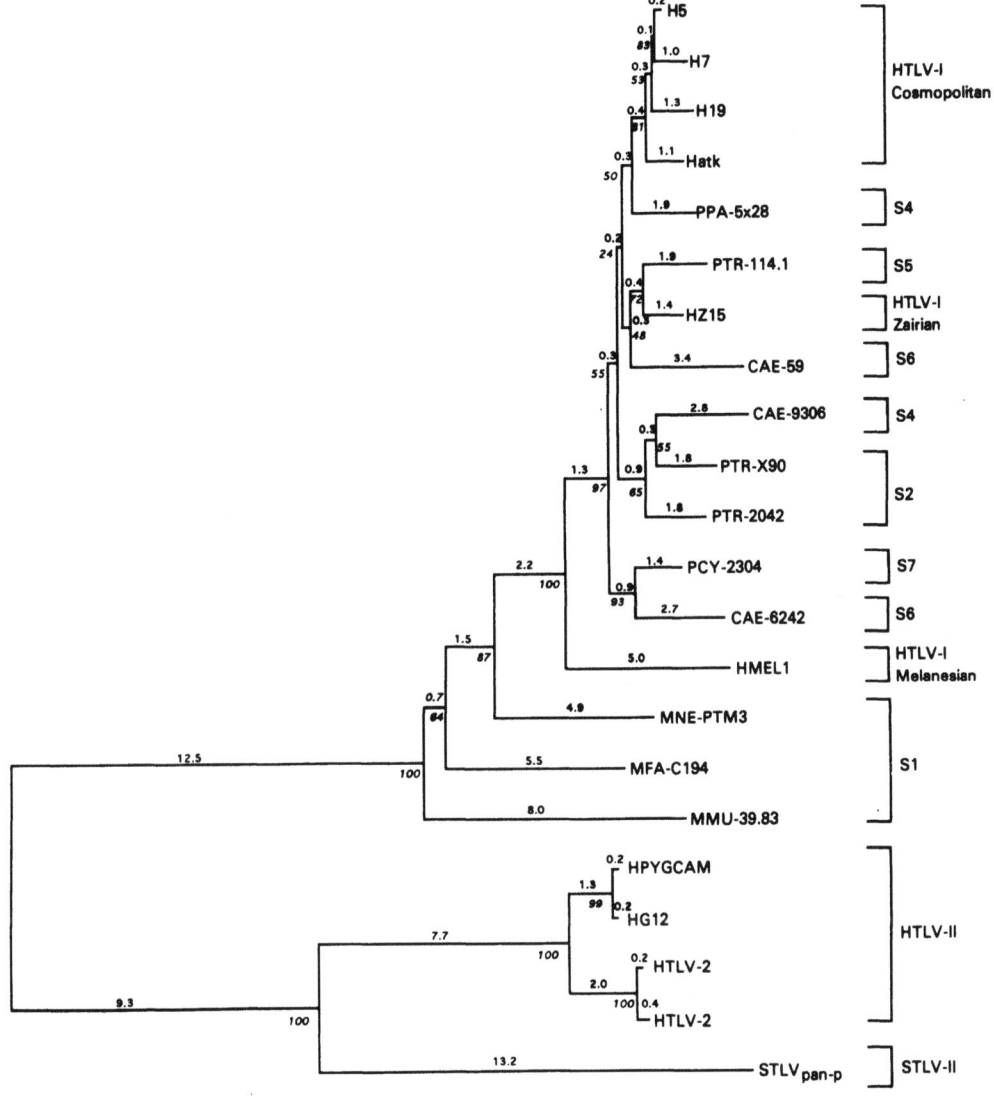

The DNA sequence of a 522 bp envelope fragment from various STLV and HTLV strains was used in a neighbour-joining analysis to define their phylogenetic relationship.
Adapted from Koralnik *et al.* (1994)

1.1.5 *Target tissue* (in vitro *and* in vivo)

HTLV-I infects CD4⁺ T-cells and occasionally CD8⁺ T-cells *in vitro* (Markham *et al.*, 1983; Popovic *et al.*, 1983) and, less efficiently, other cells including macrophages, B-cells and glial cells (Longo *et al.*, 1984; Hoffman *et al.*, 1992; Koralnik *et al.*, 1992a). *In vivo*, HTLV-I is mainly, if not exclusively, associated with CD4⁺ T-cells (Richardson *et al.*, 1990). HTLV-II infects mainly CD8⁺ T-cells *in vitro* and almost exclusively CD8⁺ T-cells *in vivo* (Rosenblatt *et al.*, 1988a; Hall *et al.*, 1994).

1.1.6 *Genomic structure and properties of gene products*

The HTLV-I genome (Seiki *et al.*, 1983) of approximately 9 kb encodes structural proteins (Gag and Env), enzymes (RT, integrase and protease) and regulatory proteins (Tax and Rex). The two long terminal repeats (LTR) located at the 5′ and 3′ ends of the viral genome contain the viral promoter and other regulatory elements. HTLV-I increases its complexity by alternative splicing of viral messenger ribonucleic acid (mRNA) in the region at the 3′ end of the genome known as pX (Seiki *et al.*, 1985; Aldovini *et al.*, 1986; Nagashima *et al.*, 1986; Furukawa *et al.*, 1991; Orita *et al.*, 1991; Berneman *et al.*, 1992a; Koralnik *et al.*, 1992b; Orita *et al.*, 1993), which contains at least four open-reading frames (Gitlin *et al.*, 1993), and possibly by the use of an internal promoter (Nosaka *et al.*, 1993). The regulatory proteins Tax and Rex are derived from this region. Rex, a post-transcriptional regulator of viral expression (Kiyokawa *et al.*, 1985; Hidaka *et al.*, 1988; Inoue *et al.*, 1991), and Tax, the viral transactivator of transcription (Sodroski *et al.*, 1984; Cann *et al.*, 1985; Felber *et al.*, 1985), are both encoded by double-spliced polycistronic mRNAs in open reading frames III and IV.

Tax, the 42 kDa viral transactivator, is a nuclear phosphoprotein which exerts its effect on the Tax-responsive elements (TRE-1 and TRE-2) located in the U3 region of the viral LTR (Sodroski *et al.*, 1984; Felber *et al.*, 1985). Tax does not bind directly to TRE-1 or TRE-2, but activates other transcriptional factors which do so. Members of the cyclic AMP (c-AMP)-responsive element-binding proteins and activating transcription factor (CREB/ATF) family (leucine zipper protein) have been shown to interact with TRE-1 (a 21-bp repeated element) (Jeang *et al.*, 1988a; Willems *et al.*, 1992a; Suzuki *et al.*, 1993; Adam *et al.*, 1994), whereas TRE-2 contains binding sites for other transcriptional factors such as Sp1, TIF-1, Ets1 and Myb (Bosselut *et al.*, 1990; Gitlin *et al.*, 1991; Bosselut *et al.*, 1992; Franchini, 1995) (reviewed in Gitlin *et al.*, 1993; Yoshida, 1994). In addition to this complex transactivation of the viral LTR U3 region, Tax also positively transactivates cellular genes. Tax-mediated transactivation pathways and the resulting effects on cellular gene expression are discussed in detail in Section 4.3.

Rex (Kiyokawa *et al.*, 1985; Nagashima *et al.*, 1986; Hidaka *et al.*, 1988; Inoue *et al.*, 1991), generated by the same double-spliced mRNA that encodes Tax, is a 27 kDa nucleolar phosphoprotein which regulates the balance of single- and double-spliced versus unspliced viral mRNAs necessary for viral replication. Rex stimulates the expression of both the single-spliced mRNA for the envelope gene and the unspliced viral genomic RNA for the Gag/Pol proteins. However, it inhibits the splicing and transport of double-spliced mRNAs which encode for Rex itself, Tax and the other alternatively spliced mRNAs in the pX region. The effect of Rex on mRNA level is exerted *in trans* on the *cis*-acting Rex response element (Rex RE), a highly stable RNA stem-loop structure in the U3/R region of the 3' LTR (Seiki *et al.*, 1985; Yoshida & Seiki, 1987; Hanly *et al.*, 1989). Since the Rex RE stem structure is present in all viral mRNAs, the differential regulation of spliced versus unspliced mRNA by Rex also relies on other *cis* elements in the viral genome (Black *et al.*, 1994a). Rex also stabilizes the mRNA for the interleukin (IL)-2Rα chain by acting *in trans* on the coding sequence of the IL-2Rα chain gene (Kanamori *et al.*, 1990), as well as indirectly potentiating IL-2 gene expression in concert with Tax (McGuire *et al.*, 1993).

1.1.7 *Other genes encoded by open reading frames I, II and III in the HTLV-I pX region*

The double-spliced mRNA that encodes Tax and Rex also encodes another protein, $p21^{rexIII}$, a cytoplasmic protein of unknown function (Furukawa *et al.*, 1991), that has been identified in several HTLV-I-infected cell lines. Transcripts for $p21^{rexIII}$ have been found to be highly expressed also in uncultured adult T-cell leukaemia/lymphoma (ATLL) samples (Berneman *et al.*, 1992b). Three other proteins are encoded by alternative splicing of the pX region and transcripts for these mRNAs have been demonstrated in infected cells *in vitro* and in *ex-vivo* samples from healthy individuals as well as from patients with ATLL and tropical spastic paraparesis/HTLV-I-associated myelopathy (TSP/HAM) (Berneman *et al.*, 1992b; Ciminale *et al.*, 1992; Koralnik *et al.*, 1992b; Orita *et al.*, 1993). Double- and single-spliced mRNAs from open reading frame I encode a single protein of 12 kDa ($p12^I$) in transfected cells (Koralnik *et al.*, 1993).

The $p13^{II}$ and $p30^{II}$ proteins, encoded by open reading frame II in the pX region, are expressed in the nucleus and nucleoli, respectively, of transfected cells (Koralnik *et al.*, 1993). Neither $p13^{II}$ nor $p30^{II}$ influences the activity of the regulatory genes *tax* and *rex* (Roithmann *et al.*, 1994).

Four additional proteins are expressed in HTLV-II from open-reading frames I, II, III and V (Ciminale *et al.*, 1995). Schematic representations of the most recent genomic maps of HTLV-I and HTLV-II are presented in Figure 4.

Spliced genes from the pX region of the bovine leukaemia virus (BLV) have also been described. This distant relative of HTLV causes B-cell leukaemia in cattle (Alexandersen *et al.*, 1993; Kettmann *et al.*, 1994), of which the clinical stages mirror those of HTLV-I-induced ATLL in humans (see Section 3.3). BLV encodes genes functionally equivalent to Tax and Rex and other proteins from the pX region. In a leukaemogenic BLV molecular clone, deletion of the R3 and G4 open reading frames (which are topologically equivalent to HTLV-I open reading frames I and II) results in an attenuated viral phenotype *in vivo* (Willems *et al.*, 1994) (see also Section 3.3.2). Whether there is a biological relationship between these proteins encoded by the BLV and HTLV-I pX region is uncertain. In the case of HTLV-II, deletion of the region encoding these proteins but sparing the *tax* and *rex* genes does not alter its ability to immortalize T-cells *in vitro* (Green *et al.*, 1995).

Figure 4. Schematic representation of the genomic structure of HTLV-I and HTLV-II

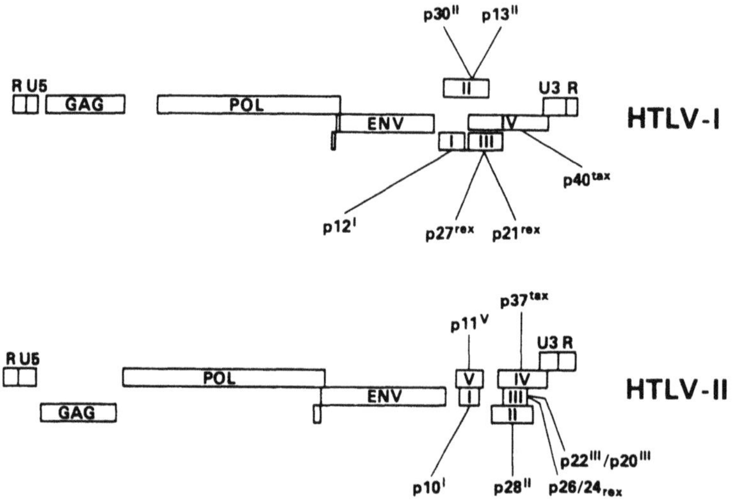

From Franchini (1995)

1.2 Methods of detection

The confirmed presence of HTLV-I or HTLV-II antibodies is considered to represent current infection, because, as with other human retroviruses, once acquired, infection is lifelong. This has been confirmed by virological and molecular studies.

1.2.1 *Serological detection of specific antibodies*

Two successive steps are generally necessary to demonstrate the presence of specific antibodies against HTLV-I or HTLV-II in serum, plasma, cerebrospinal fluid or other body fluids (Verdier *et al.*, 1990; Lal & Heinene, 1996). The first is a screening assay, while the second is a confirmatory test which can also discriminate between antibodies directed specifically against HTLV-I or HTLV-II. The screening assays include enzyme-linked immunosorbent assay (ELISA), particle agglutination assay and immunofluorescence. All three methods can be used quantitatively (Gessain *et al.*, 1988).

Commercial ELISA tests use, either alone or in combination, disrupted purified virions or specific peptides and recombinant proteins of HTLV-I or HTLV-II (Chen *et al.*, 1990; Lillehoj *et al.*, 1990; Lal *et al.*, 1991; Washitani *et al.*, 1991; Bonis *et al.*, 1993; Rudolph *et al.*, 1993, 1994; Lal, 1996). The specificity and sensitivity of these assays have been defined (Kline *et al.*, 1991; Wiktor *et al.*, 1991; Cossen *et al.*, 1992; Karopolous *et al.*, 1993; Jang *et al.* 1995). The use of additional specific peptides or recombinant proteins in earlier assays has increased their specificity.

The particle agglutination test uses gelatin particles sensitized with HTLV-I antigens (Ikeda *et al.*, 1984; Fujino *et al.*, 1991).

The indirect immunofluorescence test uses HTLV-I- and HTLV-II-producing cell lines as antigens (Aoki et al., 1985; Gallo et al., 1991).

Confirmatory assays use western blot, radioimmuno-precipitation and immunofluorescence. All commercial western blots contain disrupted purified HTLV-I virions (Gallo et al., 1994a). Generally, HTLV-I and HTLV-II induce antibodies directed against Gag proteins (p19 and p24) and their p53 precursor and Env glycoproteins (gp21 and gp46). Due to significant differences between HTLV-I and HTLV-II in the sequences of p19 and p24, HTLV-I-infected serum generally exhibits a stronger reactivity against p19 than against p24, while the opposite is true for HTLV-II (Wiktor et al., 1990). Some of these western blot assays have been supplemented by the addition of native gp46 specific to HTLV-I or recombinant gp21, recognized by both anti-HTLV-I and anti-HTLV-II antibodies (Lal et al., 1992a,b; Kleinman et al., 1994; Hadlock et al., 1995). HTLV-I and HTLV-II antibodies can be discriminated by the addition of synthetic specific peptides from the gp46 of HTLV-I (MTA1) and HTLV-II (K55) (Lipka et al., 1990; Hadlock et al., 1992; Lipka et al., 1992; Roberts et al., 1993).

A WHO working committee (WHO, 1990) proposed that confirmation of HTLV-I seropositivity must be based upon reactivity both to at least one *gag*-encoded protein (p19, p24) and to one or two *env*-encoded glycoproteins (gp21, gp46). However, more stringent criteria for HTLV-I and HTLV-II serodiagnosis have been proposed (HTLV European Research Network, 1996).

Indirect immunofluorescence has been used as a confirmatory assay to discriminate between HTLV-I and HTLV-II infection (Gallo et al., 1991).

Radioimmuno-precipitation is more sensitive than western blot, but is rarely used as a confirmatory assay because it is time-consuming, expensive and uses radioactive material. It has been useful in the detection of gp21 and gp46 seroreactivities in some unusual sero-indeterminate western blot patterns (Aboulafia et al., 1993; Gallo et al., 1994b).

Most of the immunoglobulins detected are IgG (Lal et al., 1993), but IgA and IgM can also be detected at certain periods of infection (Robert-Guroff et al., 1981; Manns et al., 1991, 1994).

Several algorithms have been used for the detection and confirmation of HTLV-I- or HTLV-II-positive serum specimens at blood banks in Japan (Aoki et al., 1985), the United States (Busch et al., 1994) and Europe (Tosswill et al., 1992; Taylor, 1996). However, some of the assays used for screening are less sensitive for HTLV-II than for HTLV-I and several studies have shown that HTLV-II may go undetected in blood donors (Hjelle et al., 1993; Weiss, 1994; Zehender et al., 1996).

1.2.2 *Detection and characterization of viral nucleic acids*

HTLV-I and HTLV-II are mainly cell-associated viruses. PCR allows the direct detection of proviral DNA sequences of HTLV-I or HTLV-II in cellular DNA (Ehrlich et al., 1990), which is usually obtained from peripheral blood mononuclear cells (PBMCs) found not only in blood but also in semen, breast milk and other body fluids (Iwahara et al., 1990). Primer pairs specific for HTLV-I and/or HTLV-II have been developed from the *pol* and *tax* regions (Ehrlich *et al.*, 1990). The genetic variability of both HTLV-I and HTLV-II is sufficiently low to permit the detection of the great majority of the existing viral strains.

Single-round PCR with 30/35 cycles can detect specific HTLV-I or HTLV-II proviral sequences in the DNA of PBMCs of persons with ATLL or TSP/HAM and in most healthy carriers. However, nested PCR is required for the detection of HTLV-I proviral sequences in a few individuals with a low viral level. The viral DNA can be sequenced either directly after PCR (Komurian *et al.*, 1991) or after cloning in one of several possible vectors (Gessain *et al.*, 1993). A simpler method to determine HTLV-I or HTLV-II viral subtype involves restriction fragment length polymorphism (RFLP) analysis of either LTR or the *env* gene (Ureta-Vidal *et al.*, 1994).

The clonal integration of provirus(es) in ATLL cells can be demonstrated by Southern blot analysis (Yamaguchi *et al.*, 1984) and/or inverse PCR (Takemoto *et al.*, 1994).

In-vivo expression of HTLV-I or HTLV-II viral antigens is very low. Detection of viral RNA can generally be achieved only by very sensitive methods such as RT/PCR or in-situ hybridization (Gessain *et al.*, 1991). In-situ PCR has recently been applied to HTLV-I infection (Levin *et al.*, 1996).

Quantification of the proviral copy number in the DNA of PBMCs can be achieved by several techniques (Tachibana *et al.*, 1992; Matsumura *et al.*, 1993; Cimarelli *et al.*, 1995; Miyata *et al.*, 1995; Morand-Joubert *et al.*, 1995) (see Section 4.3.1).

1.2.3 *Isolation of HTLV-I and HTLV-II*

Culture, in the presence of IL-2, of PBMCs from HTLV-I- or HTLV-II-infected individuals can lead, usually after several months, to the establishment of long-term T-cell lines which are either $CD4^+$ or $CD8^+$ cells expressing markers of activation (CD25, HLA-DR) (Gessain *et al.*, 1990a; Dezzutti *et al.*, 1993). These clonal T-cell lines, which can also be established by co-culture of PBMCs with phytohaemagglutinin-stimulated cord blood, produce viral particles, visible by electron microscopy, and viral antigens, as demonstrated by specific immunofluorescence using either polyclonal or monoclonal antibodies directed against p19 (Robert-Guroff *et al.*, 1981), p24 (Gessain *et al.*, 1990b) or gp46 (Edouard *et al.*, 1994). These cell lines release viral Gag antigens into the culture supernatant, detectable by an antigen capture assay. The use of the BJAB cell line is very useful to isolate HTLV-II from cultured PBMCs of a patient co-infected with HTLV-II and HIV (Hall *et al.*, 1992).

1.2.4 *Sero-indeterminate HTLV-I western blots*

There are difficulties in interpreting some western blots of HTLV-I or HTLV-II in serum specimens, particularly those from tropical areas (Weber *et al.*, 1989; Verdier *et al.*, 1990; Gessain *et al.*, 1995a). A high percentage of western blots of specimens from equatorial Africa and Melanesia exhibit indeterminate patterns, with reactivities to '*gag*-encoded proteins' p19, and/or p24 and/or p53 and/or proteins of uncertain origin (p26, p28, p32 and p36), but without reactivity to Env glycoproteins gp21 and gp46 (Garin *et al.*, 1994). As a consequence, a number of studies have overestimated the

HTLV-I seroprevalence in these regions (Biggar *et al.*, 1985; Brabin *et al.*, 1989; Garin *et al.*, 1994). In an effort to standardize results, more stringent criteria for western blot positivity have been proposed by WHO (1990) and by the Centers for Disease Control and Prevention (CDC) (1992).

With commercial HTLV-I western blot kits that contain only low amounts of native glycoprotein (gp21, gp46), only persons with high HTLV-I titres, such as patients with TSP/HAM, exhibit a clear Env reactivity. Despite significant progress in specificity of western blot assays, some problems remain; for example, the low specificity of sero-reactivity directed against the recombinant Env gp21 leads to false-positive interpretations. A modified version of this recombinant antigen with higher specificity is now available (Varma *et al.*, 1995). The WHO and the CDC diagnostic guidelines need to be further validated for samples originating from tropical areas (Gessain *et al.*, 1995b).

1.2.5 *Seronegative HTLV-I-infected individuals*

A few individuals have been described who are seronegative for both HTLV-I and HTLV-II, but in whom fragments of HTLV-I provirus in their PBMCs have been detected by PCR. In some West Indian HTLV-I-seronegative patients with a clinical TSP/HAM syndrome, some investigators have demonstrated the presence of HTLV-I-related sequences in their PBMC DNA. In most such cases, the detected sequences were small fragments of the *tax* and/or *pol* genes. Recently, an HTLV-I-seronegative TSP/HAM patient harbouring a defective HTLV-I virus in his PBMCs was reported (Daenke *et al.*, 1994). However, most studies indicate that, in healthy individuals, this is very rare, even in HTLV-I endemic areas. Thus, several studies performed in Japan, in the Caribbean region and in the United States have failed to detect HTLV-I proviral sequences in the DNA of PBMCs from seronegative subjects, even children born to HTLV-I-seropositive parents. The possibility of a cryptic infection in which HTLV-I resides elsewhere than in the peripheral blood remains, however, a possibility.

The issue of detection of proviral HTLV sequences in seronegative patients with cutaneous T-cell lymphomas other than ATLL is discussed in Section 2.1.2.

1.3 Epidemiology of HTLV infection

1.3.1 *HTLV-I transmission*

Three modes of transmission have been demonstrated for HTLV-I.

(a) *Mother-to-child transmission*

Mother-to-child transmission represents a major mode of transmission of HTLV-I in endemic areas, mainly due to breast-feeding beyond six months (Hino, 1990a; Tajima *et al.*, 1990a; Takahashi *et al.*, 1991; Monplaisir *et al.*, 1993; Wiktor *et al.*, 1993; Hino *et al.*, 1994), after which time the protective IgG maternal antibodies decline (Takahashi *et al.*, 1991). Seroconversion (the development of detectable specific antibodies to the virus in the serum) in children occurs between 18 and 24 months of age (Takahashi *et al.*, 1991). Depending on the population studied, 10–25% of breast-fed children from

HTLV-I-seropositive mothers become infected with the virus (Ando *et al.*, 1987; Hino *et al.*, 1987a,b; Hino, 1990a; Tajima *et al.*, 1990a; Takahashi *et al.*, 1991; Ando *et al.*, 1993; Monplaisir *et al.*, 1993; Hino *et al.*, 1994). This transmission is linked to the presence of HTLV-I provirus in mononuclear cells in breast milk (Kinoshita *et al.*, 1984, 1985a). Maternal factors associated with transmission, which correlate with high HTLV-I viral load, are: high HTLV-I antibody titres directed against the whole virus, presence of anti-Tax antibodies and in-vitro maternal HTLV-I antigen expression in short-term culture (Sugiyama *et al.*, 1986; Hino *et al.*, 1987a; Sawada *et al.*, 1989; Kashiwagi *et al.*, 1990; Wiktor *et al.*, 1993). Other factors include the presence of antibodies directed against certain immunogenic epitopes of the gp46 envelope glycoprotein and maternal age > 30 years (Wiktor *et al.*, 1993).

Strong evidence that breast-feeding plays the predominant role in mother-to-child transmission comes from Japanese studies in which advice to HTLV-I-seropositive mothers not to breast-feed their babies resulted in a significant decrease in mother-to-child transmission of the virus, albeit with unexplained regional variation (Ando *et al.*, 1987; Hino *et al.*, 1987a; Tsuji *et al.*, 1990; Hino *et al.*, 1994; Katamine *et al.*, 1994). Thus in Nagasaki prefecture, the risk of the maternal transmission was reduced from 20–30% to 3% by bottle feeding (Hino *et al.*, 1994; Takezaki *et al.*, 1996), whereas in Okinawa prefecture about 13% of bottle-fed children (all under 10 years of age and none transfused) born to carrier mothers were infected by HTLV-I. Evidence against transplacental transmission comes from a study in which none of seven children with HTLV-I proviral DNA-positive cord blood cells seroconverted by 24–48 months. The observation that none of the cord blood samples of nine formula-fed children, who were later confirmed to be infected, was positive for HTLV-I suggests that intrauterine infection was not the cause of viral transmission (Katamine *et al.*, 1994).

There are no data on the role of vaginal delivery in HTLV-I transmission.

(b) Sexual transmission

HTLV-I is sexually transmissible and this transmission is more efficient from men to women than the reverse (Tajima *et al.*, 1982; Kajiyama *et al.*, 1986; Stuver *et al.*, 1993; Take *et al.*, 1993; Figueroa *et al.*, 1995; Takezaki *et al.*, 1995). The risk for transmission, over 10 years, from seropositive husbands to wives has been calculated at 60%, whereas that for transmission from wives to husbands was only 0.4% (Kajiyama *et al.*, 1986). Another study reported that over 50% of the wives of HTLV-I seropositive husbands were infected within one to four years after marriage (Take *et al.*, 1993). Female prostitutes of Fukuoka (Japan) had a significantly higher seroprevalence of HTLV-I antibodies than various control populations (Nakashima *et al.*, 1995). In prostitutes in Peru, HTLV-I seropositivity was linked to duration of prostitution, lack of consistent condom use and past infection with *Chlamydia trachomatis* (Wignall *et al.*, 1992; Gotuzzo *et al.*, 1994). In a group of 409 Zairian prostitutes from Kinshasa, the annual incidence of HTLV-I was 0.7% (Delaporte *et al.*, 1995). Risk factors for HTLV-I infection in Jamaican women attending sexually transmitted disease clinics included multiple sexual partnership, a current diagnosis of syphilis and the presence of other venereal diseases (Murphy *et al.*, 1989a). Further strong evidence for sexually transmitted infection comes from a prospective study of 600 subjects over the age of 40 years tested during 1976–93; eight seroconverted, of whom five had an HTLV-I-seropositive spouse and two seroconverted after blood transfusions (Takezaki *et al.*, 1995). In Europe, HTLV-I-infected blood donors, who are usually female, are almost always from an endemic area or have had sexual intercourse with a person from an HTLV-I endemic area (The HTLV Europe Research Network, 1996; Taylor, 1996). Seroconversion in the female partner of a transplant recipient infected by blood transfusion has also been documented (Gout *et al.*, 1990).

(c) *Transmission by blood*

Infection by blood transfusion appears to be the most efficient mode of HTLV-I transmission, with a 15–60% risk of infection among recipients of a contaminated cellular blood product (Okochi *et al.*, 1984; Inaba *et al.*, 1989; Manns *et al.*, 1991; Sandler *et al.*, 1991; Manns *et al.*, 1992; Donegan *et al.*, 1994). Fresh frozen plasma, which is acellular, is not infectious. Platelets are more likely than red blood cells to transmit HTLV-I infection when transfused, probably because they are more heavily contaminated by T lymphocytes (Okochi *et al.*, 1984; Lairmore *et al.*, 1989; Manns *et al.*, 1991; Sandler *et al.*, 1991; Manns *et al.*, 1992). Infectivity decreases with increasing duration of storage at 4 °C, a temperature at which lymphocyte survival is reduced. In a study in Jamaica, immunosuppressive therapy at the time of transfusion was found to increase the risk of HTLV-I seroconversion (Manns *et al.*, 1992).

In highly endemic areas such as southern Japan and the West Indies, with a 0.5–5% HTLV-I seroprevalence among blood donors (Gessain *et al.*, 1984; Minamoto *et al.*, 1988), multi-transfused patients (Barbara, 1994) including renal transplant recipients (Linhares *et al.*, 1994) have high HTLV-I seroprevalence. Screening of blood donations has been implemented in Japan (Maeda *et al.*, 1984; Okochi *et al.*, 1984), French Guiana and the Caribbean islands of Martinique and Guadeloupe (Massari *et al.*, 1994; Pillonel *et al.*, 1994), the United States (Williams *et al.*, 1988; Lee *et al.*, 1991; Sandler *et al.*, 1991), Canada, France (Couroucé *et al.*, 1993; Massari *et al.*, 1994; Pillonel *et al.*, 1994) and Denmark (Bohn Christiansen *et al.*, 1995) and Netherlands during the last decade. The issues in relation to testing blood donors in other European countries have been discussed (Salker *et al.*, 1990; Brennan *et al.*, 1993; Soriano *et al.*, 1993; Taylor, 1996). In areas of low endemicity (0.002–0.02% among blood donors) such as metropolitan France and the United States, HTLV-I seropositivity among donors is associated mainly with birth in highly endemic regions (such as the West Indies) or with having sexual partners from endemic areas. In various African and South American countries, where HTLV-I seroprevalence in blood donors ranges from 0.2% to 1%, it has been suggested that compulsory HTLV-I screening of donors should be considered (Gutfraind *et al.*, 1994; Ferreira *et al.*, 1995).

Transmission of both HTLV-I and HTLV-II between intravenous drug users has been documented, with a higher rate for HTLV-II than for HTLV-I (Hall *et al.*, 1994; Schwebke *et al.*, 1994; Hall *et al.*, 1996).

1.3.2 *Animal models of HTLV-I transmission*

Experiments have demonstrated that HTLV-I can be transmitted to and infect several species of monkeys (Yamamoto *et al.*, 1984; Nakamura *et al.*, 1986), rabbits (Miyoshi *et al.*, 1985; Cockerell *et al.*, 1991) and rats (Ibrahim *et al.*, 1994) by either intravenous or intraperitoneal inoculation of autologous or heterologous HTLV-I-transformed cell lines. HTLV-I infection of rabbits or marmosets has been effected by intravenous or oral inoculation of HTLV-I-transformed and virus-producing cells (Kinoshita *et al.*, 1985a; Yamanouchi *et al.*, 1985; Uemura *et al.*, 1986; Iwahara *et al.*, 1990). Inoculation of rabbits with cell-free concentrated HTLV-I virions led to only a transient seroconversion, without detectable virus remaining after a few months (Miyoshi, 1994). Experimental transmission of HTLV-I by blood transfusion and from mother to offspring has also been observed in rabbits (Uemura *et al.*, 1986; Iwahara *et al.*, 1990); as little as 0.01 mL of infected blood (corresponding to 1.7×10^4 lymphocytes) was capable of transmitting the virus. Hori *et al.* (1995) have demonstrated intrauterine transmission of HTLV-I in rats, albeit at a low rate.

1.3.3 *Geographical distribution of HTLV-I*

HTLV-I is not a ubiquitous virus but is spread throughout the world with small clusters of hyperendemicity located within endemic areas (Levine *et al.*, 1988; Mueller, 1991; Blattner & Gallo, 1994). Information on seroprevalence has been based on surveys of highly variable size and quality and may not be reliable. Only in Japan have population-based studies been conducted. In endemic areas, the HTLV-I antibody prevalence in the adult population varies from 0.2% to 15% (see Figure 5). Based on strict diagnostic criteria using confirmatory assays (western blot; WHO, 1990; Gessain & Mathieux, 1995) and/or specific immunofluorescence (Gallo *et al.*, 1991), low HTLV-I seroprevalence refers to seropositivity in adults ranging from 0.2% to 2%, while higher rates in adults define highly endemic areas. The latter include the south-western islands of Japan, the Caribbean, South America, intertropical Africa, parts of the Middle East (Iran) and Melanesia.

In the Far East, the Japanese islands of Okinawa, Kyushu and Shikoku represent highly endemic areas, with an estimated one million HTLV-I carriers (Tajima *et al.*, 1982; Hino *et al.*, 1984; Ishida *et al.*, 1985; Hinuma, 1986; Tajima *et al.*, 1986, 1987; Kosaka *et al.*, 1989; Tajima & Hinuma, 1992; Morofuji-Hirata *et al.*, 1993; Tajima *et al.*, 1994; Brodine *et al.*, 1995). Most other parts of Japan have lower seroprevalence. The rest of the Far East region has a low level of HTLV-I endemicity, with sporadic cases reported in Taiwan (Wang *et al.*, 1988; Chen *et al.*, 1994), in some areas of India (Babu *et al.*, 1993; Singhal *et al.*, 1993), China (Pan *et al.*, 1991), Korea (Lee *et al.*, 1986), Nepal (Ishida *et al.*, 1992) and the Philippines (Ishida *et al.*, 1988). Few data are available relating to Siberia (Gessain *et al.*, 1996a) or Mongolia (Batsuuri *et al.*, 1993), but sporadic cases of HTLV-I infection in individuals living in the central part of Sakhalin island have been reported (Gurtsevitch *et al.*, 1995; Gessain *et al.*, 1996a). In spite of some reported cases of HTLV-I infection, circumpolar populations cannot be considered as endemically infected (Robert-Guroff *et al.*, 1985; Davidson *et al.*, 1990).

Figure 5. Estimated percentage of HTLV-I carriers among blood donors ≥ 40 years) in Japanese prefectures in 1983

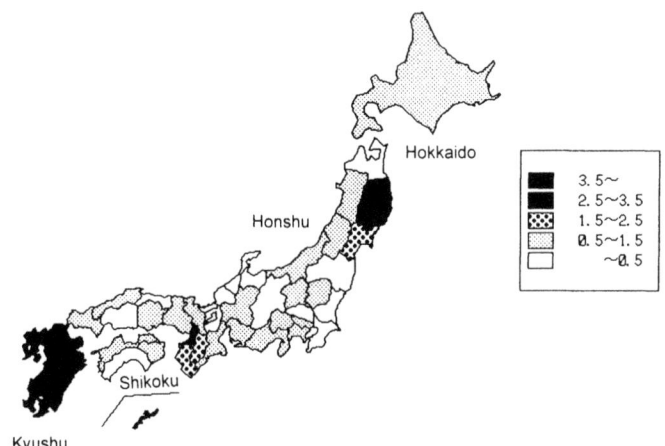

From Maeda et al. (1984)

Africa is often considered to be the largest reservoir for HTLV-I infection. It has been estimated that 5–10 million individuals may be infected (Hunsmann et al., 1984; Saxinger et al., 1984; Verdier et al., 1994), in most tropical countries including Benin, Burkina-Fasso, Equatorial Guinea, Ghana, Guinea, Guinea Bissau, Ivory Coast, Mali, Nigeria, Senegal and Tchad in west Africa (Biggar et al., 1984; Hunsmann et al., 1984; Saxinger et al., 1984; de Thé et al., 1985; de Thé & Gessain, 1986; Delaporte et al., 1989a; Ouattara et al., 1989; Verdier et al., 1989; Dumas et al., 1991; Biggar et al., 1993; Dada et al., 1993; Del Mistro et al., 1994; Verdier et al., 1994; Jeannel et al., 1995) and Cameroon, Central African Republic, the Congo, Gabon and Zaire in central Africa (Hunsmann et al., 1984; Saxinger et al., 1984; Delaporte et al., 1989b; Goubau et al., 1990; Delaporte et al., 1991; Schrijvers et al., 1991; Goubau et al., 1993a; Garin et al., 1994; Mauclere et al., 1994; Tuppin et al., 1996). While most of these countries exhibit low HTLV-I seroprevalence overall, areas of high prevalence have been detected in southern Gabon (Delaporte et al., 1989, 1991; Schrijvers et al., 1991) and northern Zaire (Goubau et al., 1990, 1993a; Garin et al., 1994). In north Africa (El-Farrash et al., 1988; Farouqi et al., 1992), east and South Africa (Hunsmann et al., 1984; Saxinger et al., 1984; Bhigjee et al., 1990, 1993; Verdier et al., 1994) and Indian Ocean islands (Mahieux et al., 1994), the level of endemicity seems very low, despite occasional clusters, such as in the Seychelles (Román et al., 1987).

In the Americas, highly endemic areas include the Caribbean islands of Haiti, Jamaica, Martinique and Trinidad (Schaffar-Deshayes et al., 1984; Clark et al., 1985a; Miller et al., 1986; Gibbs et al., 1987; Riedel et al., 1989; Blattner et al., 1990; Fréry et al., 1991; Maloney et al., 1991; Murphy et al., 1991; Ramirez et al., 1991; Allain et al., 1992; Manns et al., 1992; Miller et al., 1994) and limited areas of South America such as Tumaco in Colombia (Trujillo et al., 1992) and the Noir-Marron territory in

French Guiana (Gessain et al., 1984; Gérard et al., 1995; Tuppin et al., 1995). Low-level HTLV-I endemicity has been reported in large regions of Latin America (Ohtsu et al., 1987; Maloney et al., 1989; Cevallos et al., 1990; Pombo de Oliveira et al., 1990; Zamora et al., 1990; Guerena-Burgueno et al., 1992; Duenas-Barajas et al., 1993). In the United States and Canada, prevalence is low except in Afro-Americans and in recent immigrants from endemic areas (Weinberg et al., 1988; Williams et al., 1988; Khabbaz et al., 1990; Chadburn et al., 1991; Eble et al., 1993; Dekaban et al., 1994; Harrington et al., 1995).

There is no known HTLV-I endemic area in Europe; early reports from southern Italy (Manzari et al., 1985) are disputed (de Stasio et al., 1989; Chironna et al., 1994) and most cases of HTLV-I infection have been in immigrants from the West Indies, Africa or the Middle East, or in persons who had sexual relationships with such immigrants (Cruickshank et al., 1989; Wyld et al., 1990; Taylor, 1996). However, sporadic cases of HTLV-I infection without evidence of a link with an endemic area have been reported in Greece (Dalekos et al., 1995), Romania (Paun et al., 1994), Georgia (Senjuta et al., 1991), Sicily (Boeii et al., 1995; Mansueto et al., 1995) and the United Kingdom (Wyld et al., 1990).

While in European countries the great majority of HTLV-seropositive blood donors are infected with HTLV-I (Taylor, 1996), in the United States (Lee et al., 1991), 60–70% are infected with HTLV-II.

In the Middle East, the Mashhad region in northern Iran appears to be an important reservoir of HTLV-I infection (Achiron et al., 1993; Nerurkar et al., 1995), with seropositive emigrants from this region now living in Israel, the United States (Meytes et al., 1990) and northern Italy (Achiron et al., 1993). Furthermore, sporadic cases of HTLV-I infection have been reported in Iraq (Denic et al., 1990) and Kuwait (Voevodin et al., 1995).

In the Pacific region, isolated clusters of HTLV-I have been described, especially in two tribes of Papua New Guinea (Garruto et al., 1990; Yanagihara et al., 1990; Lal et al., 1992c; Nerurkar et al., 1992; Yanagihara, 1994) and in the Australian Aboriginal population (May et al., 1988; Bastian et al., 1993; Bolton et al., 1994). Furthermore, HTLV-I is endemic in the Solomon Islands (Garruto et al., 1990; Yanagihara et al., 1991), but seems very rare in most other Pacific islands (Garruto et al., 1990).

The origin of this puzzling geographical clustering is not well understood, but is probably linked to a founder effect in certain communities, with persistence due to a putatively high mother-to-child transmission of the virus under favourable environmental and cultural conditions (Tajima et al., 1990a; Mueller, 1991; Kaplan & Khabbaz, 1993; Blattner & Gallo, 1994; Tajima et al., 1994). Such clustering linked to the background of the population has been studied in French Guiana (Tuppin et al., 1995): among 1873 pregnant women (the HTLV-I serological status could be established for 1716 of them), the HTLV-I seroprevalence rate differed significantly between ethnic groups: 5.7% for Noir-Marron (70/1302), 6.3% for Haitian (3/50) and 0% for Creole (0/126), Amerindians (0/166) and Hmong (0/64). Thus, the Noir-Marron, descendants of fugitive slaves of African origin, with limited contact with other groups, represent a major reservoir for

HTLV-I infection (Gessain *et al.*, 1984; Gérard *et al.*, 1995; Tuppin *et al.*, 1995). In Trinidad, among a sample of persons selected from a government register, 3.2% of 1025 persons of African descent were HTLV-I-seropositive compared with 0.2% among 487 persons of Asian descent, while the prevalence of HTLV-I infection was 11.4% among persons of African ancestry in a coastal village of Tobago (Blattner *et al.*, 1990).

1.3.4 *HTLV-I prevalence and demographic features of HTLV-I infection*

It has been estimated that worldwide between 15 and 20 million individuals are infected with HTLV-I, with 2–10% developing an HTLV-I-associated disease during their lifetime (de Thé & Bomford, 1993; Blattner & Gallo, 1994) (described in Sections 1.4 and 2.1). In highly endemic areas, and despite widely different socioeconomic and cultural environments, the HTLV-I seroprevalence is low and stable among children but increases gradually with age, most markedly in women over 50 years of age, but also in men (Tajima & Hinuma, 1984; Tajima *et al.*, 1987; Maloney *et al.*, 1991; Mueller, 1991; Murphy *et al.*, 1991; Blattner & Gallo, 1994). Several explanations for this significant age-dependent increase in HTLV-I seroprevalence in women have been proposed. First, it could be the result of an accumulation of sexual exposure with increasing age. However, for most sexually transmitted infections, transmission occurs mainly during the period when sexual activity is at its peak (Mueller, 1991). Second, the apparent age-dependence may be confounded by a cohort effect (Blattner *et al.*, 1986; Chavance *et al.*, 1989; Ueda *et al.*, 1989; Chavance & Fréry, 1993; Takezaki *et al.*, 1995), suggested in some but not all cross-sectional surveys in Japan. Finally, these infections in older persons might be due to reactivation of silent infection which becomes apparent on account of immuno-dysregulation that occurs with aging. However, several studies using PCR methods have failed to detect proviral DNA sequences in the PBMCs of HTLV-I-seronegative healthy individuals (Nakashima *et al.*, 1990). Thus, there is at present no consistent explanation for the excess prevalence among older people (Figure 6).

In Kumamoto (Japan), the annual age- and sex-specific HTLV-I carrier prevalence in blood donors below 50 years of age declined between 1986 to 1990 in both sexes, and it has been suggested that the HTLV-I carrier state of individuals below the age of 50 years will become negligible in southern Japan within the first half of the next century (Oguma, 1990; Oguma *et al.*, 1992, 1995).

1.3.5 *Epidemiology of tropical spastic paraparesis/HTLV-I-associated myelopathy*

The etiological link between HTLV-I and tropical spastic paraparesis/HTLV-I-associated myelopathy (TSP/HAM) is based on: (1) observations of very high prevalence (up to 90%) of HTLV-I infection in patients with TSP, (2) the occurrence of TSP/HAM following transfusion with HTLV-I-contaminated blood and (3) the decreased incidence of TSP/HAM in transfusion recipients after the introduction of blood donor screening for HTLV-I in Japan (Gessain *et al.*, 1985; Osame *et al.*, 1986a,b; Gout *et al.*, 1990; Kaplan *et al.*, 1990).

Figure 6. Age- and sex-specific HTLV-I seroprevalence in Japan (Miyazaki cohort study) and Jamaica (applicants for food-handling licences)

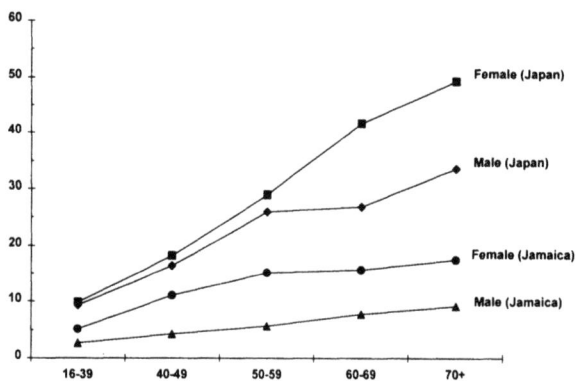

From Mueller & Blattner (1996)

The association between HTLV-I and tropical spastic paraparesis (TSP) in the French West Indies (Martinique) was described in 1985 (Gessain et al., 1985) and was soon confirmed in Jamaica (Rodgers-Johnson et al., 1988) and in Colombia (Rodgers-Johnson et al., 1985), and subsequently in Japan, where the same clinical entity was named HTLV-I-associated myelopathy (HAM) by Osame et al. (1986a). TSP/HAM is more frequent in women (sex ratio ranging from 1 : 1.5 in Japan 1 : 3.5 in Martinique) and is common in most HTLV-I endemic areas, but is very rare in children (Osame et al., 1986a; Román et al., 1987; Shibasaki et al., 1989; Kaplan et al., 1990; Kayembe et al., 1990; Janssen et al., 1991; Ramiandrisoa et al., 1991; Gessain & Gout, 1992; Jeannel et al., 1993), where it can be one of the major neurological diseases. Reliable estimates of TSP/HAM incidence and prevalence are available only for Japan, some Caribbean areas and rare clusters in Africa and South America (Gessain & Gout, 1992). Thus, the prevalence of TSP/HAM ranges from 8.6/100 000 inhabitants in Kyushu (Japan) (Shibasaki et al., 1989; Kaplan et al., 1990; Osame et al., 1990) to 128/100 000 in Mahé (Seychelles) (Gessain & Gout, 1992). Estimates of the annual incidence range from 0.04/100 000 in Kyushu (Shibasaki et al., 1989; Kaplan et al., 1990) to 3/100 000 in Lisala (Zaire) (Kayembe et al., 1990). The female predominance seems to be less marked in South America (Araújo et al., 1993), where TSP/HAM affects all racial groups (Araújo et al., 1993; Rodgers-Johnson, 1994; Domingues et al., 1995).

The prevalence of TSP/HAM varies greatly across geographical areas despite similar levels of HTLV-I seropositivity (Román et al., 1987; Kaplan et al., 1990; Kayembe et al., 1990; Trujillo et al., 1992; Jeannel et al., 1993). Thus, southern Japan and Martinique have similar seroprevalence of HTLV-I, but in Martinique, the prevalence of TSP/HAM among HTLV-I carriers (around 250 cases among 6000–10 000 HTLV-I carriers in a total population of 333 000) is estimated at 1.5–3%, while in Japan, the prevalence of TSP/HAM in HTLV-I-infected persons is estimated to be only 0.08% (Kaplan et al., 1990).

Within a particular geographical area, the prevalence of TSP/HAM can vary according to ethnic group. Thus in Inongo, Zaire (Jeannel et al., 1993), among the five major ethnic groups, the Bolia exhibit the highest prevalence of HTLV-I (6.5%) without any detected TSP/HAM cases, while six TSP/HAM cases were found among the Ntomba, whose HTLV-I prevalence rate was only 2.2%. Such findings suggest that, besides HTLV-I infection, environmental and/or genetic cofactors play a part in the development of TSP/HAM.

People infected with HTLV-I through blood transfusion have a higher risk for developing TSP/HAM than people infected by other means (Gout et al., 1990; Osame et al., 1990). In Japan and Martinique, up to 20% of TSP/HAM patients had a blood transfusion in the five years preceding onset of the disease. In the first two years of screening of the blood supply in Japan for HTLV-I, started at the end of 1986, a 16% decrease in patients with TSP/HAM was reported (Osame et al., 1990). Direct evidence for a causal relationship between HTLV-I and TSP/HAM was obtained when a seronegative cardiac graft recipient seroconverted 14 weeks after an HTLV-I-positive blood transfusion and, four weeks later, exhibited a severe disorder of the pyramidal tract identical to that seen in TSP/HAM. HTLV-I was isolated from mononuclear cell cultures from his peripheral blood and from his cerebrospinal fluid (Gout et al., 1990).

In contrast, development of ATLL after HTLV-I infection by blood transfusion seems extremely rare, if it exists (Williams et al., 1991).

1.3.6 *Natural history of HTLV-I primary infection*

Among the several dozen documented cases of HTLV-I seroconversion, no acute seroconversion illness has been reported. Following infection with HTLV-I by blood transfusion, viral IgG-specific antibodies are detectable within one to four months in most cases. In the first two months after infection, antibody to Gag protein predominates, with anti-p24 generally appearing before anti-p19. Antibody to recombinant gp21 is frequently the earliest Env reactivity detected, with anti-gp46 appearing later. Anti-Tax antibodies appear much later (Manns et al., 1991, 1994). In the first three months, IgM are the most frequent isotypes, although IgG and IgA can also be detected. HTLV-I-specific antibody responses persist in all Ig isotypes during the next four to six months and remain for many years (Manns et al., 1994).

1.3.7 *Molecular epidemiology of HTLV-I*

Based on sequence and/or RFLP analysis of more than 250 HTLV-I isolates originating from the main viral endemic areas, three major clades have emerged (Gessain et al., 1996b). Between the three clades (HTLV-I_{Cosm} or HTLV-IA, HTLV-I_{Zaire} or HTLV-IB and HTLV-I_{Mel} or HTLV-IC (see Section 1.1.2), depending on the gene, the nucleotide changes range from 0.5 to 10%. DNA sequence analyses indicate that, within the three clades, there exist molecular subgroups clearly defined by several specific mutations, but these are not always consistent with phylogenetic analyses. For example, there is evidence for two ancestral HTLV-I lineages in Japan (Mahieux et al., 1995): the classical cosmopolitan genotype, that represents around 25% of the Japanese HTLV-I and is found mainly in the southern islands, and another related subgroup called the 'Japanese' group, that differs at the nucleotide level by around 1.6% in the LTR and is evenly distributed in the Japanese archipelago (Ureta-Vidal et al., 1994). Similarly, within the central African clade (HTLV-I$_{zaire}$), there are molecular subgroups defined by specific substitutions in either the Env or the LTR sequences.

1.3.8 HTLV-II epidemiology

In 1982, HTLV-II was isolated from a cell line derived from the splenic cells of a patient with a lymphoproliferative disease originally considered to be a 'T variant of hairy-cell leukaemia' (Kalyanaraman et al., 1982).

While the modes of transmission of HTLV-II appear to be basically the same as those of HTLV-I, the global distribution of HTLV-II is very different. HTLV-II is highly endemic among some scattered Amerindian tribes including the Navajo and Pueblo in New Mexico, the Seminole in Florida, the Guaymi in Panama, the Cayapo (Kayapo) and Kraho in Brazil, the Wayu and Guahido in Colombia and the Tobas and Matacos in northern Argentina (Heneine et al., 1991; Gabbai et al., 1993; Black et al., 1994b; Bouzas et al., 1994) (reviewed in Hall et al., 1994, 1996). In these populations, HTLV-II seroprevalence varies greatly but can reach 20% of the general adult population and up to 50% in women aged over 50 years, as in Cayapo groups living in Brazil (Black et al., 1994b). HTLV-II also appears to be endemic in some pygmy tribes from Zaire and Cameroon (Goubau et al., 1993b) (reviewed in Gessain et al., 1995a; Gessain & de Thé, 1996), in contradiction to the earlier idea that HTLV-II was exclusively a 'New World virus' brought to the Americas by migrations of infected Mongoloid populations, who were the ancestors of the present-day Amerindians.

In aboriginal groups, mother-to-child transmission of HTLV-II through breast-feeding and sexual transmission appears to be important (Black et al., 1994b). In the developed countries, HTLV-II is found almost exclusively in intravenous drug users and their sexual partners (Tedder et al., 1984; Lee et al., 1989; Zella et al., 1990; Parry et al., 1991; Khabbaz et al., 1992; Al et al., 1993; Coste et al., 1993; Blomberg et al., 1994; Vallejo & Garcia-Saiz, 1994; Henrard et al., 1995); transmission occurs mainly through sharing contaminated needles (among intravenous drug users) (Lee et al., 1989; Khabbaz et al., 1992) and blood transfusion (Lee et al., 1991).

1.4 Clinical description of non-neoplastic disorders

1.4.1 HTLV-I infection

(a) Tropical spastic paraparesis/HTLV-I-associated myelopathy

TSP/HAM is a progressive form of chronic spastic myelopathy associated with demyelination of the spinal cord motor neurons (Gessain et al., 1985; Osame et al., 1986a; Dalgleish et al., 1988; Salazar-Grueso et al., 1990; Cruickshank et al., 1992; Araújo et al., 1993; Domingues et al., 1995; Harrington et al., 1995). It usually has an insidious onset but rare cases of more rapid onset have been described, particularly following blood transfusion. The main clinical manifestations are weakness and stiffness of the lower limbs, urinary bladder disturbances, paraesthesias, lumbar pain and impotence. Difficulty in walking develops several months after presentation (Cruickshank et al., 1992; Rodgers-Johnson, 1994; St Clair Morgan, 1994). Cerebellar signs, cranial nerve palsies and convulsions are rare. Neurological examination reveals spasticity and/or hyperreflexia and muscle weakness in the lower extremities; half of the patients have mild sensory abnormalities. Objective clinical criteria for the diagnosis of TSP/HAM have been published by a WHO working group (WHO, 1989). [The diagnosis of TSP/HAM requires differentiation from multiple sclerosis, spinal cord compression, spinal canal stenosis and cervical spondylosis.]

The main immuno-virological features of TSP/HAM are: the presence of high titres of anti-HTLV-I antibodies in serum and cerebrospinal fluid (Dalgleish et al., 1988); pleocytosis in the cerebrospinal fluid with intrathecal IgG synthesis with oligoclonal bands that react with HTLV-I (Gessain et al., 1988); a high proviral load in the PBMCs (Yoshida et al., 1989; Gessain et al., 1990b); ex-vivo spontaneous lymphoid proliferation (Itoyama et al., 1988); circulating activated T-cell subpopulations (Minato et al., 1989; Shibayama et al., 1992) and presence of cytotoxic T-cells which recognize epitopes of the products of the *tax* gene (Jacobson et al., 1990). All of these features except those in the cerebrospinal fluid have been described in asymptomatic carriers.

A small number of circulating abnormal 'flower-like' lymphocytes similar to those of ATLL are present in about half of the patients (Dalgleish et al., 1988; St Clair Morgan, 1994).

Magnetic resonance imaging may reveal abnormalities in the white matter of the brain and electrophysiology often demonstrates latency delays of visual, brain stem auditory and somatosensory evoked potentials with normal peripheral nerve conduction (St Clair Morgan, 1994).

Histological data are derived mainly from post-mortem examinations. The pathological changes affect the grey and white matter of the spinal cord, particularly the lateral columns; the brain is grossly normal and the leptomeninges are thickened (St Clair Morgan, 1994). The main features are marked demyelination and axonal destruction with an inflammatory mononuclear-cell infiltrate; astrocytic gliosis and meningeal thickening are common. By immunohistology, perivascular infiltrating mononuclear cells are T cells, mainly $CD4^+$ at early stages and $CD8^+$ in the later stages. Macrophages may also be found. HTLV-I has been detected in the nervous tissue by PCR with primers against *pol*, *env* and *pX* genes and by in-situ hybridization (Kira et al., 1991, 1992a; Kira, 1994; Kuroda et al., 1994; Sueyoshi et al., 1994; Umehara et al., 1994), but there is no direct evidence that HTLV-I infects neurons *in vivo* (St Clair Morgan, 1994) and it is uncertain which cell type (T lymphocytes, microglia or neural cells) is infected.

The clinical course of TSP/HAM is progressive. Oral corticosteroids may produce a transient beneficial effect, particularly when given in the early phases of the disease. Other drugs including azathioprine, danazol, intrathecal hydrocortisone and α-interferon can provide temporary relief. In addition, symptomatic treatment with diazepam or dantrolene can be used to relieve spasticity (St Clair Morgan, 1994).

The pathogenesis of TSP/HAM is uncertain, but viral load, specific molecular viral strain, specific and non-specific immune response and human leukocyte antigen (HLA) variability have been considered as potential factors in disease development (Gessain & Gout, 1992; Bangham, 1993; Bangham *et al.*, 1996). Extensive sequence studies mainly of the LTR region and the *env* gene have failed to define any specific nucleotide changes linked to disease (Mahieux *et al.*, 1995). Although Tax-specific cytotoxic T-cells were first described in the PBMCs of TSP/HAM patients (Jacobson *et al.*, 1990), their prevalence and frequency have been reported to be the same in TSP/HAM cases and asymptomatic carriers (Parker *et al.*, 1994; Daenke *et al.*, 1996). Central nervous system (CNS) inflammation is characterized by perivascular infiltration of lymphocytes (mainly $CD8^+$), but HTLV-I is rarely detected in the CNS. It has therefore been suggested that the CNS damage may be a non-specific consequence of T-cells activated by HTLV-I leaving the circulation and causing bystander damage (Bangham *et al.*, 1996).

(b) Uveitis

Uveitis is an inflammatory condition of the uveal tract. The majority of cases of uveitis are idiopathic, but some are caused by bacterial or viral infections and some are associated with autoimmune diseases, such as in Behçet's syndrome. Idiopathic uveitis in Japan is more frequent in HTLV-I endemic areas, such as southern Kyushu, and the seroprevalence of HTLV-I in these patients is significantly higher (up to 38%) than in patients with uveitis of other known etiologies (Mochizuki *et al.*, 1992, 1994). Because the seroprevalence of HTLV-I is much higher in young patients, it has been suggested that early exposure to the virus, such as at birth, is important in the development of uveitis (Mochizuki *et al.*, 1994).

HTLV-I-associated uveitis affects younger adults, usually under 50 years of age, and can be uni- or bilateral. It has a subacute onset, presenting with blurred vision but with little or no decrease in visual acuity. The main physical sign of HTLV-I uveitis is vitreous opacity (Mochizuki *et al.*, 1994). The course is progressive in the absence of treatment with topical or systemic corticosteroids. Recurrence of uveitis is common but remission may last for years (Ohba *et al.*, 1994). Familial occurrence of HTLV-I uveitis has been described (Araki *et al.*, 1993), as well as its association with TSP/HAM and hyperthyroidism (Nakao *et al.*, 1994; Ohba *et al.*, 1994).

An association between HTLV-I-associated uveitis and Graves' disease has been reported, evoking speculation that thyroid hormones may modify the host response to the virus and/or activate viral replication (Mochizuki *et al.*, 1994).

Inflammatory cellular infiltrates with HTLV-I-infected cells are present in the ocular tissues. Infiltrating lymphocytes in the vitreous and aqueous humour contain integrated proviral *tax* gene (Mochizuki *et al.*, 1994; Sagawa *et al.*, 1995) and express mRNA for HTLV-I proteins (Sagawa *et al.*, 1995). These lymphocytes display an activated T-cell phenotype ($CD3^+$, $CD4^+$, $CD25^+$) and release a variety of cytokines (such as ILs and tumour necrosis factor (TNF) α), which may be responsible for the inflammation

(Sagawa et al., 1995). Sequencing of the LTR region of HTLV-I has shown that uveitis is not associated with a specific viral strain (Ono et al., 1994). Although the etiopathogenesis is unknown, the evidence available supports an autoimmune mechanism mediated by HTLV-I-activated T cells.

(c) Other inflammatory disorders

Patients with TSP/HAM additionally have inflammation in tissues other than the CNS, that is characterized by infiltration with activated T-lymphocytes and antibodies in the relevant body fluids. HTLV-I has been detected by molecular methods in these tissues, usually in lymphocytes, but epidemiological data linking HTLV-I with these conditions are weaker than for TSP/HAM. In particular, there is ascertainment bias, with most conditions initially described in patients with TSP/HAM. These inflammatory disorders have also been reported in HTLV-I infected persons without TSP/HAM.

(i) *Infective dermatitis*

Infective dermatitis, an exudative dermatitis affecting the scalp, ears, axillae and groin, characterized by the presence of non-pathogenic bacteria, has been almost exclusively reported in HTLV-I-seropositive Jamaican children (LaGrenade et al., 1990), with an average age at onset of two years. These children require long-term antibiotic therapy. There is mild lymphocytosis in peripheral blood with an increase in $CD4^+$ cells and often polyclonal hypergammaglobulinaemia. Retrospective analysis has suggested that children with infective dermatitis may be at increased risk of later developing TSP/HAM or ATLL (Bunker et al., 1990; Pagliuca et al., 1990; Hanchard et al., 1991; LaGrenade, 1994).

(ii) *Polymyositis*

Polymyositis is an inflammatory myopathy characterized by proximal muscle weakness and wasting, raised serum levels of muscle enzymes (serum lactate dehydrogenase, creatine kinase and aminotransferase) and distinct histological changes. The cause is largely unknown, although some cases are linked to autoimmune disease or infections with viruses such as Coxsackie B. In HTLV-I-endemic areas, the prevalence of HTLV-I antibodies in patients with polymyositis has been found to be substantially higher than in corresponding control groups (85% against 8%: St Clair Morgan et al., 1989; 28% against 11.6%: Higuchi et al., 1992) (reviewed in Dalakas, 1993). HTLV-I-positive polymyositis affects women more frequently than men, appears to be more common in Caribbean than in Japanese patients and seems to be associated with TSP/HAM (St Clair Morgan et al., 1989; Smadja et al., 1993; Sherman et al., 1995). Both IgM and IgG HTLV-I antibodies are detected in most cases. Electromyography shows changes consistent with an inflammatory myopathy, such as short duration of polyphasic motor unit potentials (St Clair Morgan et al., 1989; Sherman et al., 1995).

Histological features are those of a myositis (Sherman et al., 1995), with atrophy, necrosis, oedema, fibrosis and interstitial cellular infiltrates composed of macrophages and lymphocytes (mainly $CD8^+$ with some $CD4^+$). HTLV-I sequences have not been found in the muscle cells (Higuchi et al., 1992; Sherman et al., 1995).

(iii) *Alveolitis*

In the original description, asymptomatic alveolitis was found at bronchoalveolar lavage (BAL) in patients with TSP/HAM (Sugimoto et al., 1987). Asymptomatic alveolitis may occur in HLTV-I carriers and in patients with HTLV-I-associated uveitis (Maruyama et al., 1988; Sugimoto et al., 1993). However, a few patients have a persistent cough and/or a variable degree of dyspnoea. The chest X-ray is usually normal, but localized or patchy reticular shadows, pleural thickening and/or lung fibrosis have been described. Antibodies to HTLV-I are detected in both serum and BAL fluid. BAL fluid may contain lymphocytes predominantly of the $CD4^+$ phenotype (Maruyama et al., 1988) or have a normal distribution of $CD4^+$ and $CD8^+$ cells (Sugimoto et al., 1993) and display an immune response to HTLV-I (Maruyama et al., 1988). An increased number of activated T cells ($CD3^+$, $CD4^+$ or $CD8^+$) expressing HLA-DR determinants and CD25 have been found in the blood and BAL fluid from these patients (Mukae et al., 1994). Patients with alveolitis associated with TSP/HAM have increased soluble IL-2 receptors in the BAL fluid (Sugimoto et al., 1989). Patients with alveolitis associated with uveitis have increased viral load in both blood and BAL fluid (Sugimoto et al., 1993).

(iv) *Arthritis (HTLV-I-associated arthropathy)*

HTLV-I-associated arthropathy is a chronic inflammatory oligoarthritis of large joints, which preferentially affects middle-aged or elderly female HTLV-I carriers (Nishioka et al., 1989; Ijichi et al., 1990; Nishioka et al., 1993) and is often associated with TSP/HAM (Kitajima et al., 1989). Antibodies to HTLV-I are detected in both the serum and synovial fluid. Most patients have IgG antibodies, but up to two thirds also have IgM antibodies, suggesting active replication of the virus in the synovial fluid. Rheumatoid factor and features of autoimmune disease are usually absent and X-rays of the affected joints show marginal erosions and narrowing of the joint spaces (Kitajima et al., 1989). Arthroscopy reveals synovial proliferation, while mild changes in the cartilage and subchondral bone are seen histologically, with mononuclear infiltrates composed of lymphocytes with multilobulated nuclei (Nishioka et al., 1989, 1993). Immunostaining demonstrates HLA-DR expression by the synovial cells and by lymphocytes that are mainly $CD4^+$ and $CD8^+$ T-cells expressing retroviral proteins (Nishioka et al., 1993). By PCR, HTLV-I proviral sequences have been detected in both lymphocytes and synovial cells purified by T-cell depletion (Kitajima et al., 1991). Cultured synovial cells express mRNA for HTLV-I *tax/rex* as well as HTLV-I core and envelope proteins, as detected by immunostaining (Kitajima et al., 1991; Nishioka et al., 1993). In-vitro studies have also demonstrated that synovial cells are susceptible to infection by HTLV-I, proliferate vigorously and produce large amounts of granulocyte-macrophage colony-stimulating factor (Sakai et al., 1993).

The importance of HTLV-I *tax* in the pathogenesis of this condition is supported by studies in which transgenic mice with the HTLV-I *pX* gene develop a similar polyarthritis (Iwakura et al., 1991; Yamamoto et al., 1993). Whether this is mediated by HTLV-I-infected lymphocytes secreting cytokines which stimulate the proliferation of synovial cells or by a direct stimulation of synovial cells by HTLV-I is unknown.

(v) *Thyroiditis*

An association between HTLV-I infection and Hashimoto's thyroiditis (inflammation of the thyroid gland with autoantibodies) has been reported from Japan (Kawai *et al.*, 1991, 1992; Smadja *et al.*, 1993; Mizokami *et al.*, 1995). The seroprevalence of HTLV-I in these patients was significantly higher than that in the corresponding general population (6.3% versus 2.2%) (Kawai *et al.*, 1992). This condition is often found in patients with TSP/HAM (Kawai *et al.*, 1991, 1992) and uveitis (Mizokami *et al.*, 1995).

(vi) *Sjögren's syndrome*

Sjögren's syndrome, a keratoconjunctivitis, with dryness of the eyes and mouth and hypertrophy and lymphocytic infiltration of the salivary glands, has been observed in HTLV-I carriers and in patients with HTLV-I-associated diseases (Merle *et al.*, 1994; Eguchi *et al.*, 1992; Plumelle *et al.*, 1993). As with other inflammatory diseases associated with HTLV-I, there is an increase in circulating activated cells (CD3$^+$, CD25$^+$, HLA-DR) that display spontaneous proliferation (Eguchi *et al.*, 1992). In some HTLV-I-seronegative patients with Sjögren's syndrome, HTLV-I *tax* but not *pol*, *gag* and *env* sequences have been detected in labial salivary glands (Mariette *et al.*, 1993, 1994; Sumida *et al.*, 1994).

Transgenic mice with the HTLV-I *tax* gene have been shown to develop a condition similar to Sjögren's syndrome. Lymphocytic infiltration of the salivary glands with the presence of *tax* in the epithelial cells has been demonstrated in these mice (Green *et al.*, 1989a).

(*d*) *Immune suppression*

T-cell subsets and CD4/CD8 ratios do not appear to be affected by HTLV-I infection (Matutes *et al.*, 1986; Welles *et al.*, 1994).

Evidence of mild immune suppression due to HTLV-I infection has been seen in studies of healthy carriers who had decreased delayed hypersensitivity to the purified protein derivative of tuberculin (Tachibana *et al.*, 1988) and marked suppression of T-cell control of B cells infected with Epstein–Barr virus (EBV) (Katsuki *et al.*, 1987). Indirect evidence of impaired cellular immunity has come from studies showing that HTLV-I carriers have a reduced ability to clear infection with *Strongyloides stercoralis* (Nakada *et al.*, 1987). *S. stercoralis* infection is associated with ATLL and, when present, is often severe (Nakada *et al.*, 1987; Dixon *et al.*, 1989; Phels *et al.*, 1991; Patey *et al.*, 1992; Plumelle *et al.*, 1993).

1.4.2 *HTLV-II infection*

HTLV-II has occasionally been associated with a myeloneuropathy resembling TSP/HAM with ataxia (Hjelle *et al.*, 1992; Murphy *et al.*, 1993; Harrington *et al.*, 1993; Murphy *et al.*, 1996). Few studies have attempted to investigate the association between HTLV-II and diseases in populations in which the infection is endemic.

1.4.3 *HTLV/HIV co-infection*

Co-infection with HIV and HTLV-I or HTLV-II is common among HIV-1-infected intravenous drug users and patients attending clinics for sexually transmitted diseases in areas where both viruses are endemic (Harper *et al.*, 1986; Wiley *et al.*, 1989; Manzari *et al.*, 1990; Khabaz *et al.*, 1992; Beilke *et al.*, 1994; Harrington *et al.*, 1995). Although the clinical consequences of the co-infection are largely unknown, it has been suggested that HTLV-I but not HTLV-II may accelerate the course of HIV-1 infection. Patients with HTLV-I and HIV-1 co-infection develop specific HIV-1-related disease manifestation at higher $CD4^+$ T-cell count than patients with HIV-1 infection only (Beilke *et al.*, 1994; Harrington *et al.*, 1995; Schechter *et al.*, 1994).

There have been some case reports of co-infected persons developing either associated haematological disease or inflammatory disease (Harper *et al.*, 1986).

1.5 Control and prevention

Prevention of HTLV-I and HTLV-II infection must be directed at the main modes of HTLV-I transmission: perinatal, especially postnatal though breast-feeding; parenteral, through blood transfusion or exposure to contaminated needles; and sexual, essentially male to female (Hino, 1990b; Sato & Okochi, 1990; Bentrem *et al.*, 1994).

Prevention of HTLV-I infection in neonates appears to be particularly important because of the association of ATLL with childhood infection. Maternal antibodies may protect infants during short-term (less than six months) exposure but, as this wanes, susceptibility to infection appears to increase (Takahashi *et al.*, 1991). An intervention programme to screen and counsel HTLV-I-seropositive mothers against breast-feeding began in Japan in the late 1980s and has been shown to prevent 90% of maternal infection of infants (Hino, 1990b). More recently, these recommendations have been changed to permit short-duration breast-feeding. Such a policy can be adopted only where safe and sustainable alternatives to breast-feeding are available.

Transmission of HTLV-I in cellular blood products is highly efficient, with a seroconversion rate of 63% (Bentrem *et al.*, 1994), and TSP/HAM and other inflammatory HTLV-I-linked diseases develop within a relatively short time following blood transfusion (Osame *et al.*, 1986b). Transfusion-related transmission can be prevented by systematic screening of blood donors for HTLV-I and HTLV-II antibodies, as is practised in several countries (see Section 1.3.1). Infection of a health worker with HTLV-I by puncture with a contaminated needle has been known to occur (Bentrem *et al.*, 1994), emphasizing the need for universal precautions in dealing with biological materials.

Use of condoms during sexual intercourse should be considered by couples when only one partner is infected with HTLV-I or HTLV-II.

Passive immunization has been shown to be effective in rabbits: hyperimmune IgG prepared from seropositive healthy persons given 24 h before transfusion with infected blood appeared to protect the recipient rabbit from infection (Takehara *et al.*, 1989; Kataoka *et al.*, 1990).

Although such policies may help to control the spread of HTLV-I and HTLV-II, the ideal intervention would be immunization with a preventive vaccine. Preclinical studies in animal models have suggested the feasibility of an HTLV-I vaccine. Various live recombinant pox virus vectors carrying the HTLV-I envelope protein have conferred protection against a cell-associated HTLV-I challenge in non-human primates (Shida *et al.*, 1987) and rabbits (Franchini *et al.*, 1995). Certain live recombinant envelope proteins alone have also conferred protection in non-human primates (Nakamura *et al.*, 1987). However, no trials of HTLV-I vaccines in humans have yet been undertaken.

2. Studies of Cancer in Humans

2.1 T-Cell malignancies

2.1.1 *HTLV-I-infection and adult T-cell leukaemia/lymphoma*

Adult T-cell leukaemia/lymphoma (ATLL) was described as a distinct clinicopathological entity by Uchiyama *et al.* (1977). Seroepidemiological surveys on lymphoid neoplasms and healthy populations in the early 1980s demonstrated that HTLV-I and ATLL were both clustered in south-western Japan and in Caribbean islands (Hinuma *et al.*, 1982; Blattner *et al.*, 1983). In the mid-1980s and early 1990s, a number of other HTLV-I endemic areas with evidence of ATLL were recognized, chiefly in central and west Africa, South America and the Middle East, and the disease was also found among immigrants from these countries to Europe and the United States (Catovsky *et al.*, 1982; Hahn *et al.*, 1984; Williams *et al.*, 1984; Delaporte *et al.*, 1989b; Denic *et al.*, 1990; Meytes *et al.*, 1990; Sidi *et al.*, 1990; Cabrera *et al.*, 1994; Matutes & Catovsky, 1994; Pombo de Oliveira *et al.*, 1995).

(*a*) *Clinical description*

ATLL is a mature (post-thymic) T-cell malignancy which may be considered within the leukaemia/lymphoma syndromes. The disease arises in peripheral lymphoid tissues, e.g., nodes or skin, but a leukaemic picture is frequent.

(i) *Distribution by subtype*

ATLL has been classified into four subtypes: acute type, lymphoma type, chronic type and smouldering type, according to the clinicopathological features (Shimoyama *et al.*, 1991). The distinguishing features of the various forms of ATLL are summarized in Table 1. Among 1400 cases of ATLL registered throughout Japan during 1990–1993, 914 cases (65%) were classified as the acute type (prototype of ATLL), 330 cases (24%) as the lymphoma type, 83 cases (6%) as the chronic type and 73 cases (5%) as the smouldering type (see Table 1) (T- and B-Cell Malignancy Study Group, 1996).

Table 1. Average age, sex ratio and clinical findings in patients with adult T-cell leukaemia/lymphoma by subtype in Japan (1990–93)

Subtype	No. of cases (%)	Age (± SE)	Sex ratio (male : female)	Skin lesion (%)[a]	Hypercal-caemia (%)[a,b]
Acute	914 (65.3)	58.2 ± 0.39	1.2	31.4 %	32.8
Lymphoma	330 (23.6)	59.4 ± 0.66	1.2	14.0%	15.4
Chronic	83 (5.9)	58.8 ± 1.41	0.9	31.8%	1.1[c]
Smouldering	73 (5.2)	58.5 ± 1.59	1.0	55.7%	0
Total	1400 (100)	58.6 ± 0.32	1.2	28.5%	25.0

From T- and B-Cell Malignancy Study Group (1996); SE, standard error
[a] Calculated by the Working Group
[b] Adjusted Ca^{++} value ≥ 5.5 mEq/L
[c] One case of chronic-type ATLL showed 5.8 mEq/L (unadjusted value, 5.4 mEq/L)

As the clinical spectrum of conditions now accepted as part of ATLL has extended, these conditions have become increasingly difficult to distinguish from other types of T-cell malignancy and sometimes diagnoses have depended on the identification of HTLV-I antibody or genomic material in the subjects, making the understanding of the relationship between this virus and these manifestations difficult to disentangle.

Ocular manifestations, particularly retinitis, resulting from intraocular infiltration by leukaemic cells, can precede or occur during the course of ATLL (Kohno *et al.*, 1993; Kumar *et al.*, 1994).

Acute adult T-cell leukaemia/lymphoma

This is the most frequent presentation of ATLL, corresponding to two thirds of the cases. The main clinical manifestations are organomegaly, high white blood cell count with lymphocytosis and often skin involvement. Lactate dehydrogenase levels are elevated and hypercalcaemia is frequent, although these two parameters are not essential diagnostic criteria of this clinical form. Other less frequent manifestations include CNS involvement, pleural effusions or ascites, lung infiltrates due either to opportunistic infections or to leukaemic infiltration of the lungs and, more rarely, primary involvement of the gastrointestinal tract (Hattori *et al.*, 1991; Nishimura *et al.*, 1994), the Waldeyer's ring (Ohguro *et al.*, 1993) or the cardiac valves (Gabarre *et al.*, 1993).

Lymphomatous adult T-cell leukaemia/lymphoma

This corresponds to the tissue-based ATLL with no evidence of peripheral blood involvement and no lymphocytosis at onset. Many cases develop to leukaemic status at terminal stage. Otherwise, the symptoms are identical to those of the acute (or prototype) form of ATLL, although hypercalcaemia is less common.

Chronic adult T-cell leukaemia/lymphoma

This form is characterized by persistent T-cell lymphocytosis ($> 4 \times 10^9$/L) with atypical cells, minor or no lymphoid organ or skin involvement and lack of systemic symptoms. The lactate dehydrogenase level may be elevated. In both smouldering and chronic ATLL, serum calcium levels are within the normal range.

Smouldering adult T-cell leukaemia/lymphoma

Smouldering ATLL, sometimes referred to as pre-ATLL or pre-leukaemic ATLL (Kinoshita *et al.*, 1985b), is characterized by skin lesions (which usually respond to topical corticosteroids), frequently lung infiltrates and an absence of systemic symptoms (Yamaguchi *et al.*, 1983; Takatsuki *et al.*, 1985; Shimoyama *et al.*, 1991). Patients may be asymptomatic, the disease being discovered during incidental examination. The white blood cell count is normal except for the presence of a few (< 4%) circulating abnormal lymphocytes. Abnormal lymphocytes are sometimes seen in healthy carriers of HTLV-I (Matutes *et al.*, 1986), but in smouldering ATLL, there is clonal integration of viral DNA, as demonstrated by Southern blot.

Smouldering ATLL can be considered to be an early stage of the acute and lymphoma types of ATLL. There does not seem to be a natural progression from the smouldering stage to acute ATLL within a period of months to years (Yamaguchi *et al.*, 1983; Cabrera *et al.*, 1994; Matutes & Catovsky, 1994; Pombo di Oliveira *et al.*, 1995).

Pre-leukaemic cases of ATLL with monoclonal proliferation of abnormal lymphocytes (see 'Histological characteristics' below) without clinical signs or symptoms were studied in south-western Japan (Ikeda *et al.*, 1990). The prevalence rate of pre-leukaemic ATLL among HTLV-I carriers over 30 years of age was estimated as 2% and the age distribution of pre-leukaemic cases, ranging from 30 to 77 years, was no different from that of overt cases of ATLL. The pre-leukaemic stage is presumed to be the clinical stage which precedes ATLL, but it remains possible that an HTLV-I carrier may develop symptoms of ATLL directly, without going through the pre-leukaemic stage. [The Working Group noted that the distinction between pre-ATLL and smouldering ATLL is not well defined.]

(ii) *Laboratory findings (Table 2)*

Hypercalcaemia is the most distinctive abnormality related to ATLL because it is extremely rare in other lymphoid neoplasms (Grossman *et al.*, 1981; Matutes & Catovsky, 1992; Yamaguchi, 1994). It is more frequent in the acute form with high white blood cell count and is rarely associated with osteolytic lesions. Hypercalcaemia is related to the release of cytokines (chiefly a parathyroid-hormone-related protein (PTH-rP), IL-1 and TNF-β) by the malignant cells, with serum levels of parathyroid hormone and vitamin D_3 remaining within the normal range. This cytokine-mediated mechanism is supported by the findings that the gene encoding PTH-rP is continuously transcribed in ATLL cells (Watanabe *et al.*, 1990), that the cells express a high level of PTH-rP mRNA and that, when cultured, they release PTH-rP into the medium (Honda *et al.*, 1988). Other biochemical abnormalities that are also found in other T-cell malignancies are high levels of lactate dehydrogenase and β_2-microglobulin; the latter is released either by the tumour cells or secondary to cytokine secretion by non-malignant cells. Both parameters are related to a poor outcome and survival (Shimamoto et al., 1990a; Tsuda et al., 1992).

Table 2. Diagnostic criteria of clinical subtypes of adult T-cell leukaemia/lymphoma

Feature	Smouldering	Chronic	Lymphoma	Acute
Lymphocytosis[a]	$< 4 \times 10^9$/L	$> 4 \times 10^9$/L	$< 4 \times 10^9$/L	$> 4 \times 10^9$/L
Lactate dehydrogenase	Normal or < 1.5 the normal limit	< 2 the normal limit	Variable[b]	Variable[b]
Calcium	Normal	Normal	Variable[b]	Variable[b]
Skin	Involved	Variable[b]	Variable[b]	Variable[b]
Lung	Often involved	Variable[b]	Variable[b]	Variable[b]
Systemic involvement[c]	No	No or minor	Variable[b]	Variable[b]

Adapted from Shimoyama et al. (1991) and Cann & Chen (1996)
[a] With > 5% atypical 'flower' cells except in the lymphoma form
[b] Not considered for the classification of the ATLL subtype
[c] Enlargement of lymph nodes, spleen, liver, central nervous system, gastrointestinal tract or other organ involvement

(iii) *Histological characteristics*

The diagnosis of ATLL is based on clinicopathological features and a number of laboratory parameters, including peripheral blood cell morphology, histopathology, immunological markers and demonstration of the presence of HTLV-I by serology or molecular analysis. The blood picture in the leukaemic forms of ATLL is pleomorphic, the predominant cell being a medium-sized lymphocyte with a highly irregular, frequently polylobated nucleus, that is often called a 'flower' cell. Circulating immunoblasts may be present in small numbers but they usually predominate in the lymphoid tissues. This blood picture is usually, but not always, distinguishable from that seen in Sézary syndrome, in which the cells have a hyperchromatic cerebriform nucleus (Matutes & Catovsky, 1992). The bone marrow is usually not heavily involved but trephine biopsy may show proliferation of osteoclasts and bone reabsorption, features which relate to the hypercalcaemia.

Histological analysis is essential in the lymphoma form of ATLL. However, there is no unique histological pattern of lymphoid involvement in ATLL, which may be very similar to that of other peripheral T-cell lymphomas. The lymph nodes show effacement of the normal architecture by lymphoid cells of different size, varying from small to large (mixed-cell pattern) (Lennert et al., 1985). Cases with unusual histology or even with a clinical picture resembling that of Hodgkin's disease have been described (Duggan et al., 1988; Ohshima et al., 1991a; Picard et al., 1990). The histological pattern of skin infiltration is not specific either; dermal infiltration by pleomorphic cells is often observed, but in some cases epidermotropism and Pautrier's microabscesses are seen.

These may also occur in Sézary syndrome and mycosis fungoides (Matutes & Catovsky, 1992; Whittaker et al., 1993; Arai et al., 1994; Pombo de Oliveira et al., 1995). Therefore, differentiating between Sézary syndrome or other T-cell lymphomas and ATLL can be difficult on the basis of histological results.

Immunological markers reveal that ATLL cells have a mature post-thymic T-cell phenotype. The most common phenotype of ATLL cells is $CD4^+$, $CD8^-$, but a few patients may have unusual phenotypes such as CD4 loss, CD8 expression or both. In the rare cases with $CD4^+$, $CD8^+$ T-cells, the disease appears to have a more aggressive course (Tamura et al., 1985). The thymic markers TdT and CD1a are always absent. Tumour cells are often positive for CD2 and CD5 markers but usually negative for CD7 (Matutes & Catovsky, 1992). CD3 may be absent or only weakly expressed on the membrane (Tsuda & Takatsuki, 1984) but is, as a rule, expressed in the cytoplasm (Matutes & Catovsky, 1992). A characteristic, but not specific, feature of ATLL cells is the strong expression of the p55 α-chain of the IL-2 receptor, detected by the monoclonal antibody CD25 (Uchiyama et al., 1985; Yodoi & Uchiyama, 1986; Matutes & Catovsky, 1992; Yamaguchi, 1994); other T-cell activation antigens, such as HLA-DR determinants and CD38, may also be expressed. In addition, soluble IL-2 receptors can be detected in the serum of these patients and the levels seem to relate to tumour burden (Yamaguchi et al., 1989). It has been shown that the high numbers of IL-2 receptors in the membrane of ATLL cells result from the continuous transcription of the IL-2 receptor gene (Yodoi & Uchiyama, 1986). These observations suggest that IL-2 receptors play a key role in the etiopathogenesis or progression of the disease.

In spite of the $CD4^+$, $CD8^-$ phenotype, ATLL cells are not helper cells functionally but act as potent suppressors of B-cell differentiation (Yamada, 1983; Miedema et al., 1984). It is uncertain whether this function is direct or is mediated by an indirect mechanism through a suppressor $CD8^+$ T-cell subset. One consequence may be that some patients have concomitant disease related to immune suppression.

(iv) Genetic studies

In ATLL, a range of chromosomal abnormalities occur but, unlike those seen in some lymphoid malignancies, such as Burkitt's lymphoma, they are not specific. Abnormalities may involve chromosomes 3, 7 and X, and/or affect 6q, 14q, 3q, 1q and 10p (Shimoyama et al., 1987; Kamada et al., 1990). They are often more complex and are more frequently found in the acute and lymphomatous forms than in smouldering or chronic ATLL, which suggests that they correlate with disease progression.

Familial ATLL has been documented in HTLV-I endemic regions (Kawano et al., 1984; Miyamoto et al., 1985; Matutes & Catovsky, 1994) and less frequently in countries with low HTLV-I seroprevalence such as the United Kingdom (Matutes et al., 1995a). In some families, several cases of TSP/HAM and ATLL have been seen (Uozumi et al., 1991; Plumelle et al., 1993) and the coexistence of the two diseases in the same patient has been described (Cartier et al., 1995; Harrington et al., 1995). The fact that, in the familial clusters, patients did not always share the same household suggests that it was the genetic background rather than the environment which influenced the development of ATLL. Early exposure to HTLV-I, e.g., neonatal or during childhood, seems to be important for the development of ATLL, as the disease occurs many years after the retroviral infection, in contrast to TSP/HAM, which may develop shortly after infection by HTLV-I.

(v) *Prognosis*

ATLL is an aggressive malignancy with poor prognosis and short median survival ranging from 5 to 13 months in all areas (Shimamoto *et al.*, 1990a,b; Lymphoma Study Group (1984–1987), 1991; Shih *et al.*, 1991; Plumelle *et al.*, 1993; Matutes & Catovsky, 1994; Yamaguchi, 1994). Patients respond poorly to chemotherapeutic schedules used successfully against other high-grade lymphomas (Shimamoto *et al.*, 1990b; Matutes & Catovsky, 1994; Mercieca *et al.*, 1994). Experimental approaches such as therapy with antibody against the IL-2 receptor anti-Tac have yielded only transient responses (Waldmann *et al.*, 1988, 1995). There have, however, been reports of good response to a combination of α-interferon and zidovudine (Gallo, 1995; Gill *et al.*, 1995; Hermine *et al.*, 1995). The mechanism of action of this therapy is unknown. Furthermore, the duration of the response remains to be evaluated.

Patients with the smouldering and chronic forms of ATLL usually have a stable or very slowly progressive course and, during this phase, clinical problems are easier to control than in the acute forms. Generally, such patients are not treated aggressively.

(vi) *Prevention of ATLL*

Prevention of ATLL and/or cancers associated with HTLV-I is difficult, as the secondary factors promoting the evolution from healthy carrier status to ATLL or neoplasia are unknown. Although spontaneous remission of ATLL has been reported (Shimamoto *et al.*, 1993), this appears to be extremely rare. Experimental work has shown that inhibitors of thioredoxin reductase, such as retinoic acid derivatives, are able to inhibit DNA synthesis and growth and replication of HTLV-I-infected cells and therefore have a potential role in the treatment of HTLV-I carriers (U-Taniguchi *et al.*, 1995).

(b) *Epidemiology*

Consideration of the epidemiological evidence concerning the relationship between HTLV-I and ATLL must be viewed in the light of the history of HTLV-I's discovery in ATLL-endemic parts of the world. Reports in the early 1980s from these regions (discussed above) found a very high prevalence (> 90%) of HTLV infection in ATLL patients, compared with much lower population prevalence in the area from which the cases came. A few patients with clinical features indistinguishable from those of ATLL have, however, been reported in whom HTLV-I infection cannot be demonstrated (Shimoyama *et al.*, 1986, 1987; Pombo de Oliveira *et al.*, 1995).

The concordance between HTLV-I positivity and ATLL was so high in the endemic areas that HTLV-I became widely accepted as the cause of ATLL, and the presence of HTLV-I infection was adopted as an additional diagnostic criterion for ATLL for lesions in which the clinical findings were ambiguous. This practice complicates assessment of the association between HTLV-I and ATLL.

When the clinical and laboratory features characteristic of ATLL are present, serological assays for HTLV-I antibodies almost always show a strongly reactive test. However, if the features are atypical, DNA analysis by Southern blot using probes specific to HTLV-I sequences may be needed to demonstrate the clonal integration of HTLV-I in the tumour cells. All cases of ATLL have proviral HTLV-I DNA integrated in a monoclonal fashion, according to Yoshida et al. (1984). Therefore, the absence of HTLV-I clonal integration may be construed as evidence against this diagnosis in a case. In addition, DNA analysis helps to distinguish cases of smouldering ATLL from healthy carriers.

(i) Geographical distribution

Following the first report of ATLL cases from Japan by Uchiyama et al. (1977), 10 familial cases of ATLL were reported in the south-western part of Japan (Ichimaru et al., 1979), where ATLL is highly endemic. A nationwide study, implemented in Japan soon after the original description, revealed that 50% of ATLL patients were registered in the southern Japanese island of Kyushu (see Figure 7). Only 25% were from major cities (Takatsuki et al., 1977; Uchiyama et al., 1977; Tajima et al., 1990b; T- and B-cell Malignancy Study Group, 1988; Tajima, 1990; Tajima et al., 1994), and 80% of these cases had been born in Kyushu. The sex ratio (male/female) is around 1.2 in Japan (T and B-cell Malignancy Study Group, 1996).

T-Cell leukaemia/lymphomas are not reported routinely as a separate diagnostic group in cancer incidence and mortality statistics. Their geographical distribution can, thus, be derived only from specific reports (or surveys) and the picture obtained is heavily influenced by the extent to which disease surveillance has been carried out in various areas. Studies in Brazil (Pombo de Oliveira et al., 1990; Matutes et al., 1994; Pombo de Oliveira et al., 1995), in Gabon (Delaporte et al., 1993) and in French Guiana (Gérard et al., 1995) have demonstrated that the incidence of ATLL will continue to be greatly underestimated unless a specific search is carried out. This is mainly due to the acuteness and rapid evolution of the disease, so that many patients die before diagnosis can be made, as well as to confusion of ATLL with pathologically similar diseases, such as Sézary syndrome, mycosis fungoides and other types of T-cell non-Hodgkin's lymphoma (Gessain et al., 1992b; Matutes & Catovsky, 1994; Pombo de Oliveira et al., 1995). Furthermore, serological confirmatory tests for HTLV-I, such as western blot and/or molecular analyses, are not readily available in most countries. However, the geographical distribution of ATLL appears to be similar to that of HTLV-I, with rough correspondence of the relative prevalences of the conditions in different areas (see Section 1.3). ATLL has a high incidence in the south-western regions of the Japanese archipelago (Hinuma et al., 1982; Clark et al., 1985b; T- and B-cell Malignancy Study Group, 1985; Tajima & Cartier, 1995; T- and B-cell Malignancy Study Group, 1996). It is also prevalent in most other HTLV-I-endemic areas, including intertropical Africa, South and Central America and Iran (Clark et al., 1988; Pombo de Oliveira et al., 1990; Rio et al., 1990; Gessain et al., 1992a; Blank et al., 1993; Delaporte et al., 1993; Plumelle et al., 1993; Pombo de Oliveira et al., 1995). Furthermore, sporadic cases of ATLL have been described in Europe and the United States, mostly in immigrants originating from regions of endemic HTLV-I infection (Rio et al., 1990; Patey et al., 1992; Matutes & Catovsky, 1994).

Figure 7. Estimated incidence rate of ATLL in persons (≥ 40 years) per 1 000 000 in Japanese prefectures during 1988–93

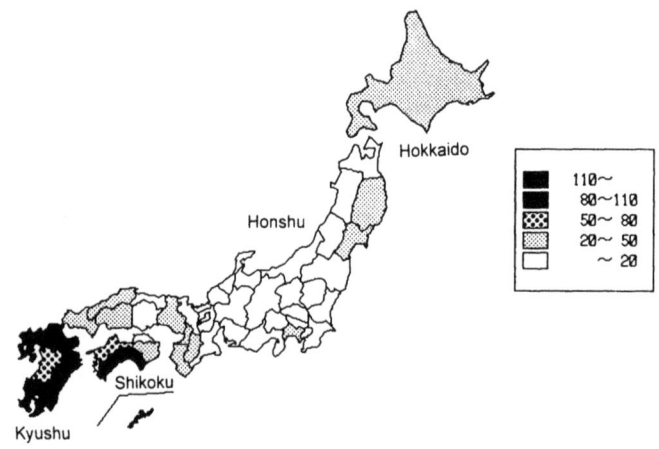

From the T- and B-cell Malignancy Study Group (1996)

Extensive reliable data concerning the occurrence of ATLL are available only for Japan and some Caribbean areas.

(ii) *Age- and sex-distribution of ATLL*

The average ages and sex ratios among ATLL cases are presented in Table 3. The average age of ATLL patients at diagnosis in Japan is 57 years (T- and B-cell Malignancy Study Group, 1988). The age pattern in Japan and the Caribbean is presented in Table 4 and Figure 8. No case of ATLL has been reported in children in Japan. In the Caribbean, South America and Africa, the mean age at ATLL onset is around 15 years younger, namely 40–45 years of age (Bartholomew et al., 1985; Gibbs et al., 1987; Gérard et al., 1995; Pombo de Oliveira et al., 1995). In addition, cases have been reported among children in Brazil (Pombo de Oliveira et al., 1995). This suggests the presence of still unknown cofactors in the pathogenesis of this disease in areas of different environmental and cultural conditions or of a cohort effect on the proportion of HTLV-I carriers infected in early childhood (Manns, 1993).

In Japan, the estimated annual incidence of ATLL lies in the range 0.6–1.5 per 1000 HTLV-I carriers aged 40–59 years (Tajima & Kuroishi, 1985; Kondo et al., 1989; Tokudome et al., 1989). The rate appears to be similar in Jamaica (Murphy et al., 1989b), but higher [6/1000] in the Noir-Marron population in French Guiana (Gérard et al., 1995). The cumulative lifetime risk for ATLL among carriers has been estimated to lie in the range of 1–5% in both sexes in Japan and Jamaica (Kondo et al., 1987, 1989;

Table 3. Average age, sex ratio and frequencies of abnormal clinical findings in patients with adult T-cell leukaemia/-lymphoma

	Japan[a] (1984–85)	Japan[b] (1992–93)	Taiwan[c] (1983–90)	USA[d] (until Dec. 1991)	Jamaica[e] (1982–85)	Trinidad[f] and Tobago (1982–83)	French Guiana[g] (1990–93)	Brazil[h] (1989–93)	UK[i] (1982–94]
Number of cases	181	712	27	102	52	12	19	53[k]	52
Average age (years)	56.9	58.9	48	~50	40	49.1	42.1	41	47
Age range (years)	24–90	25–87	28–71	7–75	20–70	22–84	21–71	2–65	19–77
Sex ratio (male versus female)	1.4	1.1	2.0	0.8	0.9	2.0	0.5	1.0	0.6
Skin lesions (%)	29.3	26.5	44	57	20	66.7	16	53	41
Hypercalcaemia (> 5.5 mEq/L)[j] (%)	17.1	23.6	37	72.5	48	58	53	34	51

Clinical findings on admission in Japanese cases in HTLV-I antibody positive cases
[a]T- and B-cell Malignancy Study Group (1988); [b]T- and B-cell Malignancy Study Group (1996); [c]Shih et al. (1992); [d]Levine et al. (1994); [e]Gibbs et al. (1987); [f]Bartholomew et al. (1985); [g]Gérard et al. (1995); [h]Pombo de Oliveira et al. (1995); [i]Matutes & Catovsky (1994); [j]In some of these series, calcium levels were measured on more than one occasion and this partially explains the variability of hypercalcaemia rates; [k]Five cases were HTLV-I negative by serology and PCR; there was 1 child and 52 adults.

Table 4. Estimated incidence of adult T-cell leukaemia/lymphoma per 1000 HTLV-I carriers per year in adult T-cell leukaemia/lymphoma endemic areas of Japan and Jamaica

Age (years)	Japan (Uwajima): Kondo et al. (1989)			Japan (Saga): Tokudome et al. (1989)			Jamaica: Murphy et al. (1989b)			Jamaica: Murphy et al. (1989b)[a]		
	Men	Women	Total	Men	Women	Total	Men	Women	Total	Men	Women	Total
20–29	0	0	0	0	0	0	[0.31]	[0.34]	[0.33]	[0.45]	[0.76]	[0.62]
30–39	0.95	0.41	0.61	0.00	0.48	[0.26]	[0.47]	[0.31]	[0.36]	[0.94]	[1.10]	[1.03]
40–49	0.83	0.66	0.72	1.19	0.63	[0.88]	[0.64]	[0.28]	[0.38]	[1.12]	[1.10]	[1.11]
50–59	2.10	0.33	0.82	1.16	0.58	[0.83]	[0.61]	[0.18]	[0.29]	[1.26]	[0.83]	[1.03]
60	[1.45]	[0.68]	[0.95]	[0.96]	[0.63]	[0.75]	[0.11]	[0.07]	[0.08]	[0.31]	[0.38]	[0.34]
>40	[1.50]	[0.58]	[0.89]	[1.06]	[0.61]	[0.93]	[0.34]	[0.15]	[0.21]	[0.80]	[0.71]	[0.75]
Cumulative rate												
(40–69)	[49.3]	[19.7]	[28.9]	[35.5]	[19.9]	[26.4]	[13.6]	[5.3]	[11.1]	[26.9]	[23.1]	[24.8]
(30–69)	[58.8]	[23.8]	[35.0]	[35.5]	[24.7]	[29.0]	[18.3]	[8.4]	[14.4]	[36.3]	[34.1]	[35.1]

[a] Calculated from HTLV-I carriers defined as people who might have been infected with HTLV-I as a newborn baby.
[ ] Calculated by the Working Group

Murphy et al., 1989b; Tokudome et al., 1989) (Table 4). The age distributions of ATLL incidence for men and women in Kyushu, Japan, are shown in Figure 9.

Figure 8. Estimated annual age-specific incidence rates (per 100 000) of adult T-cell leukaemia/lymphoma among HTLV-I carriers in Japan and Jamaica

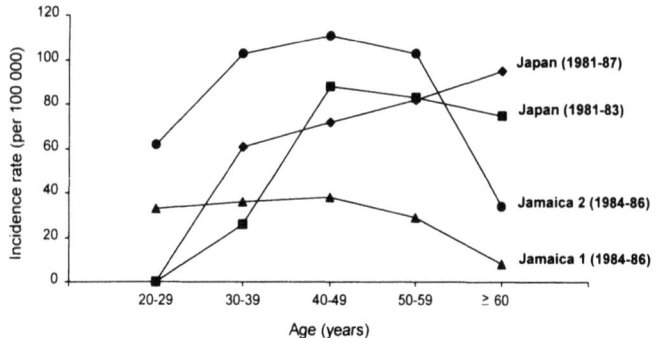

Sources: Japan, 1981–1987: Kondo et al. (1989); Japan, 1981–83: Tokudome et al. (1989); Jamaica: Murphy et al. (1989b)
Jamaica 2: calculated from HTLV-I carriers defined as people who might have been infected with HTLV-I as a newborn baby

(iii) *Cohort studies*

Tokudome et al. (1991) followed 3991 HTLV-I-seropositive blood donors aged ≥ 40 years from four blood centres in Kyushu who had donated blood between 1984 and 1987. Positivity for HTLV-I was determined by a particle agglutination antibody assay confirmed by indirect immunofluorescence in two centres. Mortality was ascertained through to August 1989; the average length of follow-up was 2.7 years for a total of 4403 person-years for men and 5591 person-years for women. The crude mortality rates for ATLL (3 deaths in men and 2 in women) were 68.1 per 100 000 for men and 35.8 for women. There were two additional deaths from malignant B-cell lymphoma (one in each sex).

Iwata et al. (1994) followed a total of 1997 individuals aged ≥ 30 years from an HTLV-I-endemic community in Nagasaki Prefecture who were screened between 1984 and 1990. Of these, 503 (25.3%) were seropositive for HTLV-I by a particle agglutination antibody assay. The cohort was followed up to mid-1992, the average follow-up being 5.3 years for a total of 2581 person-years at risk. There were two deaths from ATLL (one in each sex). The crude mortality rate was 77 per 100 000 person-years. [No expected value was given but it must be very small.]

(iv) *Case–control studies on co-factors*

In ATLL-endemic areas, almost all ATLL cases diagnosed by clinicopathological features show seropositivity for HTLV-I (see Table 5). In areas of low ATLL incidence, a small proportion of cases lack HTLV-I antibody (T- and B-Cell Malignancy Group,

1985; Pombo de Oliveira, 1995), but the vast majority (> 90%) of cases are seropositive. The majority (> 60%) of all T-cell lymphomas in Jamaica and in Trinidad and Tobago are HTLV-I-seropositive versus less than 10% of other lymphoma cases (Manns *et al.*, 1993).

Figure 9. Estimated annual sex- and age-specific incidence rates (per 1 000 000) of adult T-cell leukaemia/lymphoma in Kyushu, Japan, 1992–93

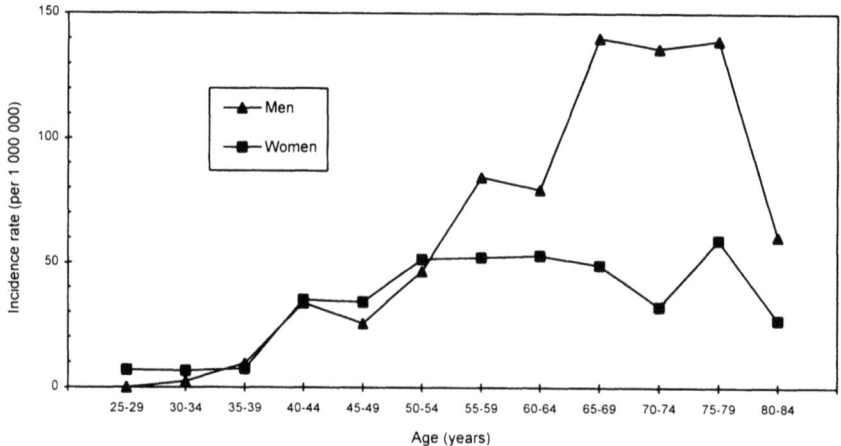

From T- and B-cell Malignancy Study Group (1996)

Several case–control studies on ATLL have been conducted in Japan (T- and B-Cell Malignancy Study Group, 1985; Tokudome *et al.*, 1993). In one, 66 cases were compared with the same number of hospital controls without cancer selected by individual matching to each case for sex and age (within five years) (T- and B-Cell Malignancy Study Group, 1985). The investigators checked factors such as blood type (A, B, O), occupation, family history of cancer, habit of raising animals and habit of eating raw meat, but found no association of ATLL with any specific environmental risk factor. They found negative associations with hepatitis and blood transfusion. Tokudome *et al.* (1993) reported that the prevalence of smoking among 141 ATLL cases from northern Kyushu (Fukuoka and Saga) (65% of 75 men, 17% of 66 women) was significantly higher than that reported in the general population (53% and 4%, respectively). [The Working Group noted that smoking data from these cases may not be directly comparable to the general population rates, and that the inverse associations reported with hepatitis and transfusion history may be due to selection bias resulting from the use of hospitalized controls.]

To examine the importance of exposure to HTLV-I during early life (presumably from breast feeding), two groups have studied mothers of patients with ATLL and TSP/HAM. In both Jamaica (Wilks *et al.*, 1996) and Trinidad (Bartholomew *et al.*, 1994), 100% of mothers of ATLL patients were HTLV-I-infected compared with

Table 5. Proportion of anti-HTLV-I antibody-positive individuals in lymphoma cases and controls in Japan and Central/South America

	Japan (Kyushu)[a]	Japan (other districts)[a]	Brazil[b]	Jamaica[d]	Trinidad & Tobago[d]
	Positive/tested (%)	Positive/tested (%)	Positive/tested (%)	Positive/tested (%)	Positive/tested (%)
T-cell lymphoma	162/192 (84.4)	60/142 (42.3)	50/188 (26.5)	41/70 (58.6)	34/43 (79.1)
ATLL	130/130 (100.0)	49/54 (90.7)	48/53 (90.5)	—	45/48 (94)[c]
Other T-cell lymphoma	32/62 (51.6)	11/88 (12.5)	1/29 (3.4)	—	—
Cutaneous T-cell lymphoma	—	—	0/54 (0)	—	—
Non-T-cell lymphoma	12/49 (24.5)	4/117 (3.4)	—	1/24 (4.2)	1/25 (4.0)
Healthy adults	241/3026 (8.0)	95/12 090 (0.8)	697/93 087 (0.7)[c]	27/376 (7.2)	20/355 (5.6)

[a]T- and B-cell Malignancy Study Group (1985)
[b]Pombo de Oliveira et al. (1995) except when noted
[c]Matutes et al. (1994)
[d]Manns et al. (1993)
[e]Cleghorn et al. (1990)

27–30% of mothers of TSP/HAM patients. The results indicate that infection early in life may be very important for the development of ATLL but that some cases of TSP/HAM occur following transmission of the virus later in life.

Studies of the role of the HLA system in relation to HTLV-I-associated disease are presented in Section 4.2.

2.1.2 *HTLV-I infection and cutaneous T-cell lymphomas*

Cutaneous T-cell lymphoma is an uncommon malignancy, with an estimated incidence of 800–1000 new cases per year in the United States (Weinstock *et al.*, 1988). It represents a small proportion (2–5%) of malignant lymphomas. A three-fold increase in the incidence of cutaneous T-cell lymphoma has occurred over the last couple of decades, although some of this increase may be due to improved diagnosis. The incidence of cutaneous T-cell lymphomas rises sharply with age and the average age of a patient at diagnosis is 52 years; the majority of new cases are over 30 years old. Men are affected more frequently than women. In the United States, cutaneous T-cell lymphoma has been found to be more prevalent in blacks than in whites (Pancake *et al.*, 1995).

When ATLL presents predominantly with cutaneous manifestations, it is sometimes indistinguishable from cutaneous T-cell lymphoma on clinical and pathological grounds (Arai *et al.*, 1994). Both are mature T-cell malignancies of $CD4^+$, $CD8^-$ phenotype and affect the skin with a similar histological pattern of infiltration (Whittaker & Luzzatto, 1993; Whittaker *et al.*, 1993).

Over the past few years, a number of reports have indicated finding of HTLV-I and/or a related or partially deleted retrovirus in a subset of cutaneous T-cell lymphomas occurring in non-endemic areas (Hall *et al.*, 1991; Zucker-Franklin *et al.*, 1991; Srivastava *et al.*, 1992; Zucker-Franklin *et al.*, 1992; Pancake & Zucker-Franklin, 1993; Zucker-Franklin & Pancake, 1994; Manca *et al.*, 1994). However, HTLV-I-related sequences have not been found in other studies (Capésius *et al.*, 1991; Bazarbachi *et al.*, 1993, 1995; Matutes *et al.*, 1995b).

Even in the studies suggesting presence of the virus, the patients either lack antibodies to HTLV-I (Hall *et al.*, 1991; Zucker-Franklin *et al.*, 1991; Pancake & Zucker-Franklin, 1993) or show an indeterminate pattern of seroreactivity by the radioimmunoprecipitation assay (RIPA) and western blot, with weak p24 (Gag) reactivity but no anti-Tax or p19 (Gag) antibodies (Srivastava *et al.*, 1992). In one notable case, Picard *et al.* (1990) described one case first described as ATLL who was initially seronegative but produced antibodies several months after chemotherapy had begun; antibody studies were carried out with immunofluorescence techniques. In cases of cutaneous T-cell lymphoma positive for some part of HTLV-I (Gag, Pol or Env) by PCR, none contained a full-length proviral DNA; only one study has shown conservation of the pX region in cutaneous T-cell lymphoma, which is considered to be essential in the pathogenesis of ATLL (Manca *et al.*, 1994). Finally, with one possible exception (Hall *et al.*, 1994), no study has documented monoclonal or oligoclonal integration of HTLV-I in the neoplastic cells, another essential feature of HTLV-associated ATLL.

It is possible that, on occasion, endogenous retroviral sequences have been amplified accidentally using HTLV-I-specific PCR primers (Bangham et al., 1988; Fujihara et al., 1994). Another possibility is that some patients may have an incorrect diagnosis and are considered as having cutaneous T-cell lymphomas, when in fact they have a cutaneous form of ATLL with partial expression of the HTLV-I genome. It is therefore doubtful whether non-ATLL T-cell lymphomas are really associated with HTLV-I sequences.

2.1.3 *HTLV-II infection*

The role of HTLV-II in the pathogenesis of lymphoid neoplasms remains uncertain (Fouchard et al., 1995). HTLV-II was first isolated from spleen cells of a patient with a T-cell malignancy diagnosed as a T-cell variant of hairy-cell leukaemia (Kalyanaraman et al., 1982). In a subsequent case (Rosenblatt et al., 1986), the patient was found to have two distinct neoplasms: a typical B-cell hairy-cell leukaemia in which HTLV-II was not detected and a $CD8^+$ T-cell disorder equivalent to large granular-lymphocyte leukaemia in which HTLV-II was oligoclonally integrated (Rosenblatt et al., 1988a,b). As the T-cell variant form of hairy-cell leukaemia is not a recognized entity among lymphoproliferative disorders, the original patient may have had a condition other than hairy-cell leukaemia.

In 1987, two groups reported finding that patients with large granular-lymphocyte leukaemia had a high prevalence (7/27 and 6/12, respectively) of antibodies against HTLV-II (Pandolfi et al., 1987; Starkebaum et al., 1987). The antibody profile seemed incomplete in most instances, prompting speculation that the response might be due to a related retrovirus. This leukaemia is a rare, chronic T-cell lymphoproliferation with a $CD8^+$, $CD4^-$ phenotype. The patients often present with splenomegaly and have an indolent course lasting for years.

Loughran et al. (1994) reported that six out of 28 patients with large granular-lymphocyte leukaemia were serologically positive for HTLV-I or HTLV-II by ELISA, although some had indeterminate patterns in which the western blot reacted only with either Gag protein or recombinant Env p21. Of these, only one patient with large granular-lymphocyte leukaemia was reported to have HTLV-II sequences in the lymphocytes, detected by PCR (using Pol and/or pX region primers) (Loughran et al., 1992). However, in other cases reported, clonal integration of the retrovirus in the lymphoma cells was not found by Martin et al. (1993) and not investigated by Loughran et al. (1992, 1994), even though the patients had HTLV-II infection. Furthermore, Heneine et al. (1994) screened 51 patients with large granular-lymphocyte leukaemia but found only one to have HTLV-II antibodies. An unusual case of HTLV-I-positive ATLL with a blood picture similar to that of large granular-lymphocyte leukaemia has been reported in Japan (Sakamoto et al., 1994).

Therefore, it remains doubtful whether HTLV-II plays a pathogenic role in large granular-lymphocyte leukaemia; undetected retroviruses or variant virus might be responsible (as proposed by Loughran et al., 1994) or an indirect and non-specific mechanism may be involved (as proposed by Martin et al., 1993).

One patient with mycosis fungoides associated with HTLV-II has been described (Zucker-Franklin et al., 1992).

2.2 Other malignancies

2.2.1 HTLV-I

(a) Case reports and case series

One approach to studying the risk of other malignancies in HTLV-I-infected persons is to look at multiple cancers in ATLL patients. Most reports of such cases come from populations in Japan, where HTLV-I infection is endemic.

Ono et al. (1989) reported that, of 43 consecutive patients with ATLL seen in northern Kyushu (Saga) between 1982 and 1987, five (all aged ≥ 70 years) had additional multiple cancers, including two persons with triple separate malignancies. This was significantly higher than the two multiple cancers seen in 36 similarly aged cases with other haematological malignancies during the same time period (not adjusted for age or sex). The other second primary cancers seen in the cases of ATLL were tumours of the colon, larynx, thyroid, stomach (three), liver and kidney. Similarly, Imamura et al. (1993) found that five of 15 ATLL cases seen at one institution between 1963 and 1985 had a second malignancy (of the thyroid, stomach, larynx, lip and lung); this was significantly higher than the 44 multiple primaries among 1156 patients with other haematological malignancies (not adjusted for age or sex).

There have been various case reports of second non-T-cell primary malignancies in cases of ATLL, including two cases of Kaposi's sarcoma (Greenberg et al., 1990; Veyssier-Belot et al., 1990), an EBV-positive B-cell lymphoma (Tobinai et al., 1991), an acute monoblastic leukaemia (Tokioka et al., 1992) and a cerebral small-cell lymphoma (Komori et al., 1995). Shibata et al. (1995) described a Japanese HTLV-I carrier with a high prevalence (13%) of circulating abnormal lymphocytes and a long history of lymphadenopathy, having a tumour diagnosed as mantle-cell lymphoma with features of mucosa-associated lymphoid tissue lymphoma. EBV genome was not detectable in this B-cell tumour. In these case reports, no integrated HTLV-I provirus was found in the non-ATLL tumour. [The Working Group noted that in the reports of Ono et al. and Veyssier-Belot et al., it is unclear whether the non-ATLL cases were tested for the presence of HTLV-I genome.]

A number of cases have been reported of HTLV-I detected by PCR in tumours other than ATLL. Since PCR will detect HTLV-I in infiltrating lymphocytes, the significance of such findings is open to question (Matsuzati et al., 1990; Imajo et al., 1993; Inoue et al., 1994a).

Several reports dealing mainly with HTLV-I-endemic populations outside Japan describe chronic lymphocytic leukaemia in HTLV-I carriers. Blattner et al. (1983) reported that, of 14 cases of chronic lymphocytic leukaemia identified among a series of haematopoietic malignancies in Jamaica, four were HTLV-I-seropositive but were negative for HTLV-I provirus. Mann et al. (1987) reported experiments using tumour cells from two HTLV-I-seropositive Jamaicans with B-cell chronic lymphocytic leukaemia. In these experiments, the cells were fused with a human B-lymphoblastoid cell line, and the secreted immunoglobulin was then characterized as to its antigen specificity for HTLV-I proteins. In one case, the antibodies reacted to the p24 Gag protein of HTLV-I, and in the other case, to the gp61 Env protein. The authors speculated that HTLV-I infection played an indirect role in the oncogenesis of antigen-committed B cells responding to the infection. [The Working Group noted that it was not clear whether the cases reported by Blattner *et al.* were of B-cell origin.]

Although there is a suggestion from case series of an excess of cancers other than ATLL among persons infected with HTLV-I, this is not supported by cohort studies (see below).

(b) Cohort studies

Tokudome *et al.* (1991) followed 3991 HTLV-I-seropositive blood donors aged ≥ 40 years from four communities in Kyushu who had donated blood between 1984 and 1987. Positivity for HTLV-I was determined by a particle agglutination antibody assay (see p. 297). Mortality was ascertained through to August 1989; the average length of follow-up was 2.7 years. Twenty-six deaths were reported in the cohort, four from malignancies (excluding those from ATLL and malignant lymphoma). Expected numbers were calculated on the basis of national age-specific rates. There was a significant deficit among HTLV-I carriers for deaths from other cancers: observed/expected, 0.32 (95% CI, 0.07–0.93) for men and 0.13 (95% CI, 0.00–0.71) for women. The authors noted that these findings are underestimates because of the healthy donor effect.

Iwata *et al.* (1994) followed up a total of 1997 individuals aged ≥ 30 years from an HTLV-I-endemic community in Nagasaki Prefecture for an average of 5.3 years (see p. 297). Population registries, death certificates and hospital records were used to identify a total of 120 deaths within the cohort; of these, 45 occurred among 503 HTLV-I carriers and included 10 non-ATLL malignancies. Based on proportionate mortality hazard, the risk for death from all other malignancies associated with HTLV-I infection was 1.2 (95% CI, 0.39–3.5) for men and 1.8 (0.61–5.2) for women.

(c) Case–control studies

In order to examine the association between HTLV-I infection and non-ATLL malignancies, Asou *et al.* (1986) identified 685 patients with malignancies other than ATLL (average age, 60 years) in 11 hospitals in central Kyushu (Kumamoto), Japan, between February and March 1985. Patients with an unknown history of blood transfusion were excluded. Seven patients had double malignancies. The comparison group included 22 726 healthy individuals who were part of a health survey by the Japanese Red Cross Health Service Center; all had lived in the Prefecture since early childhood. The two groups were compared for seroprevalence of HTLV-I as determined by ELISA, with adjustment for age and sex. The results were reported separately for cases according to whether or not they had a history of blood transfusion. The overall seroprevalence in the 394 non-transfused cases with other malignancies was 15.5% and for the 291 with a history of transfusion was 26.1%. The corresponding crude prevalence rate in the comparison population was 3.0%. The relative risk associated with HTLV-I infection for malignancies other than ATLL was 2.2 ($p < 0.01$) among the non-transfused cases and 4.2 among the transfused cases ($p < 0.03$). [The Working Group noted that the controls were likely to be more healthy than the general population and were not stratified by transfusion history.]

A series of reports described an association of HTLV-I with hepatocellular carcinoma in Japan, which is commonly due to either hepatitis B virus (HBV) or hepatitis C virus (HCV) (see IARC, 1994). Iida *et al.* (1988) evaluated the HTLV-I antibody status of 380 patients with various liver diseases including hepatocellular carcinoma in Kyushu (Kumamoto), Japan. HTLV-I seropositivity was determined by ELISA with western blot confirmation. For comparison, the overall seroprevalence rate in 62 000 blood donors from the area was 4.7%. The crude seroprevalence rate of 17.5% among the 40 cases of hepatocellular carcinoma was significantly higher than the comparison rates ($p < 0.001$); however, six of the seven seropositive cases had a history of transfusion. Among 93 cases of liver cirrhosis, a condition which almost always precedes the development of hepatocellular carcinoma, the HTLV-I seroprevalence of 10.8% was also significantly higher ($p < 0.01$), but 6 of the 10 seropositive cases had a history of transfusion. [The Working Group noted that it was unclear whether the higher HTLV-I infection rate in cases was due to disease-related transfusions or whether HTLV-I contributed to the occurrence of hepatocellular carcinoma. The data given are not sufficient to calculate age- and sex-adjusted estimates of relative risk.]

Kamihira *et al.* (1994) examined the prevalence of co-infection with HTLV-I and HCV and HBV in cases of liver disease including hepatocellular carcinoma in blood donors in Nagasaki. Cases included 181 cases of hepatocellular carcinoma seen at Nagasaki University Hospital and 228 cases of either chronic hepatitis or cirrhosis. Control data were obtained from 77 540 local blood donors. HTLV-I positivity was determined by particle agglutination assay and ELISA, with confirmation by western blot if necessary. [The Working Group noted that it was unclear whether positivity was based on either particle agglutination or ELISA or whether all sera were screened by both assays.] HBV status was detected by particle agglutination assays and HCV status by the first-generation ELISA. Among the control data, there was a significant association between HCV and HTLV-I infection (1.9% HCV-positive among 2907 HTLV-I seropositive versus 1.1% among 74 633 HTLV-I seronegative ($p = 0.04$)), but not between HBV and HTLV-I infections ($p = 0.70$). The mean age at hepatocellular carcinoma diagnosis among the 31 patients with HTLV-I antibody (61.5 years) was significantly lower than that of the 112 HTLV-I-seronegative cases (64.8 years; $p = 0.04$).

Okayama *et al.* (1995) examined the effect of HTLV-I co-infection on risk for HCV-positive hepatocellular carcinoma in comparison to HCV-positive chronic hepatitis. The cases included 43 sequentially seen hepatocellular carcinoma patients (33 men and 10 women) in southern Kyushu (Miyazaki), Japan, with a mean age of 62.4 years. The control group consisted of 127 biopsy-proven HCV-positive chronic hepatitis patients (86 men and 41 women) with a mean age of 51.7 years. All subjects were seropositive for HCV antibody and negative for HBV surface antigen. HTLV-I antibody status was determined by the particle agglutination assay, with confirmation by western blot. HCV antibody status was determined by a second-generation ELISA. The HTLV-I seroprevalence among the cases of hepatocellular carcinoma was 30.2% and that among the chronic hepatitis controls was 9.5%. Among the 41 cases aged ≥ 50 years, 31.7% were HTLV-I carriers compared with 7.3% among the 82 HCV-positive chronic hepatitis patients of the same age ($p = 0.001$). With adjustment for broad age groups, the relative risk for HCV-positive hepatocellular carcinoma associated with co-infection with HTLV-I was 12.8 (95% CI, 3.3–52.3) among men; among women, there was no significant difference (relative risk, 1.3; 0.17–10.1). In this study, the prevalence of history of transfusion was similar among cases (42.9%) and chronic hepatitis controls (38.9%).

Several studies have examined the relationship between HTLV-I infection and human papillomavirus (HPV)-associated gynaecological malignancies (see IARC, 1995).

Miyazaki et al. (1991) examined the association of HTLV-I infection with gynaecological malignancies in patients from central Kyushu, Japan. Cases included 226 patients with gynaecological malignancies newly treated between April 1986 and July 1989, excluding those with a history of blood transfusion. The case group included 153 cervical cancer patients, 28 endometrial carcinoma patients, 37 ovarian carcinoma patients and 8 vaginal carcinoma patients. For comparison, the HTLV-I seroprevalence among 6701 healthy women seen at a mass health screening was used. HTLV-I status was determined by both immunofluorescence and ELISA assays. The relative risk for HTLV-I seroprevalence associated with cervical cancer among the 88 women aged ≤ 59 years was 2.9 ($p < 0.005$) and that for older cases was 1.7. Similarly, based on eight cases of vaginal carcinoma, the relative risk was 7.4 ($p < 0.001$). One of the latter cases also had smouldering ATLL. However, for the cases of endometrial and ovarian cancer, there was no association with HTLV-I (relative risks, 0.97 and 0.87, respectively). There was no significant association between HTLV-I status and stage of cervical cancer or the presence of regional node metastases in 59 patients who had primary radical surgery. However, HTLV-I status was predictive of recurrence among the cases of cervical and vaginal cancer combined ($p < 0.05$).

Strickler et al. (1995) evaluated the association between HTLV-I infection and the degree of cervical epithelial abnormalities. Cases for this case–control study were 49 outpatients with cervical intraepithelial neoplasia (CIN)-III or invasive carcinoma of the cervix sequentially seen at a colposcopy clinic in Jamaica between March 1992 and August 1993, from whom adequate tissue for analysis was available. Controls were 120 women diagnosed with benign, atypical squamous cells of unknown significance (ASCUS), CIN I or koilocytotic atypia. HTLV-I antibody status was determined by either a whole virus or recombinant gp21 ELISA with western blot confirmation. HPV DNA was detected by PCR, with typing for 11 sub-types (low, intermediate, high risk). As expected, there was a strong association with the detection of HPV DNA: 92.1% of cases were positive versus 25.7% in benign, 50% in ASCUS and 49.2% of the CIN I and koilocytotic atypia control subjects. HTLV-I seropositivity was greater among cases, who had more advanced stage (14.3%) than the controls (2.9%) (age-adjusted relative risk, 3.8; 95% CI, 1.03–14.2).

These case–control studies are summarized in Table 6. Overall, case–control studies of HTLV-I and risk of malignancies other than ATLL are few and may be influenced by selection bias (e.g., use of blood donors as controls). Significant positive associations were found for hepatocellular carcinoma and cancers of the female lower genital tract, which showed associations with HBV and HCV and with HPV, respectively. However, since these viruses are transmissible by similar routes to HTLV-I, the reported associations may be confounded.

2.2.2 HTLV-II

The majority of studies investigating an association between HTLV-I and malignancy have used assays which would also detect HTLV-II, and none has reported an association of HTLV-II with malignancy.

3. Studies of Cancer in Animals

During the study of natural retroviral infection in non-human primates, it became apparent that many African and Asian non-human primate species had serum antibodies that cross-reacted with HTLV-I antigens. Prevalence of serum antibodies found in these populations varied from < 10 to > 80% and generally increased with age. African green monkeys (*Cercopithecus aethiops*) and macaque species generally had the highest seroprevalence (Miyoshi *et al.*, 1983; Hayami *et al.*, 1984; Ishikawa *et al.*, 1987; Fultz, 1994). A virus isolated from lymphoid cell lines established from seropositive monkeys was shown by Southern blot analysis of genomic DNA, nucleotide sequence analysis and type-specific synthetic peptide epitopes to be 90–95% homologous to HTLV-I (Komuro *et al.*, 1984; Tsujimoto *et al.*, 1985; Watanabe *et al.*, 1985; Ishikawa *et al.*, 1987; Rudolph *et al.*, 1991) and was designated as simian T-cell lymphotropic virus type I (STLV-I).

3.1 HTLV-I in animal models

3.1.1 *Non-human primates*

Six cynomolgus (*Macaca fascicularis*) and two squirrel (*Saimiri sciureus*) monkeys were infected experimentally with HTLV-I by inoculation with autologous lymphoid cell lines immortalized by and producing HTLV-I. To produce the cell lines, monkey peripheral blood mononuclear cells were co-cultivated with lethally irradiated MT-2 cells producing HTLV-I. All the cell lines had monkey karyotypes, grew continuously and expressed IL-2 and virus-specific proteins of HTLV-I. Specific antibodies against HTLV-I and transformed HTLV-I-infected peripheral blood cells were found in the inoculated monkeys. No neoplastic lesion was detected up to two years after inoculation (Nakamura *et al.*, 1986).

Table 6. Case–control studies of the association of HTLV-I infection with malignancies other than adult T-cell leukaemia/lymphoma

Reference	Cancer site		Cases	HTLV-I+ (%)	Controls	HTLV-I+ (%)	Odds ratio	Comments
Asou et al. (1986)	All sites except ATLL		394	15.5	Healthy volunteers	3.0	2.2	Excludes cases with history of blood transfusion
	Liver only		33	15.2	Healthy volunteers	3.0	2.6	
Iida et al. (1988)	Liver		40	17.5	Local blood donors	4.7	NG	6/7 HTLV-I+ cases had been transfused
Miyazaki et al. (1991)	Cervix	< 59 years	88	10.2	Healthy volunteers	[3.3]	2.9	
		> 60 years	65	16.9	Healthy volunteers	10.2	1.7	
	Ovary		37	2.7	Healthy volunteers		0.87	
	Vagina		8	50.0	Healthy volunteers		7.4	
	Endometrium		28	7.1	Healthy volunteers		0.97	
Kamihira et al. (1994)	Liver		181	20.4	Local blood donors	3.8	NG	HTLV-I seropositivity was associated with HCV seropositivity
Okayama et al. (1995)	Liver		43	30.2	HCV-positive chronic hepatitis	9.5	12.8 (males) 1.3 (females)	Transfusion prevalence similar in cases and controls
Strickler et al. (1995)	Cervix		49	14.3	Benign, ASCUS, koilocytotic atypia or CIN I	3.3	3.8	Cases had invasive carcinoma or CIN III

NG, not given; CIN, cervical intraepithelial neoplasia; ASCUS, atypical squamous cells of unknown significance

3.1.2 *Other models*

Adult T-cell leukaemia-like disease was experimentally induced by injection of an HTLV-I-transformed rabbit T-cell line into syngenic rabbits. The cell line was obtained from peripheral blood of a two-month-old virus-infected (B/J × Chbb:HM) F1 rabbit. Fifty per cent of 13 intraperitoneally inoculated newborn rabbits died or were moribund within seven days. Four rabbits surviving for four weeks had detectable cellular cytotoxic activity against transformed cells, increased leukocyte counts and abnormal lymphocytes with convoluted or lobulated nuclei. Histologically, leukaemic infiltrates, probably direct cell-line progeny, were seen in the liver, lung, spleen and mesenteric lymph nodes. The same cell line and dosage killed two syngenic adult rabbits when given intravenously. Three adult virus carriers, 8–15 months of age, were resistant to similar doses (Seto *et al.*, 1988). [The Working Group noted the incomplete description of the lymphoid infiltrates and that this system was not sufficiently characterized to be accepted as a useful model.]

LTR-*tax* transgenic and HTLV-I infected severe combined immunodeficient (SCID) mouse models are discussed in Sections 4.3.2 and 4.3.4 respectively.

3.2 STLV-I in non-human primates

3.2.1 *STLV-I-associated lymphomas* (see also Table 7)

Malignant lymphoma is the most commonly occurring neoplasm in non-human primates and is found most frequently in Old World species (reviewed in Beniashvili, 1989).

Homma *et al.* (1984) detected serum antibodies to membrane antigens of HTLV-I-infected cells in 11 of 13 macaques (*Macaca cyclopis, M. mulatta, M. fascicularis*) with malignant lymphoma or lymphoproliferative disease. In contrast, these antibodies were found in only 7 of 95 healthy macaques of the same colony.

Voevodin *et al.* (1985) reported that, among Sukhumi lymphoma-prone baboons (*Papio hamadryas*), serum antibodies to HTLV-I antigens were found by the indirect immunofluorescence test in 57 of 58 lymphomatous baboons but in only 80 of 177 healthy baboons from the same 'lymphoma-prone' colony. The prevalence of HTLV-I antibodies in baboon populations considered to be 'lymphoma-free' was 5–8%. [The Working Group noted that interpretation of these data was complicated by the introduction of human leukaemic blood into the baboon colony. This blood was not evaluated for viral infection before use (Lapin, 1969). Herpesvirus papio (HVP) was also endemic in the colony.] Later it was shown that monoclonally integrated STLV-I proviral information of rhesus origin was present in the lymphomatous tissue of these baboons (Voevodin *et al.*, 1996).

Srivastava *et al.* (1986) detected antibodies reactive against HTLV-I by several assays, including western blot analysis, in three serum samples collected over a period of approximately four years from a 24-year-old female gorilla (*Gorilla gorilla graueri*) with non-Hodgkin's lymphoma. Morphologically, the neoplasm was diagnosed as a T-cell

Table 7. Lymphoid neoplasia in STLV-I-positive nonhuman primates

Genus, species	Country	No. of animals	Neoplasm	Proviral integration	Comments	Reference
Papio spp.	Georgia	57	Lymphoma	Monoclonal	Rhesus STLV-I$^+$	Voevodin et al. (1985, 1996)
Papio spp.	USA	27	Lymphoma (11 with leukaemia)	ND	—	Hubbard et al. (1993)
Papio spp.	USA	1	Leukaemia/lymphoma	ND	—	McCarthy et al. (1990)
Cercopithecus aethiops	USA	1	Lymphoproliferative disease	Monoclonal	SIV$^+$/STLV-I$^+$	Traina-Dorge et al. (1992)
Cercopithecus aethiops	Japan	6	Leukaemia (1) Pre-leukaemic (5)	Monoclonal	STLV-I$^+$	Tsujimoto et al. (1987)
Cercopithecus aethiops	Japan	1	Lymphoma	Monoclonal	—	Sakakibara et al. (1986)
Cercopithecus aethiops	USA	1	Lymphoma	ND	—	Jayo et al. (1990)
Cercocebus atys	USA	3	Lymphocytosis (1) Leukaemia (1) Lymphoma (1)	ND	SIV$_{SM}^+$/STLV-I$^+$	McClure et al. (1992)
Macaca cyclops *Macaca mulatta* *Macaca fascicularis*	USA	3 5 3	Lymphoproliferative disease	ND	—	Homma et al. (1984)
Gorilla gorilla graueri	USA	1	Lymphoma	Monoclonal	—	Srivastava et al. (1986)

ND, not detected

histiocytic lymphoma. [The Working Group noted the lack of immunochemical information to confirm the T-cell origin of the neoplasm.] Southern blot analysis of DNA from *Bam*HI-digested neoplastic tissue using a complete HTLV-I genome probe yielded one 10-kb fragment and a 1.05-kb internal fragment common to all HTLV-I isolates. This confirmed that the gorilla was infected with HTLV-I or a closely related virus. The gorilla was also seropositive for cytomegalovirus, Epstein–Barr-like virus and Yaba virus.

Sakakibara *et al*. (1986) reported lymphoma and leukaemia in a wild-caught female green monkey (*Cercopithecus aethiops*) that was very similar to human ATLL. Neoplastic lymphocyte antigens reacted specifically with antibodies to HTLV-I and were $CD2^+$ ($Leu 2a^+$), $CD3^-$ ($Leu3a^-$) and negative for surface immunoglobulin.

Spontaneous malignant lymphomas, including 12 cases with leukaemia and lymphoma, were reported in 28 baboons and one African green monkey. All the lymphoma cases were seropositive for HTLV-I antigen, while the prevalence in the 3200-member baboon colony was about 40%. The disease in these monkeys had many similarities to ATLL in humans, including skin involvement, adult onset, generalized lymphadenopathy, hepatosplenomegaly, anaemia, leukaemia, hypercalcaemia, pulmonary involvement and similar histological and immunocytochemical features. Immunohistochemically, 24 of the lymphomas were of T-cell origin, two of B-cell lineage, two could not be identified as B- or T-cell origin and one was not evaluated (Jayo *et al*., 1990; McCarthy *et al*., 1990; Hubbard *et al*., 1993).

McClure *et al*. (1992) found T-cell leukaemia, lymphocytosis and lymphoma, respectively, in three 10–23 year-old sooty mangabeys (*Cercocebus atys*) naturally infected with SIV_{SMM} and STLV-I. Another dual infection of SIV and STLV-I together with a lymphoproliferative disease was observed in an African green monkey (Traina-Dorge *et al*., 1992).

3.2.2 *Pathological and molecular aspects*

Ishikawa *et al*. (1987) established 11 cell lines of virus-producing lymphoid cells in the presence of IL-2 from five species of STLV-I antibody-positive non-human primates. The cell lines expressed T-cell activation markers and either $CD3^+$ or $CD2^+$, expressed viral antigens that reacted with sera from human ATLL patients and monoclonal antibodies against p19 and p24 of HTLV-I core protein, and produced virus particles with RNA-dependent DNA polymerase activity. DNA from these cell lines contained proviral sequences similar to HTLV-I but with different restriction patterns.

Peripheral blood lymphocyte chromosomal DNA taken from 31 wild-caught captive STLV-I-seropositive African green monkeys was evaluated for proviral integration of STLV-I. One of these monkeys was overtly leukaemic and five were pre-leukaemic. Pre-leukaemia was diagnosed by finding abnormal lymphocytes in the peripheral blood. The monoclonal integration sites of the proviral genome in these six monkeys indicated proliferation of STLV-I-infected cells. Restriction patterns with *Pst*I and *Sst*I were the same as those for prior isolates from African green monkeys, except that three animals had deletions of one *Pst*I site, suggesting that the virus could be defective in these cases.

Lymphocytes from seropositive monkeys without leukaemic changes did not contain provirus detectable by Southern blot and were polyclonal. The development of ATLL-like disease with monoclonal integration of STLV-I proviral genome indicated that STLV-I has similar leukaemogenicity to HTLV-I (Tsujimoto et al., 1987). [The Working Group noted that the pre-leukaemic diagnosis in five animals was tentative, as abnormal lymphocytes were found in STLV-I-seronegative monkeys, and it is difficult to correlate the occurrence of abnormal lymphocytes with seropositivity.]

Lymphoproliferative disease was diagnosed in an African green monkey with monoclonally integrated STLV-I. STLV-related sequences were identified by Southern blot analysis of DNA extracted from hyperplastic lymphoid tissue. This animal was also infected with SIV and was immunodeficient, as suggested by wasting, cryptosporidial intestinal infection and relatively low levels of $CD4^+$ and high levels of $CD8^+$ lymphocytes (Traina-Dorge et al., 1992). [The Working Group noted that the immunodeficiency diagnosis was questionable.]

Moné et al. (1992) established a cell line from a non-Hodgkin's lymphoma of a baboon and detected monoclonally integrated STLV-I proviral DNA, using Southern blot assay and HTLV-I PCR.

An STLV-I rhesus strain (*M. mulatta*) has been characterized in lymphomas from Sukhumi baboons (*Papio hamadryas*). Thirty-seven STLV-I isolates were investigated by PCR which discriminated rhesus-type and baboon-type STLV-I strains. The PCR results were confirmed by DNA sequence data. Partial nucleotide sequences of both STLV-I isolates from lymphomatous baboons were 97–100% homologous to known rhesus STLV-I and 85% homologous to conventional baboon STLV-I. This macaque-to-baboon inter-species transfer of STLV-I may have initiated the outbreak and increased the incidence of lymphoma among Sukhumi baboon colonies (Voevodin et al., 1996).

3.3 Bovine leukaemia virus in sheep and cattle

Bovine leukaemia virus (BLV), HTLV-I, HTLV-II and STLV constitute a unique subgroup within the retrovirus family, characterized by a distinct genetic content, genomic organization and strategy for gene expression (Cann & Chen, 1990; Gallo & Wong-Staal, 1990; Burny et al., 1994; Kettmann et al., 1994). Although BLV is not as closely related to HTLV-I as are the STLVs, much more is known about its pathogenicity and transmission. Therefore the carcinogenicity of BLV is considered here. BLV infection has been eradicated from western European cattle. No evidence of human infection has been documented.

BLV is a transactivating retrovirus recognized as the etiological agent of enzootic bovine leukosis (reviewed in Burny et al., 1994; Kettmann et al., 1994; Schwartz & Lévy, 1994). Presence of the virus has been reported in cattle, sheep, water-buffaloes and capybaras (a South American rodent, *Hydrochoerus hydrochaeris*). Experimental induction of tumours by BLV has been carried out in cattle, sheep and goats (Kettmann et al., 1984), but it is not known if tumours can be induced in water-buffaloes and capybaras.

Replication of these viruses is regulated at the transcriptional and post-transcriptional levels by their own regulatory proteins, notably Tax and Rex. Infection is followed by a long latent period, and only a small proportion of infected individuals develop the terminal neoplastic disease. BLV virions are difficult to identify in neoplastic tissue, but can be found in normal or neoplastic lymphoid cells from BLV-infected cattle or sheep (Jensen et al., 1991; Powers & Radke, 1992). Apart from the difference in host range, a notable difference between BLV and HTLV is that infection by BLV is associated with malignancy of B cells, whereas HTLV affects T cells (Paul et al., 1977).

BLV provirus comprises 8714 bp, making up the following genes (Figure 10):

- *gag*, representing the genetic information for the matrix (p15), capsid (p24) and nucleic acid-binding (p12) proteins;
- *prt*, encoding the viral protease, p14;
- *pol*, the gene for reverse transcriptase and integrase (852 amino acids);
- *env*, the gene for gp51 (268 amino acids) and gp30 (214 amino acids), the external and transmembrane glycoproteins respectively;
- *tax*, the genetic element coding for a transactivator protein, p34 Tax;
- *rex*, the sequence coding for the Rex protein (p18), a molecule involved in the export of genomic RNA from the nucleus;
- R3 and G4, two open reading frames coding for protein products of 44 amino acids and 105 amino acids, respectively, that upregulate BLV expression in the infected host.

Figure 10. Genomic organization of BLV provirus[a]

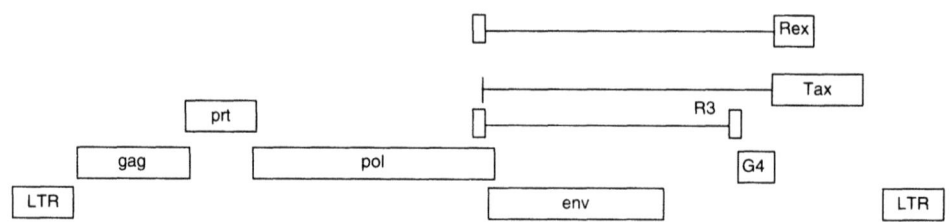

[a] From Schwarz & Lévy (1994)

Transmission of BLV occurs mainly via transfer of infected lymphocytes by contaminated needles, syringes, etc. Transmission can also occur via milk and *in utero* (Schwartz & Lévy, 1994). Infection can be experimentally transmitted to sheep, goats, pigs, rabbits, monkeys and buffalos (Kettmann et al., 1984; 1994). Tattooing, dehorning, rectal palpation and vaccination procedures can be involved in the transmission of BLV via contaminated blood (Foil & Issel, 1991). Once established, infection is lifelong. The viral load of the inoculum, the time since infection, the efficiency of virus propagation and clonal expansion of BLV-infected cells are key factors determining the number of infected cells at any given time and the probability of neoplastic transformation.

Experimental transmission via biting insects (Foil & Issel, 1991) or intradermal inoculation of BLV proviral DNA into sheep (Willems *et al.*, 1992b; 1993) has been reported.

The presence of BLV within a host is detected by agar-gel immunodiffusion and ELISA. PCR is not useful because viral propagation is slow and the immunogenicity of the virus is high. Seropositivity is detected by gp51 ELISA within two to three weeks after infection (see Kettmann *et al.*, 1994).

3.3.1 Disorders induced by BLV

BLV is associated with enzootic bovine leukosis (EBL) (also called bovine leukaemia, bovine lymphoma, bovine lymphosarcoma, bovine malignant lymphoma), which is the most common neoplastic disease of cattle. In terms of the long-term progression of BLV infection, cattle fall into three major groups (see Figure 11). The first and largest of these groups includes those animals (about 60%) that develop a persistent infection and humoral immune response but are normal in every other respect. The second group, representing 30–35% of all BLV-infected cattle, develop persistent lymphocytosis, a disorder that results from polyclonal expansion of the B-lymphocyte population (Kettmann *et al.*, 1980a,b). The third, and much smaller, group (about 5% of infected animals), includes animals that develop leukaemia/lymphosarcoma.

Figure 11. BLV-induced pathogenesis in cattle

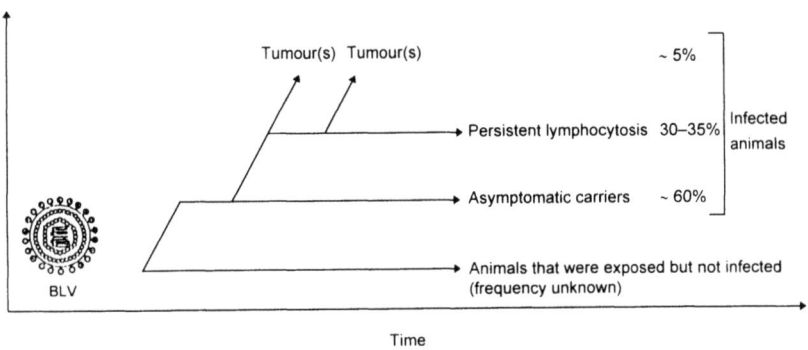

From Kettmann *et al.* (1994)

BLV is the etiological agent of not only bovine leukosis but also ovine leukosis. Although less than 5% of BLV-infected cattle go on to develop tumours, all experimentally infected sheep progress to and die in the tumour phase of the disease and after shorter latency periods than cattle (Djilali *et al.*, 1987; Djilali & Parodi, 1989; Gatei *et al.*, 1989).

(a) Cattle

Three types of EBL are clinically recognized (International Committee on Bovine Leukosis, 1968):

Calf multicentric type: This is characterized by rapidly growing generalized lymph node enlargement with bone marrow involvement. Lymphocytes infiltrate various internal organs, particularly late in the disease.

Adult multicentric type: There is usually lymph node enlargement which may be either symmetrical or asymmetrical. Any tissue in the body may be infiltrated by neoplastic cells and clinical signs depend on the organs or organ systems involved.

Skin leukosis: The first sign may be an urticaria-like change in the skin, especially on the neck, back, rump and thighs. Lymph nodes may be enlarged and the skin lesions may become covered with a thick scab. There may be complete healing of skin lesions and lymph node regression. However, the disease may take a fatal course with typical lymph node involvement and neoplastic-cell infiltration of organs.

(b) Sheep

The haematological disorders associated with BLV infection are less well defined in sheep. BLV-infected sheep do not develop a persistent lymphocytosis lasting for years, as is seen in cattle. Some infected animals develop lymphosarcoma with no previous haematological disorder (Djilali & Parodi, 1989; Ohshima *et al.*, 1991b). Lymphoid leukaemia and localized lymphosarcoma frequently occur together (Gatei *et al.*, 1989; Ohshima *et al.*, 1991a; Murakami *et al.*, 1994a).

3.3.2 Pathological and molecular aspects

(a) Cattle

BLV persists in peripheral B-lymphocytes (Paul *et al.*, 1977) and the proportion of B-lymphocytes in the peripheral blood of BLV-positive animals increases before any potential increase in the number of circulating lymphocytes (Fossum *et al.*, 1988). Persistent lymphocytosis, when it develops (Figure 11), is a polyclonal expansion of the B-cell population, including BLV-infected and BLV-uninfected cells (Kenyon & Piper, 1977). The ratio of infected to uninfected cells is roughly 1 : 3 to 1 : 4 (Kettmann *et al.*, 1980a). Animals are considered to be in persistent lymphocytosis when successive total lymphocyte counts significantly exceed normal values (International Committee on Bovine Leukosis, 1968).

Studies of the heritability of susceptibility to persistent lymphocytosis led to the conclusion that persistent lymphocytosis is familial (Abt *et al.*, 1970; Lewin & Bernoco, 1986; Lewin *et al.*, 1988). BLV-infected B-cells from cows with persistent lymphocytosis expressed high levels of major histocompatibility complex (MHC) class II, surface IgM and CD5 antigen. Cells expressing CD11b and CD11c, normally expressed by cells of the myeloid lineage were also found. $CD5^+$ cells from BLV-positive cattle, whether with persistent lymphocytosis or not, are activated, cycling cells that respond to IL-2 (Matheise *et al.*, 1992).

In persistent lymphocytosis, proviral DNA is integrated at many genomic sites in BLV-positive circulating leukocytes. In lymphosarcoma, in contrast, proviral DNA is integrated at only one or a few sites. Tumours result from a mono- or oligoclonal proliferation of cells. Integration sites, however, are not conserved from one animal to another. For example, DNAs from 25 independent hamster × bovine somatic-cell hybrids were analysed by Southern blot with probes made of unique cell DNA fragments adjacent to single-copy proviruses from three different bovine tumours. It appeared that these cellular sequences, and thus the respective proviruses, belonged to three different chromosomes in the three tumours examined (Grégoire et al., 1984). No rearrangement of cellular DNA sequences flanking a BLV provirus was found in 28 other BLV-induced tumours (Kettmann et al., 1983). It can be concluded that tumour cells can accommodate proviral DNA sequences at many sites in the genome.

Histological classification of BLV-induced lymphomas was carried out using the National Cancer Institute Working Formulation (Vernau et al., 1992). The distribution of cell types varied much more than in humans. Most of the bovine lymphomas (1067/1198; 89%) were high-grade tumours. The diffuse large-cell type and its cleaved variant comprised 66% of the lymphomas. Follicular tumours were extremely rare (4/1198; 0.3%), in marked contrast to human non-Hodgkin's lymphomas, of which at least 34% are follicular.

Seventeen BLV-induced bovine lymphoid tumours were determined to be of B-cell lineage, based on their immunoglobulin gene rearrangements (Heeney & Valli, 1990). Immunohistochemical studies of bovine lymphosarcomas using a pan-T monoclonal antibody revealed that they all lacked detectable-T cells. Although one tumour failed to react with monoclonal antibodies directed against either T- or B-cell determinants, all others were positive for various B-cell markers. The most frequent phenotype was Ia$^+$, cytoplasmic IgM$^+$ or surface IgM$^+$, with occasional concurrent appearance of the IgG isotype. Cells positive for terminal deoxynucleotidyl transferase (TdT$^+$) occurred sporadically. It follows that BLV-induced tumours are composed of relatively mature B-cells.

(b) *Sheep*

BLV infection in sheep causes increases in circulating B-lymphocytes. Tumours have been described as polymorphic centroblastic lymphosarcoma (Parodi et al., 1982; Parodi, 1987), in which more than 95% of the cells were positive for surface immunoglobulins and MHC class II (Murakami et al., 1994a,b). In one study, coexpression of CD5 and B-cell markers occurred in half of the cases (Dimmock et al., 1990).

Tumours in sheep are monoclonal or oligoclonal expansions of cells carrying proviral information. Most of the tumours tested contained one BLV provirus per genome. In contrast, peripheral blood lymphocytes from aleukaemic sheep and sheep with early lymphocytosis are characterized by polyclonally integrated provirus. Appearance of a clonal subpopulation among cells with polyclonally integrated provirus indicates the onset of leukaemia (Rovnak et al., 1993). Tumours from different sheep harbour the provirus at different sites, suggesting that the mechanisms for tumour initiation are independent of the integration site.

(c) Mechanistic studies

The mode of cell transformation by BLV remains conjectural. BLV Tax protein probably plays a central role, as it is a major determinant of the replication potential of the virus. The same is true of the protein products of the viral genes R3 and/or G4 (Willems *et al.*, 1994) and of the YXXL motifs of the transmembrane glycoprotein (Willems *et al.*, 1995). Bovine Tax protein complements activated human *ras* p21 in transforming Fischer rat embryo fibroblasts (Willems *et al.*, 1990) and the Tax/*ras* p21 cooperative effect is not hampered by a mutation that abrogates the transactivating activity of Tax protein (Willems *et al.*, 1990; 1992c). It is thus clear that transactivation by Tax and transformation by Tax in collaboration with *ras* p21 are separable functions of the Tax molecule. No data yet demonstrate whether the induction of leukaemia/lymphoma is affected by cellular oncogenes in cattle, sheep or goats.

Alterations of the *p53* tumour-suppressor gene have been examined in cattle and sheep. No *p53* mutation was found in 10 BLV-induced sheep tumours. In cattle, 5 out of 10 tumours harboured *p53* mutations, whereas only one of seven samples from animals in persistent lymphocytosis showed an alteration of the *p53* gene. It appears that *p53* genomic alterations are not frequently involved in BLV-induced leukaemogenesis in sheep (Dequiedt *et al.*, 1995).

3.3.3 *Vaccination trials*

Protection against retrovirus infection has been achieved in sheep by vaccination with recombinant vaccinia viruses expressing the BLV Env protein (Ohishi *et al.*, 1991; Portetelle *et al.*, 1991). Sheep protected against infection showed a CD4 response to Env peptide 51-70 (Gatei *et al.*, 1993) and a high neutralizing antibody titre (Portetelle *et al.*, 1991). Vaccinated sheep which become infected after challenge with the virus maintain a low viral load for several years without signs of disease.

4. Other Data Relevant to an Evaluation of Carcinogenesis and its Mechanisms

4.1 General observations on retroviral oncogenesis

Oncogenic retroviruses are naturally occurring infections of a large number of vertebrate hosts ranging from fish to humans. Retroviruses cause many types of neoplasm, including leukaemias, lymphomas, mammary and other carcinomas, and sarcomas (Weiss *et al.*, 1985; Levy, 1992–1995).

There are several distinct mechanisms by which animal retroviruses may elicit neoplasms under experimental and natural conditions. An indirect oncogenic effect occurs when neither the malignant cell nor its precursors are infected by the retrovirus. An immunodeficiency virus may permit the appearance of neoplasms as opportunistic events in the same sense as opportunistic infections occur in immunodeficient animals and humans. A directly oncogenic retrovirus inserts its provirus into a cell destined to become malignant. Such viruses may either cause cancer after a long incubation period, or do so acutely.

The majority of nonhuman retroviruses which are directly oncogenic are C-type viruses with 'simple' genomes containing the long terminal repeats (LTR) and *gag*, *pol* and *env* genes. Such viruses do not carry transforming genes but in the tumour cells, the DNA provirus is integrated adjacent to specific cellular proto-oncogenes. These cellular genes become overexpressed through *cis*-acting promoter or enhancer functions of the LTR. Oncogenesis usually depends on a period of high virus replication. The ectopic activation of the proto-oncogene by the LTR is the crucial viral step in oncogenesis. The viruses found in the tumour cells may be either replication competent or defective variants.

Acutely transforming retroviruses carry viral oncogenes originally derived from cellular oncogenes and which are not required for viral replication. These transduced oncogenes can induce the growth of tumours with a short latency (days in contrast to months or years). Acutely transforming retroviruses are usually replication-defective, as the oncogene is substituted for viral gene sequences in the genome. Their replication relies on replication-competent 'helper' viruses which provide the missing viral proteins. Despite an excess of helper virus, acutely transforming retroviruses are seldom transmitted from one host to another.

The human T-cell leukaemia viruses, together with the related STLV of primates and bovine leukosis virus, differ from both the acutely transforming, oncogene-transducing viruses and the slowly oncogenic, replication-competent viruses in having 'complex' genomes bearing regulatory genes, such as *tax* (Section 1.1.1), required for efficient viral replication. The *tax* gene encodes a protein which also activates the expression of cellular genes (transactivation) and this effect is related to the immortalizing properties of these viruses. The transactivating effect of *tax* probably plays an important role in HTLV-I oncogenesis (Section 4.3.2). While the *tax* genes of both HTLV-I and HTLV-II exert an immortalizing effect on human T-lymphocytes *in vitro* (Section 4.3.2), only HTLV-I has been strongly linked with malignancy on the basis of epidemiological evidence (Section 2). In contrast to the *cis*-acting, slowly transforming retroviruses, the HTLV-I provirus integrates at many different chromosomal sites in ATLL cells in different patients (Yoshida *et al.*, 1984). It therefore appears that the site of integration of the viral genome is not crucial for its oncogenic effect. However, the possibility that certain sites of proviral insertion predispose to malignant transformation as a multistep process requires further investigation.

4.2 Host factors

4.2.1 *The role of the HLA system in HTLV-I infection*

HTLV-I infection can result in no disease, leukaemia or one of a range of inflammatory conditions, but particular genotypes of the virus do not appear to be associated with these different manifestations (Bangham *et al.*, 1996). It is likely that host factors strongly influence the outcome of HTLV-I infection; the HLA system is a major candidate for such a host factor, because of its association with many diseases, including inflammatory and infectious diseases. The high degree of polymorphism of the HLA system necessitates large sample and control sizes in studies designed to test for a possible HLA association with disease. To date, large enough samples have not been tested to allow a firm conclusion to be drawn about possible association between HLA and HTLV-I infection, or to estimate the strength of an association (relative risk of disease) with confidence. However, there are strong suggestions that genetic factors, including HLA, influence the outcome of HTLV-I infection. Specifically, genetic factors might influence either the proviral load and/or the development of HTLV-I associated disease.

Most of the work examining HLA genotypes in relation to HTLV-I infection has been carried out in the island of Kyushu in southern Japan, where the seroprevalence of HTLV-I exceeds 10%. Furukawa et al. (1992) showed that clonal proliferation of HTLV-I-infected T cells (as shown by clonal integration of HTLV-I provirus), which is associated with a high proviral load, is commoner in TSP/HAM patients and their first-degree relatives than in unrelated healthy HTLV-I-seropositive individuals. Usuku et al. (1988) examined the HLA types of 27 patients with TSP/HAM, 12 patients with ATLL and healthy asymptomatic controls. They found a predominance of certain haplotypes. In ATLL patients, the haplotype A26Bw62Cw3DR5 appeared to occur in excess, but no statistical correction for multiple comparisons was applied. Sonoda et al. (1992) extended these observations, and again found an apparent excess of certain A25 haplotypes in ATLL patients. However, because of the way in which the study was designed, a complete statistical analysis was not made, and so these interesting observations await confirmation.

4.2.2 Immune surveillance and escape

(a) Antibodies

It seems unlikely that antibodies are effective in limiting viral replication in established human HTLV-I infections, because the viral load increases mainly by division of infected proviral-DNA-containing cells (Wattel et al., 1995). However, it appears that the antibody titre reflects the HTLV-I proviral load (Shinzato et al., 1993; Ishihara et al., 1994; Miyata et al., 1995).

(b) T-cells

The cytotoxic T-lymphocyte (CTL) is the most important antigen-specific element of the immune system for controlling most established viral infections. Kannagi et al. (1983, 1984) detected a CTL response specific to HTLV-I in patients with a diagnosis of ATLL. Notably, they reported that the CTL response was detectable only in those patients in whom the ATLL was in remission, and disappeared when the patients relapsed.

It is now clear that there is a very powerful, chronically activated CTL response to HTLV-I in the majority of both TSP/HAM patients (Jacobson et al., 1990; Parker et al., 1992, 1994; Daenke et al., 1996) and healthy carriers of the virus (Parker et al., 1992,

1994; Daenke et al., 1996). The great majority of these CTLs are specific to the Tax protein of HTLV-I. There is evidence that the Tax-specific CTLs select antigenic variants of the Tax protein (Niewiesk et al., 1995) that escape recognition by the patient's own CTLs. The selection process appears to be more efficient in healthy carriers (Niewiesk et al., 1994).

The above evidence suggests that Tax-specific CTLs play a significant part in limiting viral replication, but the precise role of CTLs in protection against HTLV-I-associated diseases, or in the pathogenesis of these conditions, is not yet clear. There appears to be little difference, if any, between healthy HTLV-I carriers and TSP/HAM patients with respect to the chronic activation state, the abundance in peripheral blood, the antigen specificity or the epitope specificity of these CTL.

The observations by Kannagi et al. (1983, 1984) suggested that the development of ATLL might be associated with inefficient immune surveillance by CTLs. This would probably be a result of the low expression of the Tax protein by leukaemic cells.

As observed in other viral infections and malignancies, natural killer (NK) cells may also play a part in surveillance of HTLV-I infection and ATLL (see Section 4.3.3).

4.2.3 Host genetic factors required during the transition to ATLL

Host genetic factors are thought to be required for the transition from HTLV-I-infection of a cell to ATLL. Chromosomal abnormalities have been described in ATLL, but no specific pattern has been identified. This topic is discussed more extensively in Section 2.1.1.

At the molecular level, mutations in three tumour-suppressor genes, *p53*, *p16* and *p15*, have been identified in ATLL samples and/or HTLV-I-transformed human T-cell lines.

p53 missense mutations have been observed in 17–40% of fresh ATLL samples (Sugito et al., 1991; Sakashita et al., 1992; Yamato et al., 1993) as well as in some HTLV-I-transformed T-cell lines. The aberrant expression of p53 protein, in the presence or absence of p53 missense mutations, has also been noted in a proportion of both fresh ATLL samples and HTLV-I-transformed T-cell lines (Sugito et al., 1991; Reid et al., 1993; Yamamoto et al., 1993). While one report noted a correlation between Tax expression and p53 expression in HTLV-I transformed T-cell lines which lacked p53 mutations, another study did not observe any difference in p53 gene expression, methylation, and chromatin structure between HTLV-I transformed and mitogen-activated human T-cells (Lübbert et al., 1989). In HTLV-I-transformed T-cells, p53 is also functionally impaired, despite an increased expression of the cell-cycle control protein $p21^{waf1/cip1}$ (Cereseto et al., 1996). Thus, p53 mutation and aberrant expression may occur in less than half of ATLL cases and could conceivably play a role in tumour progression. Tax has also been demonstrated to impair $p16^{INK}$ function (Suzuki et al., 1996). Homozygous deletions of the p15 (MTS2) and/or p16 (CDKN2/MTSI) tumour-suppressor genes have been reported in 10/37 (27%) ATLL patients and individual cases suggest a possible association of deletions in the genes and leukaemia progression (Hatta *et al.*, 1995). Deletion, mutation or aberrant expression of tumour-suppressor genes may thus play a role in the pathogenesis of ATLL.

4.3 Viral factors

4.3.1 *Proviral load and clonal integration of HTLV-I infection*

The epidemiological evidence summarized in Section 2 links HTLV-I with the emergence of ATLL in a small proportion of HTLV-I-infected individuals after a delay of several decades.

The proportion of peripheral blood mononuclear cells (PBMCs) that carry an HTLV-I provirus — the proviral load — is usually between 10 and 100 times higher in patients with HTLV-I associated inflammatory diseases such as TSP/HAM than in healthy carriers of the virus (Yoshida *et al.*, 1989; Kira *et al.*, 1991; Gessain *et al.*, 1990a,b; Kira *et al.*, 1992a,b; Kubota *et al.*, 1993; Mita *et al.*, 1993; Sugimoto *et al.*, 1993), although the ranges overlap. Typically about 10% of peripheral blood lymphocytes are provirus-positive in TSP/HAM patients, and < 1% in healthy carriers of the virus. However, the fact that TSP/HAM and ATLL appear to occur independently suggests that a high HTLV-I proviral load does not necessarily predispose to ATLL. The proviral load in ATLL is largely dependent on the number of leukaemic cells and may be very high. However, no viral genes are expressed in ATLL cells (see below). In BLV infection (Section 3.3), a high virus load early after infection is associated with an elevated risk for development of leukaemia. It will be interesting to determine whether the same is true in HTLV-I infection.

HTLV-I-infected human T-cells show clonal expansion, even in asymptomatic individuals (Furukawa *et al.*, 1992; Wattel *et al.*, 1995). It has been suggested that after infection of human T-cells by HTLV-I and following a few rounds of reverse transcription, a clonal expansion of the infected cells predominates (Wattel *et al.*, 1996). Experiments using inverse or linker-mediated PCR have indeed indicated that HTLV-I proviral copy numbers increase predominantly via mitosis rather than via reverse transcription (Cavrois *et al.*, 1996). These findings may explain the remarkable stability of the HTLV-I genome and the high proviral load present in many HTLV-I infected individuals (Wattel *et al.*, 1995, 1996). The only viral mRNA to be reproducibly detected in PBMCs of HTLV-I-infected people is the mRNA encoding Tax/Rex/p21/Rex (Koralnik *et al.*, 1992b). This could explain the predominance of chronically activated Tax-specific CTLs in these individuals (see Section 4.2.2). In HTLV-I-infected PBMCs, the level of Tax mRNA expression per infected cell is the same in asymptomatic carriers and in TSP/HAM patients, but low or absent in uncultured ATLL samples (Franchini *et al.*, 1984; Furukawa *et al.*, 1995).

Thus, although HTLV-I-infected individuals carry HTLV-I provirus in a significant proportion of clonally expanded T-cell populations, the occurrence of ATLL is comparatively rare (Chen *et al.*, 1995).

4.3.2 *The role of Tax in cellular transformation/immortalization*

Following the discovery of the Tax protein of HTLV-I (Seiki *et al.*, 1983), intense efforts have been made to demonstrate its oncogenic properties *in vitro* and in animal models. These, as well as the possible role of other viral components in the development of ATLL, are reviewed in this section.

(*a*) *Transforming/immortalizing properties of HTLV-I Tax* in vitro

   (i) *Immortalizing effects on T-cells in vitro*

In vitro, HTLV-I, as well as its close relative HTLV-II, can clearly cause human T-cells to proliferate continuously (immortalization) and, with time, acquire IL-2 independence (transformation). Co-cultivation of mitomycin-treated or lethally irradiated HTLV-I or HTLV-II producer cell lines with human peripheral blood or cord blood lymphocytes results in the immortalization of mainly $CD4^+$ and, occasionally, $CD8^+$ T-lymphocytes (Miyoshi *et al.*, 1981; Yamamoto *et al.*, 1982; Chen *et al.*, 1983; Popovic *et al.*, 1983). Several lines of evidence suggest that the viral transactivator Tax, encoded by two exons flanking the envelope gene (see Section 1.1.6), is involved in this process. Tax has immortalizing/transforming properties *in vitro*: when transduced into primary human T-cells from adult or cord blood by a retroviral vector (Akagi & Shimotohno, 1993) or a recombinant herpesvirus saimiri (Grassmann *et al.*, 1989, 1992), it is capable of altering their growth properties. Transduction of *tax* into peripheral blood T-cells by a retroviral vector leads to enhancement of the proliferation caused by IL-2 and anti-CD3 antibody (Akagi & Shimotohno, 1993). These *tax*-transduced T-cells are still dependent on IL-2, but do not require periodic restimulation with antigen and feeder cells (Akagi & Shimotohno, 1993). Transduction of cord blood cells with *tax* using a herpesvirus saimiri vector resulted in permanently growing, but still IL-2-dependent, T-cell lines (Grassmann *et al.*, 1989, 1992).

The ability of Tax to immortalize primary human T-cells may be linked to its ability to induce the expression of cellular genes which are normally involved in the early response to mitogenic and antigenic stimuli (Kelly *et al.*, 1992) as well as to a long list of cytokines and cytokine receptors (see below). However, it is possible that other viral and cellular factors contribute to the efficient immortalization of human T-cells by HTLV-I *in vitro*: whereas *tax*-transduced T-cells remain IL-2-dependent, T-cells infected in bulk culture by co-cultivation with HTLV-I producer cell lines lose their IL-2-dependence after extended passage *in vitro*. If co-cultivation is carried out with limiting numbers of HTLV-I producer cells, the resulting transformed T-cell lines can be shown to maintain their dependence on IL-2 for a longer time, and other lymphokines, such as IL-4 and IL-7, can substitute for IL-2 to some extent (Persaud *et al.*, 1995). The constitutive activation of the JAK3 and STAT kinases in HTLV-I infected T-cells could be a crucial step during the acquisition of IL-2 independence: the JAK/STAT pathway is normally required for the downstream signalling triggered by the β- and γ-chain of the IL-2 receptor and by other cytokine receptors (Migone *et al.*, 1995), suggesting that its constitutive activation would lead to IL-2 independence.

Four infectious molecular clones of HTLV-I have recently been reported (Nicot et al., 1993; Kimata et al., 1994; Derse et al., 1995; Zhao et al., 1995), some of which produce HTLV-I capable of stimulating PBMCs. However, only one of these (Zhao et al., 1995) has been used successfully *in vitro* to transform (to IL-2 independence) human peripheral blood T-cells. It is also possible to achieve transformation of human PBMCs *in vitro* with a molecular clone of HTLV-II (Green et al., 1995).

(ii) *Transforming effect of Tax on fibroblast cultures* in vitro

Transfection of *tax* into RAT-1 or NIH 3T3 fibroblasts results in colony formation in soft agar and morphological changes (transformation), and the *tax*-transfected RAT-1 cells are tumorigenic in nude mice (Tanaka et al., 1990). This ability to transform rat fibroblasts is dependent on the CREB/ATF pathway of Tax action (see Section 1.1.6), but does not require interaction of Tax with nuclear factor-κB (NF-κB) (see Section 4.3.3) (Smith & Greene, 1991), a pathway which is predominantly activated by Tax in T-cells. Continuous expression of *tax* is required to maintain the transformed phenotype of RAT-1 fibroblasts (Yamaoka et al., 1992). Fusion of *tax*-transformed rat fibroblasts with normal human fibroblasts results in suppression of the transformed phenotype even in the presence of continued *tax* expression, suggesting the existence of a dominant inhibitory human factor acting downstream of *tax* (Inoue et al., 1994b). Tax has also been shown to immortalize and, in combination with the activated Ha-ras protein, to transform primary rat embryo fibroblasts (Pozzatti et al., 1990). Some naturally occurring sequence variants of Tax which are capable of activating the NF-κB or CREB/ATF pathways and of transforming rat fibroblast cell lines lack the ability to cooperate with *ras* in this manner (Matsumoto et al., 1994).

(b) *Tumorigenic properties of* tax *in transgenic mice*

Several groups have generated transgenic mice carrying different parts of the HTLV-I genome. Transgenic mice with the *tax* gene under the control of the HTLV-I LTR (Nerenberg et al., 1987) developed thymic atrophy and mesenchymal tumours (Hinrichs et al., 1987; Nerenberg et al., 1987), proliferation of ductal epithelial cells of the salivary glands (Green et al., 1989b), muscle degeneration (Nerenberg & Wiley, 1989) and adrenal medullary tumours characterized by proliferation of undifferentiated spindle cells (Green et al., 1992). Thymic atrophy was also consistently observed in other lines of mice transgenic for *tax* under the control of the SV40 promoter, the Ig enhancer and the mouse mammary tumour virus (MMTV) LTR (Furuta et al., 1989).

Environmental variables may contribute to tumour formation in LTR-*tax* transgenic mice, as the development of tumours can be delayed by feeding a low-folate diet (Bills et al., 1992). No lymphomas or leukaemias have been seen in LTR-*tax* transgenic mice, which may be related to the fact that the LTR-*tax* transgene was most strongly expressed in muscle, bone and cartilage, brain, pituitary, skin and salivary glands, but less so in lymphoid tissue (Bieberich et al., 1993). However, the use of a Thy-1 promoter to target the *tax* expression to the thymus of transgenic mice also resulted in the formation of fibroblastic tumours accompanied by infiltration of other cell types, as in the case of the LTR-*tax* transgenic mice, but did not lead to lymphoma formation. Nor was any expansion or phenotypic alteration of circulating lymphocytes or lymphocytes of the thymus or spleen seen in these animals (Nerenberg et al., 1991).

In contrast, transgenic mice carrying the complete pX region (i.e., the genomic region containing open reading frames I, II, III and IV; see Section 1.1.6 and Figure 4) under the control of the granzyme B promoter, targeting the transgene expression to mature T-cells and NK cells, develop large granular lymphocytic leukaemia and solid tumours composed of NK-large granular lymphocytic (LGL)-like cells, which expressed FcγR, Thy 1.2, CD 44 and lacked rearranged T-cell receptor β and γ genes, and neutrophils (Grossman et al., 1995). While the phenotype of these NK-LGL-like cells is clearly different from that of ATLL cells, this experiment supports the transforming potential of Tax in lymphoid cells in vivo. The marked neutrophil infiltration of tumours in these animals has also been noted in neurofibromas of LTR-*tax* transgenic mice and may be related to the activation of granulocyte-macrophage colony-stimulating factor expression by Tax (Green et al., 1989b). LTR-*tax* transgenic mice can also exhibit marked splenomegaly and lymphadenopathy, due to a striking increase in the percentage of B-cells in these organs. This expansion of the B-lymphocyte population may also be related to cytokines secreted from *tax*-expressing fibroblastoid tumour cells, which were shown to stimulate B-cell proliferation and IgM production (Peebles et al., 1995). Transforming growth factor β1 (TGF-β1) is overexpressed in several tissues from LTR-*tax* transgenic mice and stimulates the growth of cell lines derived from neurofibromas of these animals, and it has therefore been suggested that this cytokine might be involved in the development of these tumours (Kim et al., 1991). Mammary carcinomas observed in *tax*-transgenic rats also expressed several cytokines, including the granulocyte chemoattractants *Gro* and *MIP-2*, but not TGF-β1 (Yamada et al., 1995). Similarly, the increased bone turnover and skeletal abnormalities of LTR-*tax* transgenic mice may be related to Tax-induced local expression of cytokines (Ruddle et al., 1993). Thus, in addition to a directly transforming effect of Tax are demonstrated by these in-vivo experiments, more indirect mechanisms, involving a variety of cytokines, contribute to tumour formation and may underlie other pathological effects seen in these animals.

The lymphomas described above differ from ATLL in lacking CD4 expression. Lymphomas of a $CD4^+$ phenotype were observed in 70% of bitransgenic mice carrying an LTR-c-*myc* and an Ig promoter/enhancer-*tax* construct. In addition to $CD4^+$, $CD3^+$, CD8 lymphomas, these animals develop brain tumours of neuronal lineage at very high frequency (Benvenisty et al., 1992). However, the relative contributions of overexpressed c-*myc* and *tax* to tumour development in this model remain unclear.

Transgenic mice carrying the *env* and pX region of HTLV-I [i.e., with the potential to encode the envelope proteins, Tax, Rex, $p21^{rexIII}$, $p12^I$, $p30^{II}$, $p13^{II}$; see Section 1.1] under the control of the HTLV-I LTR develop an inflammatory arthropathy resembling human rheumatoid arthritis, in addition to the thymic atrophy, mesenchymal tumours and adenocarcinomas reported in LTR-*tax* transgenic mice (Iwakura et al., 1991, 1994). In addition to increased c-*fos* and c-*jun* expression in the tumours and normal skin and muscle of these animals (Iwakura et al., 1994), a variety of inflammatory cytokines, including IL-1α, IL-1β, IL-6, TNF-α, TGF-β1, interferon-γ and IL-2, as well as MHC genes, are overexpressed in transgenic joints (Iwakura et al., 1995). This widespread activation of components of the immune system is probably related to the expression of the transgenic construct in many organs, including brain, salivary gland, spleen, thymus, skin, muscle and mammary gland (Iwakura et al., 1994, 1995).

Taken together, the evidence emerging from studies with these different lines of HTLV-I transgenic mice suggests that *tax* has a relatively weak oncogenic effect *in vivo* which is apparent only in transgenic animals with high levels of *tax* expression. Lymphoid cells are not particularly sensitive to the transforming effect of Tax and T-cell malignancies have been found only when a strong, non-HTLV-I-derived, promoter was used, or after simultaneous expression of *tax* and c-*myc*. Some aspects of the pathology induced by *tax in vivo* may be related to the aberrant expression of a variety of lymphokines, resulting in marked neutrophil infiltration of mesenchymal tumours and increased bone turnover.

4.3.3 *Pathways of Tax-mediated transactivation of cellular genes*

The transforming properties of the Tax protein, demonstrated in transgenic mice, transduced T-cells and transfected fibroblasts (see above) are the result of its ability to induce the expression of a wide variety of cellular genes in addition to the HTLV-I LTR (see Table 8). Tax negatively regulates the expression of β-polymerase, a cellular DNA repair enzyme (Jeang et al., 1990), and the tumour-suppressor genes *p53* (Uittenbogaard et al., 1995) and *p16*^{INK4A} and represses the tumour-suppressor role (Suzuki et al., 1996).

Transcriptional activation by Tax of these various cellular and viral genes requires the presence of specific target sequences in the promoter DNA. Three different such target sequences, the cyclic AMP-responsive element (CRE), the NF-κB binding site and the serum response element (SRE), are known to mediate the Tax-induced transactivation of most of the cellular genes listed above. Additional, so far unidentified, pathways probably account for the activation of a few other Tax-responsive genes.

Modified CREs are present in the HTLV-I LTR within three 21-bp repeat elements, at least two of which are required for Tax-induced transactivation (Fujisawa et al., 1986; Shimotohno et al., 1986). CRE binds members of the bZIP family of cellular transcription factors which include CRE binding protein (CREB) (Zhao & Giam, 1992; Suzuki et al., 1993), CRE modulator (CREM) (Foulkes et al., 1991), activating transcription factor (ATF) (Hai et al., 1989), Tax-responsive element binding protein (TREB) (Yoshimura et al., 1989) and HEB (21-bp binding proteins) (Béraud et al., 1991). Tax activates transcription from the HTLV-I LTR as well as the CRE-containing promoters of the *c-fos*, *c-egr* and nerve growth factor genes by binding to one or several of these transcription factors and enhancing their interaction with the target DNA (Zhao & Giam, 1992) or altering their DNA-binding specificity (Paca-Uccaralertkun et al., 1994). Tax achieves this by binding to the basic domain of bZIP transcription factors (Baranger et al., 1995; Perini et al., 1995), thus enhancing their dimerization (Wagner & Green, 1993) and stabilizing a complex consisting of DNA, bZIP and Tax (Wagner & Green, 1993; Baranger et al., 1995). As part of this process, Tax also alters the relative affinity

Table 8. Tax-activated cellular genes[a]

Interleukin (IL)-related genes	
IL-2Rα	Inoue et al. (1986)
IL-1	Sawada et al. (1992)
IL-2	Siekevitz et al. (1987)
IL-3	Wolin et al. (1993)
IL-6	Yamashita et al. (1994)
IL-8	Mori et al. (1995)
'Housekeeping' genes	
Vimentin	Lilienbaum et al. (1990)
MHC class I	Sawada et al. (1990)
Growth-factors/hormone genes	
Granulocyte-macrophage colony-stimulating factor (GM-CSF)	Miyatake et al. (1988)
Nerve growth factor (NGF)	Green (1991)
Transforming growth factor β1 (TGF-β1)	Kim et al. (1990)
Tumour necrosis factor α (TNF-α)	Dhib-Jalbut et al. (1994)
Tumour necrosis factor β (TNF-β)	Paul et al. (1993)
Parathyroid-hormone-related protein	Watanabe et al. (1990)
Proenkephalin	Joshi & Dave (1992)
Early response cellular genes	Alexandre et al. (1991); Kelly et al. (1992)
Cellular oncogenes	
c-*egr*	Fujii et al. (1991)
c-*fos*	Fujii et al. (1988)
c-*jun*	Fujii et al. (1991)
c-*myc*	Duyao et al. (1992)
c-*rel*	Li et al. (1993)
c-*sis*	Pantazis et al. (1987)
Viral promoters	
HTLV long terminal repeat	Sodroski et al. (1984); Felber et al. (1985)
HIV long terminal repeat	Jeang et al. (1988b)
Cytomegalovirus IE enhancer	Moch et al. (1992)
SV40 promoter	Fujisawa et al. (1988)

[a] Referencing is not exhaustive

of a bZIP protein for different DNA binding sites, thus modifying DNA binding site selection (Perini et al., 1995). This explains the ability of Tax to transactivate a wide range of promoters containing recognition sites for members of the bZIP family. There are, however, subtle differences between the activation of the CRE-related sequences in the HTLV-I LTR and that of cellular CREs: in the case of the viral LTR, Tax binds to unphosphorylated CREB, increases its association with the 21 bp repeats and thus promotes interaction with CREB, an essential component of the transcription factor complex (Chrivia et al., 1993; Kwok et al., 1996). In contrast, Tax does not bind directly to CREB associated with a cellular CRE (Kwok et al., 1996), and phosphorylation of CREB, which is required for its normal activation of cellular CRE-containing promoters and interaction with CREB (Chrivia et al., 1993), is also necessary for the activation of these cellular promoters by Tax. Rather, by also binding to CREB, Tax promotes its interaction with phosphorylated CREB associated with a cellular CRE (Kwok et al., 1996). Thus, for activation of the viral LTR, Tax is able to bypass a normal control mechanism of this pathway, whereas this control step is still operative in the case of Tax-activated cellular genes.

In a related manner, Tax binds to all members of the NF-κB family of transcription factors to activate transcription (Suzuki et al., 1994). The NF-κB binding site is present in several genes known to be activated by Tax, such as those encoding IL-2Rα, GM-CSF, TNF-β and the HIV LTR. In addition to binding to NF-κB in the nucleus, Tax also interacts with the NF-κB pathway at an earlier, cytoplasmic stage, in a completely different manner. Tax complexes with two proteins, I-κBα and I-κBγ, that are inhibitors of NF-κB. I-κB proteins normally bind to members of the NF-κB family in the cytoplasm and prevent their entry into the nucleus. Following stimulation of cells, I-κB proteins are phosphorylated and the NF-κB/I-κB complex dissociates, allowing the free NF-κB to enter the nucleus. Tax has been shown to bind to I-κBα and I-κBγ and it causes dissociation of NF-κB/I-κB complexes, thus increasing the turnover of NF-κB and its import into the nucleus (Hirai et al., 1994; Suzuki et al., 1995). As in the case of members of the CREB/ATF family, binding of Tax thus mimics the effect of phosphorylation and thus interferes with physiological control mechanisms of these different pathways.

The third target sequence known to be involved in Tax-mediated activation of cellular genes is the SRE. An SRE is found in the promoters of early response genes known to be activated by Tax (Kelly et al., 1992) and interacts with the transcription factor SRF. Tax binds to SRF, including unphosphorylated SRF, and the SRF/Tax complex activates transcription (Fujii et al., 1992).

An additional Tax-responsive sequence, TRE-2, is present in the HTLV-I LTR. TRE-2 alone is not sufficient to mediate a Tax response, but can do so in the presence of one single 21-bp element (Marriott et al., 1990). A 36-kDa zinc finger protein, termed TIF-1 or THP and related to the GLI family of proteins, interacts with TRE-2 (Marriott et al., 1990; Tanimura et al., 1993). Thus, cooperative binding of a CREB/ATF protein (binding to CRE in the 21-bp element) and THP may be required for Tax-mediated activation of this target sequence.

Thus, the pleiotropic effect of Tax on at least three different enhancer sequences is explained by its ability to interact with a variety of different transcription factors or inhibitors. Binding of Tax to these proteins may substitute for modifications such as phosphorylation or dimerization which normally occur in these proteins as a result of intracellular signalling. Different regions in Tax are required for the activation of individual pathways and mutants with specificity for individual pathways have been designed (Smith & Greene, 1990, 1991). There is also evidence that extracellular Tax, released from infected cells, may induce NF-κB-site-containing promoters, such as the IL-2Rα or TNF-β promoter, and thus induce the activation of uninfected cells (Lindholm *et al.*, 1992; Marriott *et al.*, 1992). However, a role of extracellular Tax in the pathogenesis of ATLL, over and above that of Tax produced within infected cells, is uncertain.

In addition to its role in cellular activation, Tax may be involved in increasing the likelihood of DNA damage in infected cells, possibly by increasing DNA instability (Saggioro *et al.*, 1994) and/or through its inhibitory effect on the expression of the repair enzyme, β-polymerase (Jeang *et al.*, 1990).

4.3.4 *Differences between HTLV-I-transformed T-cells and ATLL cells*

Although the experiments summarized above indicate that *tax* has some transforming potential *in vitro*, as well as *in vivo*, it is clear that HTLV-I-transformed T-cell lines, or T-cells transduced with *tax*, are not representative of ATLL.

Whereas HTLV-I-transformed T-cell lines (either cell lines obtained by co-cultivation of irradiated HTLV-I producer cell lines with fresh human primary T-cells, or non-ATLL cells grown from HTLV-I infected individuals) express viral mRNAs *in vitro*, cell lines originating from ATLL do not (Maeda *et al.*, 1985; Imada *et al.*, 1995). Early experiments suggested that ATLL cells *in vivo* also do not express HTLV-I mRNAs (Franchini *et al.*, 1984). While some expression of viral mRNA in fresh ATLL samples has been seen using RT-PCR (Berneman *et al.*, 1992a; Koralnik *et al.*, 1992b), it is unclear whether this occurred in ATLL cells or other HTLV-I infected T-cells. In-situ hybridization suggested some expression of *tax* mRNA in ATLL cells (Setoyama *et al.*, 1994). However, ATLL-derived cell lines which engraft in SCID mice show no, or reduced, expression of viral mRNAs (Imada *et al.*, 1995).

Leukaemic cells from ATLL patients do not usually grow in the presence of IL-2 (Maeda *et al.*, 1985), but occasionally ATLL cells have been found to respond to IL-2, and grow as permanently IL-2-dependent cell lines, suggesting that at some stage during their development ATLL cells require IL-2 to proliferate (Maeda *et al.*, 1985, 1987).

Primary cultures of ATLL cells, as well as ATLL-derived cell lines, can grow in SCID mice to form tumours with the same phenotypic profile and HTLV-I integration patterns as the ATLL samples from which they were established (Feuer *et al.*, 1993; Kondo *et al.*, 1993; Imada *et al.*, 1995). While uncultured HTLV-I-infected T-cells from a few asymptomatic individuals and those from about one third of TSP/HAM patients will persist in SCID mice, they do not form tumours (Feuer *et al.*, 1993). In contrast to ATLL cells or cell lines, HTLV-I-transformed T-cell lines not derived from ATLL cells will only grow in SCID mice which have been pretreated with antibodies to asialo GM1 (Ishihara *et al.*, 1992; Feuer *et al.*, 1995) to reduce NK cell activity. However, this distinction may not be absolute: untreated animals can be successfully engrafted using increased numbers of an HTLV-I-transformed, non-leukaemic cell line (Ohsugi *et al.*, 1994), while blocking of NK function with monoclonal antibody TM-β1 or the β-chain of the murine IL-2 receptor may enhance the rate of engraftment of fresh ATLL cells. However, taken together, these reports suggest that ATLL cells have a higher tumorigenic potential *in vivo* than HTLV-I-transformed T-cell lines because of their ability to evade NK-mediated cell lysis (Feuer *et al.*, 1995).

Thus, infection of T-cells with HTLV-I may provide some proliferative advantage and oligoclonal expansion, probably related to the pleiotropic activating properties of *tax*. NK-cell activity as well as CTL activity (see Section 4.2.3) may play an important role in limiting the expansion of HTLV-I-infected T-cells at this stage, and progression to ATLL requires a number of additional events. Whereas HTLV-I producer T-cell lines express high levels of the adhesion molecules LFA-1, LFA-3 and ICAM-1, ATLL-derived cell lines show reduced expression of these surface markers (Fukudome *et al.*, 1992). As these molecules play an important role in the recognition of tumour cells by the immune system, it is conceivable that their reduced expression on ATLL cells may facilitate their escape from immunosurveillance. At present, there is no convincing evidence that variation in viral sequences (see Section 4.2.3) will allow the emergence of more 'leukaemogenic' clones of HTLV-I-infected cells.

4.3.5 *The role of other viral and host cell proteins in lymphocyte stimulation and leukaemogenesis*

Apart from Tax, the HTLV-I envelope protein and the recently described $p12^1$ protein have been investigated with regard to their potential roles in T-cell stimulation and/or leukaemogenesis. Purified HTLV-I viruses have been reported to stimulate human T-cells via the HTLV-I envelope protein and a CD2/LFA-3-dependent pathway (Gazzolo & Duc Dodon, 1987; Duc Dodon *et al.*, 1989), but the interpretation of this phenomenon remains controversial. Recombinant HTLV-I envelope protein, expressed in a vaccinia virus vector (Cassé *et al.*, 1994) does not induce T-cell proliferation. Whereas a (YXXL/I), signalling motif in the cytoplasmic domain of the BLV envelope protein mediates activation of B-lymphocytes *in vitro* (Beaufils *et al.*, 1993), and is required for efficient replication *in vivo* (Willems *et al.*, 1995), the cytoplasmic domain of the HTLV-I envelope has only a truncated (YXXL) motif which appears functionally inactive (Beaufils *et al.*, 1993).

Several adhesion molecules, such as LFA-3, ICAM-1, LFA-1, and the cell surface markers CD28, CD69 and CD5 show increased expression on the surface of HTLV-I-infected (Fukudome *et al.*, 1992; Imai *et al.* 1993) or *tax*-transfected (Chlichlia *et al.*, 1995; Tanaka *et al.*, 1995) cells. Antibodies to CD2 and LFA-3 inhibit the mitogenic activity of HTLV-I-infected T-cell lines (Kimata *et al.*, 1993) and the spontaneous proliferation of PBMCs from HTLV-I-infected asymptomatic carriers or TSP/HAM patients (Höllsberg *et al.*, 1992; Wucherpfennig *et al.*, 1992), suggesting that these molecules contribute to the process of proliferation.

Contrary to this conclusion, results obtained with both the SCID model (see above) and the rabbit model suggest that the potential of HTLV-I-infected cell lines to stimulate lymphocyte proliferation *in vitro* does not necessarily correlate with their leukaemogenic potential *in vivo*. An experiment reported by Leno *et al.* (1995) suggests that the leukaemogenic potential of an HTLV-I-infected T-cell line could be linked to its ability to induce apoptosis, which was demonstrated in thymic cells *in vivo* and peripheral blood T-cells *in vitro*, rather than its ability to induce T-cell stimulation, and that this phenotype is due to a cellular, rather than viral, factor. However, in another report (Seto

& Kumagai, 1993), the leukaemogenic potential of individual cell lines in (B/J × Chbb:HM) F1 rabbits did correlate with their ability to induce leukocytosis *in vivo* in the parental Chbb:HM rabbit strain and this phenotype seemed to be linked to the surface expression of a cellular 65 kDa glycoprotein, the precise role of which remains to be established. While these experiments may help to identify cellular factors promoting the growth of HTLV-I-transformed cell lines in rabbits, they do not necessarily reflect events occurring in human ATLL.

The Tax protein itself has been shown to induce apoptosis in Jurkat cells (Chlichlia *et al.*, 1995), in particular when Tax-expressing Jurkat cells were stimulated via the T-cell receptor. *Tax*-transfected RAT-1 cells are also prone to apoptosis via a BCL-2-dependent pathway when cultured in the absence of serum (Yamada *et al.*, 1994). In RAT-1 cells, *tax* induces apoptosis less efficiently than the cellular oncogenes c-*myc* and c-*fos* and through a different pathway (Fujita & Shiku, 1995). The ability of Tax to induce apoptosis is probably related to its pleiotropic effect on cellular promoters (see above), and reflects an increased susceptibility of activated cells to undergo apoptosis in the absence of essential stimuli. These experiments may not explain the observations reported by Leno *et al.* (1995).

The $p12^I$ protein of HTLV-I (Koralnik *et al.* 1992b, 1993) has been shown to cooperate with the E5 protein of bovine papilloma virus in the transformation of C127 mouse cells (Franchini *et al.* 1993) and may thus have oncogenic properties. $p12^I$ and E5 share some structural similarity: both proteins localize to the cellular endomembranes and interact with another very hydrophobic protein, the 16 kDa subunit of H+ vacuolar ATPase (Schlegel *et al.*, 1986; Goldstein *et al.*, 1991; Franchini *et al.*, 1993). Both E5 and $p12^I$ interact with distinct growth factor receptors. E5 activates the platelet-derived growth factor receptor (Petti *et al.*, 1991; Goldstein *et al.*, 1994) and $p12^I$ specifically interacts with the β and γ, but not the α chains of the IL-2R (Mulloy *et al.*, 1994). Possibly, binding of $p12^I$ to the IL-2R chains could alter the receptor signalling by inducing their cytoplasmic juxtaposition, an event thought to be crucial in kinase activation and IL-2 signalling (Nelson *et al.*, 1994). In this regard, it is noteworthy that constitutive activation of STAT and JAK3 kinases has been demonstrated in HTLV-I-transformed T-cells (see Section 4.3.2). In fact, constitutive activation of the IL-2R signalling pathway is correlated with IL-2 independence (Migone *et al.*, 1995). The DNA sequence of the HTLV-I $p12^I$ gene from 21 HTLV-I positive individuals (7 healthy carriers, 8 TSP/HAM and 6 ATLL) has been found to be highly conserved (Franchini, 1995).

However, the precise role of $p12^I$ in T-cells is not yet understood. $p12^I$ is not required for the transformation of cord blood lymphocytes *in vitro* (Ratner *et al.*, 1985) and is dispensable for *tax*, *rex* or envelope expression *in vitro* (Roithmann *et al.*, 1994).

In proviral DNA extracted from ATLL, the genes encoding $p13^{II}$ and $p30^{II}$ appear to be subject to frequent mutations leading to premature translational termination codons, suggesting that these proteins might not be essential in maintaining disease (Berneman *et al.*, 1992b; Chou *et al.*, 1995).

4.3.6 *Differences between HTLV-I and HTLV-II*

As discussed in section 2.1, HTLV-I is associated with human leukaemia whereas HTLV-II is not. Section 1.1.7 summarized the differences in genomic structure between HTLV-I and HTLV-II.

It is unlikely that there is a functional homologue of HTLV-I $p12^I$ in HTLV-II, but deletions in the region between the HTLV-II *env* gene and the second *tax* exon, which would eliminate expression of any potential homologue of HTLV-I $p12^I$, $p13^{II}$ or $p30^{II}$, have no effect on virus production, envelope function or transforming potential *in vitro* (Green *et al.*, 1995). The effect of disrupting the G4 and R3 reading frames of BLV, located in a similar region of the BLV genome but of only limited similarity to HTLV-I $p12^I$, $p13^{II}$ or $p30^{II}$ (Alexandersen *et al.*, 1993), is discussed in Sections 1.1.7 and 3.3. In conclusion, it is not clear whether any of the small accessory proteins found only in HTLV-I, e.g., $p21^I$, is responsible for the leukaemogenic properties of HTLV-I in humans, and the precise roles of HTLV-I $p12^I$, $p13^{II}$ and $p30^{II}$ during in-vivo leukaemogenesis remain to be established.

It is also conceivable that as yet unidentified minor differences in the in-vitro transforming potential between HTLV-I and HTLV-II might translate into a weak oncogenic effect *in vivo* (for example, a long latency period for leukaemia development) for HTLV-I but not for HTLV-II.

5. Summary of Data Reported and Evaluation

5.1 Exposure data

Human T-lymphotropic viruses (HTLV-I and HTLV-II), the only known human *oncornavirinae*, have distinct genetic and structural features. Both HTLV-I and HTLV-II are complex retroviruses. Their genomes encode structural core and envelope proteins, regulatory proteins (Tax and Rex) and several additional proteins which may play an important role in the pathogenesis of the HTLV-I-associated diseases. Several related viruses (known as simian T-lymphotropic viruses; STLVs) have been identified in African and Asian non-human primates, and such primates appear to have been the original sources of the human retroviruses.

Serological detection of specific reactivity to Gag and Env HTLV-I or HTLV-II antigens, confirmed if necessary by western blot, is indicative of current infection. HTLV-I and HTLV-II infection can also be confirmed by amplification of viral sequences by polymerase chain reaction (PCR) from peripheral blood mononuclear cells. Three major clades of HTLV-I with distinct geographical distribution have been distinguished by PCR and sequencing or by restriction fragment length polymorphism. A higher prevalence among women, particularly over the age of 50 years, has been observed in highly endemic areas.

Three modes of transmission have been described for HTLV-I and HTLV-II: mother-to-child transmission, mainly due to breast-feeding beyond six months, sexual transmission predominantly from men to women and transmission by transfusion of cellular blood products and through intravenous drug use.

HTLV-I prevalence varies widely worldwide, with high levels in diverse geographic areas: i.e., southwest Japan, the Caribbean basin, parts of South America, Central and West Africa and parts of Melanesia. Clusters of especially high endemicity occur within these areas. HTLV-I remains endemic among emigrants from these areas.

It is estimated that worldwide between 15 and 20 million individuals are infected by HTLV-I.

Independent of the background of HTLV-I seroprevalence, geographical and ethnic differences in the prevalence of tropical spastic paraparesis/HTLV-I-associated myelopathy (TSP/HAM; a major HTLV-I-associated disease) have been reported. This is a chronic spastic myelopathy that preferentially affects middle-aged women. TSP/HAM may develop shortly after transfusion-acquired HTLV-I infection. Other inflammatory conditions associated with HTLV-I are uveitis, infective dermatitis, polymyositis, alveolitis, arthritis, thyroiditis and Sjögren's syndrome. Various combinations of these conditions may co-exist in the same patient and are often found in patients with TSP/HAM. HTLV-I-infected individuals may have impairment of the immune system, and some have reduced ability to clear *Strongyloides stercoralis*.

HTLV-II is endemic in several African pygmy and Amerindian populations and is epidemic among intravenous drug users in the Americas and parts of Europe. HTLV-II has not been clearly associated with any non-neoplastic human disease.

Control and prevention of HTLV-I and HTLV-II infection depend on reduced transmission by the three major routes: perinatal, sexual and parenteral. Perinatal transmission has been greatly reduced in Japan by avoidance of prolonged breast-feeding. Passive and active immunization is effective in animal models but no preventive vaccine is available for humans. A number of countries have introduced universal screening of blood donors to prevent transmission of HTLV-I and HTLV-II and in Japan a decline in the incidence of post-transfusion TSP/HAM has been demonstrated.

5.2 Human carcinogenicity data

Adult T-cell leukaemia/lymphoma (ATLL) occurs almost exclusively in areas where HTLV-I is endemic, such as Japan, the Caribbean and West Africa. Cases of ATLL described in Europe and the United States have mostly been in immigrants from HTLV-I endemic regions or their offspring. Evidence of HTLV-I infection was originally found in at least 90% of patients with ATLL in endemic regions. Subsequently, HTLV-I has become part of the diagnostic criteria for ATLL. In ATLL, the virus is clonally integrated into the tumour cells. ATLL develops in 2–5% of HTLV-I-infected individuals. Infection early in life appears to be important for the development of ATLL. No environmental cofactor promoting the progression to ATLL has so far been identified.

HTLV-I has been associated with non-ATLL cutaneous T-cell malignancies by a few investigators, but most studies have not found an association. Difficulties in distinguishing cutaneous T-cell lymphomas from ATLL may have contributed to these inconsistent findings. Some investigators have detected HTLV-I genome sequences in HTLV-I and HTLV-II-seronegative patients with cutaneous T-cell lymphomas, but this has not been confirmed by others.

HTLV-II antibody has been reported in a few patients with large granular lymphocyte leukaemia, but prevalence surveys and a lack of clonal integration of the virus have not supported an association.

Several case–control studies have found an association between HTLV-I seroprevalence and tumours of the vagina, cervix and liver, but confounding effects and bias could not be excluded.

5.3 Animal carcinogenicity data

In the few studies on HTLV-I infection of animals, no neoplastic disease was demonstrated.

While neoplastic disease has not been induced experimentally in non-human primates by infection with STLV-I, there is strong evidence that 'natural' infection with STLV-I is associated with lymphoid neoplasia in non-human primates. The following evidence supports this hypothesis: lymphoma is the most common malignancy in Old World non-human primates; STLV-I is endemic in Old World non-human primates; the disease in monkeys is very similar to ATLL; STLV-I is very similar biologically, morphologically, physicochemically and molecularly to HTLV-I; and STLV-I has the ability to activate and immortalize lymphocytes in culture. Monoclonally integrated provirus has been identified in all neoplastic tissues from STLV-I-infected non-human primates that have been evaluated.

Bovine leukaemia virus, which belongs to the same family as HTLV-I, is a good model for the study of lymphomas induced by viruses with *tax* and *rex* genes. This virus induces lymphomas in approximately 5% of infected cattle and in all experimentally infected sheep. Unlike HTLV-I-associated lymphomas in humans, all tumours are of B-cell origin.

5.4 Molecular mechanisms of leukaemogenesis

HTLV-I, as well as HTLV-II, is capable of immortalizing human and rabbit T-cells *in vitro*. Transfection of HTLV-I *tax* alone immortalizes and transforms primary human T-cells and transforms cells of fibroblastoid lineage. In transgenic models, HTLV-I *tax* under the control of HTLV-I long terminal repeat induces tumours of mesenchymal origin, whereas lymphomas have so far only been obtained by using a granzyme B promoter to control *tax* expression, or by producing mice transgenic for both c-*myc* and *tax*. Tax activates the expression of several cellular genes which are themselves involved in the control of cell proliferation. Tax achieves this pleiotropic effect by interfering with at least three different classes of transcription factors, at either nuclear or cytoplasmic levels. However, HTLV-I transformed cell lines, although capable of inducing lymphomas in severe combined immunodeficient mice (SCID) under certain conditions, are different from ATLL cells, for the development of which subsequent cellular changes are required. In keeping with this scenario, clonally expanded HTLV-I-infected T-cell populations can persist *in vivo* for long periods of time without progression to leukaemia. While *tax* is expressed in non-neoplastic T-cell populations, its expression is lost in ATLL cells.

Observations made in *tax*-transgenic mice suggest that cytokines secreted by *tax*-expressing cells are responsible for some aspects of the pathologies observed in these animals; whether this applies to the pathogenesis of ATLL in humans is uncertain. The expression of *tax* during the early stages of leukaemogenesis may interfere with mechanisms of DNA repair by reducing the expression of β-polymerase and *p53*, and increasing chromosomal instability.

HTLV-I and HTLV-II have similar transforming properties *in vitro*. HTLV-I is associated with leukaemia, whereas HTLV-II is not. HTLV-I and HTLV-II differ in some of their small accessory proteins. The role of some of these HTLV-I encoded viral proteins, in particular the small accessory protein p12[1], during the early stages of leukaemogenesis is still uncertain, but in-vitro experiments suggest a possible involvement. There is no indisputable evidence that these accessory proteins are expressed in ATLL cells.

Cellular alterations required during the transition from an HTLV-I-infected T-cell to a malignant ATLL cell are largely undefined, but constitutive activation of signal transduction pathways may play a role. Mutations in several tumour-suppressor genes occur in some ATLL samples and HTLV-I-transformed cell lines and may play a role during tumour progression.

Cytotoxic T-cell (CTL) immunity is directed mainly against the Tax protein and there is evidence that CTLs play a role in killing HTLV-I expressing T-cells, but not ATLL cells as these do not express *tax*. The role of natural killer cells in human HTLV-I infection remains to be established, although such cells limit the growth of HTLV-I transformed human cells in immunodeficient mice. Studies in Japan suggest an association of certain human leukocyte antigen (HLA) haplotypes with TSP/HAM and ATLL. Different genotypes of HTLV-I do not appear to be associated with different diseases.

5.5 Evaluation[1]

There is *sufficient evidence* in humans for the carcinogenicity of HTLV-I.
There is *inadequate evidence* in humans for the carcinogenicity of HTLV-II.

Overall evaluation

HTLV-I is *carcinogenic to humans (Group 1)*.
HTLV-II is *not classifiable as to its carcinogenicity to humans (Group 3)*.

---

[1]For definition of the italicized terms, see Preamble, pp. 22–25.

6. References

Aboulafia, D.M., Feigal, E., Vranzian, K., Bennett, C., Blattner, W., Moss, A. & Slamon, D. (1993) Human T cell leukemia virus (HTLV-I/II) serodiagnostic testing: disparate results among a cohort of intravenous drug users. *AIDS Res. hum. Retroviruses*, **9**, 1043–1050

Abt, D.A., Marshak, R.R., Kulp, H.W. & Pollock, R.J., Jr (1970) Studies on the relationship between lymphocytosis and bovine leukosis. *Bibl. Haematol.*, **36**, 527–536

Achiron, A., Pinhas-Hamiel, O., Doll, L., Djaldetti, R., Chen, A., Ziv, I., Avni, A., Frankel, G., Melamed, E. & Shohat, B. (1993) Spastic paraparesis associated with human T-lymphotropic virus type I: a clinical, serological, and genomic study in Iranian-born Mashhadi Jews. *Ann. Neurol.*, **34**, 670–675

Adam, E., Kerkhofs, P., Mammerickx, M., Kettmann, R., Burny, A., Droogmans, L. & Willems, L. (1994) Involvement of the cyclic AMP-responsive element binding protein in bovine leukemia virus expression *in vivo*. *J. Virol.*, **68**, 5845–5853

Akagi, T. & Shimotohno, K. (1993) Proliferative response of Tax1-transduced primary human T-cells to anti-CD3 antibody stimulation by an interleukin-2-independent pathway. *J. Virol.*, **67**, 1211–1217

Al, B., Visser, S., van den Hoek, A., van Doornum, G., Coutinho, R. & Huisman, H. (1993) Incidence of HTLV-I/II infection in seronegative high-risk individuals. *J. med. Virol.*, **39**, 260–265

Aldovini, A., De Rossi, A., Feinberg, M.B., Wong-Staal, F. & Franchini, G. (1986) Molecular analysis of a deletion mutant provirus of type 1 human T-cell lymphotropic virus: evidence for a doubly spliced *x-lor* mRNA. *Proc. natl Acad. Sci. USA*, **83**, 38–42

Alexandersen, S., Carpenter, S., Christensen, J., Storgaard, T., Viuff, B., Wannemuehler, Y., Belousov, J. & Roth, J.A. (1993) Identification of alternatively spliced mRNAs encoding potential new regulatory proteins in cattle infected with bovine leukemia virus. *J. Virol.*, **67**, 39–52

Alexandre, C., Charnay, P. & Verrier, B. (1991) Transactivation of *Krox-20* and *Krox-24* promoters by the HTLV-I Tax protein through common regulatory elements. *Oncogene*, **6**, 1851–1857

Allain, J.-P., Hodges, W., Einstein, M.H., Geisler, J., Neilly, C., Delaney, S., Hodges, B. & Lee, H. (1992) Antibody to HIV-1, HTLV-I, and HCV in three populations of rural Haitians. *J. acquir. Immune Defic. Syndr.*, **5**, 1230–1236

Ando, Y., Nakano, S., Saito, K., Shimamoto, I., Ichijo, M., Toyama, T. & Hinuma, Y. (1987) Transmission of adult T-cell leukemia retrovirus (HTLV-I) from mother to child: comparison of bottle- with breast-fed babies. *Jpn. J. Cancer Res. (Gann)*, **78**, 322–324

Ando, Y., Tanigawa, T., Ekuni, Y., Ichijo, M. & Tohyama, T. (1993) Family study of women showing development of antibody to human T-cell leukemia virus I and assessment of the risk of vertical transmission of the virus to their children. *J. Infect.*, **27**, 151–155

Aoki, T., Miyakoshi, H., Koide, H., Yoshida, T., Ishikawa, H., Sugisaki, Y., Mizukoshi, M., Tamura, K., Misawa, H., Hamada, C., Ting, R.C., Robert-Guroff, M. & Gallo, R.C. (1985) Seroepidemiology of human T-lymphotropic retrovirus type I (HTLV-I) in residents of Niigata Prefecture, Japan. Comparative studies by indirect immunofluorescence microscopy and enzyme-linked immunosorbent assay. *Int. J. Cancer*, **35**, 301–306

Arai, E., Chow, K.-C., Li, C.-Y., Tokunaga, M. & Katayama, I. (1994) Differentiation between cutaneous form of adult T cell leukemia/lymphoma and cutaneous T cell lymphoma by in situ hybridization using a human T cell leukemia virus-I DNA probe. *Am. J. Pathol.*, **144**, 15–20

Araki, S., Mochizuki, M., Yamaguchi, K., Watanabe, T., Ono, A., Yoshimura, K., Shirao, M. & Miyata, N. (1993) Familial clustering of human T lymphotropic virus type I uveitis. *Br. J. Ophthalmol.*, **77**, 747–748

Araújo, A. de Q.-C., Afonso, C.R., Schor, D., Leite, A.C. & de Andrada-Serpa, M.J. (1993) Clinical and demographic features of HTLV-I associated myelopathy/tropical spastic paraparesis (HAM/TSP) in Rio de Janeiro, Brazil. *Acta neurol. scand.*, **88**, 59–62

Asou, N., Kumagai, T., Uekihara, S., Ishii, M., Sato, M., Sakai, K., Nishimura, H., Yamaguchi, K. & Takatsuki, K. (1986) HTLV-I seroprevalence in patients with malignancy. *Cancer*, **58**, 903–907

Babu, P.G., Gnanamuthu, C., Saraswathi, N.K., Nerurkar, V.R., Yanagihara, R. & John, T.J. (1993) HTLV-I-associated myelopathy in south India (Letter to the Editor). *AIDS Res. hum. Retroviruses*, **9**, 499–500

Bangham, C.R.M. (1993) Human T-cell leukaemia virus type I and neurological disease. *Curr. Opin. Neurobiol.*, **3**, 773–778

Bangham, C.R.M., Daenke, S., Phillips, R.E., Cruickshank, J.K. & Bell, J.I. (1988) Enzymatic amplification of exogenous and endogenous retroviral sequences from DNA of patients with tropical spastic paraparesis. *EMBO J.*, **7**, 4179–4184

Bangham, C.R.M., Kermode, A.G., Hall, S.E. & Daenke, S. (1996) The cytotoxic T-lymphocyte response to HTLV-I: the main determinant of disease? *Sem. Virol.*, **7**, 41–48

Baranger, A.M., Palmer, C.R., Hamm, M.K., Giebler, H.A., Brauweiler, A., Nyborg, J.K. & Scheparz, A. (1995) Mechanism of DNA-binding enhancement by the human T-cell leukaemia virus transactivator Tax. *Nature*, **376**, 606–608

Barbara, J.A.J. (1994) HTLV-I in multiply transfused patients in Trinidad and Tobago (Letter to the Editor). *Vox Sang.*, **66**, 152

Bartholomew, C., Charles, W., Saxinger, C., Blattner, W., Robert-Guroff, M., Raju, C., Ratan, P., Ince, W., Quamina, D., Basdeo-Maharaj, K. & Gallo, R.C. (1985) Racial and other characteristics of human T cell leukaemia/lymphoma (HTLV-I) and AIDS (HTLV-III) in Trinidad. *Br. med. J.*, **290**, 1243–1246

Bartholomew, C., Edwards, J., Jack, N., Corbin, D., Murphy, J., Cleghorn, F., White, F. & Blattner, W. (1994) Studies on maternal transmission of HTLV-I in patients with adult T-cell leukaemia (ATL) in Trinidad and Tobago (Abstract no. 12). *AIDS Res. hum. Retroviruses*, **10**, 470

Bastian, I.B., Gardner, J., Webb, D. & Gardner, I. (1993) Isolation of a human T-lymphotropic virus type I strain from Australian aboriginals. *J. Virol.*, **67**, 843–851

Batsuuri, J., Dashnyam, B., Maidar, J., Battulga, D., Dorjsuren, D. & Ishida, T. (1993) Absence of human T-lymphotropic retrovirus type I (HTLV-I) in different populations of Mongolia. *Scand. J. infect. Dis.*, **25**, 398–399

Bazarbachi, A., Saal, F., Laroche, L., Flageul, B., Périès, I. & de Thé, H. (1993) HTLV-I provirus and mycosis fungoides. *Science*, **259**, 1470–1471

Bazarbachi, A., Soriano, V., Vallejo, A,. Moudgil, T., Péries, J., de Thé, H. & Gill, P.S. (1995) Mycosis fungoides and Sézary syndrome are not associated with HTLV-I infection: an international study (Abstract no. 3702). *Blood*, **86** (Suppl. 1), 928a

Beaufils, P., Choquet., D., Mamoun, R.Z. & Malissen, B. (1993) The $(YXXL/I)_2$ signalling motif found in the cytoplasmic segments of the bovine leukaemia virus envelope protein and Epstein–Barr virus latent membrane protein 2A can elicit early and late lymphocyte activation events. *EMBO J.*, **12**, 5105–5112

Beilke, M.A., Greenspan, D.L., Impey, A., Thompson, J. & Didier, P.J. (1994) Laboratory study of HIV-1 and HTLV-I/II coinfection. *J. med. Virol.*, **44**, 132–143

Beniashvili, D.S. (1989) An overview of the world literature on spontaneous tumors in non-human primates. *J. med. Primatol.*, **18**, 423–437

Bentrem, D.J., McGovern, E.E., Hammarskjöld, M.-L. & Edlich, R.F. (1994) Human T-cell lymphotropic virus type I (HTLV-I) retrovirus and human disease. *J. Emerg. Med.*, **12**, 825–832

Benvenisty, N., Ornitz, D.M., Bennett, G.L., Sahagan, B.G., Kuo, A., Cardiff, R.D. & Leder, P. (1992) Brain tumours and lymphomas in transgenic mice that carry HTLV-I LTR/c-*myc* and Ig/*tax* genes. *Oncogene*, **7**, 2399–2405

Béraud, C., Lombard-Platet, G., Michal,Y. & Jalinot, P. (1991) Binding of the HTLV-I Tax 1 transactivator to the inducible 21 bp enhancer is mediated by the cellular factor HEB1. *EMBO J.*, **10**, 3795–3803

Berneman, Z.N., Gartenhaus, R.B., Reitz, M.S., Jr, Blattner, W.A., Manns, A., Hanchard, B., Ikehara, O., Gallo, R.C. & Klotman, M.E. (1992a) Expression of alternatively spliced human T-lymphotropic virus type I pX mRNA in infected cell lines and in primary uncultured cells from patients with adult T-cell leukemia/lymphoma and healthy carriers. *Proc. natl Acad. Sci. USA*, **89**, 3005–3009

Berneman, Z.N., Gartenhaus, R.B., Reitz, M.S., Jr, Klotman, M.E. & Gallo, R.C. (1992b) cDNA sequencing confirms HTLV-I expression in adult T-cell leukemia/lymphoma and different sequence variations in *in vivo* and *in vitro*. *Leukemia*, **6** (Suppl. 3), 67S–71S

Bhigjee, A.I., Kelbe, C., Haribhai, H.C., Windsor, I.M., Hoffmann, M.H., Modi, G., Bill, P.L.A., Becker, W.B., Singh, B. & Engelbrecht, S. (1990) Myelopathy associated with human T-cell lymphotropic virus type-I (HTLV-I) in Natal, South Africa. A clinical and investigative study in 24 patients. *Brain*, **113**, 1307–1320

Bhigjee, A.I., Vinsen, C., Windsor, I.M., Gouws, E., Bill, P.L.A. & Tait, D. (1993) Prevalence and transmission of HTLV-I infection in Natal/KwaZulu. *S. Afr. med. J.*, **83**, 665–667

Bieberich, C.J., King, C.M., Tinkle, B.T. & Jay, G. (1993) A transgenic model of transactivation by the Tax protein of HTLV-I. *Virology*, **196**, 309–318

Biggar, R.J., Saxinger, C., Gardiner, C., Collins, W.E., Levine, P.H., Clark, J.W., Nkrumah, F.K. & Blattner, W.A. (1984) Type-I HTLV antibody in urban and rural Ghana, West Africa. *Int. J. Cancer*, **34**, 215–219

Biggar, R.J., Gigase, P.L., Melbye, M., Kestens, L., Sarin, P.S., Bodner, A.J., Demedts, P., Stevens, W.J., Paluku, L., Delacollette, C. & Blattner, W.A. (1985) ELISA HTLV retrovirus antibody reactivity associated with malaria and immune complexes in healthy Africans. *Lancet*, **ii**, 520–523

Biggar, R.J., Neequaye, J.E., Neequaye, A.R., Ankra-Badu, G.A., Levine, P.H., Manns, A., Taylor, M., Drummond, J. & Waters, D. (1993) The prevalence of antibodies to the human T lymphotropic virus (HTLV) in Ghana, West Africa. *AIDS Res. hum. Retroviruses*, **9**, 505–511

Biggar, R.J., Taylor, M.E., Neel, J.V., Hjelle, B., Levine, P.H., Black, F.L., Shaw, G.M., Sharp, P.M. & Hahn, B.H. (1996) Genetic variants of human T-lymphotropic virus type II in American Indian groups. *Virology*, **216**, 166–173

Bills, N.D., Hinrichs, S.H., Morgan, R. & Clifford, A.J. (1992) Delayed tumor onset in transgenic mice fed a low-folate diet. *J. natl Cancer Inst.*, **84**, 332–337

Black, A.C., Ruland, C.T., Luo, J., Bakker, A., Fraser, J.K. & Rosenblatt, J.D. (1994a) Binding of nuclear proteins to HTLV-II *cis*-acting repressive sequence (CRS) RNA correlates with CRS function. *Virology*, **200**, 29–41

Black, F.L., Biggar, R.J., Neel, J.V., Maloney, E.M. & Waters, D.J. (1994b) Endemic transmission of HTLV type II among Kayapo Indians of Brazil. *AIDS Res. hum. Retroviruses*, **10**, 1165–1171

Blank, A., Yamaguchi, K., Blank, M., Zaninovic, V., Sonoda, S. & Takatsuki, K. (1993) Six Colombian patients with adult T-cell leukemia/lymphoma. *Leuk. Lymph.*, **9**, 407–412

Blattner, W.A. & Gallo, R.C. (1994) Epidemiology of HTLV-I and HTLV-II infection. In: Takatsuki, K., ed., *Adult T-cell Leukaemia*, Oxford, Oxford University Press, pp. 45–90

Blattner, W.A., Gibbs, W.N., Saxinger, C., Robert-Guroff, M., Clark, J., Lofters, W., Hanchard, B., Campbell, M. & Gallo, R.C. (1983) Human T-cell leukemia/lymphoma virus-associated lymphoreticular neoplasia in Jamaica. *Lancet*, **ii**, 61–64

Blattner, W.A., Nomura, A., Clark, J.W., Ho, G.Y.F., Nakao, Y., Gallo, R.C. & Robert-Guroff, M. (1986) Modes of transmission and evidence for viral latency from studies of human T-cell lymphotrophic virus type I in Japanese migrant populations in Hawaii. *Proc. natl Acad. Sci. USA*, **83**, 4895–4898

Blattner, W.A., Saxinger, C., Riedel, D., Hull, B., Taylor, G., Cleghorn, F., Gallo, R.C., Blumberg, B. & Bartholomew, C. (1990) A study of HTLV-I and its associated risk factors in Trinidad and Tobago. *J. acquir. immun. Defic. Syndr.*, **3**, 1102–1108

Blomberg, J., Moestrup, T., Frimand, J., Hansson, B.-G., Krogsgaard, K., Grillner, L. & Nordenfelt, E. (1994) HTLV-I and -II in intravenous drug users from Sweden and Denmark. *Scand. J. infect. Dis.*, **26**, 23–26

Boeri, E., Abecasis, C., Varnier, O.E. & Franchini, G. (1995) Analysis of HTLV-I *env* gene sequence from an Italian polytransfused patient: evidence for a Zairian HTLV-I in Sicily. *AIDS Res. hum. Retroviruses*, **11**, 649–651

Bohn Christiansen, C., Wantzin, P. & Dickmeiss, E. (1995) Prevalence of antibodies to HTLV-I/II in high-risk patients and blood donors in Denmark (Letter to the Editor). *Vox Sang.*, **68**, 63–64

Bolton, W.V., Best, S.J., Davis, A.R., Kenrick, K.G. & Wylie, B.R. (1994) The first Australian case of human T-cell lymphotropic virus type II infection (Letter to the Editor). *Med. J. Aust.*, **161**, 451

Bonis, J., Baillou, A., Barin, F., Verdier, M., Janvier, B. & Denis, F. (1993) Discrimination between human T-cell lymphotropic virus type I and II (HTLV-I and HTLV-II) infections by using synthetic peptides representing an immunodominant region of the core protein (p19) of HTLV-I and HTLV-II. *J. clin. Microbiol.*, **31**, 1481–1485

Bosselut, R., Duvall, J.F., Gégonne, A., Bailly, M., Hémar, A., Brady, J. & Ghysdael, J. (1990) The product of the c-*ets*-1 proto-oncogene and the related Ets2 protein act as transcriptional activators of the long terminal repeat of human T cell leukemia virus HTLV-I. *EMBO J.*, **9**, 3137–3144

Bosselut, R., Lim, F., Romond, P.-C., Frampton, J., Brady, J. & Ghysdael, J. (1992) Myb protein binds to multiple sites in the human T cell lymphotropic virus type I long terminal repeat and transactivates LTR-mediated expression. *Virology*, **186**, 764–769

Bouzas, M.B., Zapiola, I., Quiruelas, S., Gorvein, D., Panzita, A., Rey, J., Carnese, F.P., Corral, R., Perez, C., Zala, C., Gallo, D., Hanson, C.V. & Muchinik, G. (1994) HTLV type I and HTLV type II infection among Indians and natives from Argentina. *AIDS Res. hum. Retroviruses*, **10**, 1567–1571

Brabin, L., Brabin, B.J., Doherty, R.R., Gust, I.D., Alpers, M.P., Fujino, R., Imai, J. & Hinuma, Y. (1989) Patterns of migration indicate sexual transmission of HTLV-I infection in non-pregnant women in Papua New Guinea. *Int. J. Cancer*, **44**, 59–62

Brennan, M., Runganga, J., Barbara, J.A.J., Contreras, M., Tedder, R.S., Garson, J.A., Tuke, P.W., Mortimer, P.P., McAlpine, L. & Tosswill, J.H.C. (1993) Prevalence of antibodies to human T cell leukaemia/lymphoma virus in blood donors in north London. *Br. med. J.*, **307**, 1235–1239

Brodine, S.K., Hyams, K.C., Molgaard, C.A., Ito, S.I., Thomas, R.J., Roberts, C.R., Golbeck, A.L., Oldfield, E.C., III & Blattner, W.A. (1995) The risk of human T cell leukemia virus and viral hepatitis infection among US Marines stationed in Okinawa, Japan. *J. infect. Dis.*, **171**, 693–696

Bunker, C.B., Whittaker, S, Luzzatto, L., Gore, M.E., Rustin, M.H.A., Smith, N.P. & Levene, G.M. (1990) Indolent cutaneous prodrome of fatal HTLV-I infection (Letter to the Editor). *Lancet*, **i**, 426

Burny, A. & Mammerickx, M., eds (1987) *Enzootic Bovine Leukosis and Bovine Leukemia Virus*, Boston, Martinus Nijhoff Publishing

Burny, A., Willems, L., Callebaut, I., Adam, E., Cludts, I., Dequiedt, F., Droogmans, L. Grimonpont, C., Kerkhofs, P., Mammerickx, M., Portetelle, D., Van den Broeke, A. & Kettmann, R. (1994) Bovine leukaemia virus: biology and mode of transformation. In: Minson, A.C., Neil, J.C. & McRae, M.A., eds, *Viruses and Cancer*, Cambridge, Cambridge University Press, pp. 213–234

Busch, M.P., Laycock, M., Kleinman, S.H., Wages, J.W., Jr, Calabro, M., Kaplan, J.E., Khabbaz, R.F., Hollingsworth, C.G. and the Retrovirus Epidemiology Donor Study (1994) Accuracy of supplementary serologic testing for human T-lymphotropic virus types I and II in US blood donors. *Blood*, **83**, 1143–1148

Cabrera, M.E., Labra, S., Catovsky, D., Ford, A.M., Colman, S.M., Greaves, M.F. & Matutes, E. (1994) HTLV-I positive adult T-cell leukaemia/lymphoma (ATLL) in Chile. *Leukemia*, **8**, 1763–1767

Cann, A.J. & Chen, I.S.Y. (1990) Human T-cell leukemia virus Types I and II. In: Fields, B.N. & Knipe, D.R., eds, *Virology*, New York, Raven Press, pp. 1501–1527

Cann, A.J. & Chen, I.S.Y. (1996) Human T-cell leukemia virus types I and II. In: Fields, B.N., Knipe, D.M., Howley, P.M., Chanock, R.M., Melnick, J.L., Monath, T.P., Roizman, B. & Straus, S.E., eds, *Fields Virology*, 3rd Ed., Vol. 2, Philadelphia, Lippincott-Raven Publishers, pp. 1849–1880

Cann, A.J., Rosenblatt, J.D., Wachsman, W., Shah, N.P. & Chen, I.S.Y. (1985) Identification of the gene responsible for human T-cell leukaemia virus transcriptional regulation. *Nature*, **318**, 571–574

Capésius, C., Saal, F., Maero, E., Bazarbachi, A., Lasneret, J., Laroche, L., Gessain, A., Hojman, F. & Périés, J. (1991) No evidence for HTLV-I infection in 24 cases of French and Portuguese mycosis fungoides and Sézary syndrome (as seen in France). *Leukemia*, **5**, 416–419

Cartier, L., Castillo, J.L., Cabrera, M.E., Araya, F., Matutes, E., Ford, A.M. & Greaves, M.F. (1995) HTLV-I positive progressive spastic paraparesis (TSP) associated with a lymphoid disorder in three Chilean patients. *Leuk. Lymph.*, **17**, 459–464

Cassé, H., Girerd, Y., Gazzolo, L. & Duc Dodon, M. (1994) Critical involvement of human T-cell leukemia virus type I virions in mediating the viral mitogenic effect. *J. gen. Virol.*, **75**, 1909–1916

Catovsky, D., Rose, M., Goolden, A.W.G., White, J.M., Bourikas, G., Brownell, A.I., Blattner, W.A., Greaves, M.F., Galton, D.A.G., McCluskey, D.R., Lampert, I., Ireland, R., Bridges, J.M. & Gallo, R.C. (1982) Adult T-cell lymphoma-leukaemia in blacks from the West Indies. *Lancet*, **i**, 639–643

Cavrois, M., Gessain, A., Wain-Hobson, S. & Wattel, E. (1996) Proliferation of HTLV-I infected circulating cells *in vivo* in all asymptomatic carriers and patients with TSP/HAM. *Oncogene* (in press)

Centers for Disease Control and Prevention (1992) Update: serologic testing for human T-lymphotropic virus type I. United States 1989 and 1990. *Morbid. Mortal. Wkly Rep.*, **41**, 259–262

Cereseto, A., Diella, F., Mulloy, J.C., Cara, A., Michieli, P., Grassmann, R., Franchini, G. & Klotman, M.E. (1996) p53 functional impairment and high $p21^{waf1/cip1}$ expression in human T-cell lymphotropic/leukemia virus type I (HTLV-I) transformed T-cells. *Blood* (in press)

Cevallos, R., Barberis, L., Evans, L., Barriga, J., Verdier, M., Bonis, J., Leonard, G. & Denis, F. (1990) HIV-1, HIV-2 and HTLV-I seroprevalence surveys in continental Ecuador and Galapagos (Letter to the Editor). *AIDS*, **4**, 1300–1301

Chadburn, A., Athan, E., Wieczorek, R. & Knowles, D.M. (1991) Detection and characterization of human T-cell lymphotropic virus type I (HTLV-I) associated T-cell neoplasms in an HTLV-I nonendemic region by polymerase chain reaction. *Blood*, **77**, 2419–2430

Chavance, M. & Fréry, N. (1993) Re: 'Declining seroprevalence and transmission of HTLV-I in Japanese families who emigrated to Hawaii' (Letter to the Editor). *Am. J. Epidemiol.*, **138**, 898–900

Chavance, M., Fréry, N., Valette, I., Monplaisir, N. & Schaffar, L. (1989) Cohort effect of HTLV-I seroprevalence in southern Japan (Letter to the Editor). *Lancet*, **ii**, 1337

Chen, I.S.Y., Quan, S.G. & Golde, D.W. (1983) Human T-cell leukemia virus type II transforms normal human lymphocytes. *Proc. natl Acad. Sci. USA*, **80**, 7006–7009

Chen, Y.-C., Wang, C.-H., Su, I.-J., Hu, C.-Y., Chou, M.-J., Lee, T.-H., Lin, D.-T., Chung, T.-Y., Liu, C.-H. & Wang, C.-S. (1989) Infection of human T-cell leukemia virus type I and development of human T-cell leukemia/lymphoma in patients with hematological neoplasms: a possible linkage to blood transfusion. *Blood*, **74**, 388–394

Chen, Y.-M., Lee, T.-H., Wiktor, S.Z., Shaw, G.M., Murphy, E.L., Blattner, W.A. & Essex, M. (1990) Type-specific antigens for serological discrimination of HTLV-I and HTLV-II infection. *Lancet*, **336**, 1153–1155

Chen, C.-J., Hsieh, S.-F. & Yang, C.-S. (1994) Seroepidemiology of human T-lymphotropic virus type I infection among intravenous drug abusers in Taiwan. *J. med. Virol.*, **42**, 264–267

Chen, Y.-X., Ikeda, S., Mori, H., Hata, T., Tsukasaki, K., Momita, S., Yamada, Y., Kamihira, S., Mine, M. & Tomonaga, M. (1995) Molecular detection of pre-ATL state among healthy HTLV-I carriers in an endemic area of Japan. *Int. J. Cancer*, **60**, 798–801

Chironna, M., Quarto, M., Sabato, V. & De Mattia, D. (1994) HTLV-I infection in a thalassemic patient from Apulia (southern Italy) (Letter to the Editor). *Vox Sang.*, **67**, 321–322

Chlichlia, K., Moldenhauer, G., Daniel, P.T., Busslinger, M., Gazzolo, L., Schirrmacher, V. & Khazaie, K. (1995) Immediate effects of reversible HTLV-1 *tax* function: T-cell activation and apoptosis. *Oncogene*, **10**, 269–277

Chou, K.S., Okayama, A., Tachibana, N., Lee, T.-H. & Essex, M. (1995) Nucleotide sequence analysis of full-length human T-cell leukemia virus type I from adult T-cell leukemia cells: a prematurely terminated pX open reading frame II. *Int. J. Cancer*, **60**, 701–706

Chrivia, J.C., Kwok, R.P., Lamb, N., Hagiwara, M., Montminy, M.R. & Goodman, R.H. (1993) Phosphorylated CREB binds specifically to the nuclear protein CBP. *Nature*, **365**, 855–859

Cimarelli, A., Duclos, C.A., Gessain, A., Cattaneo, E., Casoli, C., Biglione, M., Mauclère, P. & Bertazzoni, U. (1995) Quantification of HTLV-II proviral copies by competitive polymerase chain reaction in peripheral blood mononuclear cells of Italian injecting drug users, central Africans, and Amerindians. *J. acquir. Immune Defic. Syndr. hum. Retrovirol.*, **10**, 198–204

Ciminale, V., Pavlakis, G.N., Derse, D., Cunningham, C.P. & Felber, B.K. (1992) Complex splicing in the human T-cell leukemia virus (HTLV) family of retroviruses: novel mRNAs and proteins produced by HTLV type I. *J. Virol.*, **66**, 1737–1745

Ciminale, V., D'Agostino, D.M., Zotti, L., Franchini, G., Felber, B.K. & Chieco-Bianchi, L. (1995) Expression and characterization of proteins produced by mRNAs spliced into the X region of the human T-cell leukemia/lymphotropic virus type II. *Virology*, **209**, 445–456

Clark, J., Saxinger, C., Gibbs, W.N., Lofters, W., Lagranade, L., Deceulaer, K., Ensroth, A., Robert-Guroff, M., Gallo, R.C. & Blattner, W.A. (1985a) Seroepidemiologic studies of human T-cell leukemia/lymphoma virus type I in Jamaica. *Int. J. Cancer*, **36**, 37–41

Clark, J.W., Robert-Guroff, M., Ikehara, O., Henzan, E. & Blattner, W.A. (1985b) Human T-cell leukemia-lymphoma virus type I and adult T-cell leukemia-lymphoma in Okinawa. *Cancer Res.*, **45**, 2849–2852

Clark, J.W., Gurgo, C., Franchini, G., Gibbs, W.N., Lofters, W., Neuland, C., Mann, D., Saxinger, C., Gallo, R.C. & Blattner, W.A. (1988) Molecular epidemiology of HTLV-I-associated non-Hodgkin's lymphomas in Jamaica. *Cancer*, **61**, 1477–1482

Cleghorn, F., Charles, W., Blattner, W.A. & Bartholomew, C. (1990) Adult T-cell leukemia in Trinidad and Tobago. In: Blattner, W.A., ed., *Human Retrovirology: HTLV*, New York, Raven Press, pp. 185–190

Cockerell, G.L., Weiser, M.G., Rovnak, J., Wicks-Beard, B., Roberts, B., Post, A., Chen, I.S.Y. & Lairmore, M.D. (1991) Infectious transmission of human T-cell lymphotropic virus type II in rabbits. *Blood*, **78**, 1532–1537

Coffin, J.M. (1996) Retroviridae: the viruses and their replication. In: Fields, B.N., Knipe, P.M., Howley, P.M., Chanock, R.M., Melnick, J.L., Monath, T.P. & Roizman, B., eds, *Fields Virology*, 3rd Ed., Vol. 2, Philadelphia, Lippincott-Raven Publishers, pp. 1767–1847

Cossen, C., Hagens, S., Fukuchi, R., Forghani, B., Gallo, D. & Ascher, M. (1992) Comparison of six commercial human T-cell lymphotropic virus type I (HTLV-I) enzyme immunoassay kits for detection of antibody to HTLV-I and -II. *J. clin. Microbiol.*, **30**, 724–725

Coste, J., Lemaire, J.-M., Couroucé, A.-M., the Retrovirus Study Group of the French Society of Blood Transfusion & Canavaggio, M. (1993) Human T-lymphotropic virus (HTLV) type I and II: seroprevalence among intravenous drug users in continental France. *AIDS*, **7**, 440–441

Couroucé, A.-M., Pillonel, J., Lemaire, J.-M., Maniez, M. & Brunet, J.-B. (1993) Seroepidemiology of HTLV-I/II in universal screening of blood donations in France. *AIDS*, **7**, 841–847

Cruickshank, J.K., Rudge, P., Dalgleish, A.G., Newton, M., McLean, B.N., Barnard, R.O., Kendall, B.E. & Miller, D.H. (1989) Tropical spastic paraparesis and human T cell lymphotropic virus type I in the United Kingdom. *Brain*, **112**, 1057–1090

Cruickshank, J.K., Corbin, D.O.C., Bucher, B. & Vernant, J.C. (1992) HTLV-I and neurological disease. *Ballière's clin. Neurol.*, **1**, 61–81

Dada, A.J., Oyewole, F., Onofowokan, R., Nasidi, A., Harris, B., Levin, A., Diamondstone, L., Quinn, T.C. & Blattner, W.A. (1993) Demographic characteristics of retroviral infections (HIV-1, HIV-2, and HTLV-I) among female professional sex workers in Lagos, Nigeria. *J. acquir. Immune Defic. Syndr.*, **6**, 1358–1363

Daenke, S., Parker, C.E., Niewiesk, S., Newsom-Davis, J., Nightingale, S. & Bangham, C.R.M. (1994) Spastic paraparesis in a patient carrying defective human T cell leukemia virus type I (HTLV-I) provirus sequences but lacking a humoral or cytotoxic T cell response to HTLV-I (Letter to the Editor). *J. infect. Dis.*, **169**, 941–943

Daenke, S., Kermode, A.G., Hall, S.E., Taylor, G., Weber, J., Nightingale, S. & Bangham, C.R.M. (1996) High activated and memory cytotoxic T-cell responses to HTLV-I in healthy carriers and patients with tropical spastic paraparesis. *Virology*, **217**, 139–146

Dalakas, M.C. (1993) Retroviruses and inflammatory myopathies in humans and primates. *Ballière's clin. Neurol.*, **2**, 659–691

Dalekos, G.N., Zervou, E., Karabini, F., Elisaf, M., Bourantas, K. & Siamopoulos, K.C. (1995) Prevalence of antibodies to human T-lymphotropic virus types I and II in volunteer blood donors and high-risk groups in northwestern Greece. *Transfusion*, **35**, 503–506

Dalgleish, A., Richardson, J., Matutes, E., Cruickshank, K., Newell, A., Sinclair, A., Thorpe, R., Brasher, M., Weber, J., Catovsky, D. & Rudge, P. (1988) HTLV-I infection in tropical spastic paraparesis: lymphocyte culture and serological response. *AIDS Res. hum. Retroviruses*, **4**, 475–485

Davidson, M., Kaplan, J.E., Hartley, T.M., Lairmore, M.D. & Lanier, A.P. (1990) Prevalence of HTLV-I in Alaska Natives (Letter to the Editor). *J. infect. Dis.*, **161**, 359–360

Dekaban, G., Oger, J.J.F., Foti, D., Fing, E.E., Waters, D.J., Picard, F.J., Arp, J., Werker, D. & Rice, G.P.A. (1994) HTLV-I infection associated with disease in aboriginal Indians from British Colombia: a serological and PCR analysis. *Clin. diagn. Virol.*, **2**, 67–78

Delaporte, E., Peeters, M., Simoni, M. & Piot, P. (1989a) HTLV-I infection in western equatorial Africa (Letter to the Editor). *Lancet*, **ii**, 1226

Delaporte, E., Peeters, M., Durand, J.-P., Dupont, A., Schrijvers, D., Bedjabaga, L., Honoré, C., Ossari, S., Trebucq, A., Josse, R. & Merlin, M. (1989b) Seroepidemiological survey of HTLV-I infection among randomized populations of western central African countries. *J. acquir. Immune Defic. Syndr.*, **2**, 410–413

Delaporte, E., Monplaisir, N., Louwagie, J., Peeters, M., Martin-Prével, Y., Louis, J.-P., Trebucq, A., Bedjabaga, L., Ossari, S., Honoré, C., Larouzé, B., d'Auriol, L., Van der Goen, G. & Piot, P. (1991) Prevalence of HTLV-I and HTLV-II infection in Gabon, Africa. Comparison of the serological and PCR results. *Int. J. Cancer*, **49**, 373–376

Delaporte, E., Klotz, F., Peeters, M., Martin-Prevel, Y., Bedjabaga, L., Larouzé, B., Nguembi-Mbina, C., Walter, P. & Piot, P. (1993) Non-Hodgkin lymphoma in Gabon and its relation to HTLV-I. *Int. J. Cancer*, **53**, 48–50

Delaporte, E., Buvé, A., Nzila, N., Goeman, J., Dazza, M.-C., Henzel, D., Heyward, W., St-Louis, M., Piot, P. & Laga, M. (1995) HTLV-I infection among prostitutes and pregnant women in Kinshasa, Zaire: how important is high-risk sexual behavior? *J. acquir. Immune Defic. Syndr. hum. Retrovirol.*, **8**, 511–515

Del Mistro, A., Chotard, J., Hall, A.J., Fortuin, M., Whittle, H., De Rossi, A. & Chieco-Bianchi, L. (1994) HTLV-I/II seroprevalence in The Gambia: a study of mother-child pairs. *AIDS Res. hum. Retroviruses*, **10**, 617–620

Denic, S., Nolan, P., Doherty, J., Garson, J., Tuke, P. & Tedder, R. (1990) HTLV-I infection in Iraq (Letter to the Editor). *Lancet*, **336**, 1135–1136

Depelchin, A., Letesson, J., Lostrie, N., Mammerickx, M., Portetelle, D. & Burny, A. (1989) Bovine leukemia virus (BLV)-infected B cells express a marker similar to the CD5 T-cell marker. *Immunol. Lett.*, **20**, 69–76

Dequiedt, F., Kettmann, R., Burny, A. & Willems, L. (1995) Mutations in the p53 tumor-suppressor gene are frequently asociated with bovine leukemia virus-induced leukemogenesis in cattle but not in sheep. *Virology*, **209**, 676–683

Derse, D., Mikovits, J., Polianova, M., Felber, B.K. & Ruscetti, F. (1995) Virions released from cells transfected with a molecular clone of human T-cell leukemia virus type I give rise to primary and secondary infections of T cells. *J. Virol.*, **69**, 1907–1912

Dezzutti, C.S., Rudolph, D.L., Roberts, C.R. & Lal, R.B. (1993) Characterization of human T-lymphotropic virus type I- and II-infected T-cell lines: antigenic, phenotypic, and genotypic analysis. *Virus Res.*, **29**, 59–70

Dhib-Jalbut, S., Hoffman, P.M., Yamabe, T., Sun, D., Xia, J., Eisenberg, H., Bergey, G. & Ruscetti, F.W. (1994) Extracellular human T-cell lymphotropic virus type I Tax protein induces cytokine production in adult human microglial cells. *Ann. Neurol.*, **36**, 787–790

Dimmock, C.K., Ward, W.H. & Trueman, K.F. (1990) Lymphocyte subpopulations in sheep with lymphosarcoma resulting from experimental infection with bovine leukaemia virus. *Immunol. Cell Biol.*, **68**, 45–49

Dixon, A.C., Yanagihara, E.T., Kwock, D.W. & Nakamura, J.M. (1989) Strongyloidiasis associated with human T-cell lymphotropic virus type I infection in a nonendemic area. *West. J. Med.*, **151**, 410–413

Djilali, S. & Parodi, A.-L. (1989) The BLV-induced leukemia-lymphosarcoma complex in sheep. *Vet. Immunol. Immunopathol.*, **22**, 233–244

Djilali, S., Parodi, A.-L., Levy, D. & Cockerell, G.L. (1987) Development of leukemia and lymphosarcoma induced by bovine leukemia virus in sheep. A hematopathological study. *Leukemia*, **1**, 777–781

Domingues, R.B., Muniz, M.R., Pinho, J.R.R., Bassit, L., Jorge, M.L.C., Saez Alquezar, A., Marchiori, P.E., Chamone, D.F. & Scaff, M. (1995) Human T lymphotropic virus type I-associated myelopathy/tropical spastic paraparesis in São Paulo, Brazil. *Clin. infect. Dis.*, **20**, 1540–1542

Donegan, E., Lee, H., Operskalski, E.A., Shaw, G.M., Kleinman, S.H., Busch, M.P., Stevens, C.E., Schiff, E.R., Nowicki, M.J., Hollingsworth, C.G., Mosley, J.W. & the Transfusion Safety Study Group (1994) Transfusion transmission of retroviruses: human T-lymphotropic virus types I and II compared with human immunodeficiency virus type 1. *Transfusion*, **34**, 478–483

Dube, D.K., Sherman, M.P., Saksena, N.K., Bryz-Gornia, V., Mendelson, J., Love, J., Arnold, C.B., Spicer, T., Dube, S., Glaser, J.B., Williams, A.E., Nishimura, M., Jacobsen, S., Ferrer, J.F., Del Pino, N., Quiruelas, S. & Poiesz, B.J. (1993) Genetic heterogeneity in human T-cell leukemia/lymphoma virus type II. *J. Virol.*, **67**, 1175–1184

Duc Dodon, M., Bernard, A. & Gazzolo, L. (1989) Peripheral T-lymphocyte activation by human T-cell leukemia virus type I interferes with the CD2 but not with the CD3/TCR pathway. *J. Virol.*, **63**, 5413–5419

Duenas-Barajas, E., Bernal, J.E., Vaught, D.R., Nerurkar, V.R., Sarmiento, P., Yanagihara, R. & Gajdusek, D.C. (1993) Human retroviruses in Amerindians of Colombia: high prevalence of human T cell lymphotropic virus type II infection among the Tunebo Indians. *Am. J. trop. Med. Hyg.*, **49**, 657–663

Duggan, D.B., Ehrlich, G.D., Davey, F.P., Kwok, S., Sninsky, J., Goldberg, J., Baltrucki, L. & Poiesz, B.J. (1988) HTLV-I-induced lymphoma mimicking Hodgkin's disease. Diagnosis by polymerase chain reaction amplification of specific HTLV-I sequences in tumor DNA. *Blood*, **71**, 1027–1032

Dumas, M., Houinato, D., Verdier, M., Zohoun, T., Josse, R., Bonis, J., Zohoun, I., Massougbodji, A. & Denis, F. (1991) Seroepidemiology of human T-cell lymphotropic virus type I/II in Benin (West Africa). *AIDS Res. hum. Retroviruses*, **7**, 447–451

Duyao, M.P., Kessler, D.J., Spicer, D.B. & Sonenshein, G.E. (1992) Transactivation of the murine *c-myc* gene by HTLV-I *tax* is mediated by NFκB. *AIDS Res. hum. Retroviruses*, **8**, 752–754

Eble, B.E., Busch, M.P., Guiltinan, A.M., Khayam-Bashi, H. & Murphy, E.L. (1993) Determination of human T lymphotropic virus type by polymerase chain reaction and correlation with risk factors in northern California blood donors. *J. infect. Dis.*, **167**, 954–957

Edouard, E., Legrand, E., Astier-Gin, T., Dalibart, R., Geoffre, S., Dalbon, P., Guillemain, B. & Londos-Gagliardi, D. (1994) Characterization of monoclonal antibodies directed against the gp46 of human T-cell leukemia virus type I. *Leukemia*, **8** (Suppl. 1), S60–S64

Eguchi, K., Matsuoka, N., Ida, H., Nakashima, M., Sakai, M., Sakito, S., Kawakami, A., Terada, K., Shimada, H., Kawabe, Y., Fukuda, T., Sawada, T. & Nagataki, S. (1992) Primary Sjögren's syndrome with antibodies to HTLV-I: clinical and laboratory features. *Ann. rheum. Dis.*, **51**, 769–776

Ehrlich, G.D., Greenberg, S. & Abbott, M.A. (1990) Detection of human T-cell lymphoma/leukemia viruses. In: Innis, M.A., Gelfand, D.H., Sninsky, J.J. & White, T.J., eds, *PCR Protocols: A Guide to Methods and Applications*, San Diego, CA, Academic Press, pp. 324–336

Eiraku, N., Monken, C., Kubo, T., Zhu, S.W., Rios, M., Bianco, C., Hjelle, B., Nagashima, K. & Hall, W.W. (1995) Nucleotide sequence and restriction fragment length polymorphism analysis of the long terminal repeat of human T-cell leukemia virus type II. *AIDS Res. hum. Retroviruses*, **11**, 625–636

Eiraku, N., Novoa, P., Da Costa Ferreira, M., Monken, C., Ishak, R., Da Costa Ferreira, O., Zhu, S.W., Lorenco, R., Ishak, M., Azvedo, V., Guerreiro, J., Pombo de Oliveira, M., Loureiro, P., Hammerschlak, N., Ijichi, S. & Hall, W.W. (1996) Identification and characterization of a new and distinct molecular subtype of human T-cell lymphotropic virus type II. *J. Virol.*, **70**, 1481–1492

El-Farrash, M.A., Badr, M.F., Hawas, S.A., El-Nashar, N.M., Imai, J., Komoda, H. & Hinuma, Y. (1988) Sporadic carriers of human T-lymphotropic virus type I in northern Egypt. *Microbiol. Immunol.*, **32**, 981–984

Farouqi, B., Yahyaoui, M., Alaoui, F.M., Noraz, N., Sekkat, S., Chkili, T., Desgrange, C. & Benslimane, A. (1992) Establishment of T-lymphoid cell lines from Morroccan patients with tropical spastic paraparesis. *AIDS Res. hum. Retroviruses*, **8**, 1209–1213

Felber, B.K., Paskalis, H., Kleinman-Ewing, C., Wong-Staal, F. & Pavlakis, G.N. (1985) The pX protein of HTLV-I is a transcriptional activator of its long terminal repeats. *Science*, **229**, 675–679

Ferreira, O.C., Jr, Vaz, R.S., Carvalho, M.B., Guerra, C., Fabron, A.L., Rosemblit, J. & Hamerschlak, N. (1995) Human T-lymphotropic virus type I and type II infections and correlation with risk factors in blood donors from São Paulo, Brazil. *Transfusion*, **35**, 258–263

Feuer, G., Zack, J.A., Harrington, W.J., Jr, Valderama, R., Rosenblatt, J.D., Wachsman, W., Baird, S.M. & Chen, I.S.Y. (1993) Establishment of human T-cell leukemia virus type I T-cell lymphomas in severe combined immunodeficient mice. *Blood*, **82**, 722–731

Feuer, G., Stewart, S.A., Baird, S.M., Lee, F., Feuer, R. & Chen, I.S.Y. (1995) Potential role of natural killer cells in controlling tumorigenesis by human T-cell leukemia viruses. *J. Virol.*, **69**, 1328–1333

Figueroa, J.P., Morris, J., Brathwaite, A., Ward, E., Peruga, A., Hayes, R., Vermund, S.H. & Blattner, W. (1995) Risk factors for HTLV-I among heterosexual STD clinic attenders. *J. Acquir. Immune Defic. Syndr. hum. Retrovirol.*, **9**, 81–88

Foil, L.D. & Issel, C.J. (1991) Transmission of retroviruses by arthropods. *Annu. Rev. Entomol.*, **36**, 355–381

Fossum, C., Burny, A., Portetelle, D., Mammerickx, M. & Morein, B. (1988) Detection of T and B cells with lectins and antibodies in healthy and bovine leukemia virus-infected cattle. *Vet. Immunol. Immunopathol.*, **18**, 269–278

Fouchard, N., Flageul, B., Bagot, M., Avril, M.-F., Hermine, O., Sigaux, F., Merle-Beral, H., Troussard, X., Delfraissy, J.-F., de Thé, G. & Gessain, A. (1995) Lack of evidence of HTLV-I/II infection in T CD8 malignant or reactive lymphoproliferative disorders in France: a serological and/or molecular study of 169 cases. *Leukemia*, **9**, 2087–2092

Foulkes, N.S., Borrelli, E. & Sassone-Corsi, P. (1991) CREM gene: use of alternative DNA-binding domains generates multiple antagonists of cAMP-induced transcription. *Cell*, **64**, 739–749

Franchini, G. (1995) Molecular mechanisms of human T-cell leukemia/lymphotropic virus type I infection. *Blood*, **86**, 3619–3639

Franchini, G., Wong-Staal, F. & Gallo, R.C. (1984) Human T-cell leukemia virus (HTLV-I) transcripts in fresh and cultured cells of patients with adult T-cell leukemia. *Proc. natl Acad. Sci. USA*, **81**, 6207–6211

Franchini, G., Mulloy, J.C., Koralnik, I.J., Lo Menico, A., Sparkowski, J.J., Andresson, T., Goldstein, D.J. & Schlegel, R. (1993) The human T-cell leukemia/lymphotropic virus type I p12^I protein cooperates with the E5 oncoprotein of bovine papillomavirus in cell transformation and binds the 16-kilodalton subunit of the vacuolar H$^+$ ATPase. *J. Virol.*, **67**, 7701–7704

Franchini, G., Tartaglia, J., Markham, P., Benson, J., Fullen, J., Wills, M., Arp, J., Dekaban, G., Paoletti, E. & Gallo, R.C. (1995) Highly attenuated HTLV type I$_{env}$ poxvirus vaccines induce protection against a cell-associated HTLV type I challenge in rabbits. *AIDS Res. hum. Retroviruses*, **11**, 307–313

Fréry, N., Chavance, M., Valette, I., Schaffar, L., Neisson-Vernant, C., Jouannelle, J. & Monplaisir, N. (1991) HTLV-I infection in French West Indies: a case–control study. *Eur. J. Epidemiol.*, **7**, 175–182

Fujihara, K., Du, T.-L., Selkirk, S,. Ward, P., Pickert, M., Hohmann, P., Bisaccia, E. & Greenberg, S.J. (1994) A new human endogenous DNA sequence homologous to HTLV-I *pol*. *Genomics*, **22**, 244–246

Fujii, M., Sassone-Corsi, P. & Verma, I.M. (1988) C-*fos* promoter transactivation by the tax$_1$ protein of human T-cell leukemia virus type I. *Proc. natl Acad. Sci. USA*, **85**, 8526–8530

Fujii, M., Niki, T., Mori, T., Matsuda, T., Matsui, M., Nomura, N. & Seiki, M. (1991) HTLV-I Tax induces expression of various immediate early serum response genes. *Oncogene*, **6**, 1023–1029

Fujii, M., Tsuchiya, H., Chuhjo, T., Akizawa, T. & Seiki, M (1992) Interaction of HTLV-I Tax1 with p67^{SRF} causes the aberrant induction of cellular immediate early genes through CArG boxes. *Genes Dev.*, **6**, 2066–2076

Fujino, R., Kawato, K., Ikeda, M., Miyakoshi, H., Mizukoshi, M. & Imai, J. (1991) Improvement of gelatin particle agglutination test for detection of anti-HTLV-I antibody. *Jpn. J. Cancer Res.*, **82**, 367–370

Fujisawa, J.-I., Seiki, M., Sato, M. & Yoshida, M. (1986) A transcriptional enhancer of HTLV-I is responsible for *trans*-activation mediated by p40` of HTLV-I. *EMBO J.*, **5**, 713–718

Fujisawa, J., Seiki, M., Miyatake, S., Arai, K. & Yoshida, M. (1988) Cell-line specific activation of SV40 transcriptional enhancer by p40tax of HTLV-I. *Jpn. J. Cancer Res.*, **79**, 800–804

Fujita, M. & Shiku, H. (1995) Differences in sensitivity to induction of apoptosis among rat fibroblast cells transformed by HTLV-I *tax* gene or cellular nuclear oncogenes. *Oncogene*, **11**, 15–20

Fukudome, K., Furuse, M., Fukuhara, N., Orita, S., Imai, T., Takagi, S., Nagira, M., Hinuma, Y. & Yoshie, O. (1992) Strong induction of ICAM-1 in human T-cells transformed by human T-cell-leukemia virus type I and expression of ICAM-1 or LFA-1 in adult T-cell-leukemia-derived cell lines. *Int. J. Cancer*, **52**, 418–427

Fultz, P.N. (1994) Simian T-lymphotrophic virus type I. In: Levy, J.A., ed., *The Retroviridae*, Vol. 3, New York, Plenum Press, pp. 111–131

Furukawa, K., Furukawa, K. & Shiku, H. (1991) Alternatively spliced mRNA of the *pX* region of human T-lymphotropic virus type I proviral genome. *FEBS Lett.*, **295**, 141–145

Furukawa, Y., Fujisawa, J., Osame, M., Toita, M., Sonoda, S., Kubota, R., Ijichi, S. & Yoshida, M. (1992) Frequent clonal proliferation of human T-cell leukemia virus type I (HTLV-I)-infected T cells in HTLV-I-associated myelopathy (HAM-TSP). *Blood*, **80**, 1012–1016

Furukawa, Y., Osame, M., Kubota, R., Tara, M. & Yoshida, M. (1995) Human T-cell leukemia virus type-I (HTLV-I) Tax is expressed at the same level in infected cells of HTLV-I-associated myelopathy or tropical spastic paraparesis patients as in asymptomatic carriers but at a lower level in adult T-cell leukemia cells. *Blood*, **85**, 1865–1870

Furuta, Y., Aizawa, S., Suda, Y., Ikawa, Y., Kishimoto, H., Asano, Y., Tada, T., Hikikoshi, A., Yoshida, M. & Seiki, M. (1989) Thymic atrophy characteristic in transgenic mice that harbor pX genes of human T-cell leukemia virus type I. *J. Virol.*, **63**, 3185–3189

Gabarre, J., Gessain, A., Raphael, M., Merle-Béral, H., Dubourg, O., Fourcade, C., Gandjbakhch, I., Jault, F., Delcourt, A. & Binet, J.-L. (1993) Adult T-cell leukemia/lymphoma revealed by a surgically cured cardiac valve lymphomatous involvement in an Iranian woman: clinical, immunopathological and viromolecular studies. *Leukemia*, **7**, 1904–1909

Gabbai, A.A., Bordin, J.O., Vieira-Filho, J.P.B., Kuroda, A., Oliveira, A.S.B., Cruz, M.V., Ribeiro, A.A.F., Delaney, S.R., Henrard, D.R., Rosario, J. & Roman, G.C. (1993) Selectivity of human T lymphotropic virus type-I (HTLV-I) and HTLV-II infection among different populations in Brazil. *Am. J. trop. Med. Hyg.*, **49**, 664–671

Gallo, D., Penning, L.M. & Hanson, C.V. (1991) Detection and differentiation of antibodies to human T-cell lymphotropic virus types I and II by the immunofluorescence method. *J. clin. Microbiol.*, **29**, 2345–2347

Gallo, D., Diggs, J.L. & Hanson, C.V. (1994a) Evaluation of two commercial human T-cell lymphotropic virus western blot (immunoblot) kits with problem specimens. *J. clin. Microbiol.*, **32**, 2046–2049

Gallo, D., Penning, L.M., Diggs, J.L. & Hanson, C.V. (1994b) Sensitivities of radioimmunoprecipitation assay and PCR for detection of human T-lymphotropic type II infection. *J. clin. Microbiol.*, **32**, 2464–2467

Gallo, R.C. (1995) A surprising advance in the treatment of viral leukemia. *New Engl. J. Med.*, **332**, 1783–1784

Gallo, R. & Wong-Staal (1990) *Retrovirus Biology and Human Disease*, New York, Marcel Dekker

Gallo, R.C., Sliski, A. & Wong-Staal, F. (1983) Origin of human T-cell leukaemia-lymphoma virus (Letter to the Editor). *Lancet*, **ii**, 962–963

Garin, B., Gosselin, S., de Thé, G. & Gessain, A. (1994) HTLV-I/II infection in a high viral endemic area of Zaire, Central Africa: comparative evaluation of serology, PCR, and significance of indeterminate western blot pattern. *J. med. Virol.*, **44**, 104–109

Garruto, R.M., Slover, M., Yanagihara, R., Mora, C.A., Alexander, S.S., Asher, D.M., Rodgers-Johnson, P. & Gajdusek, D.C. (1990) High prevalence of human T-lymphotropic virus type I infection in isolated populations of the Western Pacific region confirmed by western immunoblot. *Am. J. hum. Biol.*, **2**, 439–447

Gatei, M.H., Brandon, R., Naif, H.M., Lavin, M.F. & Daniel, R.C.W. (1989) Lymphosarcoma development in sheep experimentally infected with bovine leukaemia virus. *J. vet. Med.*, **B36**, 424–432

Gatei, M.H., Naif, H.M., Kumar, S., Boyle, D.B., Daniel, R.C.W., Good, M.F. & Lavin, M.F. (1993) Protection of sheep against bovine leukemia virus (BLV) infection by vaccination with recombinant vaccinia viruses expressing BLV envelope glycoproteins: correlation of protection with CD4 T-cell response to gp51 peptide 51–70. *J. Virol.*, **67**, 1803–1810

Gazzolo, L. & Duc Dodon, M. (1987) Direct activation of resting T lymphocytes by human T-lymphotropic virus type I. *Nature*, **326**, 714–717

Gelderblom, H.R. (1991) Assembly and morphology of HIV: potential effect of structure on viral function. *AIDS*, **5**, 617–637

Gérard, Y., Lepere, J.-F., Pradinaud, R., Joly, F., Lepelletier, L., Joubert, M., Sainte Marie, D., Mahieux, R., Ureta Vidal, A., Larregain-Fournier, D., Valensi, F., Moynet, D., de Thé, G., Guillemain, B., Moreau, J.-P. & Gessain, A. (1995) Clustering and clinical diversity of adult T-cell leukemia/lymphoma associated with HTLV-I in a remote black population of French Guiana. *Int. J. Cancer*, **60**, 773–776

Gessain, A. & Gout, O. (1992) Chronic myelopathy associated with human T-lymphotropic virus type-I (HTLV-I). *Ann. intern. Med.*, **117**, 933–946

Gessain, A. & Mathieux, R. (1995) HTLV-I 'indeterminate' western blot patterns observed in sera from tropical regions: the situation revisited. *J. acquir. Immune Defic. Syndr. hum. Retrovirol.*, **9**, 316–319

Gessain, A. & de Thé, G. (1996) What is the situation of human T cell lymphotropic virus type II (HTLV-II) in Africa ? Origin and dissemination of genomic subtypes. *J. acquir. Immune Defic. Syndr. hum. Retrovirol.* (in press)

Gessain, A., Calender, A., Strobel, M., Lefait-Robin, R. & de Thé, G. (1984) High prevalence of antiHTLV-I antibodies in the Boni, an ethnic group of African origin isolated in French Guiana since the 18th century. *C. R. Acad. Sci. Paris III*, **299**, 351–353 (in French)

Gessain, A., Barin, F., Vernant, J.-C., Gout, O., Maurs, L., Calender, A. & de Thé, G. (1985) Antibody to human T-lymphotropic virus type-I in patients with tropical spastic paraparesis. *Lancet*, **ii**, 407–409

Gessain, A., Caudie, C., Gout, O., Vernant, J.-C., Maurs, L., Giordano, C., Malone, G., Tournier-Lasserve, E., Essex, M. & de Thé, G. (1988) Intrathecal synthesis of antibodies to human T lymphotropic virus type I and the presence of IgG oligoclonal bands in the cerebrospinal fluid of patients with endemic tropical spastic paraparesis. *J. infect. Dis.*, **157**, 1226–1234

Gessain, A., Saal, F., Gout, O., Daniel, M.-T., Landrin, G., de Thé, G., Périès, J. & Sigaux, F. (1990a) High human T-cell lymphotropic virus type I proviral DNA load with polyclonal integration in peripheral blood mononuclear cells of French West Indian, Guianese, and African patients with tropical spastic paraparesis. *Blood*, **75**, 428–433

Gessain, A., Saal, F., Iron, M.-L., Lasneret, J., Lagaye, S., Gout, O., de Thé, G., Sigaux, F. & Périès, J. (1990b) Cell surface phenotype and human T lymphotropic virus type I antigen expression in 12 T cell lines derived from peripheral blood and cerebrospinal fluid of West Indian, Guyanese and African patients with tropical spastic paraparesis. *J. gen. Virol.*, **71**, 333–341

Gessain, A., Louie, A., Gout, O., Gallo, R.C. & Franchini, G. (1991) Human T-cell leukemia-lymphoma virus type I (HTLV-I) expression in fresh peripheral blood mononuclear cells from patients with tropical spastic paraparesis/HTLV-I-associated myelopathy. *J. Virol.*, **65**, 1628–1633

Gessain, A., Gallo, R.C. & Franchini, G. (1992a) Low degree of human T-cell leukemia/lymphoma virus type I genetic drift *in vivo* as a means of monitoring viral transmission and movement of ancient human populations. *J. Virol.*, **66**, 2288–2295

Gessain, A., Caumes, E., Feyeux, C., d'Agay, M.F., Capesius, C., Gentilini, M. & Morel, P. (1992b) The cutaneous form of adult T-cell leukemia/lymphoma in a woman from the Ivory Coast. Clinical, immunovirologic studies and a review of the African adult T-cell leukemia/lymphoma cases. *Cancer*, **69**, 1362–1367

Gessain, A., Boeri, E., Yanagihara, R., Gallo, R.C. & Franchini, G. (1993) Complete nucleotide sequence of a highly divergent human T-cell leukemia (lymphotropic) virus type I (HTLV-I) variant from Melanesia: genetic and phylogenetic relationship to HTLV-I strains from other geographical regions. *J. Virol.*, **67**, 1015–1023

Gessain, A., Mauclère, P., Froment, A., Biglione, M., Le Hesran, J.Y., Tekaia, F., Millan, J. & de Thé, G. (1995a) Isolation and molecular characterization of a human T-cell lymphotropic virus type II (HTLV-II), subtype B, from a healthy Pygmy living in a remote area of Cameroon: an ancient origin for HTLV-II in Africa. *Proc. natl Acad. Sci. USA*, **92**, 4041–4045

Gessain, A., Mahieux, R. & de Thé, G. (1995b) HTLV-I 'indeterminate' western blot patterns observed in sera from tropical regions: the situation revisited (Letter to the Editor). *J. acquir. Immune Defic. Syndr. hum. Retrovirol.*, **9**, 316–317

Gessain, A., Malet, C., Robert-Lamblin, J., Lepère, A., David, P., Chichlo, B., Sousova, O., Stepina, V., Gurtsevitch, V., Tortevoye, P., Hubert, A. & de Thé, G. (1996a) Serological evidence of HTLV-I but not HTLV-II infection in ethnic groups of northern and eastern Siberia. *J. acquir. Immune Defic. Syndr. hum. Retrovirol.*, **11**, 413–414

Gessain, A., Mahieux, R. & de Thé, G. (1996b) Genetic variability and molecular epidemiology of human and simian T cell leukemia/lymphoma virus type I. *J. acquir. Immune Defic. Syndr. hum. Retrovirol.* (in press)

Gibbs, W.N., Lofters, W.S., Campbell, M., Hanchard, B., LaGrenade, L., Cranston, B., Hendriks, J., Jaffe, E.S., Saxinger, C., Robert-Guroff, M., Gallo, R.C., Clark, J. & Blattner, W.A. (1987) Non-Hodgkin lymphoma in Jamaica and its relation to adult T-cell leukemia-lymphoma. *Ann. intern. Med.*, **106**, 361–368

Gill, P.S., Harrington, W., Jr, Kaplan, M.H., Ribeiro, R.C., Bennett, J.M., Liebman, H.A., Bernstein-Singer, M., Espina, B.M., Cabral, L., Allen, S., Kornblau, S., Pike, M.C. & Levine, A.M. (1995) Treatment of adult T-cell leukemia-lymphoma with a combination of interferon alfa and zidovudine. *New Engl. J. Med.*, **332**, 1744–1748

Giri, A., Markham, P., Digilio, L., Hurteau, G., Gallo, R.C. & Franchini, G. (1994) Isolation of a novel simian T-cell lymphotropic virus from *Pan paniscus* that is distantly related to the human T-cell leukemia/lymphotropic virus types I and II. *J. Virol.*, **68**, 8392–8395

Gitlin, S.D., Bosselut, R., Gégonne, A., Ghysdael, J. & Brady, J.N. (1991) Sequence-specific interaction of the Ets1 protein with the long terminal repeat of the human T-lymphotropic virus type I. *J. Virol.*, **65**, 5513–5523

Gitlin, S.D., Dittmer, J., Reid, R.L. & Brady, J.N. (1993) The molecular biology of human T-cell leukemia viruses. In: Cullen. B., ed., *Frontiers in Molecular Biology*, Oxford, Oxford University Press, pp. 159–192

Goldstein, D.J., Finbow, M.E., Andresson, T., McLean, P., Smith, K., Bubb, V. & Schlegel, R. (1991) The bovine papillomavirus E5 oncoprotein binds to the 16 kilodalton component of vacuolar H^+-ATPases. *Nature*, **352**, 347–349

Goldstein, D.J., Li, W., Wang, L.-M., Heidaran, M.A., Aaronson, S., Shinn, R., Schlegel, R. & Pierce, J.H. (1994) The bovine papillomavirus type 1 E5 transforming protein specifically binds and activates the β-type receptor for the platelet-derived growth factor but not other related tyrosine kinase-containing receptors to induce cellular transformation. *J. Virol.*, **68**, 4432–4441

Gotuzzo, E., Sánchez, J., Escamilla, J., Carrillo, C., Phillips, I.A., Moreyra, L., Stamm, W., Ashley, R., Roggen, E.L., Kreiss, J., Piot, P. & Holmes, K.K. (1994) Human T cell lymphotropic virus type I infection among female sex workers in Peru. *J. infect. Dis.*, **169**, 754–759

Goubau, P., Carton, H., Kazadi, K., Muya, K.W. & Desmyter, J. (1990) HTLV seroepidemiology in a central African population with high incidence of tropical spastic paraparesis. *Trans. R. Soc. trop. Med. Hyg.*, **84**, 577–579

Goubau, P., Desmyter, J., Ghesquiere, J. & Kasereka, B. (1992) HTLV-II among pygmies (Letter to the Editor). *Nature*, **359**, 201

Goubau, P., Desmyter, J., Swanson, P., Reynders, M., Shih, J., Surmont, I., Kazadi, K. & Lee, H. (1993a) Detection of HTLV-I and HTLV-II infection in Africans using type-specific envelope peptides. *J. med. Virol.*, **39**, 28–32

Goubau, P., Liu, H.-F., De Lange, G.G., Vandamme, A.-M. & Desmyter, J. (1993b) HTLV-II seroprevalence in Pygmies across Africa since 1970. *AIDS Res. hum. Retroviruses*, **9**, 709–713

Goubau, P., Van Brussel, M., Vandamme, A.-M., Liu, H.-F. & Desmyter, J. (1994) A primate T-lymphotropic virus, PTLV-L, different from human T-lymphotropic viruses types I and II, in a wild-caught baboon (*Papio hamadryas*). *Proc. natl Acad. Sci. USA*, **91**, 2848–2852

Gout, O., Baulac, M., Gessain, A., Semah, F., Saal, F., Périès, J., Cabrol, C., Foucault-Fretz, C., Laplane, D., Sigaux, F. & de Thé, G. (1990) Rapid development of myelopathy after HTLV-I infection acquired by transfusion during cardiac transplantation. *New Eng. J. Med.*, **322**, 383–388

Grassmann, R., Dengler, C., Müller-Fleckenstein, I., Fleckenstein, B., McGuire, K., Dokhelar, M.-C., Sodroski, J.G. & Haseltine, W.A. (1989) Transformation to continuous growth of primary human T-lymphocytes by human T-cell leukemia virus type I X-region genes transduced by a *Herpesvirus saimiri* vector. *Proc. natl Acad. Sci. USA*, **86**, 3351–3355

Grassmann, R., Berchtold, S., Radant, I., Alt, M., Fleckenstein, B., Sodroski, J.G., Haseltine, W.A. & Ramstedt, U. (1992) Role of human T-cell leukemia virus type I X region proteins in immortalization of primary human T-lymphocytes in culture. *J. Virol.*, **66**, 4570–4575

Green, J.E. (1991) *trans* Activation of nerve growth factor in transgenic mice containing the human T-cell lymphotropic virus type I *tax* gene. *Mol. cell. Biol.*, **11**, 4635–4641

Green, J.E., Hinrichs, S.H., Vogel, J. & Jay, G. (1989a) Exocrinopathy resembling Sjögren's syndrome in HTLV-1 *tax* transgenic mice. *Nature*, **341**, 72–74

Green, J.E., Begley, C.G., Wagner, D.K., Waldmann, T.A. & Jay, G. (1989b) *trans* Activation of granulocyte-macrophage colony-stimulating factor and the interleukin-2 receptor in transgenic mice carrying the human T-lymphotropic virus type 1 *tax* gene. *Mol. cell. Biol.*, **9**, 4731–4737

Green, J.E., Baird, A.M., Hinrichs, S.H., Klintworth, G.K. & Jay, G. (1992) Adrenal medullary tumors and iris proliferation in a transgenic mouse model of neurofibromatosis. *Am. J. Pathol.*, **140**, 1401–1410

Green, P.L., Ross, T.M., Chen, I.S.Y. & Pettiford, S. (1995) Human T-cell leukemia virus type II nucleotide sequences between *env* and the last exon of *tax/rex* are not required for viral replication or cellular transformation. *J. Virol.*, **69**, 387–394

Greenberg, S.J., Jaffe, E.S., Ehrlich, G.D., Korman, N.J., Poiesz, B.J. & Waldmann, T.A. (1990) Kaposi's sarcoma in human T-cell leukemia virus type I-associated adult T-cell leukemia. *Blood*, **76**, 971–976

Grégoire, D., Couez, D., Deschamps, J., Heuertz, S., Hors-Cayla, M.-C., Szpirer, J., Szpirer, C., Burny, A., Huez, G. & Kettmann, R. (1984) Different bovine leukemia virus-induced tumors harbor the provirus in different chromosomes. *J. Virol.*, **50**, 275–279

Grossman, B., Schechter, G.P., Horton, J.E., Pierce, L., Jaffe, E. & Whal, L. (1981) Hypercalcaemia associated with T-cell lymphoma-leukemia. *Am. J. clin. Pathol.*, **75**, 149–155

Grossman, W.J., Kimata, J.T., Wong, F.-H., Zutter, M., Ley, T.J. & Ratner, L. (1995) Development of leukemia in mice transgenic for the *tax* gene of human T-cell leukemia virus type I. *Proc. natl Acad. Sci. USA*, **92**, 1057–1061

Guerena-Burgueno, F., Benenson, A.S., Sepulveda-Amor, J., Ascher, M.S., Vugia, D.J. & Gallo, D. (1992) Prevalence of human T cell lymphotropic virus types I and II (HTLV-I/II) in selected Tijuana subpopulations. *Am. J. trop. Med. Hyg.*, **47**, 127–132

Gurtsevitch, V., Senyuta, N., Shih, J., Stepina, V., Pavlish, O., Syrtsev, A., Susova, O., Yakovleva, L., Scherbak, L. & Hayami, M. (1995) HTLV-I infection among Nivkhi people in Sakhalin (Letter to the Editor). *Int. J. Cancer*, **60**, 432–433

Gutfraind, Z., Blejer, J.L., Saguier, M.C., Gomez Carretero, M.L., Pirola, D.A. & Carreras Vescio, L.A. (1994) Seroprevalence of HTLV-I/HTLV-II in blood donors in Buenos Aires (Argentina) (Letter to the Editor). *Vox Sang.*, **67**, 408–409

Hadlock, K.G., Lipka, J.J., Chow, T.P., Foung, S.K.H. & Reyes, G.R. (1992) Cloning and analysis of a recombinant antigen containing an epitope specific for human T-cell lymphotropic virus type II. *Blood*, **79**, 2789–2796

Hadlock, K.G., Goh, C.-J., Bradshaw, P.A., Perkins, S., Lo, J., Kaplan, J.E., Khabbaz, R. & Foung, S.K.H. (1995) Delineation of an immunodominant and human T-cell lymphotropic virus (HTLV)-specific epitope within the HTLV-I transmembrane glycoprotein. *Blood*, **86**, 1392–1399

Hahn, B.H., Shaw, G.M., Popovic, M., Lo Monico, A., Gallo, R.C. & Wong-Staal, F. (1984) Molecular cloning and analysis of a new variant of human T-cell leukemia virus (HTLV-Ib) from an African patient with adult T-cell leukemia-lymphoma. *Int. J. Cancer*, **34**, 613–618

Hai, T., Liu, F., Coukos, W.J. & Green, M.R. (1989) Transcription factor ATF cDNA clones: an extensive family of leucine zipper proteins able to selectively form DNA-binding heterodimers. *Genes Dev.*, **3**, 2083–2090

Hall, W.W., Liu, C.R., Schneewind, O., Takahashi, H., Kaplan, M.H., Röupe, G. & Vahlne, A. (1991) Deleted HTLV-I provirus in blood and cutaneous lesions of patients with mycosis fungoides. *Science*, **253**, 317–320

Hall, W.W., Takahashi, H., Liu, C., Kaplan, M.H., Scheewind, O., Ijichi, S., Nagashima, K. & Gallo, R.C. (1992) Multiple isolates and characteristics of human T-cell leukemia virus type II. *J. Virol.*, **66**, 2456–2463

Hall, W.W., Kubo, T., Ijichi, S., Takahashi, H. & Zhu, S.W. (1994) Human T-cell leukemia/lymphoma virus, type II (HTLV-II): emergence of an important newly recognized pathogen. *Sem. Virol.*, **5**, 165–178

Hall, W.W., Zhu, S.W., Novoa, P., Eiraku, N., Ishak, R., Ferreira, M.C., Acevedo, V., Ishak, M., Guerreiro, J.F., Ferreira, O.C., Monken, C. & Kurata, T. (1996) Human T lymphotrophic virus, type II (HTLV-II): epidemiology, molecular properties and clinical features of infection. *J. acquir. Immune Defic. Syndr. hum. Retrovirol.* (in press)

Hanchard, B., LaGrenade, L., Carberry, C., Fletcher, V., Williams, E., Cranston, B., Blattner, W.A. & Manns, A. (1991) Childhood infective dermatitis evolving into adult T-cell leukaemia after 17 years (Letter to the Editor). *Lancet*, **ii**, 1593–1594

Hanly, S.M., Rimsky, L.T., Malim, M.H., Kim, J.H., Hauber, J., Duc Dodon, M., Le, S.-Y., Maizel, J.V., Cullen, B.R. & Greene, W.C. (1989) Comparative analysis of the HTLV-I Rex and HIV-1 Rev *trans*-regulatory proteins and their RNA response elements. *Genes Dev.*, **3**, 1534–1544

Harper, M.E., Kaplan, M.H., Marselle, L.M., Pahwa, S.G., Chayt, K.J., Sarngadharan, M.G., Wong-Staal, F. & Gallo, R.C. (1986) Concomitant infection with HLTV-I and HTLV-III in a patient with T8 lymphoproliferative disease. *New Engl. J. Med.*, **315**, 1073–1078

Harrington, W.J., Jr, Sheremata, W., Hjelle, B., Dube, D.K., Bradshaw, P., Foung, S.K., Snodgrass, S., Toedter, G., Cabral, L. & Poiesz, B. (1993) Spastic ataxia associated with human T-cell lymphotropic virus type II infection. *Ann. Neurol.*, **33**, 411–414

Harrington, W.J., Jr, Ucar, A., Gill, P., Snodgrass, S., Sheremata, W., Cabral, L., Rabin, M., Byrne, G.E., Jr, Berger, J., Voight, W., Kemper, R., Miller, G., Whitcomb, C.C., Greenberg, A., Byrnes, J.J. & Poiesz, B. (1995) Clinical spectrum of HTLV-I in South Florida. *J. acquir. Immune Defic. Syndr. hum. Retrovirol.*, **8**, 466–473

Hatta, Y., Hirama, T., Miller, C.W., Yamada, Y., Tomonaga, M. & Koeffler, H.P. (1995) Homozygous deletions of the p15 (MTS2) and p16 (CDKN2/MTS1) genes in adult T-cell leukemia. *Blood*, **85**, 2699–2704

Hattori, T., Asou, N., Suzushima, H., Takatsuki, K., Tanaka, K., Naito, K., Natori, H. & Oizumi, K. (1991) Leukaemia of novel gastrointestinal T-lymphocyte population infected with HTLV-I. *Lancet*, **337**, 76–77

Hayami, M., Komuro, A., Nozawa, K., Shotake, T., Ishikawa, K.I., Yamamoto, K., Ishida, T., Honjo, S. & Hinuma, Y. (1984) Prevalence of antibody to adult T-cell leukemia virus-associated antigens (ATLA) in Japanese monkeys and other non-human primates. *Int. J. Cancer*, **33**, 179–183

Heeney, J.L. & Valli, V.E.O. (1990) Transformed phenotype of enzootic bovine lymphoma reflects differentiation-linked leukemogenesis. *Lab. Invest.*, **62**, 339–346

Heneine, W., Kaplan, J.E., Gracia, F., Lal, R., Roberts, B., Levine, P.H. & Reeves, W.C. (1991) HTLV-II endemicity among Guaymi indians in Panama (Letter to the Editor). *New Engl. J. Med.*, **234**, 565

Heneine, W., Chan, W.C., Lust, J.A., Sinha, S.D., Zaki, S.R., Khabbaz, R.F. & Kaplan, J.E. (1994) HTLV-II infection is rare in patients with large granular lymphocyte leukemia (Letter to the Editor). *J. acquir. Immune Defic. Syndr.*, **7**, 736–737

Henrard, D.R., Soriano, V., Robertson, E., Gutierrez, M., Stephens, J., Dronda, F., Miles, F., Pujol, E., Buytendorp, M., Castro, A., Chan, E., Vallejo, A., Llibre, J., Motley, C., Prillaman, J. & the HTLV-I and HTLV-II Spanish Study Group (1995) Prevalence of human T-cell lymphotropic virus type I (HTLV-I) and HTLV-II infection among Spanish drug users measured by HTLV-I assay and HTLV-I and -II assay. *J. clin. Microbiol.*, **33**, 1735–1738

Hermine, O., Bouscary, D., Gessain, A., Turlure, P., Leblond, V., Franck, N., Buzyn-Veil, A., Rio, B., Macintyre, E., Dreyfus, F. & Bazarbachi, A. (1995) Brief report: treatment of adult T-cell leukemia-lymphoma with zidovudine and interferon alfa. *New Engl. J. Med.*, **332**, 1749–1751

Hidaka, M., Inoue, J., Yoshida, M. & Seiki, M. (1988) Post-transcriptional regulator (*rex*) of HTLV-I initiates expression of viral structural proteins but suppresses expression of regulatory proteins. *EMBO J.*, **7**, 519–523

Higuchi, I., Nerenberg, M., Yoshimine, K., Yoshida, M., Fukunaka, H., Tajima, K. & Osame, M. (1992) Failure to detect HTLV-I by in situ hybridization in the biopsied muscles of viral carriers with polymyositis. *Muscle Nerve*, **15**, 43–47

Hino, S. (1990a) Maternal-infant transmission of HTLV-I — Implication for disease. In: Blattner, W.A., ed., *Human Retrovirology: HTLV*, New York, Raven Press, pp. 363–375

Hino, S. (1990b) Milk-borne transmission of HTLV-I from carrier mothers and its prevention. *Hematol. Rev.*, **3**, 223–233

Hino, S., Kinoshita, K. & Kitamura, T. (1984) HTLV and the propagation of christianity in Nagasaki (Letter to the Editor). *Lancet*, **ii**, 572–573

Hino, S., Sugiyama, H., Doi, H., Ishimaru, T., Yamabe, T., Tsuji, Y. & Miyamoto, T. (1987a) Breaking the cycle of HTLV-I transmission via carrier mothers' milk (Letter to the Editor). *Lancet*, **ii**, 158–159

Hino, S., Doi, H., Yoshikuni, H., Sugiyama, H., Ishimaru, T., Yamabe, T., Tsuji, Y. & Miyamoto, T. (1987b) HTLV-I carrier mothers with high-titer antibody are at high risk as a source of infection. *Jpn. J. Cancer Res. (Gann)*, **78**, 1156–1158

Hino, S., Katamine, S., Kawase, K.-I., Miyamoto, T., Doi, H., Tsuji, Y. & Yamabe, T. (1994) Intervention of maternal transmission of HTLV-I in Nagasaki, Japan. *Leukemia*, **8** (Suppl. 1), S68–S70

Hinrichs, S.H., Nerenberg, M., Reynolds, R.K., Khoury, G. & Jay, G. (1987) A transgenic mouse model for human neurofibromatosis. *Science*, **237**, 1340–1343

Hinuma, Y. (1986) Seroepidemiology of adult T-cell leukemia virus (HTLV-I/ATLV): origin of virus carriers in Japan. *AIDS Res.*, **2** (Suppl. 1), S17–S22

Hinuma, Y., Komoda, H., Chosa, T., Kondo, T., Kohakura, M., Takenaka, T., Kikuchi, M., Ichimaru, M., Yunoki, K., Sato, I., Matsuo, R., Takiuchi, Y., Uchino, H. & Hanaoka, M. (1982) Antibodies to adult T-cell leukemia-virus-associated antigen (ATLA) in sera from patients with ATL and controls in Japan: a nation-wide sero-epidemiologic study. *Int. J. Cancer*, **29**, 631–635

Hirai, H., Suzuki, T., Fujisawa, J.-I., Inoue, J.-I. & Yoshida, M. (1994) Tax protein of human T-cell leukemia virus type I binds to the ankyrin motifs of inhibitory factor κB and induces nuclear translocation of transcription factor NF-κB proteins for transcriptional activation. *Proc. natl Acad. Sci. USA*, **91**, 3584–3588

Hjelle, B., Appenzeller, O., Mills, R., Alexander, S., Torrez-Martinez, N., Jahnke, R. & Ross, G. (1992) Chronic neurodegenerative disease associated with HTLV-II infection. *Lancet*, **339**, 645–646

Hjelle, B., Wilson, C., Cyrus, S., Bradshaw, P., Lo, J., Schammel, C., Wiltbank, T. & Alexander, S. (1993) Human T-cell leukemia virus type II infection frequently goes undetected in contemporary US blood donors. *Blood*, **81**, 1641–1644

Hoffman, P.M., Dhib-Jalbut, S., Mikovits, J.A., Robbins, D.S., Wolf, A.L., Bergey, G.K., Lohrey, N.C., Weislow, O.S. & Ruscetti, F.W. (1992) Human T-cell leukemia virus type I infection of monocytes and microglial cells in primary human cultures. *Proc. natl Acad. Sci. USA*, **89**, 11784–11788

Höllsberg, P., Wucherpfennig, K.W., Ausubel, L.J., Calvo, V., Bierer, B.E. & Hafler, D.A. (1992) Characterization of HTLV-I in vivo infected T cell clones: IL-2-independent growth of nontransformed T-cells. *J. Immunol.*, **148**, 3256–3263

Homma, T., Kanki, P.J., King, N.W., Jr, Hunt, R.D., O'Connell, M.J., Letvin, N.L., Daniel, M.D., Desrosiers, R.C., Yang, C.S. & Essex, M. (1984) Lymphoma in macaques: association with virus of human T lymphotrophic family. *Science*, **225**, 716–718

Honda, S., Yamaguchi, K., Miyake, Y., Hayashi, N., Adachi, N., Kinoshita, K.-I., Ikehara, O., Kimura, S., Kinoshita, T., Shimotohno, K., Shimoyama, M. & Abe, K. (1988) Production of parathyroid hormone-related protein in adult T-cell leukemia cells. *Jpn. J. Cancer Res. (Gann)*, **79**, 1264–1268

Hori, M., Ami, Y., Kushida, S., Kobayashi, M., Uchida, K., Abe, T. & Miwa, M. (1995) Intrauterine transmission of human T-cell leukemia virus type I in rats. *J. Virol.*, **69**, 1302–1305

The HTLV European Research Network (1996) Seroepidemiology of the human T-cell leukaemia/lymphoma viruses in Europe. *J. acquir. Immune Defic. Syndr. hum. Retrovirol.*, **13**, 68–77

Hubbard, G.B., Monè, J.P., Allan, J.S., Davis, K.J., III, Leland, M.M., Banks, P.M. & Smir, B. (1993) Spontaneously generated non-Hodgkin's lymphoma in twenty-seven simian T-cell leukemia virus type I antibody-positive baboons (*Papio* species). *Lab. Anim. Sci.*, **43**, 301–309

Hunsmann, G., Bayer, H., Schneider, J., Schmitz, H., Kern, P., Dietrich, M., Büttner, D.W., Goudeau, A.M., Kulkarni, G. & Fleming, A.F. (1984) Antibodies to ATLV/HTLV-I in Africa. *Med. Microbiol. Immunol.*, **173**, 167–170

IARC (1994) *IARC Monographs on the Evaluation of Carcinogenic Risks to Humans*, Vol. 59, *Hepatitis Viruses*, Lyon

IARC (1995) *IARC Monographs on the Evaluation of Carcinogenic Risks to Humans*, Vol. 64, *Human Papillomaviruses*, Lyon

Ibrahim, F., Fiette, L., Gessain, A., Buisson, N., de Thé, G. & Bomford, R. (1994) Infection of rats with human T-cell leukemia virus type-I: susceptibility of inbred strains, antibody response and provirus location. *Int. J. Cancer*, **58**, 446–451

Ichimaru, M., Kinoshita, K., Kamihira, S., Ikeda, S., Yamada, Y. & Amagasaki, T. (1979) T-cell malignant lymphoma in Nagasaki district and its problems. *Jpn. J. clin. Oncol.*, **9** (Suppl.), 337–346

Iida, S., Fujiyama, S., Yosida, K., Morishita, T., Shibata, J., Sato, T. & Nishimura, Y. (1988) The seroprevalence of anti-HTLV-I antibodies in patients with various liver diseases. *Hepato-gastroenterology*, **35**, 242–244

Ijichi, S., Matsuda, T., Maruyama, I., Izumihara, T., Kojima, K., Niimura, T., Maruyama, Y., Sonoda, S., Yoshida, A. & Osame, M. (1990) Arthritis in a human T-lymphotropic virus type I (HTLV-I) carrier. *Ann. rheum. Dis.*, **49**, 718–721

Ikeda, M., Fujino, R., Matsui, T., Yoshida, T., Komoda, H. & Imai, J. (1984) A new agglutination test for serum antibodies to adult T-cell leukemia virus. *Gann*, **75**, 845–848

Ikeda, S., Momita, S., Amagasaki, T., Tsukasaki, K., Yamada, Y., Kusumoto, Y., Ito, M., Kanda, N., Tomonaga, M., Soda, H., Atogami, S., Kamihara, S., Hino, S., Ito, S.-I., Kinoshita, K. & Ichimaru, M. (1990) Detection of preleukemic state of adult T-cell leukemia (pre-ATL) in HTLV-I carriers. *Cancer Detect. Prev.*, **14**, 431–435

Imada, K., Takaori-Kondo, A., Akagi, T., Shimotohno, K., Sugamura, K., Hattori, T., Yamabe, H., Okuma, M. & Uchiyama, T. (1995) Tumorigenicity of human T-cell leukemia virus type I-infected cell lines in severe combined immunodeficient mice and characterization of the cells proliferating *in vivo*. *Blood*, **86**, 2350–2357

Imai, T., Tanaka, Y., Fukudome, K., Takagi, S., Araki, K. Yoshie, O. (1993) Enhanced expression of LFA-3 on human T-cell lines and leukemic cells carrying human T-cell leukemia virus type I. *Int. J. Cancer*, **55**, 811–816

Imajo, K., Shinagawa, K., Tada, S., Tsubota, T. & Kimura, I. (1993) Detection of the *pX* gene of human T-lymphotropic virus type I in respiratory diseases with diffuse interstitial pulmonary shadows and lung cancer. *Acta med. Okayama*, **47**, 363–368

Imamura, N., Inada, T., Tagaya, Y., Yodoi, J. & Kuramoto, A. (1993) Association between ATL and non-hematopoietic neoplasms. *Hematol. Oncol.*, **11**, 127–137

Inaba, S., Sato, H., Okochi, K., Fukada, K., Takakura, F., Tokunaga, K., Kiyokawa, H. & Maeda, Y. (1989) Prevention of transmission of human T-lymphotropic virus type I (HTLV-I) through transfusion, by donor screening with antibody to the virus. One-year experience. *Transfusion*, **29**, 7–11

Inoue, J.-I., Seiki, M., Taniguchi, T., Tsuru, S. & Yoshida, M. (1986) Induction of interleukin 2 receptor gene expression by p40ˣ encoded by human T-cell leukemia virus type I. *EMBO J.*, **5**, 2883–2888

Inoue, J.-I., Itoh, M., Akizawa, T., Toyoshima, H. & Yoshida, M. (1991) HTLV-I Rex protein accumulates unspliced RNA in the nucleus as well as in cytoplasm. *Oncogene*, **6**, 1753–1757

Inoue, Y., Fujii, T., Ohtsubo, T., Mori, N., Ishino, T., Hisano, H., Kaku, M., Koga, H., Kohno, S., Hara, K., Ayabe, H., Mukae, H. & Tomita, H. (1994a) A case of HTLV-I carrier associated with pulmonary cryptococcosis and thymoma. *Nippon Kyobu Shikkan Gakkai Zesshi*, **32**, 778–784 (in Japanese)

Inoue, H., Yamaoka, S., Imamura, M. & Hatanaka, M. (1994b) Suppression of the transformed phenotype in hybrids of human T-cell leukemia virus type I Tax-transformed rat fibroblasts and normal human fibroblasts. *Exp. Cell Res.*, **215**, 68–74

International Committee on Bovine Leukosis (1968) Criteria for the determination of the normal and leukotic state in cattle. *J. natl Cancer Inst.*, **41**, 243–251

Ishida, T., Yamamoto, K., Omoto, K., Iwanaga, M., Osato, T. & Hinuma, Y. (1985) Prevalence of a human retrovirus in native Japanese: evidence for a possible ancient origin. *J. Infect.*, **11**, 153–157

Ishida, T., Yamamoto, K. & Omoto, K. (1988) A seroepidemiological survey of HTLV-I in the Philippines. *Int. J. Epidemiol.*, **17**, 625–628

Ishida, T., Takayanagi, K.-I., Shotake, T., Hirai, K. & Yuasa, I. (1992) A seroepidemiological study of HTLV-I infection in Nepal. *Scand. J. infect. Dis.*, **24**, 399–400

Ishihara, S., Tachibana, N., Okayama, A., Murai, K., Tsuda, K. & Mueller, N. (1992) Successful graft of HTLV-I-transformed human T-cells (MT-2) in severe combined immunodeficiency mice treated with anti-asiolo GM-1 antibody. *Jpn. J. Cancer Res.*, **83**, 320–323

Ishihara, S., Okayama, A., Stuver, S., Horinouchi, H., Shioiri, S., Murai, K., Kubota, T., Yamashita, R., Tachibana, N., Tsubouchi, H. & Mueller, N. (1994) Association of HTLV-I antibody profile of asymptomatic cariers with proviral DNA levels of peripheral blood mononuclear cells. *J. acquir. Immune Defic. Syndr.*, **7**, 199–203

Ishikawa, K.-I., Fukasawa, M., Tsujimoto, H., Else, J.G., Isahakia, M., Ubhi, N.K., Ishida, T., Takenaka, O., Kawamoto, Y., Shotake, T., Ohsawa, H., Ivanoff, B., Cooper, R.W., Frost, E., Grant, F.C., Spriatna, Y., Sutarman, Y., Abe, K., Yamamoto, K. & Hayami, M. (1987) Serological survey and virus isolation of simian T-cell leukemia/T-lymphotropic virus type I (STLV-I) in non-human primates in their native countries. *Int. J. Cancer*, **40**, 233–239

Itoyama, Y., Minato, S., Kira, J.-I., Goto, I., Sato, H., Okochi, K. & Yamamoto, N. (1988) Spontaneous proliferation of peripheral blood lymphocytes increased in patients with HTLV-I associated myelopathy. *Neurology*, **38**, 1302–1307

Iwahara, Y., Takehara, N., Kataoka, R., Sawada, T., Ohtsuki, Y., Nakachi, H., Maehama, T., Okayama, T. & Miyoshi, I. (1990) Transmission of HTLV-I to rabbits via semen and breast milk from seropositive healthy persons. *Int. J. Cancer*, **45**, 980–983

Iwakura, Y., Tosu, M., Yoshida, E., Takiguchi, M., Sato, K., Kitajima, I., Nishioka, K., Yamamoto, K., Takeda, T., Hatanaka, M., Yamamoto, H. & Sekiguchi, T. (1991) Induction of inflammatory arthropathy resembling rheumatoid arthritis in mice transgenic for HTLV-I. *Science*, **253**, 1026–1028

Iwakura, Y., Tosu, M., Yoshida, E., Saijo, S., Nakayama-Yamada, J., Itagaki, K., Asano, M., Siomi, H., Hatanaka, M., Takeda, T., Nunoya, T., Ueda, S. & Shibuta, H. (1994) Augmentation of c-*fos* and c-*jun* expression in transgenic mice carrying the human T-cell leukemia virus type I *tax* gene. *Virus Genes*, **9**, 161–170

Iwakura, Y., Saijo, S., Kioka, Y., Nakayama-Yamada, J., Itagaki, K., Tosu, M., Asano, M., Kanai, Y. & Kakimoto, K. (1995) Autoimmunity induction by human T-cell leukemia virus type I in transgenic mice that develop chronic inflammatory arthropathy resembling rheumatoid arthritis in humans. *J. Immunol.*, **155**, 1588–1598

Iwata, K., Ito, S.-I., Saito, H., Ito, M., Nagatomo, M., Yamasaki, T., Yoshida, S., Suto, H. & Tajima, K. (1994) Mortality among inhabitants of an HTLV-I endemic area in Japan. *Jpn. J. Cancer Res.*, **85**, 231–237

Jacobson, S., Shida, H., McFarlin, D.E., Fauci, A.S. & Koenig, S. (1990) Circulating $CD8^+$ cytotoxic T lymphocytes specific for HTLV-I pX in patients with HTLV-I associated neurological disease. *Nature*, **348**, 245–248

Jang, D., Mahony, J.B., Sellors, J.W., Galli, R., Gregory, B. & Chernesky, M.A. (1995) Lack of specificity of HTLV antibody enzyme immunoassays. *J. acquir. Immune Defic. Syndr. hum. Retrovirol.*, **9**, 523–524

Janssen, R.S., Kaplan, J.E., Khabbaz, R.F., Hammond, R., Lechtenberg, R., Lairmore, M., Chiasson, M.A., Punsalang, A., Roberts, B., McKendall, R.R., Rosenblum, M., Brew, B., Farraye, J., Howley, D.J., Feraru, E., Sparr, S., Vecchio, J., Silverman, M., McHarg, M., Gorin, B., Rugg, D.R., Grenell, S., Trimble, B., Bruining, K., Guha, S., Amaraneni, P. & Price, R.W. (1991) HTLV-I-associated myelopathy/tropical spastic paraparesis in the United States. *Neurology*, **41**, 1355–1357

Jayo, M.J., Laber-Laird, K., Bullock, B.C., Tulli, H.M. & Reynolds, G.M. (1990) T-cell lymphosarcoma in a female African green monkey (*Cercopithecus aethiops*). *Lab. Anim. Sci.*, **40**, 37–41

Jeang, K.-T., Boros, I., Brady, J., Radonovich, M. & Khoury, G. (1988a) Characterization of cellular factors that interact with the human T-cell leukemia virus type I p40'- responsive 21-base-pair sequence. *J. Virol.*, **62**, 4499–4509

Jeang, K.-T., Shank, P.R. & Kumar, A. (1988b) Transcriptional activation of homologous viral long terminal repeats by the human immunodeficiency virus type I or the human T-cell leukemia virus type I Tat proteins occurs in the absence of de novo protein synthesis. *Proc. natl Acad. Sci. USA*, **85**, 8291–8295

Jeang, K.-T., Widen, S.G., Seemes, O.J., IV & Wilson, S.H. (1990) HTLV-I trans-activator protein, Tax, is a trans-repressor of the human β-polymerase gene. *Science*, **247**, 1082–1084

Jeannel, D., Garin, B., Kazadi, K., Singa, L. & de Thé, G. (1993) The risk of tropical spastic paraparesis differs according to ethnic group among HTLV-I carriers in Inongo, Zaire. *J. acquir. immune Defic. Syndr.*, **6**, 840–844

Jeannel, D., Kourouma, K., Fretz, C., Zheng, Y.M., Ureta, V.A., Dramé, L., Gessain, A., Fournel, J.J. & de Thé, G. (1995) Regional differences in human retroviral infections HIV-1, HIV-2, and HTLV-I/II in rural Guinea (West Africa) (Letter to the Editor). *J. acquir. Immune Defic. Syndr. hum. Retrovirol.*, **8**, 315–318

Jensen, W.A., Rovnak, J. & Cockerell, G.L. (1991) In vivo transcription of the bovine leukemia virus *tax/rex* region in normal and neoplastic lymphocytes of cattle and sheep. *J. Virol.*, **65**, 2484–2490

Joshi, J.B. & Dave, H.P.G. (1992) Transactivation of the proenkephalin gene promoter by the Tax$_1$ protein of human T-cell lymphotropic virus type I. *Proc. natl Acad. Sci. USA*, **89**, 1006–1010

Kajiyama, W., Kashiwagi, S., Ikematsu, H., Hayashi, J., Nomura, H. & Okochi, K. (1986) Intra-familial transmission of adult T cell leukemia virus. *J. infect. Dis.*, **154**, 851–857

Kalyanaraman, V.S., Sarngadharan, M.G., Robert-Guroff, M., Miyoshi, I., Blayney, D., Golde, D. & Gallo, R.C. (1982) A new subtype of human T-cell leukemia virus (HTLV-II) associated with a T-cell variant of hairy cell leukemia. *Science*, **218**, 571–573

Kamada, N., Tanaka, K., Takechi, M. & Kikuchi, M. (1990) Chromosome aberrations in adult T cell leukemia. *Hematol. Rev.*, **3**, 257–270

Kamihira, S., Yamada, Y., Sohda, H., Atogami, S., Tomonaga, M., Egawa, S., Fujii, M. & Chifu, K. (1994) Human T-lymphotropic virus type-I influence on hepatotropic virus infections and the subsequent development of hepatocellular carcinoma. *Cancer Detect. Prev.*, **18**, 329–334

Kanamori, H., Suzuki, N., Siomi, H., Nosaka, T., Sato, A., Sabe, H., Hatanaka, M. & Honjo, T. (1990) HTLV-1 p27^{rex} stabilizes human interleukin 2 receptor α chain mRNA. *EMBO J.*, **9**, 4161–4166

Kannagi, M., Sugamura, K., Sato, H., Okochi, K., Uchino, H. & Hinuma, Y. (1983) Establishment of human cytotoxic T cell lines specific for human adult T cell leukemia virus-bearing cells. *J. Immunol.*, **130**, 2942–2946

Kannagi, M., Sugamura, K., Kinoshita, K.-I., Uchino, H. & Hinuma, Y. (1984) Specific cytolysis of fresh tumor cells by an autologous killer T cell line derived from an adult T cell leukemia/lymphoma patient. *J. Immunol.*, **133**, 1037–1041

Kano, T. (1984) Distribution of pygmy chimpanzees (*Pan paniscus*) in the central Zaire basin. *Folia primatol.*, **43**, 36–52

Kaplan, J.E. & Khabbaz, R. (1993) The epidemiology of human T-lymphotropic virus types I and II. *Med. Virol.*, **3**, 137–148

Kaplan, J.E., Osame, M., Kubota, H., Igata, A., Nishitani, H., Maeda, Y., Khabbaz, R.F. & Janssen, R.S. (1990) The risk of development of HTLV-I-associated myelopathy/tropical spastic paraparesis among persons infected with HTLV-I. *J. acquir. immune Defic. Syndr.*, **3**, 1096–1101

Karopoulos, A., Silvester, C. & Dax, E.M. (1993) A comparison of the performance of nine commercially available anti-HTLV-I screening assays. *J. virol. Meth.*, **45**, 83–91

Kashiwagi, S., Kajiyama, W., Hayashi, J., Noguchi, A., Nakashima, K., Nomura, H., Ikematsu, H., Sawada, T., Kida, S. & Koide, A. (1990) Antibody to p40^{tax} protein of human T cell leukemia virus I and infectivity. *J. infect. Dis.*, **161**, 426–429

Katamine, S., Moriuchi, R., Yamamoto, T., Terada, K., Eguchi, K., Tsuji, Y., Yamabe, T., Miyamoto, T. & Hino, S. (1994) HTLV-I proviral DNA in umbilical cord blood of babies born to carrier mothers. *Lancet*, **343**, 1326–1327

Kataoka, R., Takehara, N., Iwahara, Y., Sawada, T., Ohtsuki, Y., Dawei, Y., Hoshino, H. & Miyoshi, I. (1990) Transmission of HTLV-I by blood transfusion and its prevention by passive immunization in rabbits. *Blood*, **76**, 1657–1661

Katsuki, T., Katsuki, K., Imai, J. & Hinuma, Y. (1987) Immune suppression in healthy carriers of adult T-cell leukemia retrovirus (HTLV-I): impairment of T-cell control of Epstein–Barr virus infected B-cells. *Jpn. J. Cancer Res. (Gann)*, **78**, 639–642

Kawai, H., Kashiwagi, S., Inui, T., Tamaki, Y., Sano, Y. & Saito, S. (1991) HTLV-I associated myelopathy (HAM/TSP) with Hashimoto's thyroiditis. *Tokushima J. exp. Med.*, **38**, 99–102

Kawai, H., Inui, T., Kashiwagi, S., Tsuchihashi, T., Masuda, K., Kondo, A., Niki, S., Iwasa, M. & Saito, S. (1992) HTLV-I infection in patients with autoimmune thyroiditis (Hashimoto's thyroiditis). *J. med. Virol.*, **38**, 138–141

Kawano, F., Tsuda, H., Yamaguchi, K., Nishimura, H., Sanada, I., Matsuzaki, H., Ishii, M. & Takatsuki, K. (1984) Unusual clinical courses of adult T-cell leukemia in siblings. *Cancer*, **54**, 131–134

Kayembe, K., Goubau, P., Desmyter, J., Vlietinck, R. & Carton, H. (1990) A cluster of HTLV-I associated tropical spastic paraparesis in Equateur (Zaire): ethnic and familial distribution. *J. Neurol. Neurosurg. Psychiat.*, **53**, 4–10

Kelly, K., Davis, P., Mitsuya, H., Irving, S., Wright, J., Grassmann, R., Fleckenstein, B., Wano, Y., Greene, W. & Siebenlist, U. (1992) A high proportion of early response genes are constitutively activated in T-cells by HTLV-I. *Oncogene*, **7**, 1463–1470

Kenyon, S.J. & Piper, C.E. (1977) Cellular basis of persistent lymphocytosis in cattle infected with bovine leukemia virus. *Infect. Immunol.*, **16**, 891–897

Kettmann, R., Cleuter, Y., Mammerickx, M., Meunier-Rotival, M., Bernardi, G., Burny, A. & Chantrenne, H. (1980a) Genomic integration of bovine leukemia provirus: comparison between persistent lymphocytosis with lymph node tumor form of enzootic bovine leukosis. *Proc. natl Acad. Sci. USA*, **77**, 2577–2581

Kettmann, R., Marbaix, G., Cleuter, Y., Portetelle, D., Mammerickx, M. & Burny, A. (1980b) Genomic integration of bovine leukemia provirus and lack of viral RNA expression in the target cells of cattle with different response to BLV infection. *Leuk. Res.*, **4**, 509–519

Kettmann, R., Deschamps, J., Couez, D., Claustriaux, J.-J., Palm, R. & Burny, A. (1983) Chromosome integration domain for bovine leukemia provirus in tumors. *J. Virol.*, **47**, 146–150

Kettmann, R., Mammerickx, M., Portetelle, D., Grégoire, D. & Burny, A. (1984) Experimental infection of sheep and goat with bovine leukemia virus: localization of proviral information in the target cells. *Leuk. Res.*, **8**, 937–944

Kettmann, R., Burny, A., Callebaut, I., Droogmans, L., Mammerickx, M., Willems, L. & Portetelle, D. (1994) Bovine leukemia virus. In: Levy, J.A., ed., *The Retroviridae*, Vol. 3, New York, Plenum Press, pp. 39–81

Khabbaz, R.F., Darrow, W.W., Hartley, T.M., Witte, J., Cohen, J.B., French, J., Gill, P.S., Potterat, J., Sikes, R.K., Reich, R., Kaplan, J.E. & Lairmore, M.D. (1990) Seroprevalence and risk factors for HTLV-I/II infection among female prostitutes in the United States. *J. Am. med. Assoc.*, **263**, 60–64

Khabbaz, R.F., Onorato, I.M., Cannon, R.O., Hartley, T.M., Roberts, B., Hosein, B. & Kaplan, J.E. (1992) Seroprevalence of HTLV-I and HTLV-II among intravenous drug users and persons in clinics for sexually transmitted diseases. *New Engl. J. Med.*, **326**, 375–380

Khono, T., Uchida, H., Inomata, H., Fukushima, S., Takeshita, M. & Kikuchi, M. (1993) Ocular manifestations of adult-T-cell leukemia/lymphoma. A clinicopathologic study. *Ophthalmology*, **100**, 1794–1799

Kim, S.-J., Kehrl, J.H., Burton, J., Tendler, C.L., Jeang, K.-T., Danielpour, D., Thevenin, C., Kim, K.Y., Sporn, M.B. & Roberts, A.B. (1990) Transactivation of the transforming growth factor $\beta 1$ (TGF-$\beta 1$) gene by human T-lymphotropic virus type I Tax: a potential mechanism for the increased production of TGF-$\beta 1$ in adult T-cell leukemia. *J. exp. Med.*, **172**, 121–129

Kim, S.-J., Winokur, T.S., Lee, H.-D., Danielpour, D., Kim, K.Y., Geiser, A.G., Chen, L.-S., Sporn, M.B., Roberts, A.B. & Jay, G. (1991) Overexpression of transforming growth factor-β in transgenic mice carrying the human T-cell lymphotropic virus type I *tax* gene. *Mol. cell. Biol.*, **11**, 5222–5228

Kimata, J.T., Palker, T.J. & Ratner, L. (1993) The mitogenic activity of Human T-cell leukemia virus type I is T-cell associated and requires the CD2/LFA-3 activation pathway. *J. Virol.*, **67**, 3134–3141

Kimata, J.T., Wong, F.-H., Wang, J.J. & Ratner, L. (1994) Construction and characterization of infectious human T-cell leukemia virus type I molecular clones. *Virology*, **204**, 656–664

Kinoshita, K., Hino, S., Amagasaki, T., Ikeda, S.-I., Yamada, Y., Suzuyama, J., Momita, S., Toriya, K., Kamihira, S. & Ichimaru, M. (1984) Demonstration of adult T-cell leukemia virus antigen in milk from three sero-positive mothers. *Gann*, 75, 103–105

Kinoshita, K., Yamanouchi, K., Ikeda, S.-I., Momita, S., Amagasaki, T., Soda, H., Ichimaru, M., Moriuchi, R., Katamine, S., Miyamoto, T. & Hino, S. (1985a) Oral infection of a common marmoset with human T-cell leukemia virus type-I (HTLV-I) by inoculating fresh human milk of HTLV-I carrier mothers. *Jpn. J. Cancer Res.*, **76**, 1147–1153

Kinoshita, K., Amagasaki, T., Ikeda, S.-I., Suzuyama, J., Toriya, K., Nishino, K., Tagawa, M., Ichimaru, M., Kamihira, S., Yamada, Y., Momita, S,. Kusano, M., Morikawa, T., Fujita, S., Umeda, Y., Ito, N. & Yoshida, M. (1985b) Preleukemic state of adult T cell leukemia: abnormal T lymphocytosis induced by human adult T cell leukemia-lymphoma virus. *Blood*, **66**, 120–127

Kira, J.-I. (1994) The presence of HTLV-I proviral DNA in the central nervous system of patients with HTLV-I-associated myelopathy/tropical spastic paraparesis. *Mol. Neurobiol.*, **8**, 139–145

Kira, J.-I., Koyanagi, Y., Yamada, T., Itoyama, Y., Goto, I., Yamamoto, N., Sasaki, H. & Sasaki, Y. (1991) Increased HTLV-I proviral DNA in HTLV-I-associated myelopathy: a quantitative polymerase chain reaction study. *Ann. Neurol.*, **29**, 194–201

Kira, J.-I., Itoyama, Y., Koyanagi, Y., Tateishi, J., Kishikawa, M., Akizuki, S.-I., Kobayashi, I., Toki, N., Sueishi, K., Sato, H., Sakaki, Y., Yamamoto, N. & Goto, I. (1992a) Presence of HTLV-I proviral DNA in central nervous system of patients with HTLV-I-associated myelopathy. *Ann. Neurol.*, **31**, 39–45

Kira, J.-I., Nakamura, M., Sawada, T., Koyanagi, Y., Ohori, N., Itoyama, Y., Yamamoto, N., Sakaki, Y. & Goto, I. (1992b) Antibody titers to HTLV-I-p40 Tax protein and gag-env hybrid protein in HTLV-I-associated myelopathy/tropical spastic paraparesis: correlation with increased HTLV-I proviral DNA load. *J. neurol. Sci*, **107**, 98–104

Kitajima, I., Maruyama, I., Maruyama, Y., Ijichi, S., Eiraku, N., Mimura, Y. & Osame, M. (1989) Polyarthrtitis in human T lymphotropic virus type I-associated myelopathy (Letter to the Editor). *Arthrit. Rheum.*, **32**, 1342–1344

Kitajima, I., Yamamoto, K., Sato, K, Nakajima, Y., Nakajima, Y., Maruyama, I., Osame, M. & Nishioka, K. (1991) Detection of human T cell lymphotropic virus type I proviral DNA and its gene expression in synovial cells in chronic inflammatory arthropathy. *J. clin. Invest.*, **88**, 1315–1322

Kiyokawa, T., Seiki, M., Iwashita, S., Imagawa, K., Shimizu, F. & Yoshida, M. (1985) p27$^{\text{x-III}}$ and p21$^{\text{x-III}}$, proteins encoded by the *pX* sequence of human T-cell leukemia virus type I. *Proc. natl Acad. Sci. USA*, **82**, 8359–8363

Kleinman, S.H., Kaplan, J.E., Khabbaz, R.F., Calabro, M.A., Thomson, R., Busch, M. & the Retrovirus Epidemiology Donor Study Group (1994) Evaluation of a p21e-spiked western blot (immunoblot) in confirming human T-cell lymphotropic virus type I or II infection in volunteer blood donors. *J. clin. Microbiol.*, **32**, 603–607

Kline, R.L., Brothers, T., Halsey, N., Boulos, R., Lairmore, M.D. & Quinn, T.C. (1991) Evaluation of enzyme immunoassays for antibody to human T-lymphotropic viruses type I/II. *Lancet*, **337**, 30–33

Kohno, T., Uchida, H., Inomata, H., Fukushima, S., Takeshita, M. & Kikuchi, M. (1993) Ocular manifestations of adult T-cell leukemia/lymphoma. A clinopathological study. *Ophthalmology*, **100**, 1794–1799

Komori, T., Kasajima, T.,Yamamoto, T., Shibata, N. & Kobayashi, M. (1995) An unclassifed cerebral small cell tumor in a patient with human T-cell lymphotropic virus type I-induced primary extranodal lymphoma. *Mod. Pathol.*, **8**, 811–816

Komurian, F., Pelloquin, F. & de Thé, G. (1991) In vivo genomic variability of human T-cell leukemia virus type I depends more upon geography than upon pathologies. *J. Virol.*, **65**, 3770–3778

Komuro, A., Watanabe, T., Miyoshi, I., Hayami, M., Tsujimoto, H., Seiki, M. & Yoshida, M. (1984) Detection and characterization of simian retroviruses homologous to human T-cell leukemia virus type I. *Virology*, **138**, 373–378

Kondo, T., Kono, H., Nonaka, H., Miyamoto, N., Yoshida, R., Bando, F., Inoue, H., Miyoshi, I., Hinuma, Y. & Hanaoka, M. (1987) Risk of adult T-cell leukaemia/lymphoma in HTLV-I carriers (Letter to the Editor). *Lancet*, **ii**, 159

Kondo, T., Kono, H., Miyamoto, N., Yoshida, R., Toki, H., Matsumoto, I., Hara, M., Inoue, H., Inatsuki, A., Funatsu, T., Yamano, N., Bando, F., Iwao, E., Miyoshi, I., Hinuma, Y. & Hanaoka, M. (1989) Age- and sex-specific cumulative rate and risk of ATLL for HTLV-I carriers. *Int. J. Cancer*, **43**, 1061–1064

Kondo, A., Imada, K., Hattori, T., Yamabe, H., Tanaka, T., Miyasaka, M., Okuma, M. & Uchiyama, T. (1993) A model of in vivo cell proliferation of adult T-cell leukemia. *Blood*, **82**, 2501–2509

Koralnik, I.J., Lemp, J.F., Jr, Gallo, R.C. & Franchini, G. (1992a) In vitro infection of human macrophages by human T-cell leukemia/lymphotropic virus type I (HTLV-I). *AIDS Res. hum. Retroviruses*, **8**, 1845–1849

Koralnik, I.J., Gessain, A., Klotman, M.E., Lo Monico, A., Berneman, Z.N. & Franchini, G. (1992b) Protein isoforms encoded by the *pX* region of human T-cell leukemia/lymphotropic virus type I. *Proc. natl Acad. Sci. USA*, **89**, 8813–8817

Koralnik, I.J., Fullen, J. & Franchini, G. (1993) The p12^I, p13^{II}, and p30^{II} proteins encoded by human T-cell leukemia/lymphotropic virus type I open reading frames I and II are localized in three different cellular compartments. *J. Virol.*, **67**, 2360–2366

Koralnik, I.J., Boeri, E., Saxinger, W.C., Lo Monico, A., Fullen, J., Gessain, A., Guo, H.-G., Gallo, R.C., Markham, P., Kalyanaraman, V., Hirsch, V., Allan, J., Murthy, K., Alford, P., Slattery, J.P., O'Brien, S.J. & Franchini, G. (1994) Phylogenetic associations of human and simian T-cell leukemia/lymphotropic virus type I strains: evidence for interspecies transmission. *J. Virol.*, **68**, 2693–2707

Kosaka, M., Iishi, Y., Horiuchi, N., Nakao, K., Okagawa, K., Saito, S., Minami, Y. & Katoh, K. (1989) A cluster of human T-lymphotropic virus type-I carriers found in the southern district of Tokushima Prefecture. *Jpn. J. clin. Oncol.*, **19**, 30–35

Kubota, R., Fujiyoshi, T., Izumo, S., Yashiki, S., Maruyama, I., Osame, M. & Sonoda, S. (1993) Fluctuation of HTLV-I proviral DNA in peripheral blood mononuclear cells of HTLV-I associated myelopathy. *J. Neuroimmunol.*, **42**, 147–154

Kumar, S.R., Gill, P.S., Wagner, D.G., Dugel, P.U., Moudgil, T. & Rao, N.A. (1994) Human T-cell lymphotropic virus type-I associated retinal lymphoma. *Arch. Ophthalmol.*, **112**, 954–959

Kuroda, Y., Matsui, M., Kikuchi, M., Kurohara, K., Endo, C., Yukitake, M., Matsuda, Y., Tokunaga, O., Komine-Sakaki, A. & Kawaguchi, R. (1994) In situ demonstration of the HTLV-I genome in the spinal cord of a patient with HTLV-I-associated myelopathy. *Neurology*, **44**, 2295–2299

Kwok, S., Lipka, J.J., McKinney, N., Kellogg, D.E., Poiesz, B., Foung, S.K. & Sninsky, J.J. (1990) Low incidence of HTLV infections in random blood donors with indeterminate western blot patterns. *Transfusion*, **30**, 491–494

Kwok, R.P.S., Laurance, M.E., Lundblad, J.R., Goldman, P.S., Shih, H.-M., Connor, L.M., Marriott, S.J. & Goodman, R.H. (1996) Control of cAMP-regulated enhancers by the viral transactivator Tax through CREB and the co-activator CBP. *Nature*, **380**, 642–646

LaGrenade, L. (1994) HTLV-I, infective dermatitis and tropical spastic paraparesis. *Mol. Neurobiol.*, **8**, 147–148

LaGrenade, L., Hanchard, B., Fletcher, V., Cranston, B. & Blattner, W. (1990) Infective dermatitis of Jamaican children: a marker for HTLV-I infection. *Lancet*, **336**, 1345–1347

Lairmore, M.D., Jason, J.M., Hartley, T.M., Khabbaz, R.F., De, B. & Evatt, B.L. (1989) Absence of human T-cell lymphotropic virus type I coinfection in human immunodeficiency virus-infected hemophilic men. *Blood*, **74**, 2596–2599

Lal, R.B. (1996) Delineation of immunodominant epitopes of human T-lymphotropic virus types-I and -II and their usefulness in developing serologic assays for detection of antibodies to HTLV-I and HTLV-II. *J. acquir. Immune Defic. Syndr. hum. Retrovirol.* (in press)

Lal, R.B. & Heinene, W. (1996) Testing for human T-lymphotropic virus type-I and -II: serological, virological and molecular detection. In: Hölsberg, P. & Hafler, D., eds, *Human T-Lymphotropic Virus Type I*, New York, John Wiley (in press)

Lal, R.B., Rudolph, D.L., Lairmore, M.D., Khabbaz, R.F., Garfield, M., Coligan, J.E. & Folks, T.M. (1991) Serologic discrimination of human T cell lymphotropic virus infection by using a synthetic peptide-based enzyme immunoassay. *J. infect. Dis.*, **163**, 41–46

Lal, R.B., Brodine, S., Kazura, J., Mbidde-Katonga, E., Yanagihara, R. & Roberts, C. (1992a) Sensitivity and specificity of a recombinant transmembrane glycoprotein (rgp21)-spiked western immunoblot for serological confirmation of human T-cell lymphotropic virus type-I and type-II infections. *J. clin. Microbiol.*, **30**, 296–299

Lal, R.B., Rudolph, D.L., Coligan, J.E., Brodine, S.K. & Roberts, C.R. (1992b) Failure to detect evidence of human T-lymphotropic virus (HTLV) type I and type II in blood donors with isolated *gag* antibodies to HTLV-I/II. *Blood*, **80**, 544–550

Lal, R.B., Rudolph, D.L., Nerurkar, V.R. & Yanagihara, R. (1992c) Humoral responses to the immunodominant *gag* and *env* epitopes of human T-lymphotropic virus type I among Melanesians. *Viral Immunol.*, **5**, 265–272

Lal, R.B., Buckner, C., Khabbaz, R.F., Kaplan, J.E., Reyes, G., Hadlock, K., Lipka, J., Foung, S.K., Chan, L. & Coligan, J.E. (1993) Isotypic and IgG subclass restriction of the humoral immune responses to human T-lymphotropic virus type-I. *Clin. Immunol. Immunopathol.*, **67**, 40–49

Lapin, B.A. (1969) Experiments in monkeys with human leukaemia. *Primates Med.*, **3**, 23–27

Lee, S.Y., Yamaguchi, K., Takatsuki, K., Kim, B.K., Park, S. & Lee, M. (1986) Seroepidemiology of human T-cell leukemia virus type-I in the Republic of Korea. *Jpn. J. Cancer Res. (Gann)*, **77**, 250–254

Lee, H., Swanson, P., Shorty, V.S., Zack, J.A., Rosenblatt, J.D. & Chen, I.S.Y. (1989) High rate of HTLV-II infection in seropositive IV drug abusers in New Orleans. *Science*, **244**, 471–475

Lee, H.H., Swanson, P., Rosenblatt, J.D., Chen, I.S.Y., Sherwood, W.C., Smith, D.E., Tegtmeier, G.E., Fernando, L.P., Fang, C.T., Osame, M. & Kleinman, S.H. (1991) Relative prevalence and risk factors of HTLV-I and HTLV-II infection in US blood donors. *Lancet*, **337**, 1435–1439

Lennert, K., Kikuchi, M., Sato, E., Suchi, T., Stansfeld, A.G., Feller, A.C., Hansmann, M.-L., Müller-Hermelink, H.K. & Gödde-Salz, E. (1985) HTLV-positive and -negative T-cell lymphomas. Morphological and immunohistochemical differences between European and HTLV-positive Japanese T-cell lymphomas. *Int. J. Cancer*, **35**, 65–72

Leno, M., Simpson, R.M., Bowers, F.S. & Kindt, T.J. (1995) Human T lymphocyte virus I from a leukemogenic cell line mediates *in vivo* and *in vitro* lymphocyte apoptosis. *J. exp. Med.*, **181**, 1575–1580

Lerche, N.W., Marx, P.A., Osborn, K.G., Maul, D.H., Lowenstine, L.J., Bleviss, M.L., Moody, P., Henrickson, R.V. & Gardner, M.B. (1987) Natural history of endemic type D retrovirus infection and acquired immune deficiency syndrome in group-housed *rhesus* monkeys. *J. natl Cancer Inst.*, **79**, 847–854

Levin, M.C., Fox, R.J., Lehky, T., Walter, M., Fox, C.H., Flerlage, N., Bamford, R. & Jacobson, S. (1996) PCR-in situ hybridization detection of human T-cell lymphotropic virus type I (HTLV-I) *tax* proviral DNA in peripheral blood lymphocytes of patients with HTLV-I-associated neurologic disease. *J. Virol.*, **70**, 924–933

Levine, P.H., Blattner, W.A., Clark, J., Tarone, R., Maloney, E.M., Murphy, E.M., Gallo, R.C., Robert-Guroff, M. & Saxinger, W.C. (1988) Geographic distribution of HTLV-I and identification of a new high-risk population. *Int. J. Cancer*, **42**, 7–12

Levine, P.H., Manns, A., Jaffe, E.S., Colclough, G., Cavallaro, A., Reddy, G. & Blattner, W.A. (1994) The effect of ethnic differences on the pattern of HTLV-I-associated T-cell leukemia/lymphoma (HATL) in the United States. *Int. J. Cancer*, **56**, 177–181

Levy, J.A., ed. (1992–95) *The Retroviridae*, Vols 1–4, New York, Plenum Press

Lewin, H.A. & Bernoco, D. (1986) Evidence for BoLA-linked resistance and susceptibility to subclinical progression of bovine leukemia virus infection. *Anim. Genet.*, **17**, 197–207

Lewin, H.A., Wu, M.-C., Stewart, J.A. & Nolan, T.J. (1988) Association between *BoLA* and subclinical bovine leukemia virus infection in a herd of Holstein-Friesian cows. *Immunogenetics*, **27**, 338–344

Li, C.-C.H., Ruscetti, F.W., Rice, N.R., Chen, E., Yang, N.-S., Mikovits, J. & Longo, D.L. (1993) Differential expression of Rel family members in human T-cell leukemia virus type I-infected cells: transcriptional activation of c-*rel* by Tax protein. *J. Virol.*, **67**, 4205–4213

Lilienbaum, A., Duc Dodon, M., Alexandre, C., Gazzolo, L. & Paulin, D. (1990) Effect of human T-cell leukemia virus type I Tax protein on activation of the human vimentin gene. *J. Virol.*, **64**, 256–263

Lillehoj, E.P., Alexander, S.S., Dubrule, C.J., Wiktor, S., Adams, R., Tai, C.-C., Manns, A. & Blattner, W.A. (1990) Development and evaluation of a human T-cell leukemia virus type I serological confirmatory assay incorporating a recombinant envelope polypeptide. *J. clin. Microbiol.*, **28**, 2653–2658

Lindholm, P.F., Reid, R.L. & Brady, J.N. (1992) Extracellular Tax1 protein stimulates tumor necrosis factor-β and immunoglobulin kappa light chain expression in lymphoid cells. *J. Virol.*, **66**, 1294–1302

Linhares, M.I.S., Eizuru, Y., de Andrade, G.P., Fonseca, I.B., Carvalho, L.B., Jr, Moreira, I.T. & Minamishima, Y. (1994) Human T cell leukemia virus type I (HTLV-I) antibodies in healthy populations and renal transplanted patients in the north-east of Brazil. *Microbiol. Immunol.*, **38**, 475–478

Lipka, J.J., Bui, K., Reyes, G.R., Moeckli, R., Wiktor, S.Z., Blattner, W.A., Murphy, E.L., Shaw, G.M., Hanson, C.V., Sninsky, J.J. & Foung, S.K.H. (1990) Determination of a unique and immunodominant epitope of human T cell lymphotropic virus type I. *J. infect. Dis.*, **162**, 353–357

Lipka, J.J., Miyoshi, I., Hadlock, K.G., Reyes, G.R., Chow, T.P., Blattner, W.A., Shaw, G.M., Hanson, C.V., Gallo, D., Chan, L. & Foung, S.K.H. (1992) Segregation of human T-cell lymphotropic virus type-I and type-II infections by antibody reactivity to unique viral epitopes. *J. infect. Dis.*, **165**, 268–272

Liu, H.-F., Vandamme, A.-M., Van Brussel, M., Desmyter, J. & Goubau, P. (1994) New retroviruses in human and simian T-lymphotropic viruses (Letter to the Editor). *Lancet*, **344**, 265–266

Longo, D.L., Gelmann, E.P., Cossman, J., Young, R.A., Gallo, R.C., O'Brien, S.J. & Matis, L.A. (1984) Isolation of HTLV-I transformed B-lymphocytes clone from a patient with HTLV-associated adult T-cell leukemia. *Nature*, **310**, 505–506

Loughran, T.P., Jr, Coyle, T., Sherman, M.P., Starkebaum, G., Ehrlich, G.D., Ruscetti, F.W. & Poiesz, B.J. (1992) Detection of human T-cell leukemia/lymphoma virus, type II, in a patient with large granular lymphocyte leukemia. *Blood*, **80**, 1116–1119

Loughran, T.P., Jr, Sherman, M.P., Ruscetti, F.W., Frey, S., Coyle, T., Montagna, R.A., Jones, B., Starkebaum, G. & Poiesz, B.J. (1994) Prototypical HTLV-I/II infection is rare in LGL leukemia. *Leuk. Res.*, **18**, 423–429

Lübbert, M., Miller, C.W., Kahan, J. & Koeffler, H.P. (1989) Expression, methylation and chromatin structure of the p53 gene in untransformed and human T-cell leukemia virus type I-transformed human T-lymphocytes. *Oncogene*, **4**, 643–651

Lymphoma Study Group (1984–1987) (1991) Major prognostic factors of patients with adult T-cell leukemia-lymphoma: a cooperative study. *Leuk. Res.*, **15**, 81–90

Maeda, Y., Furukawa, M., Takehara, Y., Yoshimura, K., Miyamoto, K., Matsuura, T., Morishima, Y., Tajima, K., Okochi, K. & Hinuma, Y. (1984) Prevalence of possible adult T-cell leukemia virus-carriers among volunteer blood donors in Japan: a nation-wide study. *Int. J. Cancer*, **33**, 717–720

Maeda, M., Shimizu, A., Ikuta, K., Okamoto, H., Kashihara, M., Uchiyama,T., Honjo, T. & Yodoi, J. (1985) Origin of human T-lymphotropic virus I-positive T cell lines in adult T cell leukemia. *J. exp. Med.*, **162**, 2169–2174

Maeda, M., Arima, N., Daitoku, Y., Kashihara, M., Okamoto, H., Uchiyama, T., Shirono, K., Matsuoka, M., Hattori, T., Takatsuki, K., Ikuta, K., Shimizu, A., Honjo, T. & Yodoi, J. (1987) Evidence for the interleukin-2 dependent expansion of leukemic cells in adult T-cell leukemia. *Blood*, **70**, 1407–1411

Mahieux, R., Gessain, A., Truffert, A., Vitrac, D., Hubert, A., Dandelot, J., Montchamp-Moreau, C., Cnudde, F., Tekaia, F. & de Thé, G. (1994) Seroepidemiology, viral isolation, and molecular characterization of human T cell leukemia/lymphoma virus type I from La Réunion Island, Indian Ocean. *AIDS Res. hum. Retroviruses*, **10**, 745–752

Mahieux, R., de Thé, G. & Gessain, A. (1995) The *tax* mutation at nucleotide 7959 of human T-cell leukemia virus type I (HTLV-I) is not associated with tropical spastic paraparesis/HTLV-1-associated myelopathy but is linked to the cosmopolitan molecular genotype (Letter to the Editor). *J. Virol.*, **69**, 5925–5927

Maloney, E.M., Ramirez, H., Levin, A. & Blattner, W.A. (1989) A survey of the human T-cell lymphotropic virus type I (HTLV-I) in south-western Colombia. *Int. J. Cancer*, **44**, 419–423

Maloney, E.M., Murphy, E.L., Figueroa, J.P., Gibbs, W.N., Cranston, B., Hanchard, B., Holding-Cobham, M., Malley, K. & Blattner, W.A. (1991) Human T-lymphotropic virus type I (HTLV-I) seroprevalence in Jamaica. II. Geographic and ecologic determinants. *Am. J. Epidemiol.*, **133**, 1125–1134

Manca, N., Piacentini, E., Gelmi, M., Calzavara, P., Manganoni, M.A., Glukhov, A., Gargiulo, F., De Francesco, M., Pirali, F., De Panfilis, G. & Turano, A. (1994) Persistence of human T cell lymphotropic virus type I (HTLV-I) sequences in peripheral blood mononuclear cells from patients with mycosis fungoides. *J. exp. Med.*, **180**, 1973–1978

Mann, D.L., DeSantis, P., Mark, G., Pfeifer, A., Newman, M., Gibbs, N., Popovic, M., Sarngadharan, M.G., Gallo, R.C., Clark, J. & Blattner, W. (1987) HTLV-I-associated B-cell CLL: indirect role for retrovirus in leukemogenesis. *Science*, **236**, 1103–1106

Manns, A. (1993) Natural history of HTLV-I infection: relationship to leukemogenesis. *Leukemia*, **7** (Suppl. 2), pp. S75–S77

Manns, A., Murphy, E.L., Wilks, R., Haynes, G., Figueroa, J.P., Hanchard, B., Barnett, M., Drummond, J., Waters, D., Cerney, M., Seals, J.R., Alexander, S.S., Lee, H. & Blattner, W.A. (1991) Detection of early human T-cell lymphotropic virus type I antibody patterns during seroconversion among transfusion recipients. *Blood*, **77**, 896–905

Manns, A., Wilks, R.J., Murphy, E.L., Haynes, G., Figueroa, J.P., Barnett, M., Hanchard, B. & Blattner, W.A. (1992) A prospective study of transmission by transfusion of HTLV-I and risk factors associated with seroconversion. *Int. J. Cancer*, **51**, 886–891

Manns, A., Cleghorn, F.R., Falk, R.T., Hanchard, B., Jaffe, E.S., Bartholomew, C., Hartge, P., Benichou, J., Blattner, W.A. & the HTLV Lymphoma Study Group (1993) Role of HTLV-I in development of non-Hodgkin lymphoma in Jamaica and Trinidad and Tobago. *Lancet*, **342**, 1447–1450

Manns, A., Wilks, R.J., Hanchard, B., St Clair Morgan, O., Rudolph, D.L. & Lal, R.B. (1994) Viral-specific humoral immune responses following transfusion-related transmission of human T cell lymphotropic virus type-I infection. *Viral Immunol.*, **7**, 113–120

Mansueto, S., Miceli, M.D., Di Blasi, P., Alleto, G., Amico, A., Mancuso, S. & Gentile, G. (1995) Antibodies anti HTLV-I/II in Sicilian residents, in drug addicts, and in African immigrants. *Eur. J. Epidemiol.*, **11**, 359–360

Manzari, V., Gradilone, A., Barillari, G., Zani, M., Collalti, E., Pandolfi, F., De Rossi, G., Liso, V., Babbo, P., Robert-Guroff, M. & Frati, L. (1985) HTLV-I is endemic in southern Italy: detection of the first infectious cluster in a white population. *Int. J. Cancer*, **36**, 557–559

Manzari, V., Modesti, M., De Marchis, L., Gradilone, A., Cifaldi, L. & Marchei, P. (1990) HTLV-I and HIV-1 infection in patients with lymphadenopathy syndrome detected during routine breast screening at a tumor prevention center. *AIDS Res. hum. Retroviruses*, **6**, 417–421

Mariette, X., Agbalika, F., Daniel, M.-T., Bisson, M., Lagrange, P., Brouet, J.-C. & Morinet, F. (1993) Detection of human T lymphotropic virus type I *tax* gene in salivary gland epithelium from two patients with Sjögren's syndrome. *Arthrit. Rheum.*, **36**, 1423–1428

Mariette, X., Cherot, P., Cazals, D., Brocheriou, C., Brouet, J.-C. & Agbalika, F. (1994) Antibodies to HTLV-I in Sjögren's syndrome (Letter to the Editor). *Lancet*, **345**, 71

Markham, P.D., Salahuddin, S.Z., Kalyanaraman, V.S., Popovic, M., Sarin, P. & Gallo, R.C. (1983) Infection and transformation of fresh human umbilical cord blood cells by multiple sources of human T-cell leukemia-lymphoma virus (HTLV). *Int. J. Cancer*, **31**, 413–420

Marriott, S.J., Boros, I., Duvall, J.F. & Brady, J.N. (1989) Indirect binding of human T-cell leukemia virus type I tax_1 to a responsive element in the viral long terminal repeat. *Mol. cell. Biol.*, **9**, 4152–4160

Marriott, S.J., Lindholm, P.F., Brown, K.M., Gitlin, S.D., Duvall, J.F., Radonovich, M.F. & Brady, J.N. (1990) A 36-kilodalton cellular transcription factor mediates an indirect interaction of human T-cell leukemia/lymphoma virus type I Tax_1 with a responsive element in the viral long terminal repeat. *Mol. cell. Biol.*, **10**, 4192–4201

Marriott, S.J., Trinh, D. & Brady, J.N. (1992) Activation of interleukin-2 receptor alpha expression by extracellular HTLV-I Tax_1 protein: a potential role in HTLV-I pathogenesis. *Oncogene*, **7**, 1749–1755

Martin, R.D. (1990) *Primate Origins and Evolution: A Phylogenic Reconstruction*, Princeton, NJ, Princeton University Press

Martin, M.P., Biggar, R.J., Hamlin-Green, G., Staal, S. & Mann, D. (1993) Large granular lymphocytosis in a patient infected with HTLV-II. *AIDS Res. hum. Retroviruses*, **9**, 715–719

Maruyama, I., Tihara, J., Sakashita, I., Mizoguti, R., Mori, S., Usuku, K., Jonosono, M., Tara, M., Niina, S., Sonoda, S., Yasaki, S. & Osame, M. (1988) HTLV-I associated bronchopneumonopathy — a new clinical entity (Abstract). *Am. Rev. respir. Dis.*, **137**, 46

Massari, V., Elghouzzi, M.H., Agis, F., Rannou, C., Gordien, E., Costagliola, D. & Lefrère, J.J. (1994) Epidemiologic comparison of human T-lymphotropic virus type I-infected blood donors from endemic and nonendemic regions over a 3-year period. *Transfusion*, **34**, 198–201

Matheise, J.P., Delcommenne, M., Mager, A., Didembourg, C.H. & Letesson, J.J. (1992) $CD5^+$ B cells from bovine leukemia virus-infected cows are activated cycling cells responsive to interleukin 2. *Leukemia*, **6**, 304–309

Matsumoto, K., Akashi, K., Shibata, H., Yutsudo, M. & Kakura, A. (1994) Single amino acid substitution (^{5x}Pro→Ser) in HTLV-I Tax results in loss of *ras* cooperative focus formation in rat embryo fibroblasts. *Virology*, **200**, 813–815

Matsumura, M., Kushida, S., Ami, Y., Suga, T., Uchida, K., Kameyama, T., Terano, A., Inoue, Y., Shiraki, H., Okochi, K., Sato, H. & Miwa, M. (1993) Quantitation of HTLV-I provirus among seropositive blood donors: relation with antibody profile using synthetic peptides. *Int. J. Cancer*, **55**, 220–222

Matsuzaki, H., Asou, N., Kawaguchi, Y., Hata, H., Yoshinaga, T., Kinuwaki, E., Ishii, T., Yamaguchi, K. & Takatsuki, K. (1990) Human T-cell leukemia virus type I associated with small cell lung cancer. *Cancer*, **66**, 1763–1768

Matutes, E. & Catovsky, D. (1992) Adult T cell leukaemia lymphoma. In: Whittaker, J.A., ed., *Leukaemia.*, 2nd Ed., London, Blackwell Scientific Publications, pp. 416–433

Matutes, E. & Catovsky, D. (1994) ATL of Carribean origin. In: Takatsuki, K., ed., *Adult T-cell Leukaemia*, Oxford, Oxford University Press, pp. 113–138

Matutes, E., Dalgleish, A.G., Weiss, R.A., Joseph, A.P. & Catovsky, D. (1986) Studies in healthy human T-cell leukemia lymphoma virus (HTLV-I) carriers from the Caribbean. *Int. J. Cancer*, **38**, 41–45

Matutes, E., Schulz, T., Serpa, M.J., de Queiroz-Campos-Araujo, A. & Pombo de Oliveira, M.S. (1994) Report of the Second International Symposium on HTLV in Brazil. *Leukemia*, **8**, 1092–1094

Matutes, E., Spittle, M.F., Smith, N.P., Eady, R.A.J. & Catovsky, D. (1995a) The first report of familial adult T-cell leukaemia lymphoma in the United Kingdom. *Br. J. Haematol.*, **89**, 615–619

Matutes, E., Schulz, T., Dyer, M., Ellis, J., Hedges, M. & Catovsky, D. (1995b) Immunoblastic transformation of a Sézary syndrome in a black Caribbean patient without evidence of HTLV-I. *Leuk. Lymph.*, **18**, 521–527

Mauclere, P., Le Hesran, J.Y., Gessain, A., Mahieux, R., Salla, R., de Thé, G. & Millan, J. (1994) Epidemiology of HTLV-I and HTLV-II in Cameroon, the situation revisited with stringent western-blot criterias (Abstract no. E-8). *AIDS Res. hum. Retroviruses*, **10**, 482

May, J.T., Stent, G. & Schnagl, R.D. (1988) Antibody to human T-cell lymphotropic virus type I in Australian aborigines (Letter to the Editor). *Med. J. Aust.*, **149**, 104

McCarthy, T.J., Kennedy, J.L., Blakeslee, J.R. & Bennett, B.T. (1990) Spontaneous malignant lymphoma and leukemia in a simian T-lymphotropic virus type I (STLV-I) antibody positive olive baboon. *Lab. Anim. Sci.*, **40**, 79–81

McClure, H.M., Anderson, D.C., Gordon, T.P., Ansari, A.A., Fultz, P.N., Klumpp, S.A., Emau, P. & Isahakia, M. (1992) Natural simian immunodeficiency virus infections in nonhuman primates. In: Matano, S, Tuttle, R.H., Ishida, H. & Goodman, M., eds, *Topics in Primatology*, Vol. 3, Tokyo, University of Tokyo Press, pp. 425–438

McGuire, K.L., Curtiss, V.E., Larson, E.L. & Haseltine, W.A. (1993) Influence of human T-cell leukemia virus type I *tax* and *rex* on interleukin-2 gene expression. *J. Virol.*, **67**, 1590–1599

Mercieca, J., Matutes, E., Dearden, C., MacLennan, K. & Catovsky, D. (1994) The role of pentostatin in the treatment of T-cell malignancies: analysis of response rate in 145 patients according to disease subtype. *J. clin. Oncol.*, **12**, 2588–2593

Merle, H., Smajda, D., Bera, O., Cabre, P. & Vernant, J.C. (1994) Ophthalmic manifestations in patients with HTLV-I associated myelopathy. A clinical study of 30 cases. *J. fr. Ophtalmol.*, **17**, 403–413 (in French)

Meytes, D., Schochat, B., Lee, H., Nadel, G., Sidi, Y., Cerney, M., Swanson, P., Shaklai, M., Kilim, Y., Elgat, M., Chin, E., Danon, Y. & Rosenblatt, J.D. (1990) Serological and molecular survey for HTLV-I infection in a high-risk Middle Eastern group. *Lancet*, **336**, 1533–1535

Miedema, F., Terpstra, F.G., Smit, J.W., Daenen, S., Gerrits, W., Hegde, U., Matutes, E., Catovsky, D., Greaves, M.F. & Melief, C.J.M. (1984) Functional properties of neoplastic T cells in adult T cell lymphoma/leukemia patients from the Caribbean. *Blood*, **63**, 477–481

Migone, T.-S., Lin, J.-X., Ceresoto, A., Mulloy, J.C., O'Shea, J.J., Franchini, G. & Leonard, W.J. (1995) Constitutively activated Jak-STAT pathway in T-cells transformed with HTLV-I. *Science*, **269**, 79–81

Miller, G.J., Pegram, S.M., Kirkwood, B.R., Beckles, G.L.A., Byam, N.T.A., Clayden, S.A., Kinlen, L.J., Chan, L.C., Carson, D.C. & Greaves, M.F. (1986) Ethnic composition, age and sex, together with location and standard of housing as determinants of HLTV-I infection in an urban Trinidadian community. *Int. J. Cancer*, **38**, 801–808

Miller, G.J., Lewis, L.L., Colman, S.M., Cooper, J.A., Lloyd, G., Scollen, N., Jones, N., Tedder, R.S. & Greaves, M.F. (1994) Clustering of human T lymphotropic virus type I seropositive in Montserrat, West Indies: evidence for an environmental factor in transmission of the virus. *J. infect. Dis.*, **170**, 44–50

Minamoto, G.Y., Gold, J.W.M., Scheinberg, D.A., Hardy, W.D., Chein, N., Zuckerman, E., Reich, L., Dietz, K., Gee, T., Hoffer, J., Mayer, K., Gabrilove, J., Clarkson, B. & Armstrong, D. (1988) Infection with human T-cell leukemia virus type I in patients with leukemia. *New Engl. J. Med.*, **318**, 219–222

Minato, S.-I., Itoyama, Y., Fujii, N., Kira, J.-I., Guo, I. & Yamamoto, N. (1989) Activated T cells in HTLV-I-associated myelopathy: autologous mixed lymphocyte reaction. *Ann. Neurol.*, **26**, 398–401

Mita, S., Sugimoto, M., Nakamura, M., Murakami, T., Tokunaga, M., Uyama, E. & Araki, S. (1993) Increased human T-lymphotropic virus type-I (HTLV-I) proviral DNA in peripheral blood mononuclear cells and bronchoalveolar lavage cells from Japanese patients with HTLV-I-associated myelopathy. *Am. J. trop. Med. Hyg.*, **48**, 170–177

Miyamoto, Y., Yamaguchi, K., Nishimura, H., Takatsuki, K., Motoori, T., Morimatsu, M., Yasaka, T., Ohya, I. & Koga, T. (1985) Familial adult T-cell leukemia. *Cancer*, **55**, 181–185

Miyata, H., Kamahora, T., Iha, S., Katamine, S., Miyamoto, T. & Hino, S. (1995) Dependency of antibody titer on provirus load in human T lymphotropic virus type I carriers: an interpretation for the minor population of seronegative carriers. *J. infec. Dis.*, **171**, 1455–1460

Miyatake, S., Seiki, M., DeWaal Malefijt, R., Heike, T., Fujisawa, J.-I., Takebe, Y., Nishida, J., Shlomai, J., Yokota, T., Yoshida, M., Arai, K.-I. & Arai, N. (1988) Activation of T cell-derived lymphokine genes in T cells and fibroblasts; effects of human T cell leukemia virus type I p40` protein and bovine papilloma virus encoded E2 protein. *Nucleic Acids Res.*, **16**, 6547–6566

Miyazaki, K., Yamaguchi, K., Tohya, T., Ohba, T., Takatsuki, K. & Okamura, H. (1991) Human T-cell leukemia virus type I infection as an oncogenic and prognostic risk factor in cervical and vaginal carcinoma. *Obstet. Gynecol.*, **77**, 107–110

Miyoshi, I. (1994) Animals models of HTLV-I infection. In: Takatsuki, K., ed., *Adult T-cell Leukaemia*, Oxford, Oxford Medical Publications, pp. 204–220

Miyoshi, I., Kubonishi, I., Yoshimoto, S., Akagi, T., Ohtsuki, Y., Shiraishi, Y., Nagata, K. & Hinuma, Y. (1981) Type C virus particles in a cord [blood] T-cell line derived by co-cultivating normal human cord leukocytes and human leukaemic T-cells. *Nature*, **294**, 770–771

Miyoshi, I., Fujishita, M., Taguchi, H., Matsubayashi, K., Miwa, N. & Tanioka, Y. (1983) Natural infection in non-human primates with adult T-cell leukemia virus or a closely related agent. *Int. J. Cancer*, **32**, 333–336

Miyoshi, I., Yoshimoto, S., Kubonishi, I., Fujishita, M., Ohtsuku, Y., Yamashita, M., Yamato, K., Hirose, S., Taguchi, H., Niiya, K. & Kobayashi, M. (1985) Infectious transmission of human T-cell leukemia virus to rabbits. *Int. J. Cancer*, **35**, 81–85

Mizokami, T., Okamura, K., Kohno, T., Sato, K., Ikenoue, H., Kuroda, T., Inokuchi, K. & Fujishima, M. (1995) Human T-lymphotropic virus type I-associated uveitis in patients with Graves' disease treated with methylmercaptoimidazole. *J. clin. Endocrinol. Metab.*, **80**, 1904–1907

Moch, H., Lang, D. & Stamminger, T. (1992) Strong *trans* activation of the human cytomegalovirus major immediate-early enhancer by p40^{tax} of human T-cell Leukemia virus type I via two repetitive Tax-responsive sequence elements. *J. Virol.*, **66**, 7346–7354

Mochizuki, M., Watanabe, T., Yamaguchi, K., Takatsuki, K., Yoshimura, K., Shirao, M., Nakashima, S., Mori, S., Araki, S. & Miyata, N. (1992) HTLV-I uveitis: a distinct clinical entity caused by HTLV-I. *Jpn. J. Cancer Res.*, **83**, 236–239

Mochizuki, M., Tajima, K., Watanabe, T. & Yamaguchi, K. (1994) Human T lymphotropic virus type I uveitis. *Br. J. Ophthalmol.*, **78**, 149–154

Moné, J., Whitehead, E., Leland, M., Hubbard, G. & Allan, J.S. (1992) Simian T-cell leukemia virus type I infection in captive baboons. *AIDS Res. hum. Retroviruses*, **8**, 1653–1661

Monplaisir, N., Neisson-Vernant, C., Bouillot, M., Duc-Dodon, M., Ugarte, E., Valette, I., Dezaphy, Y., Ouka, M., Eudaric, M.G., Gazzolo, L., Larouze, B. & D'Auriol, L. (1993) HTLV-I maternal transmission in Martinique, using serology and polymerase chain reaction. *AIDS Res. hum. Retroviruses*, **9**, 869–874

Morand-Joubert, L., Mariotti, M., Reed, D., Petit, J.-C. & Lefrere, J.-J. (1995) Correlation between viral DNA load and serum anti p19 antibody concentration in symptomless human T-lymphotropic virus type-I (HTLV-I)-infected individuals. *Int. J. Cancer*, **60**, 156–159

Mori, N., Murakami, S., Oda, S., Prager, D. & Eto, S. (1995) Production of interleukin 8 in adult T-cell leukemia cells: possible transactivation of the interleukin 8 gene by human T-cell leukemia virus type I *tax*. *Cancer Res.*, **55**, 3592–3597

Morofuji-Hirata, M., Kajiyama, W., Nakashima, K., Noguchi, A., Hayashi, J. & Kashiwagi, S. (1993) Prevalence of antibody to human T-cell lymphotropic virus type I in Okinawa, Japan, after an interval of 9 years. *Am. J. Epidemiol.*, **137**, 43–48

Mueller, N. (1991) The epidemiology of HTLV-I infection. *Cancer Causes Control*, **2**, 37–52

Mueller, N.E. & Blattner, W.A. (1996) Retroviruses: HTLV. In: Evans, A.S. & Kaslow, R., eds, *Viral Infections of Humans: Epidemiology and Control*, 4th Ed., New York, Plenum Medical Press (in press)

Mukae, H., Kohno, S., Morikawa, N., Kadota, J.-I., Matsukura, S. & Hara, K. (1994) Increase in T-cells bearing CD25 in bronchoalveolar lavage fluid from HAM/TSP patients and HTLV-I carriers. *Microbiol. Immunol.*, **38**, 55–62

Mulloy, J.C., Boeri, E., Gallo, R.C., Leonard, W.J. & Franchini, G. (1994) The HTLV-I p12^{I} protein binds to the immature forms of the IL-2 receptor β- and γ-chains: possible implication in IL2-R signalling (Abstract). *AIDS Res. hum. Retroviruses*, **10**, 443

Murai, K., Tachibana, N., Shioiri, S., Shishime, E., Okayama, A., Ishizaki, J., Tsuda, K. & Mueller, N. (1990) Suppression of delayed-type hypersensitivity to PPD and PHA in elderly HTLV-I carriers. *J. acquir. Immune Defic. Syndr.*, **3**, 1006–1009

Murakami, K., Okada, K., Ikawa, Y. & Aida, Y. (1994a) Bovine leukemia virus induces CD5$^-$ B cell lymphoma in sheep despite temporarily increasing CD5$^+$ B cells in asymptomatic stage. *Virology*, **202**, 458–465

Murakami, K., Aida, Y., Kageyama, R., Numakunai, S., Ohshima, K., Okada, K. & Ikawa, Y. (1994b) Immunopathologic study and characterization of the phenotype of transformed cells in sheep with bovine leukemia virus-induced lymphosarcoma. *Am. J. vet. Res.*, **55**, 72–80

Murphy, E.L., Figueroa, J.P., Gibbs, W.N., Brathwaite, A., Holding-Cobham, M., Waters, D., Cranston, B., Hanchard, B. & Blattner, W.A. (1989a) Sexual transmission of human T-lymphotropic virus type I (HTLV-I). *Ann. intern. Med.*, **111**, 555–560

Murphy, E.L., Hanchard, B., Figueroa, J.P., Gibbs, W.N., Lofters, W.S., Campbell, M., Goedert, J.J. & Blattner, W.A. (1989b) Modelling the risk of adult T-cell leukemia/lymphoma in persons infected with human T-lymphotropic virus type I. *Int. J. Cancer*, **43**, 250–253

Murphy, E.L., Figueroa, J.P., Gibbs, W.N., Holding-Cobham, M., Cranston, B., Malley, K., Bodner, A.J., Alexander, S.S. & Blattner, W.A. (1991) Human T-lymphotropic virus type I (HTLV-I) seroprevalence in Jamaica. I. Demographic determinants. *Am. J. Epidemiol.*, **133**, 1114–1124

Murphy, E.L., Engstrom, J.W., Miller, K., Sacher, R.A., Busch, M.P., Hollingsworth, C.G. and the REDS (Retrovirus Epidemiology in Blood Donor Study) Investigators (1993) HTLV-II associated myelopathy in 43-year-old woman (Letter to the Editor). *Lancet*, **341**, 757–758

Murphy, E.L., Smith, J.W., Sacher, R.A., Gibble, J., Thomson, B., Kaplan, J., Nemo, G., Fridey, J., Engstrom, J., Miller, K., Stevens, J., Hansma, D., Khabbaz, R. & the REDS Investigators (1996) HTLV-associated myelopathy in a cohort of HTLV-I and HTLV-II infected blood donors. *Neurology* (in press)

Myers, G., Korber, B., Wain-Hobson, S., Smith, R.F. & Pavlakis, G.N. (1993) *Human retroviruses and AIDS*, Los Alamos, NM, Los Alamos National Laboratory

Nagashima, K., Yoshida, M. & Seiki, M. (1986) A single species of *pX* mRNA of human T-cell leukemia virus type I encodes *trans*-activator p40^x and two other phosphoproteins. *J. Virol.*, **60**, 394–399

Nakada, K., Yamaguchi, K., Furugen, S., Nakasone, T., Nakasone, K., Oshiro, Y., Kohakura, M., Hinuma, Y., Seiki, M., Yoshida, M., Matutes, E., Catovsky, D., Ishi, T. & Takatsuki, K. (1987) Monoclonal integration of HTLV-I proviral DNA in patients with strongyloidiasis. *Int. J. Cancer.*, **40**, 145–148

Nakamura, H., Tanaka, Y., Komuro-Tsujimoto, A., Ishikawa, K., Takadaya, K.I., Tozawa, H., Tsujimoto, H., Honjo, S. & Hayami, M. (1986) Experimental inoculation of monkeys with autologous lymphoid cell lines immortalized by and producing human T-cell leukemia virus type-I. *Int. J. Cancer*, **38**, 867–875

Nakamura, H., Hayami, M., Ohta, Y., Ishikawa, K.-I., Tsujimoto, H., Kiyokawa, T., Yoshida, M., Sasagawa, A. & Honjo, S. (1987) Protection of cynomolgus monkeys against infection by human T-cell leukaemia virus type I by immunization with viral *env* gene products produced in *Escherichia coli*. *Int. J. Cancer*, **40**, 403–407

Nakao, K., Ohba, N., Otsuka, S., Okubo, A., Yanagita, T., Hashimoto, N. & Arimura, H. (1994) HTLV-I associated uveitis and hyperthyroidism. *Jpn. J. Ophthalmol.*, **38**, 56–61

Nakashima, M., Itagaki, A., Yamada, O., Hagari, S., Furukawa, A., Kamahora, T., Shiraki, K. & Kurimura, T. (1990) Evidence against a seronegative HTLV-I carrier rate among children (Letter to the Editor). *AIDS Res. hum. Retroviruses*, **6**, 1057–1058

Nakashima, K., Kashiwagi, S., Kajiyama, W., Hirata, M., Hayashi, J., Noguchi, A., Urabe, K., Minami, K. & Maeda, Y. (1995) Sexual transmission of human T-lymphotropic virus type I among female prostitutes and among patients with sexually transmitted diseases in Fukuoka, Kyushu, Japan. *Am. J. Epidemiol.*, **141**, 305–311

Neel, J.V., Biggar, R.J. & Sukernik, R.I. (1994) Virologic and genetic studies relate Amerind origins to the indigenous people of the Mongolia/Manchuria/southeastern Siberia region. *Proc. natl Acad. Sci. USA*, **91**, 10737–10741

Nelson, B.H., Lord, J.D. & Greenberg, P.D. (1994) Cytoplasmic domains of the interleukin-2 receptor β and γ chains mediate the signal for T-cell proliferation. *Nature*, **369**, 333–336

Nerenberg, M.I. & Wiley, C.A. (1989) Degeneration of oxidative muscle fibers in HTLV-I transgenic mice. *Am. J. Pathol.*, **135**, 1025–1033

Nerenberg, M.I., Hinrichs, S.H., Reynolds, R.K., Khoury, G. & Jay, G. (1987) The *tat* gene of human T-lymphotropic virus type I induces mesenchymal tumors in transgenic mice. *Science*, **237**, 1324–1329

Nerenberg, M.I., Minor, T., Price, J., Ernst, D.N., Shinohara, T. & Schwarz, H. (1991) Transgenic thymocytes are refractory to transformation by the human T-cell leukemia virus type I *tax* gene. *J. Virol.*, **65**, 3349–3353

Nerurkar, V.R., Miller, M.A., Leon-Monzon, M.E., Ajdukiewicz, A.B., Jenkins, C.L., Sanders, R.C., Godec, M.S., Garruto, R.M. & Yanagihara, R. (1992) Failure to isolate human T cell lymphotropic virus type I and to detect variant-specific genomic sequences by polymerase chain reaction in Melanesians with indeterminate western immunoblot. *J. gen. Virol.*, **73**, 1805–1810

Nerurkar, V.R., Achiron, A., Song, K.-J., Melland, R.R., Pinhas-Hamiel, O., Melamed, E., Shohat, B. & Yanagihara, R. (1995) Human T-cell lymphotropic virus type I in Iranian-born Mashhadi Jews: genetic and phylogenetic evidence for common source of infection. *J. med. Virol.*, **45**, 361–366

Nicot, C., Astier-Gin, T., Edouard, E., Legrand, E., Moynet, D., Vital, A., Londos-Gagliardi, D., Moreau, J.P. & Guillemain, B. (1993) Establishment of HTLV-I infected cell lines from French, Guianese and West Indian patients and isolation of a proviral clone producing viral particles. *Virus Res.*, **30**, 317–334

Niewiesk, S., Daenke, S., Parker, C.E., Taylor, G., Weber, J., Nightingale, S. & Bangham, C.R.M. (1994) The transactivator gene of human T-cell leukemia virus type I is more variable within and between healthy carriers than patients with tropical spastic paraparesis. *J. Virol.*, **68**, 6778–6781

Niewiesk, S., Daenke, S., Parker, C.E., Taylor, G., Weber, J., Nightingale, S. & Bangham, C.R.M. (1995) Naturally occurring variants of human T-cell leukaemia virus type I Tax protein impair its recognition by cytotoxic T lymphocytes and the transactivation function of Tax. *J. Virol.*, **69**, 2649–2653

Nishimura, Y., Takenaka, H., Yoshidome, K., Iwase, K., Oshima, S. & Tanaka, T. (1994) Primary mesenteric tumor of adult T-cell leukemia/lymphoma: report of a case. *Jpn. J. Surg.*, **24**, 263–267

Nishioka, K., Maruyama, I., Sato, K., Kitajima, I., Nakajima, Y. & Osame, M. (1989) Chronic inflammatory arthropathy associated with HTLV-I (Letter to the Editor). *Lancet*, **i**, 441

Nishioka, K., Nakajima, T., Hasunuma, T. & Sato, K. (1993) Rheumatic manifestation of human leukemia virus infection. *Rheum. Dis. Clin. N. Am.*, **19**, 489–503

Nomura, A.M.Y., Yanagihara, E.T., Blattner, W.A., Ho, G.Y.F., Inamasu, M.S., Severson, R.K. & Nakamura, J.M. (1990) Human T-cell lymphotropic virus type I (HTLV-I) antibodies in prediagnostic serum of patients with familial adult T-cell leukemia/lymphoma (ATL). *Hematol. Oncol.*, **8**, 169–176

Nosaka, T., Ariumi, Y., Sakurai, M., Takeuchi, R. & Hatanaka, M. (1993) Novel internal promoter/enhancer of HTLV-I for Tax expression. *Nucleic Acids Res.*, **21**, 5124–5129

Oguma, S. (1990) Simulation of dynamic changes of human T-cell leukemia virus type I carriage rates. *Jpn. J. Cancer Res.*, **81**, 15–21

Oguma, S., Imamura, Y., Kusumoto, Y., Nishimura, Y., Yamaguchi, K., Takatsuki, K., Tokudome, S. & Okuma, M. (1992) Accelerated declining tendency of human T-cell leukemia virus type I carrier rates among younger blood donors in Kumamoto, Japan. *Cancer Res.*, **52**, 2620–2623

Oguma, S., Imamura, Y., Kusumoto, Y., Nishimura, Y., Yamaguchi, K., Takatsuki, K. & Okuma, M. (1995) Stable human T-lymphotropic virus type I carrier rates for 7 years among a teenaged blood donor cohort of 1986 in Kumamoto, Japan. *Leuk. Res.*, **19**, 567–571

Ohba, N., Nakao, K., Isashiki, Y., Osame, M., Sonoda, S., Yashiki, S., Yamaguchi, K., Tajima, K. and the Study Group for HTLV-I Associated Ocular Diseases (1994) A multicenter case–control study of HTLV-I associated uveitis. *Jpn. J. Ophthalmol.*, **38**, 162–167

Ohguro, S., Himi, T., Harabuchi, Y., Suzuki, T., Asakura, K. & Kataura, A. (1993) Adult T-cell leukaemia-lymphoma in Waldeyer's ring: a report of three cases. *J. Laryngol. Otol.*, **107**, 960–962

Ohishi, K., Suzuki, H., Yamamoto, T., Maruyama, T., Miki, K., Ikawa, Y., Numakunai, S., Okada, K., Ohshima, K.-I. & Sugimoto, M. (1991) Protective immunity against bovine leukemia virus (BLV) induced in carrier sheep by inoculation with a vaccinia virus-BLV *env* recombinant: association with cell-mediated immunity. *J. gen. Virol.*, **72**, 1887–1892

Ohshima, K.-I., Kikuchi, M., Yoshida, T., Masuda, Y.-I. & Kimura, N. (1991a) Lymph nodes in incipient adult T-cell leukemia-lymphoma with Hodgkin's disease-like histological features. *Cancer*, **67**, 1622–1628

Ohshima, T., Aida, Y., Kim, J.-C., Okada, K., Chiba, T., Murakami, K. & Ikawa, Y. (1991b) Histopathology and distribution of cells harboring bovine leukemia virus (BLV) proviral sequences in ovine lymphosarcoma induced by BLV inoculation. *J. vet. med. Sci.*, **53**, 191–199

Ohsugi, T., Ishibashi, K., Shingu, M. & Nomura, T. (1994) Engraftment of HTLV-I-transformed human T-cell line into SCID mice with NK cell function. *J. vet. med. Sci.*, **56**, 601–603

Ohtsu, T., Tsugane, S., Tobinai, K., Shimoyama, M., Nanri, S. & Watanabe, S. (1987) Prevalence of antibodies to human T-cell leukemia/lymphoma virus type I and human immunodeficiency virus in Japanese immigrant colonies in Bolivia and Bolivian natives. *Jpn. J. Cancer Res. (Gann)*, **78**, 1347–1353

Okayama, A., Maruyama, T., Tachibana, N., Hayashi, K., Kitamura, T., Mueller, N. & Tsubouchi, H. (1995) Increased prevalence of HTLV-I infection in patients with hepatocellular carcinoma associated with hepatitis C virus. *Jpn. J. Cancer Res.*, **86**, 1–4

Okochi, K., Sato, H. & Hinuma, Y. (1984) A retrospective study on transmission of adult T cell leukemia virus by blood transfusion: seroconversion in recipients. *Vox Sang.*, **46**, 245–253

Ono, K., Shimamoto, Y., Suga, K., Tokioka, T., Sueoka, E., Matsuzaki, M., Sano, M., Yamaguchi, M., Suzuki, H., Sato, H. & Shimoyama, M. (1989) Cancer superimposed on adult T-cell leukemia. *Cancer*, **64**, 635–640

Ono, A., Miura, T., Araki, S., Yamaguchi, K., Takatsuki, K., Mori, S., Hayami, M., Mochizuki, M. & Watanabe, R. (1994) Subtype analysis of HTLV-I in patients with HTLV-I uveitis. *Jpn. J. Cancer Res.*, **85**, 767–770

Orita, S., Saiga, A., Takagi, S., Tanaka, I., Okumura, K., Aono, Y., Hinuma, Y. & Igarashi, H. (1991) A novel alternatively spliced viral mRNA transcribed in cells infected with human T-cell leukaemia virus type I is mainly responsible for expressing p21X protein. *FEBS Lett.*, **295**, 127–134

Orita, S., Sato, S., Aono, Y., Minoura, N., Yamashita, T., Hinuma, Y. & Igarashi, H. (1993) Identification of novel singly spliced pX mRNA transcripts common to all human T-cell leukemia virus type I-related retroviruses. *Virus Genes*, **7**, 197–204

Osame, M., Usuku, K., Izumo, S., Ijichi, N., Amitani, H., Igata, A., Matsumoto, M. & Tara, M. (1986a) HTLV-I associated myelopathy, a new clinical entity (Letter to the Editor). *Lancet*, **i**, 1031–1032

Osame, M., Izumo, S., Igata, A., Matsumoto, M., Matsumoto, T., Sonoda, S., Tara, M. & Shibata, Y. (1986b) Blood transfusion and HTLV-I associated myelopathy (Letter to the Editor). *Lancet*, **ii**, 104–105

Osame, M., Janssen, R., Kubota, H., Nishitani, H., Igata, A., Nagataki, S., Mori, M., Goto, I., Shimabukuro, H., Khabbaz, R. & Kaplan, J. (1990) Nationwide survey of HTLV-I-associated myelopathy in Japan: association with blood transfusion. *Ann. Neurol.*, **28**, 50–56

Ouattara, S.A., Gody, M. & de Thé, G. (1989) Prevalence of HTLV-I compared to HIV-1 and HIV-2 antibodies in different groups in the Ivory Coast (West Africa). *J. acquir. immune Defic. Syndr.*, **2**, 481–485

Paca-Uccaralertkun, S., Zhao, L.-J., Adya, N., Cross, J.V., Cullen, B.R., Boros, I.M. & Giam, C.-Z. (1994) In vitro selection of DNA elements highly responsive to the human T-cell lymphotropic virus type I transcriptional activator, Tax. *Mol. cell. Biol.*, **14**, 456–462

Pagliuca, A., Williams, H., Salisbury, J. & Mufty, G.J. (1990) Prodromal cutaneous lesions in adult T-cell leukaemia/lymphoma (Letter to the Editor). *Lancet.*, **335**, 733–734

Pan, X.-Z., Qiu, Z.-D., Chein, N., Gold, J.W.M., Hardy, W.D., Jr, Zuckerman, E., Wang, Q.N. & Armstrong, D. (1991) A seroepidemiological survey of HTLV-I infection in Shanghai and Chongqing cities in China. *AIDS*, **5**, 782–783

Pancake, B.A. & Zucker-Franklin, D. (1993) More on HTLV-I tax and mycosis fungoides. *Lancet*, **329**, 580

Pancake, B.A., Zucker-Franklin, D. & Coutavas, E.E. (1995) The cutaneous T cell lymphoma, mycosis fungoides, is a human T cell lymphotropic virus-associated disease. A study of 50 patients. *J. clin. Invest.*, **95**, 547–554

Pandolfi, F., Shriver, K., Scarselli, E., Fiorelli, V., Semenzato, G., Zambello, R., Chisesi, T., De Rossi, G. & Strong, D.M. (1987) HTLV-I antibodies and lymphoproliferative disease of granular lymphocytes (Letter to the Editor). *Lancet*, **ii**, 1527

Pantazis, P., Sariban, E., Bohan, C.A., Antoniades, H.N. & Kalyanaraman, V.S. (1987) Synthesis of PDGF by cultured human T-cells transformed with HTLV-I and II. *Oncogene*, **1**, 285–289

Parker, C.E., Daenke, S.D., Nightingale, S. & Bangham, C.R.M. (1992) Activated HTLV-I-specific cytotoxic T lymphocytes are found in healthy seropositives as well as in patients with tropical spastic paraparesis. *Virology*, **188**, 628–636

Parker, C.E., Nightingale, S., Taylor, G.P., Weber, J. & Bangham, C.R.M. (1994) Circulating anti-Tax cytotoxic T lymphocytes from human T-cell leukemia virus type I-infected people, with and without tropical spastic paraparesis, recognize multiple epitopes simultaneously. *J. Virol.*, **68**, 2860–2868

Parodi, A.-L. (1987) Pathology of enzootic bovine leukosis. Comparison with the sporadic form. In: Burny, A. & Mammerickx, M., eds, *Enzootic Bovine Leukosis and Bovine Leukemia Virus*, Boston, Martinus Nijhoff Publishing, pp. 15–49

Parodi, A.-L., Mialot, M., Crespeau, F., Lévy, D., Salmon, H., Noguès, G. & Gérard-Marchand, R. (1982) Attempt for a new cytological and cytoimmunological classification of bovine malignant lymphoma (BML) (lymphosarcoma). In: Straub, O.C., ed., *Fourth International Symposium on Bovine Leukosis*, Brussels-Luxembourg, European Union, pp. 561–570

Parry, C.M., Harries, A.D., Beeching, N.J., Shaw, I.M., Mutton, K.J., McAlpine, L., Tosswill, J.H., Tuke, P.W. & Garson, J.A. (1991) HTLV-II infection in a Liverpool intravenous drug user (Letter to the Editor). *J. infect. Dis.*, **23**, 337–339

Patey, O., Gessain, A., Breuil, J., Courillon-Mallet, A., Daniel, M.-T., Miclea, J.-M., Roucayrol, A.-M., Sigaux, F. & Lafaix, C. (1992) Seven years of recurrent severe strongyloidiasis in an HTLV-I-infected man who developed adult T-cell leukaemia. Short communication. *AIDS*, **6**, 575–579

Paul, P.S., Pomeroy, K.A., Castro, A.E., Johnson, D.W., Muscoplat, C.C. & Sorensen, D.K. (1977) Detection of bovine leukemia virus in B-lymphocytes by the syncytia induction assay. *J. natl Cancer Inst.*, **59**, 1269–1272

Paul, N.L., Millet, I. & Ruddle, N.H. (1993) The lymphotoxin promoter is stimulated by HTLV-I *tax* activation of NF-κB in human T-cell lines. *Cytokine*, **5**, 372–378

Paun, L., Ispas, O., Del Mistro, A. & Chieco-Bianchi, L. (1994) HTLV-I in Romania (Letter to the Editor). *Eur. J. Haematol.*, **52**, 117–118

Peebles, R.S., Maliszewski C.R., Sato, T.A., Hanley-Hyde, J., Maroulakou, I.G., Hunziker, R., Schneck, J.P. & Green, J.E. (1995) Abnormal B-cell function in HTLV-I-tax transgenic mice. *Oncogene*, **10**, 1045–1051

Perini, G., Wagner, S. & Green, M.R. (1995) Recognition of bZIP proteins by the human T-cell leukaemia virus transactivator Tax. *Nature*, **376**, 602–605

Persaud, D., Muñoz, J.L., Tarsis, S.L., Parks, E.S. & Parks, W.P. (1995) Time course and cytokine dependence of human T-cell lymphotropic virus type I T-lymphocyte transformation as revealed by a microtiter infectivity assay. *J. Virol.*, **69**, 6297–6303

Petti, L., Nilson, L.A. & DiMaio, D. (1991) Activation of the platelet-derived growth factor receptor by the bovine papillomavirus E5 transforming protein. *EMBO J,.* **10**, 845–855

Phels, K.R., Ginsberg, S.S., Cunningham, A.W., Tschachler, E. & Dosik, H. (1991) Case report: adult T-cell leukaemia/lymphoma associated with recurrent strongyloides hyperinfection. *Am. J. med. Sci.*, **302**, 224–228

Picard, F., Dreyfus, F., Le Guern, M., Tulliez, M., d'Auriol, L., Neron, S., Galibert, F., Saragosti, S. & Varet, B. (1990) Adult T-cell leukemia/lymphoma mimicking Hodgkin's disease with secondary HTLV-I seroconversion. *Cancer*, **66**, 1524–1528

Pillonel, J., Lemaire, J.M. & Courouce, A.M. (1994) Epidemiology of HTLV in blood donors resident in metropolitan France (July 1991–June 1993). *Méd. Mal. infect.*, **24**, 548–552 (in French)

Plumelle, Y., Pascaline, N., Nguyen, D., Panelatti, G., Jouannelle, A., Jouault, H. & Imbert, M. (1993) Adult T-cell leukemia-lymphoma: a clinico-pathologic study of twenty six patients from Martinique. *Hematol. Pathol.*, **7**, 251–262

Poiesz, B.J., Ruscetti, F.W., Gazdar, A.F., Bunn, P.A., Minna, J.D. & Gallo, R.C. (1980) Detection and isolation of type C retrovirus particles from fresh and cultured lymphocytes of a patient with cutaneous T-cell lymphoma. *Proc. natl Acad. Sci. USA*, **77**, 7415–7419

Pombo de Oliveira, M.S., Matutes, E., Famadas, L.C., Schultz, T.F., Calabro, M.L., Nucci, M., Andrada-Serpa, M.J., Tedder, R.S., Weiss, R.A. & Catovsky, D. (1990) Adult T-cell leukaemia/lymphoma in Brazil and its relation to HTLV-I. *Lancet*, **336**, 987–990

Pombo de Oliveira, M.S., Matutes, E., Schulz, T., Carvalho, S.M., Noronha, H., Reaves, J.D., Loureiro, P., Machado, C. & Catovsky, D. (1995) T-cell malignancies in Brazil. Clinicopathological and molecular studies of HTLV-I positive and negative cases. *Int. J. Cancer*, **60**, 823–827

Popovic, M., Lange-Wantzin, G., Sarin, P.S., Mann, D. & Gallo, R.C. (1983) Transformation of human umbilical cord blood T cells by human T-cell leukemia/lymphoma virus. *Proc. natl Acad. Sci. USA*, **80**, 5402–5406

Portetelle, D., Limbach, K., Burny, A., Mammerickx, M., Desmettre, P., Riviere, M., Zavada, J. & Paoletti, E. (1991) Recombinant vaccinia virus expression of the bovine leukemia virus envelope gene and protection of immunized sheep against infection. *Vaccine*, **9**, 194–200

Powers, M.A. & Radke, K. (1992) Activation of bovine leukemia virus transcription in lymphocytes from infected sheep: rapid transition through early to late gene expression. *J. Virol.*, **66**, 4769–4777

Pozzatti, R., Vogel, J. & Jay, G. (1990) The human T-lymphotropic virus type I *tax* gene can cooperate with the *ras* oncogene to induce neoplastic transformation of cells. *Mol. cell. Biol.*, **10**, 413–417

Ramiandrisoa, H., Dumas, M., Giordano, C., N'Diaye, I.P., Grunitzky, E.K., Kabore, J., Verdier, M., Diop, G., N'Diaye, M. & Denis, F. (1991) Human retrovirus HTLV-I, HIV-1, HIV-2 and neurological diseases in West Africa. *J. trop. geogr. Neurol.*, **1**, 39–44

Ramirez, P.H., Jimenez, R.R., Santovenia, M.B., Leyva, L.N., Matutes, E., Catovsky, D., Yamaguchi, K., Fukuyoshi, Y., Nishimura, Y., Kiyokawa, T. & Takatsuki, K. (1991) Very low seroprevalence of HTLV-I/II in Cuba: antibodies in blood donors and in hematological and nonhematological patients. *Vox Sang.*, **61**, 277–278

Ratner, L., Josephs, S.F., Starcich, B., Hahn, B., Shaw, G.M., Gallo, R.C. & Wong-Staal, F. (1985) Nucleotide sequence analysis of a variant human T-cell leukemia virus (HTLV-Ib) provirus with a deletion in pX-I. *J. Virol.*, **54**, 781–790

Reid, R.L., Lindholm, P.F., Mireskandari, A., Dittmer, J. & Brady, J.N. (1993) Stabilization of wild-type p53 in human T-lymphocytes transformed by HTLV-I. *Oncogene*, **8**, 3029–3036

Richardson, J.H., Edwards, A.J., Cruickshank, J.K., Rudge, P. & Dalgleish, A.G. (1990) In vivo cellular tropism of human T-cell leukemia virus type I. *J. Virol.*, **64**, 5682–5687

Riedel, D.A., Evans, A.S., Saxinger, C. & Blattner, W.A. (1989) A historical study of human T lymphotropic virus type I transmission in Barbados. *J. infect. Dis.*, **159**, 603–609

Rio, B., Louvet, C., Gessain, A., Dormont, D., Gisselbrecht, C., Martoia, R., Auzanneau, G., Miclea, J.M., Baumelou, E., Dombret, H., Guillevin, L., Patey, O., K'Ple Faget, P. & Zittoun, R. (1990) Adult T-cell leukaemia and non-malignant adenopathies associated with HTLV-I virus. On 17 patients born in the Caribbean region and Africa. *Presse méd.*, **19**, 746–751 (in French)

Robert-Guroff, M., Ruscetti, F.W., Posner, L.E., Poiesz, B.J. & Gallo, R.C. (1981) Detection of the human T cell lymphoma virus p19 in cells of some patients with cutaneous T cell lymphoma and leukemia using a monoclonal antibody. *J. exp. Med.*, **154**, 1957–1964

Robert-Guroff, M., Clark, J., Lanier, A.P., Beckman, G., Melbye, M., Ebbesen, P., Blattner, W.A. & Gallo, R.C. (1985) Prevalence of HTLV-I in arctic regions. *Int. J. Cancer*, **36**, 651–655

Roberts, B.D., Foung, S.K.H., Lipka, J.J., Kaplan, J.E., Hadlock, K.G., Reyes, G.R., Chan, L., Heneine, W. & Khabbaz, R.F. (1993) Evaluation of an immunoblot assay for serological confirmation and differentiation of human T-cell lymphotropic virus types I and II. *J. clin. Microbiol.*, **31**, 260–264

Rodgers-Johnson, P.E.B. (1994) Tropical spastic paraparesis/HTLV-I associated myelopathy. Etiology and clinical spectrum. *Mol. Neurobiol.*, **8**, 175–179

Rodgers-Johnson, P.E.B., Gajdusek, D.C., St Clair Morgan, O., Zaninovic, V., Sarin, P.S. & Graham, D.S. (1985) HTLV-I and HTLV-III antibodies and tropical spastic paraparesis (Letter to the Editor). *Lancet*, **ii**, 1247–1248

Rodgers-Johnson, P.E.B., St Clair Morgan, O., Mora, C., Sarin, P., Ceroni, M., Piccardo, P., Garruto, R.M., Gibbs, C.J., Jr & Gajdusek, D.C. (1988) The role of HTLV-I in tropical spastic paraparesis in Jamaica. *Ann. Neurol.*, **23** (Suppl.), S121–S126

Roithmann, S., Pique, C., Le Cesne, A., Delamarre, L., Pham, D., Tursz, T. & Dokhélar, M.-C. (1994) The open reading frame I (ORF I)/ORF II part of the human T-cell leukemia virus type I X region is dispensable for p40^{tax}, p27^{rex}, or envelope expression. *J. Virol.*, **68**, 3448–3451

Román, G.C., Schoenberg, B.S., Madden, D.L., Sever, J.L., Hugon, J., Ludolph, A. & Spencer, P.S. (1987) Human T-lymphotropic virus type I antibodies in the serum of patients with tropical spastic paraparesis in the Seychelles. *Arch. Neurol.*, **44**, 605–607

Rosenblatt, J.D., Golde, D.W., Wachsman, W., Giorgi, J.V., Jacobs, A., Schmidt, G.M., Quan, S., Gasson, J.C. & Chen, I.S.Y. (1986) A second isolate of HTLV-II associated with atypical hairy-cell leukemia. *New Engl. J. Med.*, **315**, 372–377

Rosenblatt, J.D., Gasson, J.C., Glaspy, J., Bhuta, S., Aboud, M., Chen, I.S. & Golde, D.W. (1987) Relationship between human T cell leukemia virus-II and atypical hairy cell leukemia: a serologic study of hairy cell leukemia patients. *Leukemia*, **1**, 397–401

Rosenblatt, J.D., Giorgi, J.V., Golde, D.W., Ben Ezra, J., Wu, A., Winberg, C.D., Glaspy, J., Wachsman, W. & Chen, I.S.Y. (1988a) Integrated human T-cell leukemia virus II genome in CD8$^+$ T cells from a patient with 'atypical' hairy cell leukemia: evidence for distinct T and B cell lymphoproliferative disorders. *Blood*, **71**, 363–369

Rosenblatt, J.D., Chen, I.S.Y. & Golde, D.W. (1988b) HTLV-II and human lymphoproliferative disorders. *Clin. Lab. Med.*, **8**, 85–95

Rovnak, J., Boyd, A.L., Casey, J.W., Gonda, M.A., Jensen, W.A. & Cockerell, G.L. (1993) Pathogenicity of molecularly cloned bovine leukemia virus. *J. Virol.*, **67**, 7096–7105

Ruddle, N.H., Li, C.-B., Horne, W.C., Santiago, P., Troiano, N., Jay, G., Horowitz, M. & Baron, R. (1993) Mice transgenic for HTLV-1 LTR-*tax* exhibit Tax expression in bone, skeletal alterations, and high bone turnover. *Virology*, **197**, 196–204

Rudolph, D.L., Keesling, S.S., Lerche, N., Yee, J.A. & Lal, R.B. (1991) Dominance of HTLV type I-specific antibody responsiveness in Old World monkeys. *AIDS Res. hum. Retroviruses*, **7**, 721–722

Rudolph, D.L., Khabbaz, R.F., Folks, T.M. & Lal, R.B. (1993) Detection of human T-lymphotropic virus type-I/II *env* antibodies by immunoassays using recombinant fusion proteins. *Diag. microbiol. infect. Dis.*, **17**, 35–39

Rudolph, D.L., Coligan, J.E. & Lal, R.B. (1994) Detection of antibodies to *trans*-activator protein (p40^{tax}) of human T-lymphotropic virus type-I by a synthetic peptide-based assay. *Clin. Diag. Lab. Immunol.*, **1**, 176–181

Sagawa, K., Mochizuki, M., Masuoka, K., Katagiri, K., Katayama, T., Maeda, T., Tanimoto, A., Sugita, S., Watanabe, T. & Itoh, K. (1995) Immunopathological mechanisms of human T cell lymphotropic virus type I (HTLV-I) uveitis. Detection of HTLV-I-infected T cells in the eye and their constitutive cytokine production. *J. clin. Invest.*, **95**, 852–858

Saggioro, D., Majone, F., Forino, M., Turchetto, L., Leszl, A. & Chieco-Bianchi, L. (1994) Tax protein of human T-lymphotropic virus type I triggers DNA damage. *Leuk. Lymph.*, **12**, 281–286

Sakai, M., Eguchi, K., Terada, K., Nakashima, M., Yamashita, I., Ida, H,. Kawabe, Y., Aoyagi, T., Takino, H., Nakamura, T. & Nagatika, S. (1993) Infection of human synovial cells by human T cell lymphotropic virus type I. Proliferation and granulocyte/macrophage colony-stimulating factor production by synovial cells. *J. clin Invest.*, **92**, 1957–1966

Sakakibara, I., Sugimoto, Y., Sasagawa, A., Honjo, S., Tsujimoto, H., Nakamura, H. & Hayami, M. (1986) Spontaneous malignant lymphoma in an African green monkey naturally infected with simian T-lymphotropic virus (STLV). *J. med. Primatol.*, **15**, 311–318

Sakamoto, Y., Kawachi, Y., Uchida, Y., Abe, T. & Mori, M. (1994) Adult T-cell leukaemia/-lymphoma featuring a large granular lymphocyte leukaemia morphologically. *Br. J. Haematol.*, **86**, 383–385

Sakashita, A., Hattori, T., Miller, C.W., Suzushima, H., Asou, N., Takatsuki, K. & Koeffler, H.P. (1992) Mutations of the p53 gene in adult T-cell leukemia. *Blood*, **79**, 477–480

Saksena, N., Herve, V., Durand, J.P., Mathiot, C., Love, J., Saksena, M., Barre-Sinoussi, F. & Poiesz, B. (1994) Experimental intraspecies transmission of STLV-I into non-human primates (Abstract no. A-106). *AIDS Res. hum. Retroviruses*, **10**, 458

Salazar-Grueso, E.F., Holzer, T.J., Gutierrez, R.A., Casey, J.M., Desai, S.M., Devare, S.G., Dawson, G. & Roos, R.P. (1990) Familial spastic paraparesis syndrome associated with HTLV-I infection. *New Engl. J. Med.*, **323**, 732–737

Salker, R., Tosswill, J.H.C., Barbara, J.A.J., Runganga, J., Contreras, M., Tedder, R.S., Parra-Mejia, N. & Mortimer, P.P. (1990) HTLV-I/II antibodies in UK blood donors (Letter to the Editor). *Lancet*, **336**, 317

Sandler, S.G., Fang, C.T. & Williams, A.E. (1991) Human T-cell lymphotropic virus type I and II in transfusion medicine. *Transfus. med. Rev.*, **5**, 93–107

Sato, H. & Okochi, K. (1990) Transmission of HTLV-I through blood transfusion and its prevention. *Hematol. Rev.*, **3**, 235–245

Sawada, T., Tohmatsu, J., Obara, T., Koide, A., Kamihira, S., Ichimaru, M., Kashiwagi, S., Kajiyama, W., Matsumura, N., Kinoshita, K., Yano, M., Yamaguchi, K., Kiyokawa, T., Takatsuki, K., Taguchi, H. & Miyoshi, I. (1989) High risk of mother-to-child transmission of HTLV-I in p40^{tax} antibody-positive mothers. *Jpn. J. Cancer Res.*, **80**, 506–508

Sawada, M., Suzumura, A., Yoshida, M. & Marunouchi, T. (1990) Human T-cell leukemia virus type I *trans* activator induces class I major histocompatibility complex antigen expression in glial cells. *J. Virol.*, **64**, 4002–4006

Sawada, M., Suzumura, A., Kondo, N. & Marunouchi, T. (1992) Induction of cytokines in glial cells by *trans* activator of human T-cell lymphotropic virus type I. *FEBS Lett.*, **313**, 47–50

Saxinger, W., Blattner, W.A., Levine, P.H., Clark, J., Biggar, R., Hoh, M., Moghissi, J., Jacobs, P., Wilson, L., Jacobson, R., Crookes, R., Strong, M., Ansari, A.A., Dean, A.G., Nkrumah, F.K., Mourali, N. & Gallo, R.C. (1984) Human T-cell leukemia virus (HTLV-I) antibodies in Africa. *Science*, **225**, 1473–1476

Schaffar-Deshayes, L., Chavance, M., Monplaisir, N., Courouce, A.-M., Gessain, A., Blesonski, S., Valette, I., Feingold, N. & Levy, J.-P. (1984) Antibodies to HTLV-I p24 in sera of blood donors, elderly people and patients with hemopoietic diseases in France and in French West Indies. *Int. J. Cancer*, **34**, 667–670

Schechter, M., Harrison, L.H., Halsey, N.A., Trade, G., Santino, M., Moulton, L.H. & Quinn, T.C. (1994) Coinfection with human T-cell lymphotropic virus type I and HIV in Brazil. Impact on markers of HIV disease progression. *J. Am. med. Assoc.*, **271**, 353–357

Schlegel, R., Wade-Glass, M., Rabson, M.S. & Yang, Y.-C. (1986) The E5 transforming gene of bovine papillomavirus encodes a small, hydrophobic polypeptide. *Science*, **233**, 464–467

Schrijvers, D., Delaporte, E., Peeters, M., Dupont, A. & Meheus, A. (1991) Seroprevalence of retroviral infection in women with different fertility statuses in Gabon, Western Equatorial Africa. *J. acquir. Immune Defic. Syndr.*, **4**, 468–470

Schwartz, I. & Lévy, D. (1994) Pathobiology of bovine leukemia virus. *Vet. Res.*, **25**, 521-536

Schwebke, J., Calsyn, D., Shriver, K., Saxon, A., Kleyn, J., Oluoch-Mitchell, E., Olmsted, L., Fisher, L.D., Krone, M., Ashley, R., Stamm, W., Swenson, P. & Holmes, K.K. (1994) Prevalence and epidemiologic correlates of human T cell lymphotropic virus infection among intravenous drug users. *J. infect. Dis.*, **169**, 962–967

Seiki, M., Hattori, S., Hirayama, Y. & Yoshida, M. (1983) Human adult T-cell leukemia virus: complete nucleotide sequence of the provirus genome integrated in leukemia cell DNA. *Proc. natl Acad. Sci. USA*, **80**, 3618–3622

Seiki, M., Hikikoshi, A., Taniguchi, T. & Yoshida, M. (1985) Expression of the *pX* gene of HTLV-I: general splicing mechanism in the HTLV family. *Science*, **228**, 1532–1534

Senjuta, N., Pavlish, O. & Gurtsevitch, V. (1991) Case of adult T-cell leukaemia in HTLV-I infected family in Georgia, USSR (Letter to the Editor). *Lancet*, **338**, 1394

Seto, A. & Kumagai, K. (1993) Leukemogenesis-associated antigen in HTLV-I transformed rabbit cells. *Leuk. Res.*, **17**, 567–572

Seto, A., Kawanishi, M., Matsuda, S., Ogawa, K. & Miyoshi, I. (1988) Adult T cell leukemia-like disease experimentally induced in rabbits. *Jpn. J. Cancer Res. (Gann)*, **79**, 335–341

Setoyama, M., Fujiyoshi, T., Mizoguchi, S., Katahira, Y., Yashiki, S., Tara, M., Kanzaki, T. & Sonoda, S. (1994) HTLV-I messenger RNA is expressed *in vivo* in adult T-cell leukemia/lymphoma patients: an in situ hybridization study. *Int. J. Cancer*, **57**, 760–764

Sherman, M.P., Amin, R.M., Rodgers-Johnson, P.E.B., Morgan, O.S.C., Char, G., Mora, C.A., Iannone, R., Collins, G.H., Papsidero, L., Gibbs, C.J., Jr & Poiesz, B.J. (1995) Identification of human T cell leukemia/lymphoma virus type I antibodies, DNA and protein in patients with polymyositis. *Arthrit. Rheum.*, **38**, 690–698

Shibasaki, H., Tokudome, S., Kuroda, Y., Yanagawa, T. & Yoshihara, M. (1989) Prevalence of HTLV-I-associated myelopathy among HTLV-I carriers in Saga, Japan. *Neuroepidemiology*, **8**, 124–127

Shibata, K., Shimamoto, Y., Nakano, S., Miyahara, M., Nakano, H. & Yamaguchi, M. (1995) Mantle cell lymphoma with the features of mucosa-associated lymphoid tissue (MALT) lymphoma in an HTLV-I-seropositive patient. *Ann. Hematol.*, **70**, 47–51

Shibayama, K., Nakamura, T., Kinoshita, I., Ueki, Y., Nakao, H,. Eguchi, K., Tsujihata, M. & Nagataki, S. (1992) Remarkable increase in CD26-positive T-cells in patients with human T lymphotropic virus type I (HTLV-I) associated myelopathy. *Intern. Med.*, **31**, 1081–1083

Shida, M., Tochikura, T., Sato, T., Konno, T., Hirayoshi, K., Seki, M., Ito, Y., Hatanaka, M., Hinuma, Y., Sugimoto, M., Takahashi-Nishimaki, F., Maruyama, T., Miki, K., Suzuki, K., Morita, M., Sashiyama, H. & Hayami, M. (1987) Effect of the recombinant vaccinia viruses that express HTLV-I envelope gene on HTLV-I infection. *EMBO J.*, **6**, 3379–3384

Shih, L.-Y., Kuo, T.-T., Dunn, P. & Liaw, S.-J. (1991) Human T-cell lymphotropic virus type I associated adult T-cell leukaemia/lymphoma in Taiwan Chinese. *Br. J. Haematol.*, **79**, 156–161

Shih, L.-Y., Kuo, T.-T., Dunn, P. & Liaw, S.-J. (1992) HTLV-I-positive and HTLV-I-negative peripheral T-cell lymphomas in Taiwan Chinese. *Int. J. Cancer*, **50**, 186–191

Shimamoto, Y., Suga, K., Nishimura, J., Nawata, H. & Yamaguchi, M. (1990a) Major prognostic factors of Japanese patients with lymphoma-type adult T-cell leukemia. *Am. J. Hematol.*, **35**, 232–237

Shimamoto, Y., Suga, K., Shimojo, M., Nishimura, J., Nawata, H. & Yamaguchi, M. (1990b) Comparison of CHOP versus VEPA therapy in patients with lymphoma type of adult T-cell leukemia. *Leuk. Lymph.*, **2**, 335–340

Shimamoto, Y., Kikuchi, M., Funai, N., Suga, K., Matsuzaki, M. & Yamaguchi, M. (1993) Spontaneous regression in adult T-cell leukemia/lymphoma. *Cancer*, **72**, 735–740

Shimotohno, K., Takano, M., Teruuchi, T. & Miwa, M. (1986) Requirement of multiple copies of a 21-nucleotide sequence in the *U3* regions of human T-cell leukemia virus type I and type II long terminal repeats for trans-acting activation of transcription. *Proc. natl Acad. Sci. USA*, **83**, 8112–8116

Shimoyama, M., Kagami, Y., Shimotohno, K., Miwa, M., Minato, K., Tobinai, K., Suemasu, K. & Sugimura, T. (1986) Adult T-cell leukemia/lymphoma not associated with human T-cell leukemia virus type I. *Proc. natl Acad Sci. USA*, **83**, 4524–4528

Shimoyama, M., Abe, T., Miyamoto, K., Minato, K., Tobinai, K., Nagoshi, H., Matsunaga, M., Nomura, T., Tsubota, T., Ohnoshi, T., Kimura, I. & Suemasu, K. (1987) Chromosome aberrations and clinical features of adult T-cell leukemia-lymphoma not associated with human T cell leukemia virus type I. *Blood*, **69**, 984–989

Shimoyama, M. & Members of The Lymphoma Study Group (1984–1987) (1991) Diagnostic criteria and classification of clinical subtypes of adult T-cell leukaemia-lymphoma. *Br. J. Haematol.*, **79**, 428–437

Shinzato, O., Kamihira, S., Ikeda, S., Kondo, H., Kanda, T., Nagata, Y., Nakayama, E. & Shiku, H. (1993) Relationship between the anti-HTLV-I antibody level, the number of abnormal lymphocytes and the viral-genome dose in HTLV-I-infected individuals. *Int. J. Cancer*, **54**, 208–212

Sidi, Y., Meytes, D., Shohat, B., Fenig, E., Weisbort, Y., Lee, H., Pinkhas, J. & Rosenblatt, J.D. (1990) Adult T-cell lymphoma in Israeli patients of Iranian origin. *Cancer*, **65**, 590–593

Siekevitz, M., Feinberg, M.B., Holbrook, N., Wong-Staal, F. & Greene, W.C. (1987) Activation of interleukin 2 and interleukin 2 receptor (Tac) promoter expression by the trans-activator (*tat*) gene product of human T-cell leukemia virus, type I. *Proc. natl Acad. Sci. USA*, **84**, 5389–5393

Singhal, B.S., Lalkaka, J.A., Sonoda, S., Hashimoto, K., Nomoto, M., Kubota, R. & Osame, M. (1993) Human T-lymphotropic virus type I infections in western India (Letter to the Editor). *AIDS*, **7**, 138–139

Smadja, D., Cabre, P., Bellance, R. & Vernant, J.-C. (1993) HTLV-I-associated paraplegia in Martinique. A study of 271 cases including 70 with neuromuscular involvement. *Bull. Soc. Pathol. exot.*, **86**, 433–438 (in French)

Smith, M.R. & Greene, W.C. (1990) Identification of HTLV-I *tax trans*-activator mutants exhibiting novel transcriptional phenotypes. *Genes Dev.*, **4**, 1875–1885

Smith, M.R. & Greene, W.C. (1991) Type I human T-cell leukemia virus Tax protein transforms rat fibroblasts through the cyclic adenosine monophosphate response element binding protein/-activating transcription factor pathway. *J. clin. Invest.*, **88**, 1038–1042

Sodroski, J.G., Rosen, C.A. & Haseltine, W.A. (1984) *Trans*-acting transcriptional activation of the long terminal repeat of human T lymphotropic viruses in infected cells. *Science*, **225**, 381–385

Sonoda, S., Yashiki, S., Fujiyoshi, T., Arima, N., Tanaka, H., Eiraku, N., Izumo, S. & Osame, M. (1992) Immunogenetic factors involved in the pathogenesis of adult T-cell leukemia and HTLV-I-associated myelopathy. *Gann Monogr. Cancer Res.*, **39**, 81–93

Soriano, V., Calderón, E., Esparza, B., Cilla, G., Aguilera, A., Gutiérrez, M., Tor, J., Pujol, E., Merino, F., Pérez-Trallero, E., Leal, M. & Gonzalez-Lahoz, J. from The HTLV-I/II Spanish Study Group (1993) HTLV-I/II infections in Spain. *Int. J. Epidemiol.*, **22**, 716–719

Srivastava, B.I.S., Wong-Staal, F. & Getchell, J.P. (1986) Human T-cell leukemia virus I provirus and antibodies in a captive gorilla with non-Hodgkin's lymphoma. *Cancer Res.*, **46**, 4756–4758

Srivastava, B.I.S., Banki, K. & Perl, A. (1992) Human T-cell leukemia virus type I or a related retrovirus in patients with mycosis fungoides/Sézary syndrome and Kaposi's sarcoma. *Cancer Res.*, **52**, 4391–4395

Starkebaum, G., Loughran, T.P., Jr, Kalyanaraman, V.S., Kadin, M.E., Kidd, P.G., Singer, J.W. & Ruscetti, F.W. (1987) Serum reactivity to human T-cell leukaemia/lymphoma virus type I proteins in patients with large granular lymphocytic leukaemia. *Lancet*, **i**, 596–598

de Stasio, G., Lattanzio, A., Rizzi, L., Lancieri, M., Canavaggio, M., Shreiber, L. & Lee, H. (1989) HTLV-I infection is not endemic in Apulia (southern Italy) (Letter to the Editor). *Int. J. Cancer*, **44**, 1132–1133

St Clair Morgan, O. (1994) The myeloneuropathies of Jamaica. *Mol. Neurobiol.*, **8**, 149–153

St Clair Morgan, O., Rodgers-Johnson, P., Mora, C. & Char, G. (1989) HTLV-I and polymyositis in Jamaica. *Lancet*, **ii**, 1184–1187

Strickler, H.D., Rattray, C., Escoffery, C., Manns, A., Schiffman, M.H., Brown, C., Cranston, B., Hanchard, B., Palefsky, J.M. & Blattner, W.A. (1995) Human T-cell lymphotropic virus type I and severe neoplasia of the cervix in Jamaica. *Int. J. Cancer*, **61**, 23–26

Stuver, S.O., Tachibana, N., Okayama, A., Shioiri, S., Tsunetoshi, Y., Tsuda, K. & Mueller, N.E. (1993) Heterosexual transmission of human T cell leukemia/lymphoma virus type I among married couples in southwestern Japan: an initial report from the Miyazaki Cohort Study. *J. infect. Dis.*, **167**, 57–65

Sueyoshi, K., Goto, M., Johnsono, M., Sato, E. & Shibata, D. (1994) Anatomical distribution of HTLV-I proviral sequence in an autopsy case of HTLV-I associated myelopathy: a polymerase chain reaction study. *Pathol. int.*, **44**, 27–33

Sugimoto, M., Nakashima, H., Watanabe, S., Uyama, E., Tanaka, F., Ando, M., Araki, S. & Kawasaki, S. (1987) T-lymphocyte alveolitis in HTLV-I associated myelopathy (Letter to the Editor). *Lancet*, **ii**, 1220

Sugimoto, M., Nakashima, H., Matsumoto, M., Uyama, E., Ando, M. & Araki, S. (1989) Pulmonary involvement in patients with HTLV-I-associated myelopathy: increased soluble IL-2 receptors in bronchoalveolar lavage fluid. *Am. Rev. respir. Dis.*, **139**, 1329–1335

Sugimoto, M., Mita, S., Tokunaga, M., Yamaguchi, K., Cho, I., Matsumoto, M., Mochizuki, M., Araki, S., Takatsuki, K. & Ando, M. (1993) Pulmonary involvement in human T-cell lymphotropic virus type-I uveitis: T-lymphocytosis and high proviral DNA load in bronchoalveolar lavage fluid. *Eur. respir. J.*, **6**, 938–943

Sugito, S., Yamato, K., Sameshima, Y., Yokota, J., Yano, S. & Miyoshi, I. (1991) Adult T-cell leukemia: structures and expression of the *p53* gene. *Int. J. Cancer*, **49**, 880–885

Sugiyama, H., Doi, H., Yamaguchi, K., Tsuji, Y., Miyamoto, T. & Hino, S. (1986) Significance of postnatal mother-to-child transmission of human T-lymphotropic virus type-I on the development of adult T-cell leukemia/lymphoma. *J. med. Virol.*, **20**, 253–260

Sumida, T., Yonaha, F., Maeda, T., Kita, Y., Iwamoto, I., Koike, T. & Yoshida, S. (1994) Expression of sequences homologous to HTLV-I *tax* gene in the labial salivary glands of Japanese patients with Sjögren's syndrome. *Arthrit. Rheum.*, **37**, 545–550

Suzuki, T., Fujisawa, J.-I., Toita, M. & Yoshida, M. (1993) The *trans*-activator Tax of human T-cell leukemia virus type I (HTLV-I) interacts with cAMP-responsive element (CRE) binding and CRE modulator proteins that bind to the 21-base-pair enhancer of HTLV-I. *Proc. natl Acad. Sci. USA*, **90**, 610–614

Suzuki, T., Hirai, H. & Yoshida, M. (1994) Tax protein of HTLV-I interacts with the Rel homology domain of NF-κB p65 and c-Rel proteins bound to the NF-κB binding site and activates transcription. *Oncogene*, **9**, 3099–3105

Suzuki, T., Hirai, H., Murakami, T. & Yoshida, M. (1995) Tax protein of HTLV-I destabilizes the complexes of NF-κB and IκB-α and induces nuclear translocation of NF-κB for transcriptional activation. *Oncogene*, **10**, 1199–1207

Suzuki, T., Kitao, S., Matsushime, H. & Yoshida, M. (1996) HTLV-I Tax protein interacts with cyclin-dependent kinase inhibitor p16[INK4A] and counteracts its inhibitory activity towards CDK4. *EMBO J.*, **15**, 1607–1614

Switzer, W.M., Pieniazek, D., Swanson, P., Samdal, H.H., Soriano, V., Khabbaz, R.F., Kaplan, J.E., Lal, R.B. & Heneine, W. (1995) Phylogenetic relationship and geographic distribution of multiple human T-cell lymphotropic virus type II subtypes. *J. Virol.*, **69**, 621–632

Tachibana, N., Okayama, A., Ishizaki, J., Yokota, T., Shishime, E., Murai, K., Shioiri, S., Tsuda, K., Essex, M. & Mueller, N. (1988) Suppression of tuberculin skin reaction in healthy HTLV-I carriers from Japan. *Int. J. Cancer*, **42**, 829–831

Tachibana, N., Okayama, A., Ishihara, S., Shioiri, S., Murai, K., Tsuda, K., Goya, N., Matsuo, Y., Essex, M., Stuver, S. & Mueller, N. (1992) High HTLV-I proviral DNA level associated with abnormal lymphocytes in peripheral blood from asymptomatic carriers. *Int. J. Cancer*, **51**, 593–595

Tajima, K. (1990) The 4th nation-wide study of adult T-cell leukemia/lymphoma (ATL) in Japan: estimates of risk of ATL and its geographical and clinical features. The T- and B-cell Malignancy Study Group. *Int. J. Cancer*, **45**, 237–243

Tajima, K. & Cartier, L. (1995) Epidemiological features of HTLV-I and adult T cell leukemia. *Intervirology*, **38**, 238–246

Tajima, K. & Hinuma, Y. (1984) Epidemiological features of adult T cell leukemia. In: Mathe, G. & Rizenstein, P., eds, *Pathophysiological Aspects of Cancer Epidemiology*, Oxford, Pergamon Press, pp. 75–87

Tajima, K. & Hinuma, Y. (1992) Epidemiology of HTLV-I/II in Japan and the world. *Gann Monogr. Cancer Res.*, **39**, 129–149

Tajima, K. & Kuroishi, T. (1985) Estimation of rate of incidence of ATL among ATLV (HTLV-I) carriers in Kyushu, Japan. *Jpn. J. clin. Oncol.*, **15**, 423–430

Tajima, K., Tominaga, S., Suchi, T., Kawagoe, T., Komoda, H., Hinuma, Y., Oda, T. & Fujita, K. (1982) Epidemiological analysis of the distribution of antibody to adult T-cell leukemia-virus-associated antigen: possible horizontal transmission of adult T-cell leukemia virus. *Gann*, **73**, 893–901

Tajima, K., Tominaga, S., Suchi, T., Fukui, H., Komoda, H. & Hinuma, Y. (1986) HTLV-I carriers among migrants from an ATL-endemic area to ATL non-endemic metropolitan areas in Japan. *Int. J. Cancer*, **37**, 383–387

Tajima, K., Kamura, S., Ito, S.-I., Ito, M., Nagatomo, M., Kinoshita, K.-I. & Ikeda, S. (1987) Epidemiological features of HTLV-I carriers and incidence of ATL in an ATL-endemic island: a report of the community-based co-operative study in Tsushima, Japan. *Int. J. Cancer*, **40**, 741–746

Tajima, K., Ito, S.-I., Tsushima & Tsushima ATL Study Group (1990a) Prospective studies of HTLV-I and associated diseases in Japan. In: Blattner,W.A., ed., *Human Retrovirology: HTLV*, New York, Raven Press, pp. 267–279

Tajima, K., The T- and B-cell Malignancy Study Group & Co-authors (1990b) The 4th nation-wide study of adult T-cell leukemia/lymphoma (ATL) in Japan: estimates of risk of ATL and its geographical and clinical features. *Int. J. Cancer*, **45**, 237–243

Tajima, K., Inoue, M., Takesaki, T., Ito, M. & Ito, S.-I. (1994) Ethnoepidemiology of ATL in Japan with special reference to the Mongoloid dispersal. In: Takatsuki, K., ed., *Adult T-cell Leukemia*, Oxford, Oxford University Press, pp. 91–112

Takahashi, K., Takezaki, T., Oki, T., Kawakami, K., Yashiki, S., Fujiyoshi, T., Usuku, K., Mueller, N., the Mother-to-child Transmission Study Group, Osame, M., Miyata, K., Nagata, Y. & Sonoda, S. (1991) Inhibitory effect of maternal antibody on mother-to-child transmission of human T-cell lymphotropic virus type I. *Int. J. Cancer*, **49**, 673–677

Takatsuki, K., Uchiyama, T., Sagawa, K. & Yodoi, J. (1977) Adult T-cell leukemia in Japan. In: Seno, S., Takaku, S. & Irino, S., eds, *Topics in Hematology*, Amsterdam, Excerpta Medica, pp. 73–77

Takatsuki, K., Yamaguchi, K., Kawano, F., Hattori, T., Nishimura, H., Tsuda, H., Sanada, I., Nakada, K. & Itai, Y. (1985) Clinical diversity in adult T-cell leukemia-lymphoma. *Cancer Res.*, **45** (Suppl.), 4644s–4645s

Take, H., Umemoto, M., Kusuhara, K. & Kuraya, K. (1993) Transmission routes of HTLV-I: an analysis of 66 families. *Jpn. J. Cancer Res.*, **84**, 1265–1267

Takehara, N., Iwahara, Y., Uemura, Y., Sawada, T., Ohtsuki, Y., Iwai, H., Hoshino, H. & Miyoshi, I. (1989) Effect of immunisation on HTLV-I infection in rabbits. *Int. J. Cancer*, **44**, 332–336

Takemoto, S., Matsuoka, M., Yamaguchi, K. & Takatsuki, K. (1994) A novel diagnostic method of adult T-cell leukemia: monoclonal integration of human T-cell lymphotropic virus type I provirus DNA detected by inverse polymerase chain reaction. *Blood*, **84**, 3080–3085

Takezaki, T., Tajima, K., Komoda, H. & Imai, J. (1995) Incidence of human T lymphotropic virus type I seroconversion after age 40 among Japanese residents in an area where the virus is endemic. *J. infect. Dis.*, **171**, 559–565

Takezaki, T., Tajima, K., Ito, M., Ito, S.-I., Kinoshita, K.-I., Tachibana, K., Yamashita, Y. & The Tsushima ATL Sudy Group (1996) Short-term breast-feeding may reduce the risk of vertical transmission of HTLV-I. *Leukemia Res.* (in press)

Tamura, K., Unoki, T., Sagawa, K., Aratake, Y., Kitamura, T., Tachibana, N., Ohtaki, S., Yamaguchi, K. & Seita, M. (1985) Clinical features of OKT4$^+$/OKT8$^+$ adult T-cell leukemia. *Leuk. Res.*, **9**, 1353–1359

Tanaka, A., Takahashi, C., Yamaoka, S., Nosaka, T., Maki, M. & Hatanaka, M. (1990) Oncogenic transformation by the *tax* gene of human T-cell leukemia virus type I *in vitro*. *Proc. natl Acad. Sci. USA*, **87**, 1071–1075

Tanaka, Y., Fukudome, K., Hayashi, M., Takagi, S. & Yoshie, O. (1995) Induction of ICAM-1 and LFA-3 by Tax1 of human T-cell leukemia virus type I and mechanism of down-regulation of ICAM-1 or LFA-1 in adult T-cell leukemia cell lines. *Int. J. Cancer*, **60**, 554–561

T- and B-Cell Malignancy Study Group (1985) Statistical analyses of clinico-pathological, virological and epidemiological data on lymphoid malignancies with special reference to adult T-cell leukemia/lymphoma: a report of the second nationwide study of Japan. *Jpn. J. clin. Oncol.*, **15**, 517–535

T- and B-cell Malignancy Study Group (1988) The third nation-wide study on adult T-cell leukemia/lymphoma (ATL) in Japan: characteristic patterns of HLA antigen and HTLV-I infection in ATL patients and their relatives. *Int. J. Cancer*, **41**, 505–512

T- and B-cell Malignancy Study Group (1996) A report from the 7th nationwide study of adult T-cell leukemia/lymphoma (ATL in Japan). *Jpn. J. Cancer Clin.*, **42**, 231–247 (in Japanese)

Tanimura, A., Teshima, H., Fujisawa, J.I. & Yoshida, M. (1993) A new regulatory element that augments the Tax-dependent enhancer of human T-cell leukemia virus type I and cloning of cDNAs encoding its binding proteins. *J. Virol.*, **67**, 5375–5382

Taylor, G.P. (1996) The epidemiology of HTLV-I in Europe. *J. acquir. Immune Defic. Syndr. hum. Retrovirol.*, **13** (Suppl. 1), S8–S14

Tedder, R.S., Shanson, D.C., Jeffries, D.J., Cheingsong-Popov, R., Clapham, P., Dalgleish, A., Nagy, K. & Weiss, R.A. (1984) Low prevalence in the UK of HTLV-I and HTLV-II infection in subjects with AIDS, with extended lymphadenopathy, and at risk of AIDS. *Lancet*, **ii**, 125–128

de Thé, G. & Bomford, R. (1993) An HTLV-I vaccine: why, how, for whom? *AIDS Res. hum. Retroviruses*, **9**, 381–386

de Thé, G. & Gessain, A. (1986) Seroepidemiologic data on viral infections (HTLV-I and LAV/HTLV-III) in the Caribbean region and intertropical Africa. *Ann. Pathol.*, **6**, 261–264 (in French)

de Thé, G., Gessain, A., Gazzolo, L., Robert-Guroff, M., Najberg, G., Calender, A., Peti, M'P., Brubaker, G., Bensliman, A., Fabry, F., Strobel, M., Robin, Y. & Fortune, R. (1985) Comparative seroepidemiology of HTLV-I and HTLV-III in the French West Indies and some African countries. *Cancer Res.*, **45** (Suppl.), 4633s–4636s

Tobinai, K., Ohtsu, T., Hayashi, M., Kinoshita, T., Matsuno, Y., Mukai, K. & Shimoyama, M. (1991) Epstein–Barr virus (EBV) genome carrying monoclonal B-cell lymphoma in a patient with adult T-cell leukemia-lymphoma. *Leuk. Res.*, **15**, 837–846

Tokioka, T., Shimamoto, Y., Funai, N., Nagumo, F., Motoyoshi, K., Tadano, J. & Yamaguchi, M. (1992) Coexistence of acute monoblastic leukemia and adult T-cell leukemia: possible association with HTLV-I infection in both cases? *Leuk. Lymph.*, **8**, 147–155

Tokudome, S., Tokunaga, O., Shimamoto, Y., Miyamoto, Y., Sumida, I., Kikuchi, M., Takeshita, M., Ikeda, T., Fujiwara, K., Yoshihara, M., Yanagawa, T. & Nishizumi, M. (1989) Incidence of adult T-cell leukemia/lymphoma among human T-lymphotropic virus type I carriers in Saga, Japan. *Cancer Res.*, **49**, 226–228

Tokudome, S., Maeda, Y., Fukada, K., Teshima, D., Asakura, T., Sueoka, E., Motomura, Y., Kusumoto, Y., Imamura, Y., Kiyokawa, T., Ikeda, M. & Tokunaga, O. (1991) Follow-up of asymptomatic HTLV-I carriers among blood donors in Kyushu, Japan. *Cancer Causes Control*, **2**, 75–78

Tokudome, S., Shimamoto, Y. & Sumida, I. (1993) Smoking and adult T-cell leukemia/-lymphoma. *Eur. J. Cancer Prev.*, **2**, 84–85

Tosswill, J.H.C., Parry, J.V. & Weber, J.N. (1992) Application of screening and confirmatory assays for anti-HTLV-I/II in U.K. populations. *J. med. Virol.*, **36**, 167–171

Traina-Dorge, V., Blanchard, J., Martin, L. & Murphey-Corb, M. (1992) Immunodeficiency and lymphoproliferative disease in an African green monkey dually infected with SIV and STLV-1. *AIDS Res. hum. Retroviruses*, **8**, 97–100

Trujillo, J.M., Concha, M., Muñoz, A., Bergonzoli, G., Mora, C., Borrero, I., Gibbs, C.J., Jr & Arango, C. (1992) Seroprevalence and cofactors of HTLV-I infection in Tumaco, Colombia. *AIDS Res. hum. Retroviruses*, **8**, 651–657

Tsuda, H. & Takatsuki, K. (1984) Specific decrease in T3 antigen density in adult T-cell leukaemia cells: I. Flow microfluorometric analysis. *Br. J. Cancer*, **50**, 843–845

Tsuda, H., Sawada, T., Sakata, K.-M. & Takatsuki, K. (1992) Possible mechanisms for the elevation of serum beta-2 microglobulin levels in adult T-cell leukemia. *Int. J. Hematol.*, **55**, 179–187

Tsuji, Y., Doi, H., Yamabe, T., Ishimaru, T., Miyamoto, T. & Hino, S. (1990) Prevention of mother-to-child transmission of human T-lymphotropic virus type-I. *Pediatrics*, **86**, 11–17

Tsujimoto, H., Komuro, A., Iijima, K., Miyamoto, J., Ishikawa, K.-I. & Hayami, M. (1985) Isolation of simian retroviruses closely related to human T-cell leukemia virus by establishment of lymphoid cell lines from various non-human primates. *Int. J. Cancer*, **35**, 377–384

Tsujimoto, H., Noda, Y., Ishikawa, K.-I., Nakamura, H., Fukasawa, M., Sakakibara, I., Sasagawa, A., Honjo, S. & Hayami, M. (1987) Development of adult T-cell leukemia-like disease in African green monkey associated with clonal integration of simian T-cell leukemia virus type I. *Cancer Res.*, **47**, 269–274

Tuppin, P., Lepère, J.-F., Carles, G., Ureta-Vidal, A., Gérard, Y., Peneau, C., Tortevoye, P., de Thé, G., Moreau, J.-P. & Gessain, A. (1995) Risk factors for maternal HTLV-I infection in French Guiana: high HTLV-I prevalence in the Noir Marron population. *J. acquir. Immune Defic. Syndr. hum. Retrovirol.*, **8**, 420–425

Tuppin, P., Makuwa, M., Guerma, T., Bazabana, M.M., Loukaka, J.-C., Jeannel, D., M'Pelé, P. & de Thé, G. (1996) Low HTLV-I/II seroprevalence in pregnant women in Congo and a geographic cluster of an HTLV-like indeterminate western blot pattern (Letter to the Editor). *J. acquir. Immune Defic. Syndr. hum. Retrovirol.*, **11**, 105–107

Uchiyama, T., Yodoi, J., Sagawa, K., Takatsuki, K. & Uchino, H. (1977) Adult T-cell leukemia: clinical and hematologic features of 16 cases. *Blood*, **50**, 481–492

Uchiyama, T., Hori, T., Tsudo, M., Wano, Y., Umadome, H., Tamori, S., Yodoi, J., Maeda, M., Sawami, H. & Uchino, H. (1985) Interleukin-2 receptor (Tac antigen) expressed on adult T cell leukemia cells. *J. clin. Invest.*, **76**, 446–453

Ueda, K., Kusuhara, K., Tokugawa, K., Miyazaki, C., Yoshida, C., Tokumura, K., Sonoda, S. & Takahashi, K. (1989) Cohort effect on HTLV-I seroprevalence in southern Japan (Letter to the Editor). *Lancet*, **ii**, 979

Uematsu, T., Hanada, S., Saito, T., Otsuka, M., Komidori, K., Osaki, K., Uemura, S., Ueda, H., Harada, R. & Hashimoto, S. (1989) Adult T cell leukemia in hemodialysis patients from the Kagoshima district, an area in which human T cell leukemia virus type I is highly endemic. *Nephron*, **51**, 257–260

Uemura, Y., Kotani, S., Yoshimoto, S., Fujishita, M., Yano, S., Ohtsuki, Y. & Miyoshi, I. (1986) Oral transmission of human T-cell leukemia virus type I in the rabbit. *Jpn. J. Cancer Res. (Gann)*, **77**, 970–973

Uittenbogaard, M.N., Giebler, H.A., Reisman, D. & Nyborg, J.K. (1995) Transcriptional repression of *p53* by human T-cell leukemia virus type I Tax protein. *J. biol. Chem.*, **270**, 28503–28506

Umehara, F., Nakamura, A., Izumo, S., Kubota, R., Ijichi, S., Kashio, N., Hashimoto,K.-I., Usuku, K., Sato, E. & Osame, M. (1994) Apoptosis of T lymphocytes in the spinal cord lesions in HTLV-I associated myelopathy: a possible mechanism to control viral infection in the central nervous system. *J. Neuropathol. exp. Neurol.*, **53**, 617–624

Uozumi, K., Iwahashi, M., Ueda, H., Otsuka, M., Ishibashi, K., Hanada, S. & Arima, T. (1991) Adult T-cell leukaemia and HTLV-I associated myelopathy in a family (Letter to the Editor). *Lancet*, **338**, 572

Ureta-Vidal, A., Gessain, A., Yoshida, M., Mahieux, R., Nishioka, K., Tekaia, F., Rosen, L. & de Thé, G. (1994) Molecular epidemiology of HTLV type I in Japan: evidence for two distinct ancestral lineages with a particular geographical distribution. *AIDS Res. hum. Retroviruses*, **10**, 1557–1566

Usuku, K., Sonoda, S., Osame, M., Yashiki, S., Takahashi, K., Matsumoto, M., Sawada, T., Tsuji, K., Tara, M. & Igata, A. (1988) HLA haplotype-linked high immune responsiveness against HTLV-I in HTLV-I-associated myelopathy: comparison with adult T-cell leukemia/-lymphoma. *Ann. Neurol.*, **23** (Suppl.), S143–S150

U-Taniguchi, Y., Furuke, K., Masutani, H., Nakamura, H. & Yodoi, J. (1995) Cell cycle inhibition of HTLV-I transformed T cell lines by retinoic acid: the possible therapeutic use of thioredoxin reductase inhibitors. *Oncol. Res.*, **7**, 183–189

Vallejo, A. & Garcia-Saiz, A. (1994) Isolation and nucleotide sequence analysis of human T-cell lymphotropic virus type II in Spain (Letter to the Editor). *J. acquir. Immune Defic. Syndr.*, **7**, 517–519

Vandamme, A.-M., Liu, H.-F., Van Brussel, M., De Meurichy, W., Desmyter, J. & Goubau, P. (1996) The presence of a divergent T-lymphotropic virus in a wild-caught pygmy chimpanzee (*Pan paniscus*) supports an African origin for the human T-lymphotropic/simian T-lymphotropic group of viruses. *J. gen. Virol.*, **77**, 1089–1099

Varma, M., Rudolph, D.L., Knuchel, M., Switzer, W., Hadlock, K.G., Velligan, M., Chan, L., Foung, S.K.H. & Lal, R.B. (1995) Enhanced specificity of truncated transmembrane protein for serological confirmation of human T-cell lymphotropic virus type I (HTLV-I) and HTLV-II infections by western blot (immunoblot) assay containing recombinant envelope glycoproteins. *J. clin. Microbiol.*, **33**, 3239–3244

Verdier, M., Denis, F., Sangaré, A., Barin, F., Gershy-Damet, G., Rey, J.-L., Soro, B., Léonard, G., Mounier, M. & Hugon, J. (1989) Prevalence of antibody to human T cell leukemia virus type I (HTLV-I) in populations of Ivory Coast, West Africa. *J. infect. Dis.*, **160**, 363–370

Verdier, M., Denis, F., Leonard, G., Sangare, A., Patillaud, S., Prince-David, M. & Essex, M. (1990) Comparison of immunofluorescence, particle agglutination, and enzyme immunoassays for detection of human T-cell leukemia virus type I antibody in African sera. *J. clin. Microbiol.*, **28**, 1988–1993

Verdier, M., Bonis, J. & Denis, F. (1994) The prevalence and incidence of HTLVs in Africa. In: Essex, M., Mboup, S., Kanki, P.J., & Kalengayi, M.R., eds, *AIDS in Africa*, New York, Raven Press, pp. 173–193

Vernau, W., Valli, V.E.O., Dukes, T.W., Jacobs, R.M., Shoukri, M. & Heeney, J.L. (1992) Classification of 1,198 cases of bovine lymphoma using the National Cancer Institute Working Formulation for human non-Hodgkin's lymphomas. *Vet. Pathol.*, **29**, 183–195

Veyssier-Belot, C., Couderc, L.J., Desgranges, C., Leblond, V., Dairou, F., Caubarrere, I. & de Gennes, J.L. (1990) Kaposi's sarcoma and HTLV-I infection (Letter to the Editor). *Lancet*, **336**, 575

Voevodin, A.F., Lapin, B.A., Yakovleva, L.A., Ponomaryeva, T.I., Oganyan, T.E. & Razmadze, E.N. (1985) Antibodies reacting with human T-lymphotropic retrovirus (HTLV-I) or related antigens in lymphomatous and healthy hamadryas baboons. *Int. J. Cancer*, **36**, 579–584

Voevodin, A., Al-Mufti, S., Farah, S., Khan, R. & Miura, T. (1995) Molecular characterization of human T-lymphotropic virus, type I (HTLV-I) found in Kuwait: close similarity with HTLV-I isolates originating from Mashhad, Iran. *AIDS Res. hum. Retroviruses*, **11**, 1255–1259

Voevodin, A., Samilchuk, E., Schätzl, H., Boerl, E. & Franchini, G. (1996) Interspecies transmission of macaque simian T-cell leukemia/lymphoma virus type I in baboons resulted in an outbreak of malignant lymphoma. *J. Virol.*, **70**, 1633–1639

de Waal, F.B.M. (1995) Bonobo sex and society. The behavior of a close relative challenges assumptions about male supremacy in human evolution. *Sci. Am.*, **272**, 82–88

Wagner, S. & Green, M.R. (1993) HTLV-I Tax protein stimulation of DNA binding of bZIP proteins by enhancing dimerization. *Science*, **262**, 395–399

Waldmann, T.A., Goldman, C.K., Bongiovanni, K.F., Sharrow, S.O., Davey, M.P., Cease, K.B., Greenberg, S.J. & Longo, D.L. (1988) Therapy of patients with human T-cell lymphotropic virus I-induced adult T-cell leukemia with anti-Tac, a monoclonal antibody to the receptor for interleukin-2. *Blood*, **72**, 1805–1816

Waldmann, T.A., White, J.D., Carrasquillo, J.A., Reynolds, J.C., Paik, C.H., Gansow, O.A., Brechbield, M.W., Jaffe, E.S., Fleisher, T.A., Goldman, C.K., Top, L.E., Bamford, R., Zaknoen, S., Roessler, E., Kasten-Sportes, C., England, R., Litou, H., Johnson, J.A., Jackson-White, T., Manns, A., Hanchard, B., Junghans, R.P. & Nelson, D.L. (1995) Radioimmunotherapy of interleukin-2Rα-expressing adult T-cell leukemia with yttrium-90-labeled anti-Tac. *Blood*, **86**, 4063–4075

Wang, C.-H., Chen, C.-J., Hu, C.-Y., You, S.-L., Chu, C.-T., Chou, M.-J., Essex, M., Blattner, W.A., Liu, C.-H. & Yang, C.-S. (1988) Seroepidemiology of human T-cell lymphotropic virus type I infection in Taiwan. *Cancer Res.*, **48**, 5042–5044

Washitani, Y., Kuroda, N., Shiraki, H., Nishimura, Y., Yamaguchi, K., Takatsuki, K., Fernando, L.P., Fang, C.T., Kiyokawa, H. & Maeda, Y. (1991) Serological discrimination between HTLV-I and HTLV-II antibodies by ELISA using synthetic peptides as antigens. *Int. J. Cancer*, **49**, 173–177

Watanabe, T., Seiki, M., Tsujimoto, H., Miyoshi, I., Hayami, M. & Yoshida, M. (1985) Sequence homology of the simian retrovirus genome with human T-cell leukemia virus type I. *Virology*, **144**, 59–65

Watanabe, T., Yamaguchi, K., Takatsuki, K., Osame, M. & Yoshida, M. (1990) Constitutive expression of parathyroid hormone-related protein gene in human T cell leukemia virus type I (HTLV-I) carriers and adult T cell leukemia patients that can be *trans*-activated by HTLV-I *tax* gene. *J. exp. Med.*, **172**, 759–765

Wattel, E., Vartanian, J.-P., Pannetier, C. & Wain-Hobson, S. (1995) Clonal expansion of human T-cell leukemia virus type I-infected cells in asymptomatic and symptomatic carriers without malignancy. *J. Virol.*, **69**, 2863–2868

Wattel, E., Cavrois, M., Gessain, A. & Wain-Hobson, S. (1996) Clonal expansion of infected cells — A way of life for HTLV-I. *J. acquir. Immune Defic. Syndr. hum. Retrovirol.* (in press)

Weber, J.N., Banatvala, N., Clayden, S., McAdam, K.P.W.J., Palmer, S., Moulsdale, H., Tosswill, J., Dilger, P., Thorpe, R. & Amann, S. (1989) HTLV-I infection in Papua New Guinea: evidence for serologic false positivity. *J. infect. Dis.*, **159**, 1025–1028

Weinberg, J.B., Spiegel, R.A., Blazey, D.L., Janssen, R.S., Kaplan, J.E., Robert-Guroff, M., Popovic, M., Matthews, T.J., Haynes, B.F. & Palker, T.J. (1988) Human T-cell lymphotropic virus I and adult T-cell leukemia: report of a cluster in North Carolina. *Am. J. Med.*, **85**, 51–58

Weinstock, M.A. & Horm, J.W. (1988) Mycosis fungoides in the United States. Increasing incidence and descriptive epidemiology. *J. Am. med. Assoc.*, **260**, 42–46

Weiss, S.H. (1994) The evolving epidemiology of human T lymphotropic virus type II. *J. infect. Dis.*, **169**, 1080–1083

Weiss, R.A., Teich, N.M., Varmus, H.E. & Coffin, J. (1985) *RNA Tumor Viruses*, New York, Cold Spring Harbor Laboratory Press

Welles, S.L., Tachibana, N., Okayama, A., Murai, K., Shioiri, S., Sagawa, K., Katagiri, K. & Mueller, N.E. (1994) The distribution of T-cell subsets among HTLV-I carriers in Japan. *J. acquir. Immune Defic. Syndr.*, **7**, 509–516

Whittaker, S.J. & Luzzatto, L. (1993) HTLV-I provirus and mycosis fungoides. *Science*, **259**, 1470

Whittaker, S.J., Ng, Y.L., Rustin, M., Levene, G., McGibbon, D.H. & Smith, N.P. (1993) HTLV-I associated cutaneous disease: a clinicopathological and molecular study of patients from the UK. *Br. J. Dermatol.*, **128**, 483–492

WHO (1989) Diagnostic Guidelines of HAM/TSP. Virus diseases. Human lymphotropic virus type I, HTLV-I. *Wkly Epidemiol. Rec.*, **49**, 382–383

WHO (1990) Acquired immunodeficiency syndrome. Proposed WHO criteria for interpreting results from western blot assays for HIV-1, HIV-2 and HTLV-I/HTLV-II. *Wkly Epidemiol. Rec.*, **65**, 281–283

Wignall, F.S., Hyams, K.C., Phillips, I.A., Escamilla, J., Tejada, A., Li, O., Lopez, F., Chauca, G., Sanchez, S. & Roberts, C.R. (1992) Sexual transmission of human T-lymphotropic virus type-I in Peruvian prostitutes. *J. med. Virol.*, **38**, 44–48

Wiktor, S.Z., Alexander, S.S., Shaw, G.M., Weiss, S.H., Murphy, E.L., Wilks, R.J., Shortly, V.J., Hanchard, B. & Blattner, W.A. (1990) Distinguishing between HTLV-I and HTLV-II by western blot (Letter to the Editor). *Lancet*, **335**, 1533

Wiktor, S.Z., Pate, E.J., Weiss, S.H., Gohd, R.S., Correa, P., Fontham, E.T., Hanchard, B., Biggar, R.J. & Blattner, W.A. (1991) Sensitivity of HTLV-I antibody assays for HTLV-II (Letter to the Editor). *Lancet*, **338**, 512–513

Wiktor, S.Z., Pate, E.J., Murphy, E.L., Palker, T.J., Champegnie, E., Ramlal, A., Cranston, B., Hanchard, B. & Blattner, W.A. (1993) Mother-to-child transmission of human T-cell lymphotropic virus type I (HTLV-I) in Jamaica: association with antibodies to envelope glycoprotein (gp46) epitopes. *J. acquir. immune Defic. Syndr.*, **6**, 1162–1167

Wiley, C.A., Nerenberg, M., Cros, D. & Soto-Aguilar, M.C. (1989) HTLV-I polymyositis in a patient also infected with the human immunodeficiency virus. *New Engl. J. Med.*, **320**, 992–995

Wilks, R., Hanchard, B., Morgan, O., Williams, E., Cranston, B., Smith, M.L., Rogers-Johnson, P. & Manns, A. (1996) Patterns of HTLV-I infection among family members of patients with adult T-cell leukemia/lymphoma and HTLV-I associated myelopathy/tropical spastic paraparesis. *Int. J. Cancer*, **65**, 272–273

Willems, L., Heremans, H., Chen, G., Portetelle, D., Billiau, A., Burny, A. & Kettmann, R. (1990) Cooperation between bovine leukemia virus transactivator protein and Ha-*ras* oncogene in cellular transformation. *EMBO J.*, **9**, 1577–1581

Willems, L., Kettmann, R., Chen, G., Portetelle, D., Burny, A. & Derse, D. (1992a) A cyclic AMP-responsive DNA-binding protein (CREB2) is a cellular transactivator of the bovine leukemia virus long terminal repeat. *J. Virol.*, **66**, 766–772

Willems, L., Portetelle, D., Kerkhofs, P., Chen, G., Burny, A., Mammerickx, M. & Kettmann, R. (1992b) In vivo transfection of bovine leukemia provirus into sheep. *Virology*, **189**, 775–777

Willems, L., Grimonpont, C., Heremans, H., Rebeyrotte, N., Chen, G., Portetelle, D., Burny, A. & Kettmann, R. (1992c) Mutations in the bovine leukemia virus Tax protein can abrogate the long terminal repeat-directed transactivating activity without concomitant loss of transforming potential. *Proc. natl Acad. Sci. USA*, **89**, 3957–3961

Willems, L., Kettmann, R., Dequiedt, F., Portetelle, D., Vonèche, V., Cornil, I., Kerkhofs, P., Burny, A. & Mammerickx, M. (1993) In vivo infection of sheep by bovine leukemia virus mutants. *J. Virol.*, **67**, 4078–4085

Willems, L., Kerkhofs, P., Dequiedt, F., Portetelle, D., Mammerickx, M., Burny, A. & Kettmann, R. (1994) Attenuation of bovine leukemia virus by deletion of R3 and G4 open reading frames. *Proc. natl Acad. Sci. USA*, **91**, 11532–11536

Willems, L., Gatot, J.S., Mammerickx, M., Portetelle, D., Burny, A., Kerkhofs, P. & Kettmann, R. (1995) The YXXL signalling motifs of the bovine leukemia virus transmembrane protein are required for in vivo infection and maintenance of high viral loads. *J. Virol.*, **69**, 4137–4141

Williams, C.K.O., Alabi, G.O., Junaid, T.A., Saxinger, C., Gallo, R.C., Blayney, D.W., Blattner, W.A. & Greaves, M.F. (1984) Human T cell leukaemia virus associated lymphoproliferative disease: report of two cases in Nigeria. *Br. med. J.*, **288**, 1495–1496

Williams, A.E., Fang, C.T., Slamon, D.J., Poiesz, B.J., Sandler, S.G., Darr, W.F., II, Shulman, G., McGowan, E.I., Douglas, D.K., Bowman, R.J., Peetoom, F., Kleinman, S.H., Lenes, B. & Dodd, R.Y. (1988) Seroprevalence and epidemiological correlates of HTLV-I infection in U.S. blood donors. *Science*, **240**, 643–646

Williams, N.P., Tsuda, H., Yamaguchi, K., Takeya, M., Watanabe, T., Ishii, T., Hamaguchi, I., Tsuruta, J., Ishimaru, Y. & Takatsuki, K. (1991) Blood transfusion induced opportunistic adult T-cell leukemia/lymphoma after Hodgkin's disease. *Leuk. Lymph.*, **5**, 435–439

Wolin, M., Kornuc, M., Hong, C., Shin, S.-K., Lee, F., Lau, R. & Nimer, S. (1993) Differential effect of HTLV infection and HTLV Tax on interleukin 3 expression. *Oncogene*, **8**, 1905–1911

Wucherpfennig, K.W., Höllsberg, P., Richardson, J.H., Benjamin, D. & Hafler, D.A. (1992) T-cell activation by autologous human T-cell leukemia virus type I-infected T-cell clones. *Proc. natl Acad. Sci. USA*, **89**, 2110–2114

Wyld, P.J., Tosswill, J.H.C., Mortimer, P.P. & Weber, J.N. (1990) Sporadic HTLV-I associated adult T-cell leukaemia (ATL) in the UK. *Br. J. Haematol.*, **76**, 149–150

Yamada, Y. (1983) Phenotypic and functional analysis of leukemic cells from 16 patients with adult T-cell leukemia/lymphoma. *Blood*, **61**, 192–199

Yamada, T., Yamaoka, S., Goto, T., Nakai, M., Tsujimoto, Y. & Hatanaka, M. (1994) The human T-cell leukemia virus type I Tax protein induces apoptosis which is blocked by the Bcl-2 protein. *J. Virol.*, **68**, 3374–3379

Yamada, S., Ikeda, H., Tamazaki, H., Shikishima, H., Kikuchi, K., Wakisaka, A., Kasai, N., Shimotohno, K. & Yoshiki, T. (1995) Cytokine-producing mammary carcinomas in transgenic rats carrying the *pX* gene of human T-lymphotropic virus type I. *Cancer Res.*, **55**, 2524–2527

Yamaguchi, K. (1994) Human T-lymphotropic virus in Japan. *Lancet*, **343**, 213–216

Yamaguchi, K., Nishimura, H., Kohrogi, H., Jono, M., Miyamoto, Y. & Takatsuki, K. (1983) A proposal for smoldering adult T-cell leukemia: a clinicopathologic study of five cases. *Blood*, **62**, 758–766

Yamaguchi, K., Seiki, M., Yoshida, M., Nishimura, H., Kawano, F. & Takatsuki, K. (1984) The detection of human T cell leukemia virus proviral DNA and its application for classification and diagnosis of T cell malignancy. *Blood*, **63**, 1235–1240

Yamaguchi, K., Nishimura, Y., Kiyokama, T. & Takatsuki, K. (1989) Elevated serum levels of soluble interleukin-2 receptors in HTLV-I-associated myelopathy. *J. Lab. clin. Med.*, **114**, 407–410

Yamamoto, N., Okada, M., Koyanagi, Y., Kannagi, M. & Hinuma, Y. (1982) Transformation of human leukocytes by cocultivation with an adult T cell leukemia virus producer cell line. *Science*, **217**, 737–739

Yamamoto, N., Hayami, M., Komuro, A., Schneider, J., Hunsmann, G., Okada, M. & Hinuma, Y. (1984) Experimental infection of cynomolgus monkeys with a human retrovirus, adult T-cell leukemia virus. *Med. Microbiol. Immunol.*, **172**, 57–64

Yamamoto, H., Sekiguchi, T., Itagaki, K., Saijo, S. & Iwakura, Y. (1993) Inflammatory polyarthritis in mice transgenic for human T cell leukemia virus type I. *Arthrit. Rheum.*, **36**, 1612–1620

Yamanouchi, K., Kinoshita, K., Moriuchi, R., Katamine, S., Amagasaki, T., Ikeda, S., Ichimaru, M., Miyamoto, T. & Hino, S. (1985) Oral transmission of human T-cell leukemia virus type-I into a common marmoset (*Callithrix jacchus*) as an experimental model for milk-borne transmission. *Jpn. J. Cancer Res. (Gann)*, **76**, 481–487

Yamaoka, S., Tobe, T. & Hatanaka, M. (1992) Tax protein of human T-cell leukemia virus type I is required for maintenance of the transformed phenotype. *Oncogene*, **7**, 433–437

Yamashita, I., Katamine,S., Moriuchi,R., Nakamura, Y., Miyamoto, T., Eguchi, K. & Nagataki, S. (1994) Transactivation of the human interleukin-6 gene by human T-lymphotropic virus type I Tax protein. *Blood*, **84**, 1573–1578

Yamato, K., Oka, T., Hiroi, M., Iwahara, Y., Sugito, S., Tsuchida, N. & Miyoshi, I. (1993) Aberrant expression of the p53 tumor suppressor gene in adult T-cell leukemia and HTLV-I-infected cells. *Jpn. J. Cancer Res.*, **84**, 4–8

Yanagihara, R. (1994) Geographic-specific genotypes or topotypes of human T-cell lymphotropic virus type I as markers for early and recent migrations of human populations. *Adv. Virus Res.*, **43**, 147–186

Yanagihara, R., Jenkins, C.L., Alexander, S.S., Mora, C.A. & Garruto, R.M. (1990) Human T-lymphotropic virus type-I infection in Papua New Guinea: high prevalence among the Hagahai confirmed by western analysis. *J. infect. Dis.*, **162**, 649–654

Yanagihara, R., Ajdukiewicz, A.B., Garruto, R.M., Sharlow, E.R., Wu, X.-Y., Alemaena, O., Sale, H., Alexander, S.S. & Gajudusek, D.C. (1991) Human T-lymphotropic virus type I infection in the Solomon Islands. *Am. J. trop. Med. Hyg.*, **44**, 122–130

Yodoi, J. & Uchiyama, T. (1986) IL-2 receptor dysfunction and adult T-cell leukemia. *Immunol. Rev.*, **92**, 135–156

Yoshida, M. (1994) Tenth anniversary perspectives on AIDS. Host-HTLV type I interaction at the molecular level. *AIDS Res. hum. Retroviruses*, **10**, 1193–1197

Yoshida, M. & Seiki, M. (1987) Recent advances in the molecular biology of HTLV-I: *trans*-activation of viral and cellular genes. *Ann. Rev. Immunol.*, **5**, 541–559

Yoshida, M., Seiki, N., Yamaguchi, K. & Takatsuki, K. (1984) Monoclonal integration of human T-cell leukemia provirus in all primary tumors of adult T-cell leukemia suggests causative role of human T-cell virus in the disease. *Proc. natl Acad. Sci. USA*, **81**, 2534–2537

Yoshida, M., Osame, M., Kawai, H., Toita, M., Kuwasaki, N., Nishida, Y., Hiraki, Y., Takahashi, K., Nomura, K., Sonoda, S., Eiraku, N., Ijichi, S. & Usuku, K. (1989) Increased replication of HTLV-I in HTLV-I-associated myelopathy. *Ann. Neurol.*, **26**, 331–335

Yoshiki, T., Kondo, N., Chubachi, T., Tateno, M., Togashi, T. & Itoh, T. (1987) Rat lymphoid cell lines with HTLV-I production. III. Transmission of HTLV-I into rats and analysis of cell surface antigens associated with HTLV-I. *Arch. Virol.*, **97**, 181–196

Yoshimura, T., Fujisawa, J.-I. & Yoshida, M. (1989) Multiple cDNA clones encoding nuclear proteins that bind to the *tax*-dependent enhancer of HTLV-I: all contain a leucine zipper structure and basic amino acid domain. *EMBO J.*, **9**, 2537–2542

Zamora, T., Zaninovic, V., Kajiwara, M., Komoda, H., Hayami, M. & Tajima, K. (1990) Antibody to HTLV-I in indigenous inhabitants of the Andes and Amazon regions in Colombia. *Jpn. J. Cancer Res.*, **81**, 715–719

Zehender, G., Girotto, M., de Maddalena, C., Francisco, G., Moroni, M. & Galli, M. (1996) HTLV infection in ELISA-negative blood donors. *AIDS Res. hum. Retroviruses*, **12**, 737–740

Zella, D., Mori, L., Sala, M., Ferrante, P., Casoli, C., Magnani, G., Achilli, G., Cattaneo, E., Lori, F. & Bertazzoni, U. (1990) HTLV-II infection in Italian drug abusers (Letter to the Editor). *Lancet*, **336**, 575–576

Zhao, L.-J. & Giam, C.-Z. (1992) Human T-cell lymphotropic virus type I (HTLV-I) transcriptional activator, Tax, enhances CREB binding to HTLV-I 21-base-pair-repeats by protein-protein interaction. *Proc. natl Acad. Sci. USA*, **89**, 7070–7074

Zhao, T.M., Robinson, M.A., Bowers, F.S. & Kindt, T.J. (1995) Characterization of an infectious molecular clone of human T-cell leukemia virus type I. *J. Virol.*, **69**, 2024–2030

Zucker-Franklin, D. & Pancake, B.A. (1994) The role of human T-cell lymphotropic viruses (HTLV-I and II) in cutaneous T-cell lymphomas. *Sem. Dermatol.*, **13**, 160–165

Zucker-Franklin, D., Coutavas, E.E., Rush, M.G. & Zouzias, D.C. (1991) Detection of human T-lymphotropic virus-like particles in cultures of peripheral blood lymphocytes from patients with mycosis fungoides. Proc. natl Acad. Sci. USA, 88, 7630–7634

Zucker-Franklin, D., Hooper, W.C. & Evatt, B.L. (1992) Human lymphotropic retroviruses associated with mycosis fungoides: evidence that human T-cell lymphotropic virus type II (HTLV-II) as well as HTLV-I may play a role in the disease. *Blood*, **80**, 1537–1545

Abbreviations

AIDS — acquired immunodeficiency syndrome
AIDS/ARC — AIDS-related complex
AIN — anal intraepithelial neoplasia
ALCL — anaplastic large cell lymphoma
ALV — avian leukosis/sarcoma virus
AML — acute myeloid leukaemia
AP1 — activation protein 1
ASCUS — atypical squamous cells of unknown significance
ASIL — anal squamous intraepithelial lesion
ATF — activating transcription factor
ATLL — adult T-cell leukaemia/lymphoma
ATPase — adenosine triphosphatase
AZT — azidothymidine = zidovudine
BAL — bronchoalveolar lavage
BCBL — body cavity-based lymphoma
BCC — basal cell carcinoma of the skin
bFGF — basic fibroblast growth factor
BL — Burkitt's lymphoma
BLV — bovine leukaemia virus
bp — base pair
BPV — bovine papillomavirus
c-AMP — cyclic AMP
CA — capsid
CDC Centers for Disease Control and Prevention (The CDC changed its name from Centers for Disease Control to Centers for Disease Control and Prevention on November 15, 1992)
CI — confidence interval
CIN — cervical intraepithelial neoplasia
CMV — cytomegalovirus
CNF — central nervous fluid
CNS — central nervous system
CPE — cytopathic effect
CRE — cyclic AMP-responsive element
CREB — cyclic AMP responsive element-binding protein
CREM — cyclic AMP responsive element modulator
CSF — cerebrospinal fluid (in HIV monograph); colony stimulating factor (in HTLV monograph)
CTL — cytotoxic T-lymphocyte
ddC — dideoxycytidine = zalcitabine

ddI — dideoxyinosine = didanosine
DLCL — diffuse large-cell lymphoma
EBER — Epstein–Barr encoded RNA
EBL — enzootic bovine leukosis
EBNA — Epstein–Barr nuclear antigen
EBV — Epstein–Barr virus
ECFG — endothelial cell growth factor
EGF — epidermal growth factor
EIA — enzyme immunoassay
ELISA — enzyme-linked immunosorbent assay
ENAADS — European non-aggregate AIDS data set
FDC — follicular dendritic cells
FeLV — feline leukaemia virus
FGF — fibroblast growth factor
FIV — feline immunodeficiency virus
GALV — gibbon ape leukaemia virus
GICAT — Italian Cooperative Group for AIDS-Related Tumours
Gla-8 — Glasgow-8 strain
GM — granulocyte-macrophage
GVHD — graft versus hot disease
HCG — human chorionic gonadotropin
HBV — hepatitis B virus
HCV — hepatitis C virus
HFV — human foamy virus
HHV — human herpesvirus
HIV — human immunodeficiency virus
HLA — human leukocyte antigen
HPV — human papillomavirus
HTLV — human T-cell lymphotropic virus
HVP — herpesvirus papio
HVS — herpesvirus saimiri
IBL — immunoblastic lymphoma
ICD — International Classification of Disease
Ig — immunoglobulin
IL — interleukin
IN — integrase
IOAC — insertive oroanal contact
ISH — in-situ hybridization
IVDU — intravenous drug user
kb — kilobase
kDa — kilodalton
KS — Kaposi's sarcoma
KSHV — Kaposi's sarcoma-associated herpes virus
LAM — leukocyte adhesion molecule

LAV — lymphadenopathy-associated virus
LCDL — large cell diffuse lymphoma
LCG — human chronic gonadotropin
LCR — long control region
LDH — lactose dehydrogenase
LGL — large granular lymphocytic
LMP — latent membrane protein
LTR — long terminal repeat
MA — matrix
MACS — multicentre AIDS cohort study
MCD — multicentric angiofollicular dysplasia
MHC — major histocompatibility complex
MLV — murine leukaemia virus
MMSV — Moloney murine sarcoma virus
MMTV — mouse mammary tumour virus
MoMV — Moloney murine virus
MPMV — Mason–Pfizer monkey virus
mRNA — messenger ribonucleic acid
MVV — maedi-visna virus
NC — nucleocapsid
NCSU1 — North Carolina State University 1 strain
NF — nuclear factor
NGF — nerve growth factor
NHL — non-Hodgkin's lymphoma
NK — natural killer
NSP — non-spastic paraparesis
OR — odds ratio
PAI — plasminogen activator inhibitor
Pattern II countries — countries in which extensive spread of HIV began in the mid-to-late 1970s or early 1980s and in which heterosexual transmission has predominated and continues to
PBL — peripheral blood lymphocyte
PBMC — peripheral blood mononuclear cell
PCP — *Pneumocystis carinii* pneumonia
PCR — polymerase chain reaction
PDGF — platelet-derived growth factor
PGL — persistent generalized lymphadenopathy
PHA — phytohaemagglutinin
PIDS — public information data set
PIR — proportionate incidence rate
PR — protease
pRB — retinoblastoma tumour suppressor protein
PTH-rP — parathyroid hormone-related protein
PTLV — primate T-cell lymphoma virus

Rex RE — Rex response element
RFLP — restriction fragment length polymorphism
RIPA — radioimmunoprecipitation assay
RIR — relative incidence ratio
RR — relative risk
RRE — Rev response element
RT — reverse transcriptase
SCC — squamous-cell carcinoma of the skin
SCID — severe combined immunodeficient
SEER — Surveillance, Epidemiology and End Results
SFV — simian foamy virus
SIL — squamous intraepithelial lesion
SIR — standardized incidence ratio
SIV — simian immunodeficiency virus
SNCCL — small non-cleaved-cell lymphoma
SNV — spleen necrosis virus
SPF — specific pathogen free
SPI — subclinical papillomavirus infection
SRE — serum response element
SRF — serum response factor
SRV — simian retrovirus
SRV-2 — simian immunosuppressive type D retrovirus
SSAV — simian sarcoma-associated virus
STD — sexually transmitted disease
STLV — simian T-cell lymphotropic virus
SU — surface
TAR — transactivation response
Tat protein — transcriptional transactivating protein
Tax protein — transcriptional activating protein
TdT⁺ — terminal deoxynucleotidyl transferase
TGF — transforming growth factor
TM — transmembrane
TNF — tumour necrosis factor
TRE — Tax-responsive element
TREB — Tax-responsive element binding protein
TSP — tropical spastic paraparesis
TSP/HAM — tropical spastic paraparesis/HTLV-I-associated myelopathy
uPA — urokinase plasminogen activator
vWF — von Willebrand factor
WF — international working formulation for non-Hodgkin's lymphomas

SUPPLEMENTARY CORRIGENDA TO VOLUMES 1–67

Volume 49

pp. 352–353 Nickel salts, *replace* 'lung tumours' *by* 'local tumours' in the work cited by Pott *et al.* (1989, 1990)

CUMULATIVE CROSS INDEX TO *IARC MONOGRAPHS ON THE EVALUATION OF CARCINOGENIC RISKS TO HUMANS*

The volume, page and year of publication are given. References to corrigenda are given in parentheses.

A

A-α-C	40, 245 (1986); *Suppl. 7*, 56 (1987)
Acetaldehyde	36, 101 (1985) (*corr. 42*, 263); *Suppl. 7*, 77 (1987)
Acetaldehyde formylmethylhydrazone (*see* Gyromitrin)	
Acetamide	7, 197 (1974); *Suppl. 7*, 389 (1987)
Acetaminophen (*see* Paracetamol)	
Acridine orange	16, 145 (1978); *Suppl. 7*, 56 (1987)
Acriflavinium chloride	13, 31 (1977); *Suppl. 7*, 56 (1987)
Acrolein	19, 479 (1979); 36, 133 (1985); *Suppl. 7*, 78 (1987); 63, 337 (1995) (*corr. 65*, 549)
Acrylamide	39, 41 (1986); *Suppl. 7*, 56 (1987); 60, 389 (1994)
Acrylic acid	19, 47 (1979); *Suppl. 7*, 56 (1987)
Acrylic fibres	19, 86 (1979); *Suppl. 7*, 56 (1987)
Acrylonitrile	19, 73 (1979); *Suppl. 7*, 79 (1987)
Acrylonitrile-butadiene-styrene copolymers	19, 91 (1979); *Suppl. 7*, 56 (1987)
Actinolite (*see* Asbestos)	
Actinomycins	10, 29 (1976) (*corr. 42*, 255); *Suppl. 7*, 80 (1987)
Adriamycin	10, 43 (1976); *Suppl. 7*, 82 (1987)
AF-2	31, 47 (1983); *Suppl. 7*, 56 (1987)
Aflatoxins	1, 145 (1972) (*corr. 42*, 251); 10, 51 (1976); *Suppl. 7*, 83 (1987); 56, 245 (1993)
Aflatoxin B_1 (*see* Aflatoxins)	
Aflatoxin B_2 (*see* Aflatoxins)	
Aflatoxin G_1 (*see* Aflatoxins)	
Aflatoxin G_2 (*see* Aflatoxins)	
Aflatoxin M_1 (*see* Aflatoxins)	
Agaritine	31, 63 (1983); *Suppl. 7*, 56 (1987)
Alcohol drinking	44 (1988)
Aldicarb	53, 93 (1991)
Aldrin	5, 25 (1974); *Suppl. 7*, 88 (1987)
Allyl chloride	36, 39 (1985); *Suppl. 7*, 56 (1987)
Allyl isothiocyanate	36, 55 (1985); *Suppl. 7*, 56 (1987)
Allyl isovalerate	36, 69 (1985); *Suppl. 7*, 56 (1987)
Aluminium production	34, 37 (1984); *Suppl. 7*, 89 (1987)

Amaranth	8, 41 (1975); *Suppl. 7*, 56 (1987)
5-Aminoacenaphthene	16, 243 (1978); *Suppl. 7*, 56 (1987)
2-Aminoanthraquinone	27, 191 (1982); *Suppl. 7*, 56 (1987)
para-Aminoazobenzene	8, 53 (1975); *Suppl. 7*, 390 (1987)
ortho-Aminoazotoluene	8, 61 (1975) (*corr. 42*, 254); *Suppl. 7*, 56 (1987)
para-Aminobenzoic acid	16, 249 (1978); *Suppl. 7*, 56 (1987)
4-Aminobiphenyl	1, 74 (1972) (*corr. 42*, 251); *Suppl. 7*, 91 (1987)
2-Amino-3,4-dimethylimidazo[4,5-*f*]quinoline (*see* MeIQ)	
2-Amino-3,8-dimethylimidazo[4,5-*f*]quinoxaline (*see* MeIQx)	
3-Amino-1,4-dimethyl-5*H*-pyrido[4,3-*b*]indole (*see* Trp-P-1)	
2-Aminodipyrido[1,2-*a*:3′,2′-*d*]imidazole (*see* Glu-P-2)	
1-Amino-2-methylanthraquinone	27, 199 (1982); *Suppl. 7*, 57 (1987)
2-Amino-3-methylimidazo[4,5-*f*]quinoline (*see* IQ)	
2-Amino-6-methyldipyrido[1,2-*a*:3′.2′-*d*]imidazole (*see* Glu-P-1)	
2-Amino-1-methyl-6-phenylimidazo[4,5-*b*]pyridine (*see* PhIP)	
2-Amino-3-methyl-9*H*-pyrido[2,3-*b*]indole (*see* MeA-α-C)	
3-Amino-1-methyl-5*H*-pyrido[4,3-*b*]indole (*see* Trp-P-2)	
2-Amino-5-(5-nitro-2-furyl)-1,3,4-thiadiazole	7, 143 (1974); *Suppl. 7*, 57 (1987)
2-Amino-4-nitrophenol	57, 167 (1993)
2-Amino-5-nitrophenol	57, 177 (1993)
4-Amino-2-nitrophenol	16, 43 (1978); *Suppl. 7*, 57 (1987)
2-Amino-5-nitrothiazole	31, 71 (1983); *Suppl. 7*, 57 (1987)
2-Amino-9*H*-pyrido[2,3-*b*]indole (*see* A-α-C)	
11-Aminoundecanoic acid	39, 239 (1986); *Suppl. 7*, 57 (1987)
Amitrole	7, 31 (1974); 41, 293 (1986) (*corr. 52*, 513; *Suppl. 7*, 92 (1987)
Ammonium potassium selenide (*see* Selenium and selenium compounds)	
Amorphous silica (*see also* Silica)	42, 39 (1987); *Suppl. 7*, 341 (1987)
Amosite (*see* Asbestos)	
Ampicillin	50, 153 (1990)
Anabolic steroids (*see* Androgenic (anabolic) steroids)	
Anaesthetics, volatile	11, 285 (1976); *Suppl. 7*, 93 (1987)
Analgesic mixtures containing phenacetin (*see also* Phenacetin)	*Suppl. 7*, 310 (1987)
Androgenic (anabolic) steroids	*Suppl. 7*, 96 (1987)
Angelicin and some synthetic derivatives (*see also* Angelicins)	40, 291 (1986)
Angelicin plus ultraviolet radiation (*see also* Angelicin and some synthetic derivatives)	*Suppl. 7*, 57 (1987)
Angelicins	*Suppl. 7*, 57 (1987)
Aniline	4, 27 (1974) (*corr. 42*, 252); 27, 39 (1982); *Suppl. 7*, 99 (1987)
ortho-Anisidine	27, 63 (1982); *Suppl. 7*, 57 (1987)
para-Anisidine	27, 65 (1982); *Suppl. 7*, 57 (1987)
Anthanthrene	32, 95 (1983); *Suppl. 7*, 57 (1987)
Anthophyllite (*see* Asbestos)	
Anthracene	32, 105 (1983); *Suppl. 7*, 57 (1987)
Anthranilic acid	16, 265 (1978); *Suppl. 7*, 57 (1987)
Antimony trioxide	47, 291 (1989)
Antimony trisulfide	47, 291 (1989)
ANTU (*see* 1-Naphthylthiourea)	
Apholate	9, 31 (1975); *Suppl. 7*, 57 (1987)
Aramite®	5, 39 (1974); *Suppl. 7*, 57 (1987)
Areca nut (*see* Betel quid)	
Arsanilic acid (*see* Arsenic and arsenic compounds)	

Arsenic and arsenic compounds	*1*, 41 (1972); *2*, 48 (1973); *23*, 39 (1980); *Suppl. 7*, 100 (1987)
Arsenic pentoxide (*see* Arsenic and arsenic compounds)	
Arsenic sulfide (*see* Arsenic and arsenic compounds)	
Arsenic trioxide (*see* Arsenic and arsenic compounds)	
Arsine (*see* Arsenic and arsenic compounds)	
Asbestos	*2*, 17 (1973) (*corr. 42*, 252); *14* (1977) (*corr. 42*, 256); *Suppl. 7*, 106 (1987) (*corr. 45*, 283)
Atrazine	*53*, 441 (1991)
Attapulgite	*42*, 159 (1987); *Suppl. 7*, 117 (1987)
Auramine (technical-grade)	*1*, 69 (1972) (*corr. 42*, 251); *Suppl. 7*, 118 (1987)
Auramine, manufacture of (*see also* Auramine, technical-grade)	*Suppl. 7*, 118 (1987)
Aurothioglucose	*13*, 39 (1977); *Suppl. 7*, 57 (1987)
Azacitidine	*26*, 37 (1981); *Suppl. 7*, 57 (1987); *50*, 47 (1990)
5-Azacytidine (*see* Azacitidine)	
Azaserine	*10*, 73 (1976) (*corr. 42*, 255); *Suppl. 7*, 57 (1987)
Azathioprine	*26*, 47 (1981); *Suppl. 7*, 119 (1987)
Aziridine	*9*, 37 (1975); *Suppl. 7*, 58 (1987)
2-(1-Aziridinyl)ethanol	*9*, 47 (1975); *Suppl. 7*, 58 (1987)
Aziridyl benzoquinone	*9*, 51 (1975); *Suppl. 7*, 58 (1987)
Azobenzene	*8*, 75 (1975); *Suppl. 7*, 58 (1987)

B

Barium chromate (*see* Chromium and chromium compounds)	
Basic chromic sulfate (*see* Chromium and chromium compounds)	
BCNU (*see* Bischloroethyl nitrosourea)	
Benz[*a*]acridine	*32*, 123 (1983); *Suppl. 7*, 58 (1987)
Benz[*c*]acridine	*3*, 241 (1973); *32*, 129 (1983); *Suppl. 7*, 58 (1987)
Benzal chloride (*see also* -Chlorinated toluenes)	*29*, 65 (1982); *Suppl. 7*, 148 (1987)
Benz[*a*]anthracene	*3*, 45 (1973); *32*, 135 (1983); *Suppl. 7*, 58 (1987)
Benzene	*7*, 203 (1974) (*corr. 42*, 254); *29*, 93, 391 (1982); *Suppl. 7*, 120 (1987)
Benzidine	*1*, 80 (1972); *29*, 149, 391 (1982); *Suppl. 7*, 123 (1987)
Benzidine-based dyes	*Suppl. 7*, 125 (1987)
Benzo[*b*]fluoranthene	*3*, 69 (1973); *32*, 147 (1983); *Suppl. 7*, 58 (1987)
Benzo[*j*]fluoranthene	*3*, 82 (1973); *32*, 155 (1983); *Suppl. 7*, 58 (1987)
Benzo[*k*]fluoranthene	*32*, 163 (1983); *Suppl. 7*, 58 (1987)
Benzo[*ghi*]fluoranthene	*32*, 171 (1983); *Suppl. 7*, 58 (1987)
Benzo[*a*]fluorene	*32*, 177 (1983); *Suppl. 7*, 58 (1987)
Benzo[*b*]fluorene	*32*, 183 (1983); *Suppl. 7*, 58 (1987)
Benzo[*c*]fluorene	*32*, 189 (1983); *Suppl. 7*, 58 (1987)
Benzofuran	*63*, 431 (1995)
Benzo[*ghi*]perylene	*32*, 195 (1983); *Suppl. 7*, 58 (1987)
Benzo[*c*]phenanthrene	*32*, 205 (1983); *Suppl. 7*, 58 (1987)

Benzo[a]pyrene	3, 91 (1973); 32, 211 (1983); Suppl. 7, 58 (1987)
Benzo[e]pyrene	3, 137 (1973); 32, 225 (1983); Suppl. 7, 58 (1987)
para-Benzoquinone dioxime	29, 185 (1982); Suppl. 7, 58 (1987)
Benzotrichloride (see also α-Chlorinated toluenes)	29, 73 (1982); Suppl. 7, 148 (1987)
Benzoyl chloride	29, 83 (1982) (corr. 42, 261); Suppl. 7, 126 (1987)
Benzoyl peroxide	36, 267 (1985); Suppl. 7, 58 (1987)
Benzyl acetate	40, 109 (1986); Suppl. 7, 58 (1987)
Benzyl chloride (see also α-Chlorinated toluenes)	11, 217 (1976) (corr. 42, 256); 29, 49 (1982); Suppl. 7, 148 (1987)
Benzyl violet 4B	16, 153 (1978); Suppl. 7, 58 (1987)
Bertrandite (see Beryllium and beryllium compounds)	
Beryllium and beryllium compounds	1, 17 (1972); 23, 143 (1980) (corr. 42, 260); Suppl. 7, 127 (1987); 58, 41 (1993)
Beryllium acetate (see Beryllium and beryllium compounds)	
Beryllium acetate, basic (see Beryllium and beryllium compounds)	
Beryllium-aluminium alloy (see Beryllium and beryllium compounds)	
Beryllium carbonate (see Beryllium and beryllium compounds)	
Beryllium chloride (see Beryllium and beryllium compounds)	
Beryllium-copper alloy (see Beryllium and beryllium compounds)	
Beryllium-copper-cobalt alloy (see Beryllium and beryllium compounds)	
Beryllium fluoride (see Beryllium and beryllium compounds)	
Beryllium hydroxide (see Beryllium and beryllium compounds)	
Beryllium-nickel alloy (see Beryllium and beryllium compounds)	
Beryllium oxide (see Beryllium and beryllium compounds)	
Beryllium phosphate (see Beryllium and beryllium compounds)	
Beryllium silicate (see Beryllium and beryllium compounds)	
Beryllium sulfate (see Beryllium and beryllium compounds)	
Beryl ore (see Beryllium and beryllium compounds)	
Betel quid	37, 141 (1985); Suppl. 7, 128 (1987)
Betel-quid chewing (see Betel quid)	
BHA (see Butylated hydroxyanisole)	
BHT (see Butylated hydroxytoluene)	
Bis(1-aziridinyl)morpholinophosphine sulfide	9, 55 (1975); Suppl. 7, 58 (1987)
Bis(2-chloroethyl)ether	9, 117 (1975); Suppl. 7, 58 (1987)
N,N-Bis(2-chloroethyl)-2-naphthylamine	4, 119 (1974) (corr. 42, 253); Suppl. 7, 130 (1987)
Bischloroethyl nitrosourea (see also Chloroethyl nitrosoureas)	26, 79 (1981); Suppl. 7, 150 (1987)
1,2-Bis(chloromethoxy)ethane	15, 31 (1977); Suppl. 7, 58 (1987)
1,4-Bis(chloromethoxymethyl)benzene	15, 37 (1977); Suppl. 7, 58 (1987)
Bis(chloromethyl)ether	4, 231 (1974) (corr. 42, 253); Suppl. 7, 131 (1987)
Bis(2-chloro-1-methylethyl)ether	41, 149 (1986); Suppl. 7, 59 (1987)
Bis(2,3-epoxycyclopentyl)ether	47, 231 (1989)
Bisphenol A diglycidyl ether (see Glycidyl ethers)	
Bisulfites (see Sulfur dioxide and some sulfites, bisulfites and metabisulfites)	
Bitumens	35, 39 (1985); Suppl. 7, 133 (1987)
Bleomycins	26, 97 (1981); Suppl. 7, 134 (1987)
Blue VRS	16, 163 (1978); Suppl. 7, 59 (1987)
Boot and shoe manufacture and repair	25, 249 (1981); Suppl. 7, 232 (1987)
Bracken fern	40, 47 (1986); Suppl. 7, 135 (1987)

Brilliant Blue FCF, disodium salt	*16*, 171 (1978) (*corr. 42*, 257); *Suppl. 7*, 59 (1987)
Bromochloroacetonitrile (*see* Halogenated acetonitriles)	
Bromodichloromethane	*52*, 179 (1991)
Bromoethane	*52*, 299 (1991)
Bromoform	*52*, 213 (1991)
1,3-Butadiene	*39*, 155 (1986) (*corr. 42*, 264 *Suppl. 7*, 136 (1987); *54*, 237 (1992)
1,4-Butanediol dimethanesulfonate	*4*, 247 (1974); *Suppl. 7*, 137 (1987)
n-Butyl acrylate	*39*, 67 (1986); *Suppl. 7*, 59 (1987)
Butylated hydroxyanisole	*40*, 123 (1986); *Suppl. 7*, 59 (1987)
Butylated hydroxytoluene	*40*, 161 (1986); *Suppl. 7*, 59 (1987)
Butyl benzyl phthalate	*29*, 193 (1982) (*corr. 42*, 261); *Suppl. 7*, 59 (1987)
β-Butyrolactone	*11*, 225 (1976); *Suppl. 7*, 59 (1987)
γ-Butyrolactone	*11*, 231 (1976); *Suppl. 7*, 59 (1987)

C

Cabinet-making (*see* Furniture and cabinet-making)	
Cadmium acetate (*see* Cadmium and cadmium compounds)	
Cadmium and cadmium compounds	*2*, 74 (1973); *11*, 39 (1976) (*corr. 42*, 255); *Suppl. 7*, 139 (1987); *58*, 119 (1993)
Cadmium chloride (*see* Cadmium and cadmium compounds)	
Cadmium oxide (*see* Cadmium and cadmium compounds)	
Cadmium sulfate (*see* Cadmium and cadmium compounds)	
Cadmium sulfide (*see* Cadmium and cadmium compounds)	
Caffeic acid	*56*, 115 (1993)
Caffeine	*51*, 291 (1991)
Calcium arsenate (*see* Arsenic and arsenic compounds)	
Calcium chromate (see Chromium and chromium compounds)	
Calcium cyclamate (*see* Cyclamates)	
Calcium saccharin (*see* Saccharin)	
Cantharidin	*10*, 79 (1976); *Suppl. 7*, 59 (1987)
Caprolactam	*19*, 115 (1979) (*corr. 42*, 258); *39*, 247 (1986) (*corr. 42*, 264); *Suppl. 7*, 390 (1987)
Captafol	*53*, 353 (1991)
Captan	*30*, 295 (1983); *Suppl. 7*, 59 (1987)
Carbaryl	*12*, 37 (1976); *Suppl. 7*, 59 (1987)
Carbazole	*32*, 239 (1983); *Suppl. 7*, 59 (1987)
3-Carbethoxypsoralen	*40*, 317 (1986); *Suppl. 7*, 59 (1987)
Carbon black	*3*, 22 (1973); *33*, 35 (1984); *Suppl. 7*, 142 (1987); *65*, 149 (1996)
Carbon tetrachloride	*1*, 53 (1972); *20*, 371 (1979); *Suppl. 7*, 143 (1987)
Carmoisine	*8*, 83 (1975); *Suppl. 7*, 59 (1987)
Carpentry and joinery	*25*, 139 (1981); *Suppl. 7*, 378 (1987)
Carrageenan	*10*, 181 (1976) (*corr. 42*, 255); *31*, 79 (1983); *Suppl. 7*, 59 (1987)
Catechol	*15*, 155 (1977); *Suppl. 7*, 59 (1987)
CCNU (*see* 1-(2-Chloroethyl)-3-cyclohexyl-1-nitrosourea)	
Ceramic fibres (see Man-made mineral fibres)	

Chemotherapy, combined, including alkylating agents (see MOPP and
    other combined chemotherapy including alkylating agents)
Chloral   63, 245 (1995)
Chloral hydrate   63, 245 (1995)
Chlorambucil   9, 125 (1975); 26, 115 (1981);
                                                                     Suppl. 7, 144 (1987)

Chloramphenicol   10, 85 (1976); Suppl. 7, 145 (1987);
                                                                     50, 169 (1990)
Chlordane (see also Chlordane/Heptachlor)   20, 45 (1979) (corr. 42, 258)
Chlordane/Heptachlor   Suppl. 7, 146 (1987); 53, 115 (1991)
Chlordecone   20, 67 (1979); Suppl. 7, 59 (1987)
Chlordimeform   30, 61 (1983); Suppl. 7, 59 (1987)
Chlorendic acid   48, 45 (1990)
Chlorinated dibenzodioxins (other than TCDD)   15, 41 (1977); Suppl. 7, 59 (1987)
Chlorinated drinking-water   52, 45 (1991)
Chlorinated paraffins   48, 55 (1990)
α-Chlorinated toluenes   Suppl. 7, 148 (1987)
Chlormadinone acetate (see also Progestins; Combined oral   6, 149 (1974); 21, 365 (1979)
    contraceptives)
Chlornaphazine (see N,N-Bis(2-chloroethyl)-2-naphthylamine)
Chloroacetonitrile (see Halogenated acetonitriles)
para-Chloroaniline   57, 305 (1993)
Chlorobenzilate   5, 75 (1974); 30, 73 (1983);
                                                                     Suppl. 7, 60 (1987)
Chlorodibromomethane   52, 243 (1991)
Chlorodifluoromethane   41, 237 (1986) (corr. 51, 483);
                                                                     Suppl. 7, 149 (1987)
Chloroethane   52, 315 (1991)
1-(2-Chloroethyl)-3-cyclohexyl-1-nitrosourea (see also Chloroethyl   26, 137 (1981) (corr. 42, 260);
    nitrosoureas)   Suppl. 7, 150 (1987)
1-(2-Chloroethyl)-3-(4-methylcyclohexyl)-1-nitrosourea (see also   Suppl. 7, 150 (1987)
    Chloroethyl nitrosoureas)
Chloroethyl nitrosoureas   Suppl. 7, 150 (1987)
Chlorofluoromethane   41, 229 (1986); Suppl. 7, 60 (1987)
Chloroform   1, 61 (1972); 20, 401 (1979)
                                                                     Suppl. 7, 152 (1987)
Chloromethyl methyl ether (technical-grade) (see also   4, 239 (1974); Suppl. 7, 131 (1987)
    Bis(chloromethyl)ether)
(4-Chloro-2-methylphenoxy)acetic acid (see MCPA)
1-Chloro-2-methylpropene   63, 315 (1995)
3-Chloro-2-methylpropene   63, 325 (1995)
2-Chloronitrobenzene   65, 263 (1996)
3-Chloronitrobenzene   65, 263 (1996)
4-Chloronitrobenzene   65, 263 (1996)
Chlorophenols   Suppl. 7, 154 (1987)
Chlorophenols (occupational exposures to)   41, 319 (1986)
Chlorophenoxy herbicides   Suppl. 7, 156 (1987)
Chlorophenoxy herbicides (occupational exposures to)   41, 357 (1986)
4-Chloro-ortho-phenylenediamine   27, 81 (1982); Suppl. 7, 60 (1987)
4-Chloro-meta-phenylenediamine   27, 82 (1982); Suppl. 7, 60 (1987)
Chloroprene   19, 131 (1979); Suppl. 7, 160 (1987)
Chloropropham   12, 55 (1976); Suppl. 7, 60 (1987)
Chloroquine   13, 47 (1977); Suppl. 7, 60 (1987)
Chlorothalonil   30, 319 (1983); Suppl. 7, 60 (1987)

para-Chloro-*ortho*-toluidine and its strong acid salts (*see also* Chlordimeform)	*16*, 277 (1978); *30*, 65 (1983); *Suppl. 7*, 60 (1987); *48*, 123 (1990)
Chlorotrianisene (*see also* Nonsteroidal oestrogens)	*21*, 139 (1979)
2-Chloro-1,1,1-trifluoroethane	*41*, 253 (1986); *Suppl. 7*, 60 (1987)
Chlorozotocin	*50*, 65 (1990)
Cholesterol	*10*, 99 (1976); *31*, 95 (1983); *Suppl. 7*, 161 (1987)
Chromic acetate (*see* Chromium and chromium compounds)	
Chromic chloride (*see* Chromium and chromium compounds)	
Chromic oxide (*see* Chromium and chromium compounds)	
Chromic phosphate (*see* Chromium and chromium compounds)	
Chromite ore (*see* Chromium and chromium compounds)	
Chromium and chromium compounds	*2*, 100 (1973); *23*, 205 (1980); *Suppl. 7*, 165 (1987); *49*, 49 (1990) (*corr. 51*, 483)
Chromium carbonyl (*see* Chromium and chromium compounds)	
Chromium potassium sulfate (*see* Chromium and chromium compounds)	
Chromium sulfate (*see* Chromium and chromium compounds)	
Chromium trioxide (*see* Chromium and chromium compounds)	
Chrysazin (*see* Dantron)	
Chrysene	*3*, 159 (1973); *32*, 247 (1983); *Suppl. 7*, 60 (1987)
Chrysoidine	*8*, 91 (1975); *Suppl. 7*, 169 (1987)
Chrysotile (*see* Asbestos)	
CI Acid Orange 3	*57*, 121 (1993)
CI Acid Red 114	*57*, 247 (1993)
CI Basic Red 9	*57*, 215 (1993)
Ciclosporin	*50*, 77 (1990)
CI Direct Blue 15	*57*, 235 (1993)
CI Disperse Yellow 3 (see Disperse Yellow 3)	
Cimetidine	*50*, 235 (1990)
Cinnamyl anthranilate	*16*, 287 (1978); *31*, 133 (1983); *Suppl. 7*, 60 (1987)
CI Pigment Red 3	*57*, 259 (1993)
CI Pigment Red 53:1 (*see* D&C Red No. 9)	
Cisplatin	*26*, 151 (1981); *Suppl. 7*, 170 (1987)
Citrinin	*40*, 67 (1986); *Suppl. 7*, 60 (1987)
Citrus Red No. 2	*8*, 101 (1975) (*corr. 42*, 254) *Suppl. 7*, 60 (1987)
Clofibrate	*24*, 39 (1980); *Suppl. 7*, 171 (1987); *66*, 391 (1996)
Clomiphene citrate	*21*, 551 (1979); *Suppl. 7*, 172 (1987)
Clonorchis sinensis (infection with)	*61*, 121 (1994)
Coal gasification	*34*, 65 (1984); *Suppl. 7*, 173 (1987)
Coal-tar pitches (*see also* Coal-tars)	*35*, 83 (1985); *Suppl. 7*, 174 (1987)
Coal-tars	*35*, 83 (1985); *Suppl. 7*, 175 (1987)
Cobalt[III] acetate (*see* Cobalt and cobalt compounds)	
Cobalt-aluminium-chromium spinel (*see* Cobalt and cobalt compounds)	
Cobalt and cobalt compounds	*52*, 363 (1991)
Cobalt[II] chloride (*see* Cobalt and cobalt compounds)	
Cobalt-chromium alloy (*see* Chromium and chromium compounds)	
Cobalt-chromium-molybdenum alloys (*see* Cobalt and cobalt compounds)	
Cobalt metal powder (*see* Cobalt and cobalt compounds)	
Cobalt naphthenate (*see* Cobalt and cobalt compounds)	
Cobalt[II] oxide (*see* Cobalt and cobalt compounds)	

Cobalt[II,III] oxide (see Cobalt and cobalt compounds)
Cobalt[II] sulfide (see Cobalt and cobalt compounds)

Coffee	51, 41 (1991) (corr. 52, 513)
Coke production	34, 101 (1984); Suppl. 7, 176 (1987)
Combined oral contraceptives (see also Oestrogens, progestins and combinations)	Suppl. 7, 297 (1987)
Conjugated oestrogens (see also Steroidal oestrogens)	21, 147 (1979)
Contraceptives, oral (see Combined oral contraceptives; Sequential oral contraceptives)	
Copper 8-hydroxyquinoline	15, 103 (1977); Suppl. 7, 61 (1987)
Coronene	32, 263 (1983); Suppl. 7, 61 (1987)
Coumarin	10, 113 (1976); Suppl. 7, 61 (1987)
Creosotes (see also Coal-tars)	35, 83 (1985); Suppl. 7, 177 (1987)
meta-Cresidine	27, 91 (1982); Suppl. 7, 61 (1987)
para-Cresidine	27, 92 (1982); Suppl. 7, 61 (1987)
Crocidolite (see Asbestos)	
Crotonaldehyde	63, 373 (1995) (corr. 65, 549)
Crude oil	45, 119 (1989)
Crystalline silica (see also Silica)	42, 39 (1987); Suppl. 7, 341 (1987)
Cycasin	1, 157 (1972) (corr. 42, 251); 10, 121 (1976); Suppl. 7, 61 (1987)
Cyclamates	22, 55 (1980); Suppl. 7, 178 (1987)
Cyclamic acid (see Cyclamates)	
Cyclochlorotine	10, 139 (1976); Suppl. 7, 61 (1987)
Cyclohexanone	47, 157 (1989)
Cyclohexylamine (see Cyclamates)	
Cyclopenta[cd]pyrene	32, 269 (1983); Suppl. 7, 61 (1987)
Cyclopropane (see Anaesthetics, volatile)	
Cyclophosphamide	9, 135 (1975); 26, 165 (1981); Suppl. 7, 182 (1987)

D

2,4-D (see also Chlorophenoxy herbicides; Chlorophenoxy herbicides, occupational exposures to)	15, 111 (1977)
Dacarbazine	26, 203 (1981); Suppl. 7, 184 (1987)
Dantron	50, 265 (1990) (corr. 59, 257)
D&C Red No. 9	8, 107 (1975); Suppl. 7, 61 (1987); 57, 203 (1993)
Dapsone	24, 59 (1980); Suppl. 7, 185 (1987)
Daunomycin	10, 145 (1976); Suppl. 7, 61 (1987)
DDD (see DDT)	
DDE (see DDT)	
DDT	5, 83 (1974) (corr. 42, 253); Suppl. 7, 186 (1987); 53, 179 (1991)
Decabromodiphenyl oxide	48, 73 (1990)
Deltamethrin	53, 251 (1991)
Deoxynivalenol (see Toxins derived from Fusarium graminearum, F. culmorum and F. crookwellense)	
Diacetylaminoazotoluene	8, 113 (1975); Suppl. 7, 61 (1987)
N,N'-Diacetylbenzidine	16, 293 (1978); Suppl. 7, 61 (1987)
Diallate	12, 69 (1976); 30, 235 (1983); Suppl. 7, 61 (1987)
2,4-Diaminoanisole	16, 51 (1978); 27, 103 (1982); Suppl. 7, 61 (1987)

4,4'-Diaminodiphenyl ether	*16*, 301 (1978); *29*, 203 (1982); Suppl. *7*, 61 (1987)
1,2-Diamino-4-nitrobenzene	*16*, 63 (1978); Suppl. *7*, 61 (1987)
1,4-Diamino-2-nitrobenzene	*16*, 73 (1978); Suppl. *7*, 61 (1987); *57*, 185 (1993)
2,6-Diamino-3-(phenylazo)pyridine (*see* Phenazopyridine hydrochloride)	
2,4-Diaminotoluene (*see also* Toluene diisocyanates)	*16*, 83 (1978); Suppl. *7*, 61 (1987)
2,5-Diaminotoluene (*see also* Toluene diisocyanates)	*16*, 97 (1978); Suppl. *7*, 61 (1987)
ortho-Dianisidine (*see* 3,3'-Dimethoxybenzidine)	
Diazepam	*13*, 57 (1977); Suppl. *7*, 189 (1987); *66*, 37 (1996)
Diazomethane	*7*, 223 (1974); Suppl. *7*, 61 (1987)
Dibenz[*a,h*]acridine	*3*, 247 (1973); *32*, 277 (1983); Suppl. *7*, 61 (1987)
Dibenz[*a,j*]acridine	*3*, 254 (1973); *32*, 283 (1983); Suppl. *7*, 61 (1987)
Dibenz[*a,c*]anthracene	*32*, 289 (1983) (*corr. 42*, 262); Suppl. *7*, 61 (1987)
Dibenz[*a,h*]anthracene	*3*, 178 (1973) (*corr. 43*, 261); *32*, 299 (1983); Suppl. *7*, 61 (1987)
Dibenz[*a,j*]anthracene	*32*, 309 (1983); Suppl. *7*, 61 (1987)
7*H*-Dibenzo[*c,g*]carbazole	*3*, 260 (1973); *32*, 315 (1983); Suppl. *7*, 61 (1987)
Dibenzodioxins, chlorinated (other than TCDD) [*see* Chlorinated dibenzodioxins (other than TCDD)]	
Dibenzo[*a,e*]fluoranthene	*32*, 321 (1983); Suppl. *7*, 61 (1987)
Dibenzo[*h,rst*]pentaphene	*3*, 197 (1973); Suppl. *7*, 62 (1987)
Dibenzo[*a,e*]pyrene	*3*, 201 (1973); *32*, 327 (1983); Suppl. *7*, 62 (1987)
Dibenzo[*a,h*]pyrene	*3*, 207 (1973); *32*, 331 (1983); Suppl. *7*, 62 (1987)
Dibenzo[*a,i*]pyrene	*3*, 215 (1973); *32*, 337 (1983); Suppl. *7*, 62 (1987)
Dibenzo[*a,l*]pyrene	*3*, 224 (1973); *32*, 343 (1983); Suppl. *7*, 62 (1987)
Dibromoacetonitrile (*see* Halogenated acetonitriles)	
1,2-Dibromo-3-chloropropane	*15*, 139 (1977); *20*, 83 (1979); Suppl. *7*, 191 (1987)
Dichloroacetic acid	*63*, 271 (1995)
Dichloroacetonitrile (*see* Halogenated acetonitriles)	
Dichloroacetylene	*39*, 369 (1986); Suppl. *7*, 62 (1987)
ortho-Dichlorobenzene	*7*, 231 (1974); *29*, 213 (1982); Suppl. *7*, 192 (1987)
para-Dichlorobenzene	*7*, 231 (1974); *29*, 215 (1982); Suppl. *7*, 192 (1987)
3,3'-Dichlorobenzidine	*4*, 49 (1974); *29*, 239 (1982); Suppl. *7*, 193 (1987)
trans-1,4-Dichlorobutene	*15*, 149 (1977); Suppl. *7*, 62 (1987)
3,3'-Dichloro-4,4'-diaminodiphenyl ether	*16*, 309 (1978); Suppl. *7*, 62 (1987)
1,2-Dichloroethane	*20*, 429 (1979); Suppl. *7*, 62 (1987)
Dichloromethane	*20*, 449 (1979); *41*, 43 (1986); Suppl. *7*, 194 (1987)
2,4-Dichlorophenol (*see* Chlorophenols; Chlorophenols, occupational exposures to)	
(2,4-Dichlorophenoxy)acetic acid (*see* 2,4-D)	

2,6-Dichloro-*para*-phenylenediamine	*39*, 325 (1986); *Suppl. 7*, 62 (1987)
1,2-Dichloropropane	*41*, 131 (1986); *Suppl. 7*, 62 (1987)
1,3-Dichloropropene (technical-grade)	*41*, 113 (1986); *Suppl. 7*, 195 (1987)
Dichlorvos	*20*, 97 (1979); *Suppl. 7*, 62 (1987); *53*, 267 (1991)
Dicofol	*30*, 87 (1983); *Suppl. 7*, 62 (1987)
Dicyclohexylamine (*see* Cyclamates)	
Dieldrin	*5*, 125 (1974); *Suppl. 7*, 196 (1987)
Dienoestrol (*see also* Nonsteroidal oestrogens)	*21*, 161 (1979)
Diepoxybutane	*11*, 115 (1976) (*corr. 42*, 255); *Suppl. 7*, 62 (1987)
Diesel and gasoline engine exhausts	*46*, 41 (1989)
Diesel fuels	*45*, 219 (1989) (*corr. 47*, 505)
Diethyl ether (*see* Anaesthetics, volatile)	
Di(2-ethylhexyl)adipate	*29*, 257 (1982); *Suppl. 7*, 62 (1987)
Di(2-ethylhexyl)phthalate	*29*, 269 (1982) (*corr. 42*, 261); *Suppl. 7*, 62 (1987)
1,2-Diethylhydrazine	*4*, 153 (1974); *Suppl. 7*, 62 (1987)
Diethylstilboestrol	*6*, 55 (1974); *21*, 173 (1979) (*corr. 42*, 259); *Suppl. 7*, 273 (1987)
Diethylstilboestrol dipropionate (*see* Diethylstilboestrol)	
Diethyl sulfate	*4*, 277 (1974); *Suppl. 7*, 198 (1987); *54*, 213 (1992)
Diglycidyl resorcinol ether	*11*, 125 (1976); *36*, 181 (1985); *Suppl. 7*, 62 (1987)
Dihydrosafrole	*1*, 170 (1972); *10*, 233 (1976) *Suppl. 7*, 62 (1987)
1,8-Dihydroxyanthraquinone (*see* Dantron)	
Dihydroxybenzenes (*see* Catechol; Hydroquinone; Resorcinol)	
Dihydroxymethylfuratrizine	*24*, 77 (1980); *Suppl. 7*, 62 (1987)
Diisopropyl sulfate	*54*, 229 (1992)
Dimethisterone (*see also* Progestins; Sequential oral contraceptives)	*6*, 167 (1974); *21*, 377 (1979))
Dimethoxane	*15*, 177 (1977); *Suppl. 7*, 62 (1987)
3,3'-Dimethoxybenzidine	*4*, 41 (1974); *Suppl. 7*, 198 (1987)
3,3'-Dimethoxybenzidine-4,4'-diisocyanate	*39*, 279 (1986); *Suppl. 7*, 62 (1987)
para-Dimethylaminoazobenzene	*8*, 125 (1975); *Suppl. 7*, 62 (1987)
para-Dimethylaminoazobenzenediazo sodium sulfonate	*8*, 147 (1975); *Suppl. 7*, 62 (1987)
trans-2-[(Dimethylamino)methylimino]-5-[2-(5-nitro-2-furyl)-vinyl]-1,3,4-oxadiazole	*7*, 147 (1974) (*corr. 42*, 253); *Suppl. 7*, 62 (1987)
4,4'-Dimethylangelicin plus ultraviolet radiation (*see also* Angelicin and some synthetic derivatives)	*Suppl. 7*, 57 (1987)
4,5'-Dimethylangelicin plus ultraviolet radiation (*see also* Angelicin and some synthetic derivatives)	*Suppl. 7*, 57 (1987)
2,6-Dimethylaniline	*57*, 323 (1993)
N,N-Dimethylaniline	*57*, 337 (1993)
Dimethylarsinic acid (*see* Arsenic and arsenic compounds)	
3,3'-Dimethylbenzidine	*1*, 87 (1972); *Suppl. 7*, 62 (1987)
Dimethylcarbamoyl chloride	*12*, 77 (1976); *Suppl. 7*, 199 (1987)
Dimethylformamide	*47*, 171 (1989)
1,1-Dimethylhydrazine	*4*, 137 (1974); *Suppl. 7*, 62 (1987)
1,2-Dimethylhydrazine	*4*, 145 (1974) (*corr. 42*, 253); *Suppl. 7*, 62 (1987)
Dimethyl hydrogen phosphite	*48*, 85 (1990)
1,4-Dimethylphenanthrene	*32*, 349 (1983); *Suppl. 7*, 62 (1987)
Dimethyl sulfate	*4*, 271 (1974); *Suppl. 7*, 200 (1987)

3,7-Dinitrofluoranthene	46, 189 (1989); 65, 297 (1996)
3,9-Dinitrofluoranthene	46, 195 (1989); 65, 297 (1996)
1,3-Dinitropyrene	46, 201 (1989)
1,6-Dinitropyrene	46, 215 (1989)
1,8-Dinitropyrene	33, 171 (1984); Suppl. 7, 63 (1987); 46, 231 (1989)
Dinitrosopentamethylenetetramine	11, 241 (1976); Suppl. 7, 63 (1987)
2,4-Dinitrotoluene	65, 309 (1996) (corr. 66, 485)
2,6-Dinitrotoluene	65, 309 (1996) (corr. 66, 485)
3,5-Dinitrotoluene	65, 309 (1996)
1,4-Dioxane	11, 247 (1976); Suppl. 7, 201 (1987)
2,4'-Diphenyldiamine	16, 313 (1978); Suppl. 7, 63 (1987)
Direct Black 38 (see also Benzidine-based dyes)	29, 295 (1982) (corr. 42, 261)
Direct Blue 6 (see also Benzidine-based dyes)	29, 311 (1982)
Direct Brown 95 (see also Benzidine-based dyes)	29, 321 (1982)
Disperse Blue 1	48, 139 (1990)
Disperse Yellow 3	8, 97 (1975); Suppl. 7, 60 (1987); 48, 149 (1990)
Disulfiram	12, 85 (1976); Suppl. 7, 63 (1987)
Dithranol	13, 75 (1977); Suppl. 7, 63 (1987)
Divinyl ether (see Anaesthetics, volatile)	
Doxefazepam	66, 97 (1996)
Droloxifene	66, 241 (1996)
Dry cleaning	63, 33 (1995)
Dulcin	12, 97 (1976); Suppl. 7, 63 (1987)

E

Endrin	5, 157 (1974); Suppl. 7, 63 (1987)
Enflurane (see Anaesthetics, volatile)	
Eosin	15, 183 (1977); Suppl. 7, 63 (1987)
Epichlorohydrin	11, 131 (1976) (corr. 42, 256); Suppl. 7, 202 (1987)
1,2-Epoxybutane	47, 217 (1989)
1-Epoxyethyl-3,4-epoxycyclohexane (see 4-Vinylcyclohexene diepoxide)	
3,4-Epoxy-6-methylcyclohexylmethyl-3,4-epoxy-6-methyl-cyclohexane carboxylate	11, 147 (1976); Suppl. 7, 63 (1987)
cis-9,10-Epoxystearic acid	11, 153 (1976); Suppl. 7, 63 (1987)
Erionite	42, 225 (1987); Suppl. 7, 203 (1987)
Estazolam	66, 105 (1996)
Ethinyloestradiol (see also Steroidal oestrogens)	6, 77 (1974); 21, 233 (1979)
Ethionamide	13, 83 (1977); Suppl. 7, 63 (1987)
Ethyl acrylate	19, 57 (1979); 39, 81 (1986); Suppl. 7, 63 (1987)
Ethylene	19, 157 (1979); Suppl. 7, 63 (1987); 60, 45 (1994)
Ethylene dibromide	15, 195 (1977); Suppl. 7, 204 (1987)
Ethylene oxide	11, 157 (1976); 36, 189 (1985) (corr. 42, 263); Suppl. 7, 205 (1987); 60, 73 (1994)
Ethylene sulfide	11, 257 (1976); Suppl. 7, 63 (1987)
Ethylene thiourea	7, 45 (1974); Suppl. 7, 207 (1987)
2-Ethylhexyl acrylate	60, 475 (1994)
Ethyl methanesulfonate	7, 245 (1974); Suppl. 7, 63 (1987)

N-Ethyl-N-nitrosourea	1, 135 (1972); 17, 191 (1978); Suppl. 7, 63 (1987)
Ethyl selenac (see also Selenium and selenium compounds)	12, 107 (1976); Suppl. 7, 63 (1987)
Ethyl tellurac	12, 115 (1976); Suppl. 7, 63 (1987)
Ethynodiol diacetate (see also Progestins; Combined oral contraceptives)	6, 173 (1974); 21, 387 (1979)
Eugenol	36, 75 (1985); Suppl. 7, 63 (1987)
Evans blue	8, 151 (1975); Suppl. 7, 63 (1987)

F

Fast Green FCF	16, 187 (1978); Suppl. 7, 63 (1987)
Fenvalerate	53, 309 (1991)
Ferbam	12, 121 (1976) (corr. 42, 256); Suppl. 7, 63 (1987)
Ferric oxide	1, 29 (1972); Suppl. 7, 216 (1987)
Ferrochromium (see Chromium and chromium compounds)	
Fluometuron	30, 245 (1983); Suppl. 7, 63 (1987)
Fluoranthene	32, 355 (1983); Suppl. 7, 63 (1987)
Fluorene	32, 365 (1983); Suppl. 7, 63 (1987)
Fluorescent lighting (exposure to) (see Ultraviolet radiation)	
Fluorides (inorganic, used in drinking-water)	27, 237 (1982); Suppl. 7, 208 (1987)
5-Fluorouracil	26, 217 (1981); Suppl. 7, 210 (1987)
Fluorspar (see Fluorides)	
Fluosilicic acid (see Fluorides)	
Fluroxene (see Anaesthetics, volatile)	
Formaldehyde	29, 345 (1982); Suppl. 7, 211 (1987); 62, 217 (1995) (corr. 65, 549; corr. 66, 485)
2-(2-Formylhydrazino)-4-(5-nitro-2-furyl)thiazole	7, 151 (1974) (corr. 42, 253); Suppl. 7, 63 (1987)
Frusemide (see Furosemide)	
Fuel oils (heating oils)	45, 239 (1989) (corr. 47, 505)
Fumonisin B$_1$ (see Toxins derived from Fusarium moniliforme)	
Fumonisin B$_2$ (see Toxins derived from Fusarium moniliforme)	
Furan	63, 393 (1995)
Furazolidone	31, 141 (1983); Suppl. 7, 63 (1987)
Furfural	63, 409 (1995)
Furniture and cabinet-making	25, 99 (1981); Suppl. 7, 380 (1987)
Furosemide	50, 277 (1990)
2-(2-Furyl)-3-(5-nitro-2-furyl)acrylamide (see AF-2)	
Fusarenon-X (see Toxins derived from Fusarium graminearum, F. culmorum and F. crookwellense)	
Fusarenone-X (see Toxins derived from Fusarium graminearum, F. culmorum and F. crookwellense)	
Fusarin C (see Toxins derived from Fusarium moniliforme)	

G

Gasoline	45, 159 (1989) (corr. 47, 505)
Gasoline engine exhaust (see Diesel and gasoline engine exhausts)	
Gemfibrozil	66, 427 (1996)
Glass fibres (see Man-made mineral fibres)	

Glass manufacturing industry, occupational exposures in	58, 347 (1993)
Glasswool (see Man-made mineral fibres)	
Glass filaments (see Man-made mineral fibres)	
Glu-P-1	40, 223 (1986); Suppl. 7, 64 (1987)
Glu-P-2	40, 235 (1986); Suppl. 7, 64 (1987)
L-Glutamic acid, 5-[2-(4-hydroxymethyl)phenylhydrazide] (see Agaritine)	
Glycidaldehyde	11, 175 (1976); Suppl. 7, 64 (1987)
Glycidyl ethers	47, 237 (1989)
Glycidyl oleate	11, 183 (1976); Suppl. 7, 64 (1987)
Glycidyl stearate	11, 187 (1976); Suppl. 7, 64 (1987)
Griseofulvin	10, 153 (1976); Suppl. 7, 391 (1987)
Guinea Green B	16, 199 (1978); Suppl. 7, 64 (1987)
Gyromitrin	31, 163 (1983); Suppl. 7, 391 (1987)

H

Haematite	1, 29 (1972); Suppl. 7, 216 (1987)
Haematite and ferric oxide	Suppl. 7, 216 (1987)
Haematite mining, underground, with exposure to radon	1, 29 (1972); Suppl. 7, 216 (1987)
Hairdressers and barbers (occupational exposure as)	57, 43 (1993)
Hair dyes, epidemiology of	16, 29 (1978); 27, 307 (1982);
Halogenated acetonitriles	52, 269 (1991)
Halothane (see Anaesthetics, volatile)	
HC Blue No. 1	57, 129 (1993)
HC Blue No. 2	57, 143 (1993)
α-HCH (see Hexachlorocyclohexanes)	
β-HCH (see Hexachlorocyclohexanes)	
γ-HCH (see Hexachlorocyclohexanes)	
HC Red No. 3	57, 153 (1993)
HC Yellow No. 4	57, 159 (1993)
Heating oils (see Fuel oils)	
Helicobacter pylori (infection with)	61, 177 (1994)
Hepatitis B virus	59, 45 (1994)
Hepatitis C virus	59, 165 (1994)
Hepatitis D virus	59, 223 (1994)
Heptachlor (see also Chlordane/Heptachlor)	5, 173 (1974); 20, 129 (1979)
Hexachlorobenzene	20, 155 (1979); Suppl. 7, 219 (1987)
Hexachlorobutadiene	20, 179 (1979); Suppl. 7, 64 (1987)
Hexachlorocyclohexanes	5, 47 (1974); 20, 195 (1979) (corr. 42, 258); Suppl. 7, 220 (1987)
Hexachlorocyclohexane, technical-grade (see Hexachlorocyclohexanes)	
Hexachloroethane	20, 467 (1979); Suppl. 7, 64 (1987)
Hexachlorophene	20, 241 (1979); Suppl. 7, 64 (1987)
Hexamethylphosphoramide	15, 211 (1977); Suppl. 7, 64 (1987)
Hexoestrol (see Nonsteroidal oestrogens)	
Human immunodeficiency viruses	67, 31 (1996)
Human papillomaviruses	64 (1995) (corr. 66, 485)
Human T-cell lymphotropic viruses	67, 261 (1996)
Hycanthone mesylate	13, 91 (1977); Suppl. 7, 64 (1987)
Hydralazine	24, 85 (1980); Suppl. 7, 222 (1987)
Hydrazine	4, 127 (1974); Suppl. 7, 223 (1987)
Hydrochloric acid	54, 189 (1992)
Hydrochlorothiazide	50, 293 (1990)

Hydrogen peroxide	36, 285 (1985); Suppl. 7, 64 (1987)
Hydroquinone	15, 155 (1977); Suppl. 7, 64 (1987)
4-Hydroxyazobenzene	8, 157 (1975); Suppl. 7, 64 (1987)
17α-Hydroxyprogesterone caproate (see also Progestins)	21, 399 (1979) (corr. 42, 259)
8-Hydroxyquinoline	13, 101 (1977); Suppl. 7, 64 (1987)
8-Hydroxysenkirkine	10, 265 (1976); Suppl. 7, 64 (1987)
Hypochlorite salts	52, 159 (1991)

I

Indeno[1,2,3-cd]pyrene	3, 229 (1973); 32, 373 (1983); Suppl. 7, 64 (1987)
Inorganic acids (see Sulfuric acid and other strong inorganic acids, occupational exposures to mists and vapours from)	
Insecticides, occupational exposures in spraying and application of	53, 45 (1991)
IQ	40, 261 (1986); Suppl. 7, 64 (1987); 56, 165 (1993)
Iron and steel founding	34, 133 (1984); Suppl. 7, 224 (1987)
Iron-dextran complex	2, 161 (1973); Suppl. 7, 226 (1987)
Iron-dextrin complex	2, 161 (1973) (corr. 42, 252); Suppl. 7, 64 (1987)
Iron oxide (see Ferric oxide)	
Iron oxide, saccharated (see Saccharated iron oxide)	
Iron sorbitol-citric acid complex	2, 161 (1973); Suppl. 7, 64 (1987)
Isatidine	10, 269 (1976); Suppl. 7, 65 (1987)
Isoflurane (see Anaesthetics, volatile)	
Isoniazid (see Isonicotinic acid hydrazide)	
Isonicotinic acid hydrazide	4, 159 (1974); Suppl. 7, 227 (1987)
Isophosphamide	26, 237 (1981); Suppl. 7, 65 (1987)
Isoprene	60, 215 (1994)
Isopropanol	15, 223 (1977); Suppl. 7, 229 (1987)
Isopropanol manufacture (strong-acid process) (see also Isopropanol; Sulfuric acid and other strong inorganic acids, occupational exposures to mists and vapours from)	Suppl. 7, 229 (1987)
Isopropyl oils	15, 223 (1977); Suppl. 7, 229 (1987)
Isosafrole	1, 169 (1972); 10, 232 (1976); Suppl. 7, 65 (1987)

J

Jacobine	10, 275 (1976); Suppl. 7, 65 (1987)
Jet fuel	45, 203 (1989)
Joinery (see Carpentry and joinery)	

K

Kaempferol	31, 171 (1983); Suppl. 7, 65 (1987)
Kepone (see Chlordecone)	

L

Lasiocarpine	10, 281 (1976); Suppl. 7, 65 (1987)

Lauroyl peroxide	36, 315 (1985); Suppl. 7, 65 (1987)
Lead acetate (see Lead and lead compounds)	
Lead and lead compounds	1, 40 (1972) (corr. 42, 251); 2, 52, 150 (1973); 12, 131 (1976); 23, 40, 208, 209, 325 (1980); Suppl. 7, 230 (1987)
Lead arsenate (see Arsenic and arsenic compounds)	
Lead carbonate (see Lead and lead compounds)	
Lead chloride (see Lead and lead compounds)	
Lead chromate (see Chromium and chromium compounds)	
Lead chromate oxide (see Chromium and chromium compounds)	
Lead naphthenate (see Lead and lead compounds)	
Lead nitrate (see Lead and lead compounds)	
Lead oxide (see Lead and lead compounds)	
Lead phosphate (see Lead and lead compounds)	
Lead subacetate (see Lead and lead compounds)	
Lead tetroxide (see Lead and lead compounds)	
Leather goods manufacture	25, 279 (1981); Suppl. 7, 235 (1987)
Leather industries	25, 199 (1981); Suppl. 7, 232 (1987)
Leather tanning and processing	25, 201 (1981); Suppl. 7, 236 (1987)
Ledate (see also Lead and lead compounds)	12, 131 (1976)
Light Green SF	16, 209 (1978); Suppl. 7, 65 (1987)
d-Limonene	56, 135 (1993)
Lindane (see Hexachlorocyclohexanes)	
Liver flukes (see Clonorchis sinensis, Opisthorchis felineus and Opisthorchis viverrini)	
Lumber and sawmill industries (including logging)	25, 49 (1981); Suppl. 7, 383 (1987)
Luteoskyrin	10, 163 (1976); Suppl. 7, 65 (1987)
Lynoestrenol (see also Progestins; Combined oral contraceptives)	21, 407 (1979)

M

Magenta	4, 57 (1974) (corr. 42, 252); Suppl. 7, 238 (1987); 57, 215 (1993)
Magenta, manufacture of (see also Magenta)	Suppl. 7, 238 (1987); 57, 215 (1993)
Malathion	30, 103 (1983); Suppl. 7, 65 (1987)
Maleic hydrazide	4, 173 (1974) (corr. 42, 253); Suppl. 7, 65 (1987)
Malonaldehyde	36, 163 (1985); Suppl. 7, 65 (1987)
Maneb	12, 137 (1976); Suppl. 7, 65 (1987)
Man-made mineral fibres	43, 39 (1988)
Mannomustine	9, 157 (1975); Suppl. 7, 65 (1987)
Mate	51, 273 (1991)
MCPA (see also Chlorophenoxy herbicides; Chlorophenoxy herbicides, occupational exposures to)	30, 255 (1983)
MeA-α-C	40, 253 (1986); Suppl. 7, 65 (1987)
Medphalan	9, 168 (1975); Suppl. 7, 65 (1987)
Medroxyprogesterone acetate	6, 157 (1974); 21, 417 (1979) (corr. 42, 259); Suppl. 7, 289 (1987)
Megestrol acetate (see also Progestins; Combined oral contraceptives)	
MeIQ	40, 275 (1986); Suppl. 7, 65 (1987); 56, 197 (1993)
MeIQx	40, 283 (1986); Suppl. 7, 65 (1987); 56, 211 (1993)

Melamine	39, 333 (1986); Suppl. 7, 65 (1987)
Melphalan	9, 167 (1975); Suppl. 7, 239 (1987)
6-Mercaptopurine	26, 249 (1981); Suppl. 7, 240 (1987)
Mercuric chloride (see Mercury and mercury compounds)	
Mercury and mercury compounds	58, 239 (1993)
Merphalan	9, 169 (1975); Suppl. 7, 65 (1987)
Mestranol (see also Steroidal oestrogens)	6, 87 (1974); 21, 257 (1979) (corr. 42, 259)
Metabisulfites (see Sulfur dioxide and some sulfites, bisulfites and metabisulfites)	
Metallic mercury (see Mercury and mercury compounds)	
Methanearsonic acid, disodium salt (see Arsenic and arsenic compounds)	
Methanearsonic acid, monosodium salt (see Arsenic and arsenic compounds	
Methotrexate	26, 267 (1981); Suppl. 7, 241 (1987)
Methoxsalen (see 8-Methoxypsoralen)	
Methoxychlor	5, 193 (1974); 20, 259 (1979); Suppl. 7, 66 (1987)
Methoxyflurane (see Anaesthetics, volatile)	
5-Methoxypsoralen	40, 327 (1986); Suppl. 7, 242 (1987)
8-Methoxypsoralen (see also 8-Methoxypsoralen plus ultraviolet radiation)	24, 101 (1980)
8-Methoxypsoralen plus ultraviolet radiation	Suppl. 7, 243 (1987)
Methyl acrylate	19, 52 (1979); 39, 99 (1986); Suppl. 7, 66 (1987)
5-Methylangelicin plus ultraviolet radiation (see also Angelicin and some synthetic derivatives)	Suppl. 7, 57 (1987)
2-Methylaziridine	9, 61 (1975); Suppl. 7, 66 (1987)
Methylazoxymethanol acetate	1, 164 (1972); 10, 131 (1976); Suppl. 7, 66 (1987)
Methyl bromide	41, 187 (1986) (corr. 45, 283); Suppl. 7, 245 (1987)
Methyl carbamate	12, 151 (1976); Suppl. 7, 66 (1987)
Methyl-CCNU [see 1-(2-Chloroethyl)-3-(4-methylcyclohexyl)-1-nitrosourea]	
Methyl chloride	41, 161 (1986); Suppl. 7, 246 (1987)
1-, 2-, 3-, 4-, 5- and 6-Methylchrysenes	32, 379 (1983); Suppl. 7, 66 (1987)
N-Methyl-N,4-dinitrosoaniline	1, 141 (1972); Suppl. 7, 66 (1987)
4,4'-Methylene bis(2-chloroaniline)	4, 65 (1974) (corr. 42, 252); Suppl. 7, 246 (1987); 57, 271 (1993)
4,4'-Methylene bis(N,N-dimethyl)benzenamine	27, 119 (1982); Suppl. 7, 66 (1987)
4,4'-Methylene bis(2-methylaniline)	4, 73 (1974); Suppl. 7, 248 (1987)
4,4'-Methylenedianiline	4, 79 (1974) (corr. 42, 252); 39, 347 (1986); Suppl. 7, 66 (1987)
4,4'-Methylenediphenyl diisocyanate	19, 314 (1979); Suppl. 7, 66 (1987)
2-Methylfluoranthene	32, 399 (1983); Suppl. 7, 66 (1987)
3-Methylfluoranthene	32, 399 (1983); Suppl. 7, 66 (1987)
Methylglyoxal	51, 443 (1991)
Methyl iodide	15, 245 (1977); 41, 213 (1986); Suppl. 7, 66 (1987)
Methylmercury chloride (see Mercury and mercury compounds)	
Methylmercury compounds (see Mercury and mercury compounds)	
Methyl methacrylate	19, 187 (1979); Suppl. 7, 66 (1987); 60, 445 (1994)
Methyl methanesulfonate	7, 253 (1974); Suppl. 7, 66 (1987)

2-Methyl-1-nitroanthraquinone	*27*, 205 (1982); *Suppl. 7*, 66 (1987)
N-Methyl-N-nitro-N-nitrosoguanidine	*4*, 183 (1974); *Suppl. 7*, 248 (1987)
3-Methylnitrosaminopropionaldehyde [*see* 3-(N-Nitrosomethylamino)-propionaldehyde]	
3-Methylnitrosaminopropionitrile [*see* 3-(N-Nitrosomethylamino)-propionitrile]	
4-(Methylnitrosamino)-4-(3-pyridyl)-1-butanal [*see* 4-(N-Nitrosomethylamino)-4-(3-pyridyl)-1-butanal]	
4-(Methylnitrosamino)-1-(3-pyridyl)-1-butanone [*see* 4-(-Nitrosomethylamino)-1-(3-pyridyl)-1-butanone]	
N-Methyl-N-nitrosourea	*1*, 125 (1972); *17*, 227 (1978); *Suppl. 7*, 66 (1987)
N-Methyl-N-nitrosourethane	*4*, 211 (1974); *Suppl. 7*, 66 (1987)
N-Methylolacrylamide	*60*, 435 (1994)
Methyl parathion	*30*, 131 (1983); *Suppl. 7*, 392 (1987)
1-Methylphenanthrene	*32*, 405 (1983); *Suppl. 7*, 66 (1987)
7-Methylpyrido[3,4-c]psoralen	*40*, 349 (1986); *Suppl. 7*, 71 (1987)
Methyl red	*8*, 161 (1975); *Suppl. 7*, 66 (1987)
Methyl selenac (*see also* Selenium and selenium compounds)	*12*, 161 (1976); *Suppl. 7*, 66 (1987)
Methylthiouracil	*7*, 53 (1974); *Suppl. 7*, 66 (1987)
Metronidazole	*13*, 113 (1977); *Suppl. 7*, 250 (1987)
Mineral oils	*3*, 30 (1973); *33*, 87 (1984) (*corr. 42*, 262); *Suppl. 7*, 252 (1987)
Mirex	*5*, 203 (1974); *20*, 283 (1979) (*corr. 42*, 258); *Suppl. 7*, 66 (1987)
Mists and vapours from sulfuric acid and other strong inorganic acids	*54*, 41 (1992)
Mitomycin C	*10*, 171 (1976); *Suppl. 7*, 67 (1987)
MNNG [*see* N-Methyl-N-nitro-N-nitrosoguanidine]	
MOCA [*see* 4,4'-Methylene bis(2-chloroaniline)]	
Modacrylic fibres	*19*, 86 (1979); *Suppl. 7*, 67 (1987)
Monocrotaline	*10*, 291 (1976); *Suppl. 7*, 67 (1987)
Monuron	*12*, 167 (1976); *Suppl. 7*, 67 (1987); *53*, 467 (1991)
MOPP and other combined chemotherapy including alkylating agents	*Suppl. 7*, 254 (1987)
Morpholine	*47*, 199 (1989)
5-(Morpholinomethyl)-3-[(5-nitrofurfurylidene)amino]-2-oxazolidinone	*7*, 161 (1974); *Suppl. 7*, 67 (1987)
Musk ambrette	*65*, 477 (1996)
Musk xylene	*65*, 477 (1996)
Mustard gas	*9*, 181 (1975) (*corr. 42*, 254); *Suppl. 7*, 259 (1987)
Myleran (*see* 1,4-Butanediol dimethanesulfonate)	

N

Nafenopin	*24*, 125 (1980); *Suppl. 7*, 67 (1987)
1,5-Naphthalenediamine	*27*, 127 (1982); *Suppl. 7*, 67 (1987)
1,5-Naphthalene diisocyanate	*19*, 311 (1979); *Suppl. 7*, 67 (1987)
1-Naphthylamine	*4*, 87 (1974) (*corr. 42*, 253); *Suppl. 7*, 260 (1987)
2-Naphthylamine	*4*, 97 (1974); *Suppl. 7*, 261 (1987)
1-Naphthylthiourea	*30*, 347 (1983); *Suppl. 7*, 263 (1987)
Nickel acetate (*see* Nickel and nickel compounds)	

Nickel ammonium sulfate (*see* Nickel and nickel compounds)	
Nickel and nickel compounds	2, 126 (1973) (*corr.* 42, 252); *11*, 75 (1976); *Suppl. 7*, 264 (1987) (*corr.* 45, 283); 49, 257 (1990)
Nickel carbonate (*see* Nickel and nickel compounds)	
Nickel carbonyl (*see* Nickel and nickel compounds)	
Nickel chloride (*see* Nickel and nickel compounds)	
Nickel-gallium alloy (*see* Nickel and nickel compounds)	
Nickel hydroxide (*see* Nickel and nickel compounds)	
Nickelocene (*see* Nickel and nickel compounds)	
Nickel oxide (*see* Nickel and nickel compounds)	
Nickel subsulfide (*see* Nickel and nickel compounds)	
Nickel sulfate (*see* Nickel and nickel compounds)	
Niridazole	*13*, 123 (1977); *Suppl. 7*, 67 (1987)
Nithiazide	*31*, 179 (1983); *Suppl. 7*, 67 (1987)
Nitrilotriacetic acid and its salts	48, 181 (1990)
5-Nitroacenaphthene	*16*, 319 (1978); *Suppl. 7*, 67 (1987)
5-Nitro-*ortho*-anisidine	27, 133 (1982); *Suppl. 7*, 67 (1987)
2-Nitroanisole	65, 369 (1996)
9-Nitroanthracene	*33*, 179 (1984); *Suppl. 7*, 67 (1987)
7-Nitrobenz[*a*]anthracene	46, 247 (1989)
Nitrobenzene	65, 381 (1996)
6-Nitrobenzo[*a*]pyrene	*33*, 187 (1984); *Suppl. 7*, 67 (1987); 46, 255 (1989)
4-Nitrobiphenyl	4, 113 (1974); *Suppl. 7*, 67 (1987)
6-Nitrochrysene	*33*, 195 (1984); *Suppl. 7*, 67 (1987); 46, 267 (1989)
Nitrofen (technical-grade)	30, 271 (1983); *Suppl. 7*, 67 (1987)
3-Nitrofluoranthene	*33*, 201 (1984); *Suppl. 7*, 67 (1987)
2-Nitrofluorene	46, 277 (1989)
Nitrofural	7, 171 (1974); *Suppl. 7*, 67 (1987); *50*, 195 (1990)
5-Nitro-2-furaldehyde semicarbazone (*see* Nitrofural)	
Nitrofurantoin	*50*, 211 (1990)
Nitrofurazone (*see* Nitrofural)	
1-[(5-Nitrofurfurylidene)amino]-2-imidazolidinone	7, 181 (1974); *Suppl. 7*, 67 (1987)
N-[4-(5-Nitro-2-furyl)-2-thiazolyl]acetamide	*1*, 181 (1972); 7, 185 (1974); *Suppl. 7*, 67 (1987)
Nitrogen mustard	9, 193 (1975); *Suppl. 7*, 269 (1987)
Nitrogen mustard *N*-oxide	9, 209 (1975); *Suppl. 7*, 67 (1987)
1-Nitronaphthalene	46, 291 (1989)
2-Nitronaphthalene	46, 303 (1989)
3-Nitroperylene	46, 313 (1989)
2-Nitro-*para*-phenylenediamine (*see* 1,4-Diamino-2-nitrobenzene)	
2-Nitropropane	29, 331 (1982); *Suppl. 7*, 67 (1987)
1-Nitropyrene	*33*, 209 (1984); *Suppl. 7*, 67 (1987); 46, 321 (1989)
2-Nitropyrene	46, 359 (1989)
4-Nitropyrene	46, 367 (1989)
N-Nitrosatable drugs	24, 297 (1980) (*corr.* 42, 260)
N-Nitrosatable pesticides	30, 359 (1983)
N-Nitrosoanabasine	37, 225 (1985); *Suppl. 7*, 67 (1987)
N-Nitrosoanatabine	37, 233 (1985); *Suppl. 7*, 67 (1987)
N-Nitrosodi-*n*-butylamine	4, 197 (1974); *17*, 51 (1978); *Suppl. 7*, 67 (1987)

N-Nitrosodiethanolamine	17, 77 (1978); Suppl. 7, 67 (1987)
N-Nitrosodiethylamine	1, 107 (1972) (corr. 42, 251); 17, 83 (1978) (corr. 42, 257); Suppl. 7, 67 (1987)
N-Nitrosodimethylamine	1, 95 (1972); 17, 125 (1978) (corr. 42, 257); Suppl. 7, 67 (1987)
N-Nitrosodiphenylamine	27, 213 (1982); Suppl. 7, 67 (1987)
para-Nitrosodiphenylamine	27, 227 (1982) (corr. 42, 261); Suppl. 7, 68 (1987)
N-Nitrosodi-n-propylamine	17, 177 (1978); Suppl. 7, 68 (1987)
N-Nitroso-N-ethylurea (see N-Ethyl-N-nitrosourea)	
N-Nitrosofolic acid	17, 217 (1978); Suppl. 7, 68 (1987)
N-Nitrosoguvacine	37, 263 (1985); Suppl. 7, 68 (1987)
N-Nitrosoguvacoline	37, 263 (1985); Suppl. 7, 68 (1987)
N-Nitrosohydroxyproline	17, 304 (1978); Suppl. 7, 68 (1987)
3-(N-Nitrosomethylamino)propionaldehyde	37, 263 (1985); Suppl. 7, 68 (1987)
3-(N-Nitrosomethylamino)propionitrile	37, 263 (1985); Suppl. 7, 68 (1987)
4-(N-Nitrosomethylamino)-4-(3-pyridyl)-1-butanal	37, 205 (1985); Suppl. 7, 68 (1987)
4-(N-Nitrosomethylamino)-1-(3-pyridyl)-1-butanone	37, 209 (1985); Suppl. 7, 68 (1987)
N-Nitrosomethylethylamine	17, 221 (1978); Suppl. 7, 68 (1987)
N-Nitroso-N-methylurea (see N-Methyl-N-nitrosourea)	
N-Nitroso-N-methylurethane (see N-Methyl-N-nitrosourethane)	
N-Nitrosomethylvinylamine	17, 257 (1978); Suppl. 7, 68 (1987)
N-Nitrosomorpholine	17, 263 (1978); Suppl. 7, 68 (1987)
N-Nitrosonornicotine	17, 281 (1978); 37, 241 (1985); Suppl. 7, 68 (1987)
N-Nitrosopiperidine	17, 287 (1978); Suppl. 7, 68 (1987)
N-Nitrosoproline	17, 303 (1978); Suppl. 7, 68 (1987)
N-Nitrosopyrrolidine	17, 313 (1978); Suppl. 7, 68 (1987)
N-Nitrososarcosine	17, 327 (1978); Suppl. 7, 68 (1987)
Nitrosoureas, chloroethyl (see Chloroethyl nitrosoureas)	
5-Nitro-ortho-toluidine	48, 169 (1990)
2-Nitrotoluene	65, 409 (1996)
3-Nitrotoluene	65, 409 (1996)
4-Nitrotoluene	65, 409 (1996)
Nitrous oxide (see Anaesthetics, volatile)	
Nitrovin	31, 185 (1983); Suppl. 7, 68 (1987)
Nivalenol (see Toxins derived from Fusarium graminearum, F. culmorum and F. crookwellense)	
NNA [see 4-(N-Nitrosomethylamino)-4-(3-pyridyl)-1-butanal]	
NNK [see 4-(N-Nitrosomethylamino)-1-(3-pyridyl)-1-butanone]	
Nonsteroidal oestrogens (see also Oestrogens, progestins and combinations)	Suppl. 7, 272 (1987)
Norethisterone (see also Progestins; Combined oral contraceptives)	6, 179 (1974); 21, 461 (1979)
Norethynodrel (see also Progestins; Combined oral contraceptives)	6, 191 (1974); 21, 461 (1979) (corr. 42, 259)
Norgestrel (see also Progestins, Combined oral contraceptives)	6, 201 (1974); 21, 479 (1979)
Nylon 6	19, 120 (1979); Suppl. 7, 68 (1987)

O

Ochratoxin A	10, 191 (1976); 31, 191 (1983) (corr. 42, 262); Suppl. 7, 271 (1987); 56, 489 (1993)

Oestradiol-17β (see also Steroidal oestrogens)	6, 99 (1974); 21, 279 (1979)
Oestradiol 3-benzoate (see Oestradiol-17β)	
Oestradiol dipropionate (see Oestradiol-17β)	
Oestradiol mustard	9, 217 (1975); Suppl. 7, 68 (1987)
Oestradiol-17β-valerate (see Oestradiol-17β)	
Oestriol (see also Steroidal oestrogens)	6, 117 (1974); 21, 327 (1979); Suppl. 7, 285 (1987)
Oestrogen-progestin combinations (see Oestrogens, progestins and combinations)	
Oestrogen-progestin replacement therapy (see also Oestrogens, progestins and combinations)	Suppl. 7, 308 (1987)
Oestrogen replacement therapy (see also Oestrogens, progestins and combinations)	Suppl. 7, 280 (1987)
Oestrogens (see Oestrogens, progestins and combinations)	
Oestrogens, conjugated (see Conjugated oestrogens)	
Oestrogens, nonsteroidal (see Nonsteroidal oestrogens)	
Oestrogens, progestins and combinations	6 (1974); 21 (1979); Suppl. 7, 272 (1987)
Oestrogens, steroidal (see Steroidal oestrogens)	
Oestrone (see also Steroidal oestrogens)	6, 123 (1974); 21, 343 (1979) (corr. 42, 259)
Oestrone benzoate (see Oestrone)	
Oil Orange SS	8, 165 (1975); Suppl. 7, 69 (1987)
Opisthorchis felineus (infection with)	61, 121 (1994)
Opisthorchis viverrini (infection with)	61, 121 (1994)
Oral contraceptives, combined (see Combined oral contraceptives)	
Oral contraceptives, investigational (see Combined oral contraceptives)	
Oral contraceptives, sequential (see Sequential oral contraceptives)	
Orange I	8, 173 (1975); Suppl. 7, 69 (1987)
Orange G	8, 181 (1975); Suppl. 7, 69 (1987)
Organolead compounds (see also Lead and lead compounds)	Suppl. 7, 230 (1987)
Oxazepam	13, 58 (1977); Suppl. 7, 69 (1987); 66, 115 (1996)
Oxymetholone [see also Androgenic (anabolic) steroids]	13, 131 (1977)
Oxyphenbutazone	13, 185 (1977); Suppl. 7, 69 (1987)

P

Paint manufacture and painting (occupational exposures in)	47, 329 (1989)
Panfuran S (see also Dihydroxymethylfuratrizine)	24, 77 (1980); Suppl. 7, 69 (1987)
Paper manufacture (see Pulp and paper manufacture)	
Paracetamol	50, 307 (1990)
Parasorbic acid	10, 199 (1976) (corr. 42, 255); Suppl. 7, 69 (1987)
Parathion	30, 153 (1983); Suppl. 7, 69 (1987)
Patulin	10, 205 (1976); 40, 83 (1986); Suppl. 7, 69 (1987)
Penicillic acid	10, 211 (1976); Suppl. 7, 69 (1987)
Pentachloroethane	41, 99 (1986); Suppl. 7, 69 (1987)
Pentachloronitrobenzene (see Quintozene)	
Pentachlorophenol (see also Chlorophenols; Chlorophenols, occupational exposures to)	20, 303 (1979); 53, 371 (1991)
Permethrin	53, 329 (1991)
Perylene	32, 411 (1983); Suppl. 7, 69 (1987)

Petasitenine	31, 207 (1983); Suppl. 7, 69 (1987)
Petasites japonicus (see Pyrrolizidine alkaloids)	
Petroleum refining (occupational exposures in)	45, 39 (1989)
Petroleum solvents	47, 43 (1989)
Phenacetin	13, 141 (1977); 24, 135 (1980); Suppl. 7, 310 (1987)
Phenanthrene	32, 419 (1983); Suppl. 7, 69 (1987)
Phenazopyridine hydrochloride	8, 117 (1975); 24, 163 (1980) (corr. 42, 260); Suppl. 7, 312 (1987)
Phenelzine sulfate	24, 175 (1980); Suppl. 7, 312 (1987)
Phenicarbazide	12, 177 (1976); Suppl. 7, 70 (1987)
Phenobarbital	13, 157 (1977); Suppl. 7, 313 (1987)
Phenol	47, 263 (1989) (corr. 50, 385)
Phenoxyacetic acid herbicides (see Chlorophenoxy herbicides)	
Phenoxybenzamine hydrochloride	9, 223 (1975); 24, 185 (1980); Suppl. 7, 70 (1987)
Phenylbutazone	13, 183 (1977); Suppl. 7, 316 (1987)
meta-Phenylenediamine	16, 111 (1978); Suppl. 7, 70 (1987)
para-Phenylenediamine	16, 125 (1978); Suppl. 7, 70 (1987)
Phenyl glycidyl ether (see Glycidyl ethers)	
N-Phenyl-2-naphthylamine	16, 325 (1978) (corr. 42, 257); Suppl. 7, 318 (1987)
ortho-Phenylphenol	30, 329 (1983); Suppl. 7, 70 (1987)
Phenytoin	13, 201 (1977); Suppl. 7, 319 (1987); 66, 175 (1996)
PhIP	56, 229 (1993)
Pickled vegetables	56, 83 (1993)
Picloram	53, 481 (1991)
Piperazine oestrone sulfate (see Conjugated oestrogens)	
Piperonyl butoxide	30, 183 (1983); Suppl. 7, 70 (1987)
Pitches, coal-tar (see Coal-tar pitches)	
Polyacrylic acid	19, 62 (1979); Suppl. 7, 70 (1987)
Polybrominated biphenyls	18, 107 (1978); 41, 261 (1986); Suppl. 7, 321 (1987)
Polychlorinated biphenyls	7, 261 (1974); 18, 43 (1978) (corr. 42, 258); Suppl. 7, 322 (1987)
Polychlorinated camphenes (see Toxaphene)	
Polychloroprene	19, 141 (1979); Suppl. 7, 70 (1987)
Polyethylene	19, 164 (1979); Suppl. 7, 70 (1987)
Polymethylene polyphenyl isocyanate	19, 314 (1979); Suppl. 7, 70 (1987)
Polymethyl methacrylate	19, 195 (1979); Suppl. 7, 70 (1987)
Polyoestradiol phosphate (see Oestradiol-17β)	
Polypropylene	19, 218 (1979); Suppl. 7, 70 (1987)
Polystyrene	19, 245 (1979); Suppl. 7, 70 (1987)
Polytetrafluoroethylene	19, 288 (1979); Suppl. 7, 70 (1987)
Polyurethane foams	19, 320 (1979); Suppl. 7, 70 (1987)
Polyvinyl acetate	19, 346 (1979); Suppl. 7, 70 (1987)
Polyvinyl alcohol	19, 351 (1979); Suppl. 7, 70 (1987)
Polyvinyl chloride	7, 306 (1974); 19, 402 (1979); Suppl. 7, 70 (1987)
Polyvinyl pyrrolidone	19, 463 (1979); Suppl. 7, 70 (1987)
Ponceau MX	8, 189 (1975); Suppl. 7, 70 (1987)
Ponceau 3R	8, 199 (1975); Suppl. 7, 70 (1987)
Ponceau SX	8, 207 (1975); Suppl. 7, 70 (1987)
Potassium arsenate (see Arsenic and arsenic compounds)	

Potassium arsenite (see Arsenic and arsenic compounds)
Potassium bis(2-hydroxyethyl)dithiocarbamate   *12*, 183 (1976); *Suppl. 7*, 70 (1987)
Potassium bromate   *40*, 207 (1986); *Suppl. 7*, 70 (1987)
Potassium chromate (see Chromium and chromium compounds)
Potassium dichromate (see Chromium and chromium compounds)
Prazepam   *66*, 143 (1996)
Prednimustine   *50*, 115 (1990)
Prednisone   *26*, 293 (1981); *Suppl. 7*, 326 (1987)
Printing processes and printing inks   *65*, 33 (1996)
Procarbazine hydrochloride   *26*, 311 (1981); *Suppl. 7*, 327 (1987)
Proflavine salts   *24*, 195 (1980); *Suppl. 7*, 70 (1987)
Progesterone (see also Progestins; Combined oral contraceptives)   *6*, 135 (1974); *21*, 491 (1979)
                                                                          (*corr. 42*, 259)
Progestins (see also Oestrogens, progestins and combinations)   *Suppl. 7*, 289 (1987)
Pronetalol hydrochloride   *13*, 227 (1977) (*corr. 42*, 256);
                                                                          Suppl. 7, 70 (1987)
1,3-Propane sultone   *4*, 253 (1974) (*corr. 42*, 253);
                                                                          Suppl. 7, 70 (1987)
Propham   *12*, 189 (1976); *Suppl. 7*, 70 (1987)
β-Propiolactone   *4*, 259 (1974) (*corr. 42*, 253);
                                                                          Suppl. 7, 70 (1987)
n-Propyl carbamate   *12*, 201 (1976); *Suppl. 7*, 70 (1987)
Propylene   *19*, 213 (1979); *Suppl. 7*, 71 (1987);
                                                                          60, 161 (1994)
Propylene oxide   *11*, 191 (1976); *36*, 227 (1985)
                                                                          (*corr. 42*, 263); *Suppl. 7*, 328
                                                                          (1987); *60*, 181 (1994)
Propylthiouracil   *7*, 67 (1974); *Suppl. 7*, 329 (1987)
Ptaquiloside (see also Bracken fern)   *40*, 55 (1986); *Suppl. 7*, 71 (1987)
Pulp and paper manufacture   *25*, 157 (1981); *Suppl. 7*, 385 (1987)
Pyrene   *32*, 431 (1983); *Suppl. 7*, 71 (1987)
Pyrido[3,4-c]psoralen   *40*, 349 (1986); *Suppl. 7*, 71 (1987)
Pyrimethamine   *13*, 233 (1977); *Suppl. 7*, 71 (1987)
Pyrrolizidine alkaloids (see Hydroxysenkirkine; Isatidine; Jacobine;
   Lasiocarpine; Monocrotaline; Retrorsine; Riddelliine; Seneciphylline;
   Senkirkine)

Q

Quercetin (see also Bracken fern)   *31*, 213 (1983); *Suppl. 7*, 71 (1987)
para-Quinone   *15*, 255 (1977); *Suppl. 7*, 71 (1987)
Quintozene   *5*, 211 (1974); *Suppl. 7*, 71 (1987)

R

Radon   *43*, 173 (1988) (*corr. 45*, 283)
Reserpine   *10*, 217 (1976); *24*, 211 (1980)
                                                                          (*corr. 42*, 260); *Suppl. 7*, 330 (1987)
Resorcinol   *15*, 155 (1977); *Suppl. 7*, 71 (1987)
Retrorsine   *10*, 303 (1976); *Suppl. 7*, 71 (1987)
Rhodamine B   *16*, 221 (1978); *Suppl. 7*, 71 (1987)
Rhodamine 6G   *16*, 233 (1978); *Suppl. 7*, 71 (1987)
Riddelliine   *10*, 313 (1976); *Suppl. 7*, 71 (1987)

Rifampicin	24, 243 (1980); *Suppl. 7*, 71 (1987)
Ripazepam	66, 157 (1996)
Rockwool (*see* Man-made mineral fibres)	
Rubber industry	28 (1982) (*corr. 42*, 261); *Suppl. 7*, 332 (1987)
Rugulosin	40, 99 (1986); *Suppl. 7*, 71 (1987)

S

Saccharated iron oxide	2, 161 (1973); *Suppl. 7*, 71 (1987)
Saccharin	22, 111 (1980) (*corr. 42*, 259); *Suppl. 7*, 334 (1987)
Safrole	1, 169 (1972); 10, 231 (1976); *Suppl. 7*, 71 (1987)
Salted fish	56, 41 (1993)
Sawmill industry (including logging) [*see* Lumber and sawmill industry (including logging)]	
Scarlet Red	8, 217 (1975); *Suppl. 7*, 71 (1987)
Schistosoma haematobium (infection with)	61, 45 (1994)
Schistosoma japonicum (infection with)	61, 45 (1994)
Schistosoma mansoni (infection with)	61, 45 (1994)
Selenium and selenium compounds	9, 245 (1975) (*corr. 42*, 255); *Suppl. 7*, 71 (1987)
Selenium dioxide (*see* Selenium and selenium compounds)	
Selenium oxide (*see* Selenium and selenium compounds)	
Semicarbazide hydrochloride	12, 209 (1976) (*corr. 42*, 256); *Suppl. 7*, 71 (1987)
Senecio jacobaea L. (*see* Pyrrolizidine alkaloids)	
Senecio longilobus (*see* Pyrrolizidine alkaloids)	
Seneciphylline	10, 319, 335 (1976); *Suppl. 7*, 71 (1987)
Senkirkine	10, 327 (1976); 31, 231 (1983); *Suppl. 7*, 71 (1987)
Sepiolite	42, 175 (1987); *Suppl. 7*, 71 (1987)
Sequential oral contraceptives (*see also* Oestrogens, progestins and combinations)	*Suppl. 7*, 296 (1987)
Shale-oils	35, 161 (1985); *Suppl. 7*, 339 (1987)
Shikimic acid (*see also* Bracken fern)	40, 55 (1986); *Suppl. 7*, 71 (1987)
Shoe manufacture and repair (*see* Boot and shoe manufacture and repair)	
Silica (*see also* Amorphous silica; Crystalline silica)	42, 39 (1987)
Simazine	53, 495 (1991)
Slagwool (*see* Man-made mineral fibres)	
Sodium arsenate (*see* Arsenic and arsenic compounds)	
Sodium arsenite (*see* Arsenic and arsenic compounds)	
Sodium cacodylate (*see* Arsenic and arsenic compounds)	
Sodium chlorite	52, 145 (1991)
Sodium chromate (*see* Chromium and chromium compounds)	
Sodium cyclamate (*see* Cyclamates)	
Sodium dichromate (*see* Chromium and chromium compounds)	
Sodium diethyldithiocarbamate	12, 217 (1976); *Suppl. 7*, 71 (1987)
Sodium equilin sulfate (*see* Conjugated oestrogens)	
Sodium fluoride (*see* Fluorides)	
Sodium monofluorophosphate (*see* Fluorides)	

Sodium oestrone sulfate (*see* Conjugated oestrogens)
Sodium *ortho*-phenylphenate (*see also* ortho-Phenylphenol)   *30*, 329 (1983); *Suppl. 7*, 392 (1987)
Sodium saccharin (*see* Saccharin)
Sodium selenate (*see* Selenium and selenium compounds)
Sodium selenite (*see* Selenium and selenium compounds)
Sodium silicofluoride (*see* Fluorides)
Solar radiation   *55* (1992)
Soots   *3*, 22 (1973); *35*, 219 (1985); *Suppl. 7*, 343 (1987)
Spironolactone   *24*, 259 (1980); *Suppl. 7*, 344 (1987)
Stannous fluoride (*see* Fluorides)
Steel founding (*see* Iron and steel founding)
Sterigmatocystin   *1*, 175 (1972); *10*, 245 (1976); *Suppl. 7*, 72 (1987)
Steroidal oestrogens (*see also* Oestrogens, progestins and combinations)   *Suppl. 7*, 280 (1987)
Streptozotocin   *4*, 221 (1974); *17*, 337 (1978); *Suppl. 7*, 72 (1987)
Strobane® (*see* Terpene polychlorinates)
Strong-inorganic-acid mists containing sulfuric acid (*see* Mists and vapours from sulfuric acid and other strong inorganic acids)
Strontium chromate (*see* Chromium and chromium compounds)
Styrene   *19*, 231 (1979) (*corr. 42*, 258); *Suppl. 7*, 345 (1987); *60*, 233 (1994) (*corr. 65*, 549)
Styrene-acrylonitrile-copolymers   *19*, 97 (1979); *Suppl. 7*, 72 (1987)
Styrene-butadiene copolymers   *19*, 252 (1979); *Suppl. 7*, 72 (1987)
Styrene-7,8-oxide   *11*, 201 (1976); *19*, 275 (1979); *36*, 245 (1985); *Suppl. 7*, 72 (1987); *60*, 321 (1994)
Succinic anhydride   *15*, 265 (1977); *Suppl. 7*, 72 (1987)
Sudan I   *8*, 225 (1975); *Suppl. 7*, 72 (1987)
Sudan II   *8*, 233 (1975); *Suppl. 7*, 72 (1987)
Sudan III   *8*, 241 (1975); *Suppl. 7*, 72 (1987)
Sudan Brown RR   *8*, 249 (1975); *Suppl. 7*, 72 (1987)
Sudan Red 7B   *8*, 253 (1975); *Suppl. 7*, 72 (1987)
Sulfafurazole   *24*, 275 (1980); *Suppl. 7*, 347 (1987)
Sulfallate   *30*, 283 (1983); *Suppl. 7*, 72 (1987)
Sulfamethoxazole   *24*, 285 (1980); *Suppl. 7*, 348 (1987)
Sulfites (*see* Sulfur dioxide and some sulfites, bisulfites and metabisulfites)
Sulfur dioxide and some sulfites, bisulfites and metabisulfites   *54*, 131 (1992)
Sulfur mustard (*see* Mustard gas)
Sulfuric acid and other strong inorganic acids, occupational exposures to mists and vapours from   *54*, 41 (1992)
Sulfur trioxide   *54*, 121 (1992)
Sulphisoxazole (*see* Sulfafurazole)
Sunset Yellow FCF   *8*, 257 (1975); *Suppl. 7*, 72 (1987)
Symphytine   *31*, 239 (1983); *Suppl. 7*, 72 (1987)

T

2,4,5-T (*see also* Chlorophenoxy herbicides; Chlorophenoxy herbicides, occupational exposures to)   *15*, 273 (1977)
Talc   *42*, 185 (1987); *Suppl. 7*, 349 (1987)

Tamoxifen	66, 253 (1996)
Tannic acid	10, 253 (1976) (corr. 42, 255); Suppl. 7, 72 (1987)
Tannins (see also Tannic acid)	10, 254 (1976); Suppl. 7, 72 (1987)
TCDD (see 2,3,7,8-Tetrachlorodibenzo-*para*-dioxin)	
TDE (see DDT)	
Tea	51, 207 (1991)
Temazepam	66, 161 (1996)
Terpene polychlorinates	5, 219 (1974); Suppl. 7, 72 (1987)
Testosterone (see also Androgenic (anabolic) steroids)	6, 209 (1974); 21, 519 (1979)
Testosterone oenanthate (see Testosterone)	
Testosterone propionate (see Testosterone)	
2,2′,5,5′-Tetrachlorobenzidine	27, 141 (1982); Suppl. 7, 72 (1987)
2,3,7,8-Tetrachlorodibenzo-*para*-dioxin	15, 41 (1977); Suppl. 7, 350 (1987)
1,1,1,2-Tetrachloroethane	41, 87 (1986); Suppl. 7, 72 (1987)
1,1,2,2-Tetrachloroethane	20, 477 (1979); Suppl. 7, 354 (1987)
Tetrachloroethylene	20, 491 (1979); Suppl. 7, 355 (1987); 63, 159 (1995) (corr. 65, 549)
2,3,4,6-Tetrachlorophenol (see Chlorophenols; Chlorophenols, occupational exposures to)	
Tetrachlorvinphos	30, 197 (1983); Suppl. 7, 72 (1987)
Tetraethyllead (see Lead and lead compounds)	
Tetrafluoroethylene	19, 285 (1979); Suppl. 7, 72 (1987)
Tetrakis(hydroxymethyl) phosphonium salts	48, 95 (1990)
Tetramethyllead (see Lead and lead compounds)	
Tetranitromethane	65, 437 (1996)
Textile manufacturing industry, exposures in	48, 215 (1990) (corr. 51, 483)
Theobromine	51, 421 (1991)
Theophylline	51, 391 (1991)
Thioacetamide	7, 77 (1974); Suppl. 7, 72 (1987)
4,4′-Thiodianiline	16, 343 (1978); 27, 147 (1982); Suppl. 7, 72 (1987)
Thiotepa	9, 85 (1975); Suppl. 7, 368 (1987); 50, 123 (1990)
Thiouracil	7, 85 (1974); Suppl. 7, 72 (1987)
Thiourea	7, 95 (1974); Suppl. 7, 72 (1987)
Thiram	12, 225 (1976); Suppl. 7, 72 (1987); 53, 403 (1991)
Titanium dioxide	47, 307 (1989)
Tobacco habits other than smoking (see Tobacco products, smokeless)	
Tobacco products, smokeless	37 (1985) (corr. 42, 263; 52, 513); Suppl. 7, 357 (1987)
Tobacco smoke	38 (1986) (corr. 42, 263); Suppl. 7, 357 (1987)
Tobacco smoking (see Tobacco smoke)	
ortho-Tolidine (see 3,3′-Dimethylbenzidine)	
2,4-Toluene diisocyanate (see also Toluene diisocyanates)	19, 303 (1979); 39, 287 (1986)
2,6-Toluene diisocyanate (see also Toluene diisocyanates)	19, 303 (1979); 39, 289 (1986)
Toluene	47, 79 (1989)
Toluene diisocyanates	39, 287 (1986) (corr. 42, 264); Suppl. 7, 72 (1987)
Toluenes, α-chlorinated (see α-Chlorinated toluenes)	
ortho-Toluenesulfonamide (see Saccharin)	
ortho-Toluidine	16, 349 (1978); 27, 155 (1982); Suppl. 7, 362 (1987)

Toremifene	66, 367 (1996)
Toxaphene	20, 327 (1979); Suppl. 7, 72 (1987)
T-2 Toxin (see Toxins derived from *Fusarium sporotrichioides*)	
Toxins derived from *Fusarium graminearum*, *F. culmorum* and *F. crookwellense*	11, 169 (1976); 31, 153, 279 (1983); Suppl. 7, 64, 74 (1987); 56, 397 (1993)
Toxins derived from *Fusarium moniliforme*	56, 445 (1993)
Toxins derived from *Fusarium sporotrichioides*	31, 265 (1983); Suppl. 7, 73 (1987); 56, 467 (1993)
Tremolite (see Asbestos)	
Treosulfan	26, 341 (1981); Suppl. 7, 363 (1987)
Triaziquone [see Tris(aziridinyl)-*para*-benzoquinone]	
Trichlorfon	30, 207 (1983); Suppl. 7, 73 (1987)
Trichlormethine	9, 229 (1975); Suppl. 7, 73 (1987); 50, 143 (1990)
Trichloroacetic acid	63, 291 (1995) (corr. 65, 549)
Trichloroacetonitrile (see Halogenated acetonitriles)	
1,1,1-Trichloroethane	20, 515 (1979); Suppl. 7, 73 (1987)
1,1,2-Trichloroethane	20, 533 (1979); Suppl. 7, 73 (1987); 52, 337 (1991)
Trichloroethylene	11, 263 (1976); 20, 545 (1979); Suppl. 7, 364 (1987); 63, 75 (1995) (corr. 65, 549)
2,4,5-Trichlorophenol (see also Chlorophenols; Chlorophenols, occupational exposures to)	20, 349 (1979)
2,4,6-Trichlorophenol (see also Chlorophenols; Chlorophenols, occupational exposures to)	20, 349 (1979)
(2,4,5-Trichlorophenoxy)acetic acid (see 2,4,5-T)	
1,2,3-Trichloropropane	63, 223 (1995)
Trichlorotriethylamine-hydrochloride (see Trichlormethine)	
T₂-Trichothecene (see Toxins derived from *Fusarium sporotrichioides*)	
Triethylene glycol diglycidyl ether	11, 209 (1976); Suppl. 7, 73 (1987)
Trifluralin	53, 515 (1991)
4,4',6-Trimethylangelicin plus ultraviolet radiation (see also Angelicin and some synthetic derivatives)	Suppl. 7, 57 (1987)
2,4,5-Trimethylaniline	27, 177 (1982); Suppl. 7, 73 (1987)
2,4,6-Trimethylaniline	27, 178 (1982); Suppl. 7, 73 (1987)
4,5',8-Trimethylpsoralen	40, 357 (1986); Suppl. 7, 366 (1987)
Trimustine hydrochloride (see Trichlormethine)	
2,4,6-Trinitrotoluene	65, 449 (1996)
Triphenylene	32, 447 (1983); Suppl. 7, 73 (1987)
Tris(aziridinyl)-*para*-benzoquinone	9, 67 (1975); Suppl. 7, 367 (1987)
Tris(1-aziridinyl)phosphine-oxide	9, 75 (1975); Suppl. 7, 73 (1987)
Tris(1-aziridinyl)phosphine-sulphide (see Thiotepa)	
2,4,6-Tris(1-aziridinyl)-*s*-triazine	9, 95 (1975); Suppl. 7, 73 (1987)
Tris(2-chloroethyl) phosphate	48, 109 (1990)
1,2,3-Tris(chloromethoxy)propane	15, 301 (1977); Suppl. 7, 73 (1987)
Tris(2,3-dibromopropyl)phosphate	20, 575 (1979); Suppl. 7, 369 (1987)
Tris(2-methyl-1-aziridinyl)phosphine-oxide	9, 107 (1975); Suppl. 7, 73 (1987)
Trp-P-1	31, 247 (1983); Suppl. 7, 73 (1987)
Trp-P-2	31, 255 (1983); Suppl. 7, 73 (1987)
Trypan blue	8, 267 (1975); Suppl. 7, 73 (1987)
Tussilago farfara L. (see Pyrrolizidine alkaloids)	

U

Ultraviolet radiation	40, 379 (1986); 55 (1992)
Underground haematite mining with exposure to radon	1, 29 (1972); Suppl. 7, 216 (1987)
Uracil mustard	9, 235 (1975); Suppl. 7, 370 (1987)
Urethane	7, 111 (1974); Suppl. 7, 73 (1987)

V

Vat Yellow 4	48, 161 (1990)
Vinblastine sulfate	26, 349 (1981) (corr. 42, 261); Suppl. 7, 371 (1987)
Vincristine sulfate	26, 365 (1981); Suppl. 7, 372 (1987)
Vinyl acetate	19, 341 (1979); 39, 113 (1986); Suppl. 7, 73 (1987); 63, 443 (1995)
Vinyl bromide	19, 367 (1979); 39, 133 (1986); Suppl. 7, 73 (1987)
Vinyl chloride	7, 291 (1974); 19, 377 (1979) (corr. 42, 258); Suppl. 7, 373 (1987)
Vinyl chloride-vinyl acetate copolymers	7, 311 (1976); 19, 412 (1979) (corr. 42, 258); Suppl. 7, 73 (1987)
4-Vinylcyclohexene	11, 277 (1976); 39, 181 (1986) Suppl. 7, 73 (1987); 60, 347 (1994)
4-Vinylcyclohexene diepoxide	11, 141 (1976); Suppl. 7, 63 (1987); 60, 361 (1994)
Vinyl fluoride	39, 147 (1986); Suppl. 7, 73 (1987); 63, 467 (1995)
Vinylidene chloride	19, 439 (1979); 39, 195 (1986); Suppl. 7, 376 (1987)
Vinylidene chloride-vinyl chloride copolymers	19, 448 (1979) (corr. 42, 258); Suppl. 7, 73 (1987)
Vinylidene fluoride	39, 227 (1986); Suppl. 7, 73 (1987)
N-Vinyl-2-pyrrolidone	19, 461 (1979); Suppl. 7, 73 (1987)
Vinyl toluene	60, 373 (1994)

W

Welding	49, 447 (1990) (corr. 52, 513)
Wollastonite	42, 145 (1987); Suppl. 7, 377 (1987)
Wood dust	62, 35 (1995)
Wood industries	25 (1981); Suppl. 7, 378 (1987)

X

Xylene	47, 125 (1989)
2,4-Xylidine	16, 367 (1978); Suppl. 7, 74 (1987)
2,5-Xylidine	16, 377 (1978); Suppl. 7, 74 (1987)
2,6-Xylidine (see 2,6-Dimethylaniline)	

Y

Yellow AB   8, 279 (1975); *Suppl. 7*, 74 (1987)
Yellow OB   8, 287 (1975); *Suppl. 7*, 74 (1987)

Z

Zearalenone (*see* Toxins derived from *Fusarium graminearum*,
    F. culmorum and *F. crookwellense*)
Zectran   *12*, 237 (1976); *Suppl. 7*, 74 (1987)
Zinc beryllium silicate (*see* Beryllium and beryllium compounds)
Zinc chromate (*see* Chromium and chromium compounds)
Zinc chromate hydroxide (*see* Chromium and chromium compounds)
Zinc potassium chromate (*see* Chromium and chromium
    compounds)
Zinc yellow (*see* Chromium and chromium compounds)
Zineb   *12*, 245 (1976); *Suppl. 7*, 74 (1987)
Ziram   *12*, 259 (1976); *Suppl. 7*, 74 (1987);
                                            53, 423 (1991)

IARC Monographs on the Evaluation of Carcinogenic Risks to Humans

Volume 1
Some Inorganic Substances, Chlorinated Hydrocarbons, Aromatic Amines, N-Nitroso Compounds, and Natural Products
1972; 184 pages; ISBN 92 832 1201 0
(out of print)

Volume 2
Some Inorganic and Organometallic Compounds
1973; 181 pages; ISBN 92 832 1202 9
(out of print)

Volume 3
Certain Polycyclic Aromatic Hydrocarbons and Heterocyclic Compounds
1973; 271 pages; ISBN 92 832 1203 7
(out of print)

Volume 4
Some Aromatic Amines, Hydrazine and Related Substances, N-Nitroso Compounds and Miscellaneous Alkylating Agents
1974; 286 pages; ISBN 92 832 1204 5

Volume 5
Some Organochlorine Pesticides
1974; 241 pages; ISBN 92 832 1205 3
(out of print)

Volume 6
Sex Hormones
1974; 243 pages; ISBN 92 832 1206 1
(out of print)

Volume 7
Some Anti-Thyroid and Related Substances, Nitrofurans and Industrial Chemicals
1974; 326 pages; ISBN 92 832 1207 X
(out of print)

Volume 8
Some Aromatic Azo Compounds
1975; 357 pages; ISBN 92 832 1208 8

Volume 9
Some Aziridines, N-, S- and O-Mustards and Selenium
1975; 268 pages; ISBN 92 832 1209 6

Volume 10
Some Naturally Occurring Substances
1976; 353 pages; ISBN 92 832 1210 X
(out of print)

Volume 11
Cadmium, Nickel, Some Epoxides, Miscellaneous Industrial Chemicals and General Considerations on Volatile Anaesthetics
1976; 306 pages; ISBN 92 832 1211 8
(out of print)

Volume 12
Some Carbamates, Thiocarbamates and Carbazides
1976; 282 pages; ISBN 92 832 1212 6

Volume 13
Some Miscellaneous Pharmaceutical Substances
1977; 255 pages; ISBN 92 832 1213 4

Volume 14
Asbestos
1977; 106 pages; ISBN 92 832 1214 2
(out of print)

Volume 15
Some Fumigants, the Herbicides 2,4-D and 2,4,5-T, Chlorinated Dibenzodioxins and Miscellaneous Industrial Chemicals
1977; 354 pages; ISBN 92 832 1215 0
(out of print)

Volume 16
Some Aromatic Amines and Related Nitro Compounds – Hair Dyes, Colouring Agents and Miscellaneous Industrial Chemicals
1978; 400 pages; ISBN 92 832 1216 9

Volume 17
Some N-Nitroso Compounds
1978; 365 pages; ISBN 92 832 1217 7

Volume 18
Polychlorinated Biphenyls and Polybrominated Biphenyls
1978; 140 pages; ISBN 92 832 1218 5

Volume 19
Some Monomers, Plastics and Synthetic Elastomers, and Acrolein
1979; 513 pages; ISBN 92 832 1219 3
(out of print)

Volume 20
Some Halogenated Hydrocarbons
1979; 609 pages; ISBN 92 832 1220 7
(out of print)

Volume 21
Sex Hormones (II)
1979; 583 pages; ISBN 92 832 1521 4

Volume 22
Some Non-Nutritive Sweetening Agents
1980; 208 pages; ISBN 92 832 1522 2

Volume 23
Some Metals and Metallic Compounds
1980; 438 pages; ISBN 92 832 1523 0
(out of print)

Volume 24
Some Pharmaceutical Drugs
1980; 337 pages; ISBN 92 832 1524 9

Volume 25
Wood, Leather and Some Associated Industries
1981; 412 pages; ISBN 92 832 1525 7

Volume 26
Some Antineoplastic and Immunosuppressive Agents
1981; 411 pages; ISBN 92 832 1526 5

Volume 27
Some Aromatic Amines, Anthraquinones and Nitroso Compounds, and Inorganic Fluorides Used in Drinking Water and Dental Preparations
1982; 341 pages; ISBN 92 832 1527 3

Volume 28
The Rubber Industry
1982; 486 pages; ISBN 92 832 1528 1

Volume 29
Some Industrial Chemicals and Dyestuffs
1982; 416 pages; ISBN 92 832 1529 X

Volume 30
Miscellaneous Pesticides
1983; 424 pages; ISBN 92 832 1530 3

Volume 31
Some Food Additives, Feed Additives and Naturally Occurring Substances
1983; 314 pages; ISBN 92 832 1531 1

Volume 32
Polynuclear Aromatic Compounds, Part 1: Chemical, Environmental and Experimental Data
1983; 477 pages; ISBN 92 832 1532 X

Volume 33
Polynuclear Aromatic Compounds, Part 2: Carbon Blacks, Mineral Oils and Some Nitroarenes
1984; 245 pages; ISBN 92 832 1533 8
(out of print)

Volume 34
Polynuclear Aromatic Compounds, Part 3: Industrial Exposures in Aluminium Production, Coal Gasification, Coke Production, and Iron and Steel Founding
1984; 219 pages; ISBN 92 832 1534 6

Volume 35
Polynuclear Aromatic Compounds: Part 4: Bitumens, Coal-Tars and Derived Products, Shale-Oils and Soots
1985; 271 pages; ISBN 92 832 1535 4

Volume 36
Allyl Compounds, Aldehydes, Epoxides and Peroxides
1985; 369 pages; ISBN 92 832 1536 2

Volume 37
Tobacco Habits Other than Smoking; Betel-Quid and Areca-Nut Chewing; and Some Related Nitrosamines
1985; 291 pages; ISBN 92 832 1537 0

Volume 38
Tobacco Smoking
1986; 421 pages; ISBN 92 832 1538 9

Volume 39
Some Chemicals Used in Plastics and Elastomers
1986; 403 pages; ISBN 92 832 1239 8

Volume 40
Some Naturally Occurring and Synthetic Food Components, Furocoumarins and Ultraviolet Radiation
1986; 444 pages; ISBN 92 832 1240 1

Volume 41
Some Halogenated Hydrocarbons and Pesticide Exposures
1986; 434 pages; ISBN 92 832 1241 X

Volume 42
Silica and Some Silicates
1987; 289 pages; ISBN 92 832 1242 8

Volume 43
Man-Made Mineral Fibres and Radon
1988; 300 pages; ISBN 92 832 1243 6

Volume 44
Alcohol Drinking
1988; 416 pages; ISBN 92 832 1244 4

Volume 45
Occupational Exposures in Petroleum Refining; Crude Oil and Major Petroleum Fuels
1989; 322 pages; ISBN 92 832 1245 2

Volume 46
Diesel and Gasoline Engine Exhausts and Some Nitroarenes
1989; 458 pages; ISBN 92 832 1246 0

Volume 47
Some Organic Solvents, Resin Monomers and Related Compounds, Pigments and Occupational Exposures in Paint Manufacture and Painting
1989; 535 pages; ISBN 92 832 1247 9

Volume 48
Some Flame Retardants and Textile Chemicals, and Exposures in the Textile Manufacturing Industry
1990; 345 pages; ISBN: 92 832 1248 7

Volume 49
Chromium, Nickel and Welding
1990; 677 pages; ISBN: 92 832 1249 5

Volume 50
Some Pharmaceutical Drugs
1990; 415 pages; ISBN: 92 832 1259 9

Volume 51
Coffee, Tea, Mate, Methylxanthines and Methylglyoxal
1991; 513 pages; ISBN: 92 832 1251 7

Volume 52
Chlorinated Drinking-Water; Chlorination By-products; Some other Halogenated Compounds; Cobalt and Cobalt Compounds
1991; 544 pages; ISBN: 92 832 1252 5

Volume 53
Occupational Exposures in Insecticide Application, and Some Pesticides
1991; 612 pages; ISBN 92 832 1253 3

Volume 54
Occupational Exposures to Mists and Vapours from Strong Inorganic Acids; and other Industrial Chemicals
1992; 336 pages; ISBN 92 832 1254 1

Volume 55
Solar and Ultraviolet Radiation
1992; 316 pages; ISBN 92 832 1255 X

Volume 56
Some Naturally Occurring Substances: Food Items and Constituents, Heterocyclic Aromatic Amines and Mycotoxins
1993; 600 pages; ISBN 92 832 1256 8

Volume 57
Occupational Exposures of Hairdressers and Barbers and Personal Use of Hair Colourants; Some Hair Dyes, Cosmetic Colourants, Industrial Dyestuffs and Aromatic Amines
1993; 428 pages; ISBN 92 832 1257 6

Volume 58
Beryllium, Cadmium, Mercury and Exposures in the Glass Manufacturing Industry
1994; 444 pages; ISBN 92 832 1258 4

Volume 59
Hepatitis Viruses
1994; 286 pages; ISBN 92 832 1259 2

Volume 60
Some Industrial Chemicals
1994; 560 pages; ISBN 92 832 1260 6

Volume 61
Schistosomes, Liver Flukes and *Helicobacter pylori*
1994; 280 pages; ISBN 92 832 1261 4

Volume 62
Wood Dusts and Formaldehyde
1995; 405 pages; ISBN 92 832 1262 2

Volume 63
Dry cleaning, Some Chlorinated Solvents and Other Industrial Chemicals
1995; 558 pages; ISBN 92 832 1263 0

Volume 64
Human Papillomaviruses
1995; 409 pages; ISBN 92 832 1264 9

Volume 65
Printing Processes, Printing Inks, Carbon Blacks and Some Nitro Compounds
1996; 578 pages; ISBN 92 832 1265 7

Volume 66
Some Pharmaceutical Drugs
1996; 514 pages; ISBN 92 832 1266 5

Supplements

Supplement No.1
Chemicals and Industrial Processes Associated with Cancer in Humans (IARC Monographs, Volumes 1 to 20)
1979; 71 pages; ISBN 92 832 1404 8
(out of print)

Supplement No. 2
Long-Term and Short-Term Screening Assays for Carcinogens: A Critical Appraisal
1980; 426 pages; ISBN 92 832 1404 8

Supplement No. 3
Cross Index of Synonyms and Trade Names in Volumes 1 to 26
1982; 199 pages; ISBN 92 832 1405 6
(out of print)

Supplement No.4
Chemicals, Industrial Processes and Industries Associated with Cancer in Humans (IARC Monographs, Volumes 1 to 29)
1982; 292 pages; ISBN 92 832 1407 2
(out of print)

Supplement No. 5
Cross Index of Synonyms and Trade Names in Volumes 1 to 36
1985; 259 pages; ISBN 92 832 1408 0
(out of print)

Supplement No. 6
Genetic and Related Effects: An Updating of Selected IARC Monographs from Volumes 1 to 42
1987; 729 pages; ISBN 92 832 1409 9

Supplement No. 7
Overall Evaluations of Carcinogenicity: An Updating of IARC Monographs Volumes 1 to 42
1987; 440 pages; ISBN 92 832 1411 0

Supplement No. 8
Cross Index of Synonyms and Trade Names in Volumes 1 to 46
1989; 346 pages; ISBN 92 832 1417 X

IARC Scientific Publications

No. 1
Liver Cancer
1971; 176 pages; ISBN 0 19 723000 8

No. 2
Oncogenesis and Herpesviruses
Edited by P.M. Biggs, G. de Thé and L.N. Payne
1972; 515 pages; ISBN 0 19 723001 6

No. 3
N-Nitroso Compounds: Analysis and Formation
Edited by P. Bogovski, R. Preussman and E.A. Walker
1972; 140 pages; ISBN 0 19 723002 4

No. 4
Transplacental Carcinogenesis
Edited by L. Tomatis and U. Mohr
1973; 181 pages; ISBN 0 19 723003 2

No. 5/6
Pathology of Tumours in Laboratory Animals. Volume 1: Tumours of the Rat
Edited by V.S. Turusov
1973/1976; 533 pages; ISBN 92 832 1410 2

No. 7
Host Environment Interactions in the Etiology of Cancer in Man
Edited by R. Doll and I. Vodopija
1973; 464 pages; ISBN 0 19 723006 7

No. 8
Biological Effects of Asbestos
Edited by P. Bogovski, J.C. Gilson, V. Timbrell and J.C. Wagner
1973; 346 pages; ISBN 0 19 723007 5

No. 9
N-Nitroso Compounds in the Environment
Edited by P. Bogovski and E.A. Walker
1974; 243 pages; ISBN 0 19 723008 3

No. 10
Chemical Carcinogenesis Essays
Edited by R. Montesano and L. Tomatis
1974; 230 pages; ISBN 0 19 723009 1

No. 11
Oncogenesis and Herpes-viruses II
Edited by G. de-Thé, M.A. Epstein and H. zur Hausen
1975; Two volumes, 511 pages and 403 pages; ISBN 0 19 723010 5

No. 12
Screening Tests in Chemical Carcinogenesis
Edited by R. Montesano, H. Bartsch and L. Tomatis
1976; 666 pages; ISBN 0 19 723051 2

No. 13
Environmental Pollution and Carcinogenic Risks
Edited by C. Rosenfeld and W. Davis
1975; 441 pages; ISBN 0 19 723012 1

No. 14
Environmental N-Nitroso Compounds. Analysis and Formation
Edited by E.A. Walker, P. Bogovski and L. Griciute
1976; 512 pages; ISBN 0 19 723013 X

No. 15
Cancer Incidence in Five Continents, Volume III
Edited by J.A.H. Waterhouse, C. Muir, P. Correa and J. Powell
1976; 584 pages; ISBN 0 19 723014 8

No. 16
Air Pollution and Cancer in Man
Edited by U. Mohr, D. Schmähl and L. Tomatis
1977; 328 pages; ISBN 0 19 723015 6

No. 17
Directory of On-Going Research in Cancer Epidemiology 1977
Edited by C.S. Muir and G. Wagner
1977; 599 pages; ISBN 92 832 1117 0
(out of print)

No. 18
Environmental Carcinogens. Selected Methods of Analysis. Volume 1: Analysis of Volatile Nitrosamines in Food
Editor-in-Chief: H. Egan
1978; 212 pages; ISBN 0 19 723017 2

No. 19
Environmental Aspects of N-Nitroso Compounds
Edited by E.A. Walker, M. Castegnaro, L. Griciute and R.E. Lyle
1978; 561 pages; ISBN 0 19 723018 0

No. 20
Nasopharyngeal Carcinoma: Etiology and Control
Edited by G. de Thé and Y. Ito
1978; 606 pages; ISBN 0 19 723019 9

No. 21
Cancer Registration and its Techniques
Edited by R. MacLennan, C. Muir, R. Steinitz and A. Winkler
1978; 235 pages; ISBN 0 19 723020 2

No. 22
Environmental Carcinogens: Selected Methods of Analysis. Volume 2: Methods for the Measurement of Vinyl Chloride in Poly(vinyl chloride), Air, Water and Foodstuffs
Editor-in-Chief: H. Egan
1978; 142 pages; ISBN 0 19 723021 0

No. 23
Pathology of Tumours in Laboratory Animals. Volume II: Tumours of the Mouse
Editor-in-Chief: V.S. Turusov
1979; 669 pages; ISBN 0 19 723022 9

No. 24
Oncogenesis and Herpesviruses III
Edited by G. de-Thé, W. Henle and F. Rapp
1978; Part I: 580 pages, Part II: 512 pages; ISBN 0 19 723023 7

No. 25
Carcinogenic Risk: Strategies for Intervention
Edited by W. Davis and C. Rosenfeld
1979; 280 pages; ISBN 0 19 723025 3

No. 26
Directory of On-going Research in Cancer Epidemiology 1978
Edited by C.S. Muir and G. Wagner
1978; 550 pages; ISBN 0 19 723026 1
(out of print)

No. 27
Molecular and Cellular Aspects of Carcinogen Screening Tests
Edited by R. Montesano, H. Bartsch and L. Tomatis
1980; 372 pages; ISBN 0 19 723027 X

No. 28
Directory of On-going Research in Cancer Epidemiology 1979
Edited by C.S. Muir and G. Wagner
1979; 672 pages; ISBN 92 832 1128 6
(out of print)

No. 29
Environmental Carcinogens. Selected Methods of Analysis. Volume 3: Analysis of Polycyclic Aromatic Hydrocarbons in Environmental Samples
Editor-in-Chief: H. Egan
1979; 240 pages; ISBN 0 19 723028 8

No. 30
Biological Effects of Mineral Fibres
Editor-in-Chief: J.C. Wagner
1980; Two volumes, 494 pages & 513 pages; ISBN 0 19 723030 X

No. 31
N-Nitroso Compounds: Analysis, Formation and Occurrence
Edited by E.A. Walker, L. Griciute, M. Castegnaro and M. Börzsönyi
1980; 835 pages; ISBN 0 19 723031 8

No. 32
Statistical Methods in Cancer Research. Volume 1: The Analysis of Case-control Studies
By N.E. Breslow and N.E. Day
1980; 338 pages; ISBN 92 832 0132 9

No. 33
Handling Chemical Carcinogens in the Laboratory
Edited by R. Montesano, H. Bartsch, E. Boyland, G. Della Porta, L. Fishbein, R.A. Griesemer, A.B. Swan and L. Tomatis
1979; 32 pages; ISBN 0 19 723033 4
(out of print)

No. 34
Pathology of Tumours in Laboratory Animals. Volume III: Tumours of the Hamster
Editor-in-Chief: V.S. Turusov
1982; 461 pages; ISBN 0 19 723034 2

No. 35
Directory of On-going Research in Cancer Epidemiology 1980
Edited by C.S. Muir and G. Wagner
1980; 660 pages; ISBN 0 19 723035 0
(out of print)

No. 36
Cancer Mortality by Occupation and Social Class 1851–1971
Edited by W.P.D. Logan
1982; 253 pages; ISBN 0 19 723036 9

No. 37
Laboratory Decontamination and Destruction of Aflatoxins B1, B2, G1, G2 in Laboratory Wastes
Edited by M. Castegnaro, D.C. Hunt, E.B. Sansone, P.L. Schuller, M.G. Siriwardana, G.M. Telling, H.P. van Egmond and E.A. Walker
1980; 56 pages; ISBN 0 19 723037 7

No. 38
Directory of On-going Research in Cancer Epidemiology 1981
Edited by C.S. Muir and G. Wagner
1981; 696 pages; ISBN 0 19 723038 5
(out of print)

No. 39
Host Factors in Human Carcinogenesis
Edited by H. Bartsch and B. Armstrong
1982; 583 pages;
ISBN 0 19 723039 3

No. 40
Environmental Carcinogens: Selected Methods of Analysis. Volume 4: Some Aromatic Amines and Azo Dyes in the General and Industrial Environment
Edited by L. Fishbein, M. Castegnaro, I.K. O'Neill and H. Bartsch
1981; 347 pages; ISBN 0 19 723040 7

No. 41
N-Nitroso Compounds: Occurrence and Biological Effects
Edited by H. Bartsch, I.K. O'Neill, M. Castegnaro and M. Okada
982; 755 pages; ISBN 0 19 723041 5

No. 42
Cancer Incidence in Five Continents Volume IV
Edited by J. Waterhouse, C. Muir, K. Shanmugaratnam and J. Powell
1982; 811 pages; ISBN 0 19 723042 3

No. 43
Laboratory Decontamination and Destruction of Carcinogens in Laboratory Wastes: Some N-Nitrosamines
Edited by M. Castegnaro, G. Eisenbrand, G. Ellen, L. Keefer, D. Klein, E.B. Sansone, D. Spincer, G. Telling and K. Webb
1982; 73 pages; ISBN 0 19 723043 1

No. 44
Environmental Carcinogens: Selected Methods of Analysis. Volume 5: Some Mycotoxins
Edited by L. Stoloff, M. Castegnaro, P. Scott, I.K. O'Neill and H. Bartsch
1983; 455 pages; ISBN 0 19 723044 X

No. 45
Environmental Carcinogens: Selected Methods of Analysis. Volume 6: N-Nitroso Compounds
Edited by R. Preussmann, I.K. O'Neill, G. Eisenbrand, B. Spiegelhalder and H. Bartsch
1983; 508 pages; ISBN 0 19 723045 8

No. 46
Directory of On-going Research in Cancer Epidemiology 1982
Edited by C.S. Muir and G. Wagner
1982; 722 pages; ISBN 0 19 723046 6
(out of print)

No. 47
Cancer Incidence in Singapore 1968–1977
Edited by K. Shanmugaratnam, H.P. Lee and N.E. Day
1983; 171 pages; ISBN 0 19 723047 4

No. 48
Cancer Incidence in the USSR (2nd Revised Edition)
Edited by N.P. Napalkov, G.F. Tserkovny, V.M. Merabishvili, D.M. Parkin, M. Smans and C.S. Muir
1983; 75 pages; ISBN 0 19 723048 2

No. 49
Laboratory Decontamination and Destruction of Carcinogens in Laboratory Wastes: Some Polycyclic Aromatic Hydrocarbons
Edited by M. Castegnaro, G. Grimmer, O. Hutzinger, W. Karcher, H. Kunte, M. Lafontaine, H.C. Van der Plas, E.B. Sansone and S.P. Tucker
1983; 87 pages; ISBN 0 19 723049 0

No. 50
Directory of On-going Research in Cancer Epidemiology 1983
Edited by C.S. Muir and G. Wagner
1983; 731 pages; ISBN 0 19 723050 4
(out of print)

No. 51
Modulators of Experimental Carcinogenesis
Edited by V. Turusov and R. Montesano
1983; 307 pages; ISBN 0 19 723060 1

No. 52
Second Cancers in Relation to Radiation Treatment for Cervical Cancer: Results

of a Cancer Registry Collaboration
Edited by N.E. Day and J.C. Boice, Jr
1984; 207 pages; ISBN 0 19 723052 0

No. 53
Nickel in the Human Environment
Editor-in-Chief: F.W. Sunderman, Jr
1984; 529 pages; ISBN 0 19 723059 8

No. 54
Laboratory Decontamination and
Destruction of Carcinogens in
Laboratory Wastes: Some Hydrazines
Edited by M. Castegnaro, G. Ellen,
M. Lafontaine, H.C. van der Plas,
E.B. Sansone and S.P. Tucker
1983; 87 pages; ISBN 0 19 723053

No. 55
Laboratory Decontamination and
Destruction of Carcinogens in
Laboratory Wastes: Some
N-Nitrosamides
Edited by M. Castegnaro,
M. Bernard, L.W. van Broekhoven,
D. Fine, R. Massey, E.B. Sansone,
P.L.R. Smith, B. Spiegelhalder,
A. Stacchini, G. Telling and J.J. Vallon
1984; 66 pages; ISBN 0 19 723054 7

No. 56
Models, Mechanisms and Etiology of
Tumour Promotion
Edited by M. Börzsönyi, N.E. Day,
K. Lapis and H. Yamasaki
1984; 532 pages; ISBN 0 19 723058 X

No. 57
N-Nitroso Compounds: Occurrence,
Biological Effects and Relevance to
Human Cancer
Edited by I.K. O'Neill, R.C. von Borstel,
C.T. Miller, J. Long and H. Bartsch
1984; 1013 pages; ISBN 0 19 723055 5

No 58
Age-related Factors in
Carcinogenesis
Edited by A. Likhachev, V. Anisimov and
R. Montesano
1985; 288 pages; ISBN 92 832 1158 8

No. 59
Monitoring Human Exposure to
Carcinogenic and Mutagenic Agents
Edited by A. Berlin, M. Draper,
K. Hemminki and H. Vainio
1984; 457 pages; ISBN 0 19 723056 3

No. 60
Burkitt's Lymphoma: A Human
Cancer Model
Edited by G. Lenoir, G. O'Conor and
C.L.M. Olweny
1985; 484 pages; ISBN 0 19 723057 1

No. 61
Laboratory Decontamination
and Destruction of Carcinogens in
Laboratory Wastes: Some Haloethers
Edited by M. Castegnaro, M. Alvarez,
M. Iovu, E.B. Sansone, G.M. Telling and
D.T. Williams
1985; 55 pages; ISBN 0 19 723061 X

No. 62
Directory of On-going Research in
Cancer Epidemiology 1984
Edited by C.S. Muir and G. Wagner
1984; 717 pages; ISBN 0 19 723062 8
(out of print)

No. 63
Virus-associated Cancers in Africa
Edited by A.O. Williams, G.T. O'Conor,
G.B. de Thé and C.A. Johnson
1984; 773 pages; ISBN 0 19 723063 6

No. 64
Laboratory Decontamination and
Destruction of Carcinogens in
Laboratory Wastes: Some Aromatic
Amines and 4-Nitrobiphenyl
Edited by M. Castegnaro, J. Barek,
J. Dennis, G. Ellen, M. Klibanov,
M. Lafontaine, R. Mitchum,
P. van Roosmalen, E.B. Sansone,
L.A. Sternson and M. Vahl
1985; 84 pages; ISBN: 92 832 1164 2

No. 65
Interpretation of Negative
Epidemiological Evidence for
Carcinogenicity
Edited by N.J. Wald and R. Doll
1985; 232 pages; ISBN 92 832 1165 0

No. 66
The Role of the Registry in Cancer
Control
Edited by D.M. Parkin, G. Wagner and
C.S. Muir
1985; 152 pages; ISBN 92 832 0166 3

No. 67
Transformation Assay of Established
Cell Lines: Mechanisms and
Application
Edited by T. Kakunaga and H. Yamasaki
1985; 225 pages; ISBN 92 832 1167 7

No. 68
Environmental Carcinogens: Selected
Methods of Analysis. Volume 7: Some
Volatile Halogenated Hydrocarbons
Edited by L. Fishbein and I.K. O'Neill
1985; 479 pages; ISBN 92 832 1168 5

No. 69
Directory of On-going Research in
Cancer Epidemiology 1985

Edited by C.S. Muir and G. Wagner
1985; 745 pages; ISBN 92 823 1169 3
(out of print)

No. 70
The Role of Cyclic Nucleic Acid Adducts
in Carcinogenesis and Mutagenesis
Edited by B. Singer and H. Bartsch
1986; 467 pages; ISBN 92 832 1170 7

No. 71
Environmental Carcinogens: Selected
Methods of Analysis. Volume 8: Some
Metals: As, Be, Cd, Cr, Ni, Pb, Se, Zn
Edited by I.K. O'Neill, P. Schuller and
L. Fishbein
1986; 485 pages; ISBN 92 832 1171 5

No. 72
Atlas of Cancer in Scotland, 1975–1980:
Incidence and Epidemiological
Perspective
Edited by I. Kemp, P. Boyle, M. Smans
and C.S. Muir
1985; 285 pages; ISBN 92 832 1172 3

No. 73
Laboratory Decontamination and
Destruction of Carcinogens in Laboratory
Wastes: Some Antineoplastic Agents
Edited by M. Castegnaro, J. Adams,
M.A. Armour, J. Barek, J. Benvenuto,
C. Confalonieri, U. Goff, G. Telling
1985; 163 pages; ISBN 92 832 1173 1

No. 74
Tobacco: A Major International Health
Hazard
Edited by D. Zaridze and R. Peto
1986; 324 pages; ISBN 92 832 1174 X

No. 75
Cancer Occurrence in Developing
Countries
Edited by D.M. Parkin
1986; 339 pages; ISBN 92 832 1175 8

No. 76
Screening for Cancer of the Uterine
Cervix
Edited by M. Hakama, A.B. Miller and
N.E. Day
1986; 315 pages; ISBN 92 832 1176 6

No. 77
Hexachlorobenzene: Proceedings of
an International Symposium
Edited by C.R. Morris and J.R.P. Cabral
1986; 668 pages; ISBN 92 832 1177 4

No. 78
Carcinogenicity of Alkylating
Cytostatic Drugs
Edited by D. Schmähl and J.M. Kaldor
1986; 337 pages; ISBN 92 832 1178 2

No. 79
Statistical Methods in Cancer Research. Volume III: The Design and Analysis of Long-term Animal Experiments
By J.J. Gart, D. Krewski, P.N. Lee, R.E. Tarone and J. Wahrendorf
1986; 213 pages; ISBN 92 832 1179 0

No. 80
Directory of On-going Research in Cancer Epidemiology 1986
Edited by C.S. Muir and G. Wagner
1986; 805 pages; ISBN 92 832 1180 4
(out of print)

No. 81
Environmental Carcinogens: Methods of Analysis and Exposure Measurement. Volume 9: Passive Smoking
Edited by I.K. O'Neill, K.D. Brunnemann, B. Dodet and D. Hoffmann
1987; 383 pages; ISBN 92 832 1181 2

No. 82
Statistical Methods in Cancer Research. Volume II: The Design and Analysis of Cohort Studies
By N.E. Breslow and N.E. Day
1987; 404 pages; ISBN 92 832 0182 5

No. 83
Long-term and Short-term Assays for Carcinogens: A Critical Appraisal
Edited by R. Montesano, H. Bartsch, H. Vainio, J. Wilbourn and H. Yamasaki
1986; 575 pages; ISBN 92 832 1183 9

No. 84
The Relevance of N-Nitroso Compounds to Human Cancer: Exposure and Mechanisms
Edited by H. Bartsch, I.K. O'Neill and R. Schulte-Hermann
1987; 671 pages; ISBN 92 832 1184 7

No. 85
Environmental Carcinogens: Methods of Analysis and Exposure Measurement. Volume 10: Benzene and Alkylated Benzenes
Edited by L. Fishbein and I.K. O'Neill
1988; 327 pages; ISBN 92 832 1185 5

No. 86
Directory of On-going Research in Cancer Epidemiology 1987
Edited by D.M. Parkin and J. Wahrendorf
1987; 685 pages; ISBN: 92 832 1186 3
(out of print)

No. 87
International Incidence of Childhood Cancer
Edited by D.M. Parkin, C.A. Stiller, C.A. Bieber, G.J. Draper. B. Terracini and J.L. Young
1988; 401 page; ISBN 92 832 1187 1
(out of print)

No. 88
Cancer Incidence in Five Continents, Volume V
Edited by C. Muir, J. Waterhouse, T. Mack, J. Powell and S. Whelan
1987; 1004 pages; ISBN 92 832 1188 X

No. 89
Methods for Detecting DNA Damaging Agents in Humans: Applications in Cancer Epidemiology and Prevention
Edited by H. Bartsch, K. Hemminki and I.K. O'Neill
1988; 518 pages; ISBN 92 832 1189 8
(out of print)

No. 90
Non-occupational Exposure to Mineral Fibres
Edited by J. Bignon, J. Peto and R. Saracci
1989; 500 pages; ISBN 92 832 1190 1

No. 91
Trends in Cancer Incidence in Singapore 1968–1982
Edited by H.P. Lee, N.E. Day and K. Shanmugaratnam
1988; 160 pages; ISBN 92 832 1191 X

No. 92
Cell Differentiation, Genes and Cancer
Edited by T. Kakunaga, T. Sugimura, L. Tomatis and H. Yamasaki
1988; 204 pages; ISBN 92 832 1192 8

No. 93
Directory of On-going Research in Cancer Epidemiology 1988
Edited by M. Coleman and J. Wahrendorf
1988; 662 pages; ISBN 92 832 1193 6
(out of print)

No. 94
Human Papillomavirus and Cervical Cancer
Edited by N. Muñoz, F.X. Bosch and O.M. Jensen
1989; 154 pages; ISBN 92 832 1194 4

No. 95
Cancer Registration: Principles and Methods
Edited by O.M. Jensen, D.M. Parkin, R. MacLennan, C.S. Muir and R. Skeet
1991; 296 pages; ISBN 92 832 1195 2

No. 96
Perinatal and Multigeneration Carcinogenesis
Edited by N.P. Napalkov, J.M. Rice, L. Tomatis and H. Yamasaki
1989; 436 pages; ISBN 92 832 1196 0

No. 97
Occupational Exposure to Silica and Cancer Risk
Edited by L. Simonato, A.C. Fletcher, R. Saracci and T. Thomas
1990; 124 pages; ISBN 92 832 1197 9

No. 98
Cancer Incidence in Jewish Migrants to Israel, 1961-1981
Edited by R. Steinitz, D.M. Parkin, J.L. Young, C.A. Bieber and L. Katz
1989; 320 pages; ISBN 92 832 1198 7

No. 99
Pathology of Tumours in Laboratory Animals, Second Edition, Volume 1, Tumours of the Rat
Edited by V.S. Turusov and U. Mohr
1990; 740 pages; ISBN 92 832 1199 5
For Volumes 2 and 3 (Tumours of the Mouse and Tumours of the Hamster), see IARC Scientific Publications Nos. 111 and 126.

No. 100
Cancer: Causes, Occurrence and Control
Editor-in-Chief: L. Tomatis
1990; 352 pages; ISBN 92 832 0110 8

No. 101
Directory of On-going Research in Cancer Epidemiology 1989–1990
Edited by M. Coleman and J. Wahrendorf
1989; 828 pages; ISBN 92 832 2101 X

No. 102
Patterns of Cancer in Five Continents
Edited by S.L. Whelan, D.M. Parkin and E. Masuyer
1990; 160 pages; ISBN 92 832 2102 8

No. 103
Evaluating Effectiveness of Primary Prevention of Cancer
Edited by M. Hakama, V. Beral, J.W. Cullen and D.M. Parkin
1990; 206 pages; ISBN 92 832 2103 6

No. 104
Complex Mixtures and Cancer Risk
Edited by H. Vainio, M. Sorsa and A.J. McMichael
1990; 441 pages; ISBN 92 832 2104 4

No. 105
Relevance to Human Cancer of N-Nitroso Compounds, Tobacco Smoke and Mycotoxins
Edited by I.K. O'Neill, J. Chen and H. Bartsch
1991; 614 pages; ISBN 92 832 2105 2

No. 106
Atlas of Cancer Incidence in the Former German Democratic Republic
Edited by W.H. Mehnert, M. Smans, C.S. Muir, M. Möhner and D. Schön
1992; 384 pages; ISBN 92 832 2106 0

No. 107
Atlas of Cancer Mortality in the European Economic Community
Edited by M. Smans, C. Muir and P. Boyle
1992; 213 pages + 44 coloured maps; ISBN 92 832 2107 9

No. 108
Environmental Carcinogens: Methods of Analysis and Exposure Measurement. Volume 11: Polychlorinated Dioxins and Dibenzofurans
Edited by C. Rappe, H.R. Buser, B. Dodet and I.K. O'Neill
1991; 400 pages; ISBN 92 832 2108 7

No. 109
Environmental Carcinogens: Methods of Analysis and Exposure Measurement. Volume 12: Indoor Air
Edited by B. Seifert, H. van de Wiel, B. Dodet and I.K. O'Neill
1993; 385 pages; ISBN 92 832 2109 5

No. 110
Directory of On-going Research in Cancer Epidemiology 1991
Edited by M.P. Coleman and J. Wahrendorf
1991; 753 pages; ISBN 92 832 2110 9

No. 111
Pathology of Tumours in Laboratory Animals, Second Edition. Volume 2: Tumours of the Mouse
Edited by V. Turusov and U. Mohr
1994; 800 pages; ISBN 92 832 2111 1

No. 112
Autopsy in Epidemiology and Medical Research
Edited by E. Riboli and M. Delendi
1991; 288 pages; ISBN 92 832 2112 5

No. 113
Laboratory Decontamination and Destruction of Carcinogens in Laboratory Wastes: Some Mycotoxins
Edited by M. Castegnaro, J. Barek, J.M. Frémy, M. Lafontaine, M. Miraglia, E.B. Sansone and G.M. Telling
1991; 63 pages; ISBN 92 832 2113 3

No. 114
Laboratory Decontamination and Destruction of Carcinogens in Laboratory Wastes: Some Polycyclic Heterocyclic Hydrocarbons
Edited by M. Castegnaro, J. Barek, J. Jacob, U. Kirso, M. Lafontaine, E.B. Sansone, G.M. Telling and T. Vu Duc
1991; 50 pages; ISBN 92 832 2114 1

No. 115
Mycotoxins, Endemic Nephropathy and Urinary Tract Tumours
Edited by M. Castegnaro, R. Plestina, G. Dirheimer, I.N. Chernozemsky and H. Bartsch
1991; 340 pages; ISBN 92 832 2115 X

No. 116
Mechanisms of Carcinogenesis in Risk Identification
Edited by H. Vainio, P. Magee, D. McGregor and A.J. McMichael
1992; 615 pages; ISBN 92 832 2116 8

No. 117
Directory of On-going Research in Cancer Epidemiology 1992
Edited by M. Coleman, E. Demaret and J. Wahrendorf
1992; 773 pages; ISBN 92 832 2117 6

No. 118
Cadmium in the Human Environment: Toxicity and Carcinogenicity
Edited by G.F. Nordberg, R.F.M. Herber and L. Alessio
1992; 470 pages; ISBN 92 832 2118 4

No. 119
The Epidemiology of Cervical Cancer and Human Papillomavirus
Edited by N. Muñoz, F.X. Bosch, K.V. Shah and A. Meheus
1992; 288 pages; ISBN 92 832 2119 2

No. 120
Cancer Incidence in Five Continents, Vol. VI
Edited by D.M. Parkin, C.S. Muir, S.L. Whelan, Y.T. Gao, J. Ferlay and J. Powell
1992; 1020 pages; ISBN 92 832 2120 6

No. 121
Time Trends in Cancer Incidence and Mortality
By M. Coleman, J. Estéve, P. Damiecki, A. Arslan and H. Renard
1993; 820 pages; ISBN 92 832 2121 4

No. 122
International Classification of Rodent Tumours.
Part I. The Rat
Editor-in-Chief: U. Mohr
1992–1996; 10 fascicles of 60–100 pages; ISBN 92 832 2122 2

No. 123
Cancer in Italian Migrant Populations
Edited by M. Geddes, D.M. Parkin, M. Khlat, D. Balzi and E. Buiatti
1993; 292 pages; ISBN 92 832 2123 0

No. 124
Postlabelling Methods for the Detection of DNA Damage
Edited by D.H. Phillips, M. Castegnaro and H. Bartsch
1993; 392 pages; ISBN 92 832 2124 9

No. 125
DNA Adducts: Identification and Biological Significance
Edited by K. Hemminki, A. Dipple, D.E.G. Shuker, F.F. Kadlubar, D. Segerbäck and H. Bartsch
1994; 478 pages; ISBN 92 832 2125 7

No. 126
Pathology of Tumours in Laboratory Animals, Second Edition. Volume 3: Tumours of the Hamster
Edited by V. Turusov and U. Mohr
1996; 464 pages; ISBN 92 832 2126 5

No. 128
Statistical Methods in Cancer Research. Volume IV. Descriptive Epidemiology
By J. Estève, E. Benhamou and L. Raymond
1994; 302 pages; ISBN 92 832 2128 1

No. 129
Occupational Cancer in Developing Countries
Edited by N. Pearce, E. Matos, H. Vainio, P. Boffetta and M. Kogevinas
1994; 191 pages; ISBN 92 832 2129 X

No. 130
Directory of On-going Research in Cancer Epidemiology 1994
Edited by R. Sankaranarayanan, J. Wahrendorf and E. Démaret
1994; 800 pages; ISBN 92 832 2130 3

No. 132
Survival of Cancer Patients in Europe: The EUROCARE Study
Edited by F. Berrino, M. Sant, A. Verdecchia, R. Capocaccia, T. Hakulinen and J. Estève
1995; 463 pages; ISBN 92 832 2132 X

No. 134
Atlas of Cancer Mortality in Central Europe
W. Zatonski, J. Estéve, M. Smans, J. Tyczynski and P. Boyle
1996; 300 pages; ISBN 92 832 2134 6

No. 135
Methods for Investigating Localized Clustering of Disease
Edited by F.E. Alexander and P. Boyle
1996; 235 pages; ISBN 92 832 2135 4

No. 136
Chemoprevention in Cancer Control
Edited by M. Hakama, V. Beral,
E. Buiatti, J. Faivre and D.M. Parkin
1996; 160 pages; ISBN 92 832 2136 2

No. 137
Directory of On-going Research in Cancer Epidemiology 1996
Edited by R. Sankaranarayan, J. Warendorf and E. Démaret
1996; 810 pages; ISBN 92 832 2137 0

No. 139
Principles of Chemoprevention
Edited by B.W. Stewart, D. McGregor and P. Kleihues
1996; 360 pages;
ISBN 92 832 2139 7

No. 140
Mechanisms of Fibre Carcinogenesis
Edited by A.B. Kane, P. Boffetta, R. Saracci and J.D. Wilbourn
1996; 135 pages; ISBN 92 832 2140 0

No. 141
EUCAN90: Cancer in the European Union in 1990
By J. Ferlay, R.J. Black, P. Pisani, M.T. Valdivieso and D.M. Parkin
1996; Software on IBM diskette + user's guide, 49 pages; ISBN 92 832 2141 9

IARC Technical Reports

No. 1
Cancer in Costa Rica
Edited by R. Sierra, R. Barrantes,
G. Muñoz Leiva, D.M. Parkin,
C.A. Bieber and N. Muñoz Calero
1988; 124 pages; ISBN 92 832 1412 9

No. 2
SEARCH: A Computer Package to Assist the Statistical Analysis of Case-Control Studies
Edited by G.J. Macfarlane, P. Boyle and P. Maisonneuve
1991; 80 pages; ISBN 92 832 1413 7

No. 3
Cancer Registration in the European Economic Community
Edited by M.P. Coleman and E. Démaret
1988; 188 pages; ISBN 92 832 1414 5

No. 4
Diet, Hormones and Cancer: Methodological Issues for Prospective Studies
Edited by E. Riboli and R. Saracci
1988; 156 pages; ISBN 92 832 1415 3

No. 5
Cancer in the Philippines
Edited by A.V. Laudico, D. Esteban and D.M. Parkin
1989; 186 pages; ISBN 92 832 1416 1

No. 6
La genèse du Centre international de recherche sur le cancer
By R. Sohier and A.G.B. Sutherland
1990, 102 pages; ISBN 92 832 1418 8

No. 7
Epidémiologie du cancer dans les pays de langue latine
1990, 292 pages; ISBN 92 832 1419 6

No. 8
Comparative Study of Anti-smoking Legislation in Countries of the European Economic Community
By A. J. Sasco, P. Dalla-Vorgia and P. Van der Elst
1992; 82 pages; ISBN: 92 832 1421 8
Etude comparative des Législations de Contrôle du Tabagisme dans les Pays de la Communauté économique européenne
1995; 82 pages; ISBN 92 832 2402 7

No. 9
Epidémiologie du cancer dans les pays de langue latine
1991; 346 pages; ISBN 92 832 1423 4

No. 10
Manual for Cancer Registry Personnel
Edited by D. Esteban, S. Whelan,
A. Laudico and D.M. Parkin
1995; 400 pages; ISBN 92 832 1424 2

No. 11
Nitroso Compounds: Biological Mechanisms, Exposures and Cancer Etiology
Edited by I. O'Neill and H. Bartsch
1992; 150 pages; ISBN 92 832 1425 X

No. 12
Epidémiologie du cancer dans les pays de langue latine
1992; 375 pages; ISBN 92 832 1426 9

No. 13
Health, Solar UV Radiation and Environmental Change
By A. Kricker, B.K. Armstrong,
M.E. Jones and R.C. Burton
1993; 213 pages; ISBN 92 832 1427 7

No. 14
Epidémiologie du cancer dans les pays de langue latine
1993; 400 pages; ISBN 92 832 1428 5

No. 15
Cancer in the African Population of Bulawayo, Zimbabwe, 1963–1977
By M.E.G. Skinner, D.M. Parkin,
A.P. Vizcaino and A. Ndhlovu
1993; 120 pages; ISBN 92 832 1429 3

No. 16
Cancer in Thailand 1984–1991
By V. Vatanasapt, N. Martin,
H. Sriplung, K. Chindavijak, S. Sontipong,
S. Sriamporn, D.M. Parkin and
J. Ferlay
1993; 164 pages; ISBN 92 832 1430 7

No. 18
Intervention Trials for Cancer Prevention
By E. Buiatti
1994; 52 pages; ISBN 92 832 1432 3

No. 19
Comparability and Quality Control in Cancer Registration
By D.M. Parkin, V.W. Chen, J. Ferlay,
J. Galceran, H.H. Storm and
S.L. Whelan
1994; 110 pages plus diskette;
ISBN 92 832 1433 1

No. 20
Epidémiologie du cancer dans les pays de langue latine
1994; 346 pages; ISBN 92 832 1434 X

No. 21
ICD Conversion Programs for Cancer
By J. Ferlay
1994; 24 pages plus diskette;
ISBN 92 832 1435 8

No. 22
Cancer in Tianjin
By Q.S. Wang, P. Boffetta,
M. Kogevinas and D.M. Parkin
1994; 96 pages; ISBN 92 832 1433 1

No. 23
An Evaluation Programme for Cancer Preventive Agents
By Bernard W. Stewart
1995; 40 pages; ISBN 92 832 1438 2

No. 24
Peroxisome Proliferation and its Role in Carcinogenesis
1995; 85 pages;
ISBN 92 832 1439 0

No. 25
Combined Analysis of Cancer Mortality in Nuclear Workers in Canada, the United Kingdom and the United States of America
By E. Cardis, E.S. Gilbert, L. Carpenter, G. Howe, I. Kato, J. Fix, L. Salmon, G. Cowper, B.K. Armstrong, V. Beral, A. Douglas, S.A. Fry, J. Kaldor, C. Lavé, P.G. Smith, G. Voelz and L. Wiggs
1995; 160 pages; ISBN 92 832 1440 4

Directories of Agents being Tested for Carcinogenicity
Edited by M.-J. Ghess, J.D. Wilbourn and H. Vainio

No. 15
1992; 317 pages; ISBN 92 832 1315 7

No. 16
1994; 294 pages; ISBN 92 832 1316 5

No. 17
1996; 360 pages; ISBN 92 832 1317 3

Non-serial publications
Alcool et Cancer
By A. Tuyns
1978; 48 pages

Cancer Morbidity and Causes of Death among Danish Brewery Workers
By O.M. Jensen
1980; 143 pages

Directory of Computer Systems Used in Cancer Registries
By H.R. Menck and D.M. Parkin
1986; 236 pages

Facts and Figures of Cancer in the European Community
By J. Estève, A. Kricker, J. Ferlay and D.M. Parkin
1993; 52 pages; ISBN 92 832 1437 4

All IARC Publications are available directly from
IARCPress, 150 Cours Albert Thomas, F-69372 Lyon cedex 08, France
(Fax: +33 4 72 73 83 02; E-mail: press@iarc.fr).

IARC Monographs and Technical Reports are also available from the
World Health Organization Distribution and Sales, CH-1211 Geneva 27
(Fax: +41 22 791 4857)
and from WHO Sales Agents worldwide.

IARC Scientific Publications are also available from
Oxford University Press, Walton Street, Oxford, UK OX2 6DP
(Fax: +44 1865 267782).

www.ingramcontent.com/pod-product-compliance
Ingram Content Group UK Ltd.
Pitfield, Milton Keynes, MK11 3LW, UK
UKHW051258180426
11947UKWH00020B/1774